Diagnostic Medical Sonography

THE VASCULAR SYSTEM

Diagnostic Medical Sonography

THE VASCULAR SYSTEM

First Edition

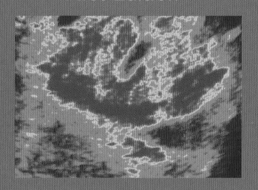

Ann Marie Kupinski, PhD, RVT, RDMS, FSVU

Technical Director, North Country Vascular Diagnostics, Inc.
Clinical Associate Professor of Radiology
Albany Medical College
Albany, NY

Wolters Kluwer | Lippincott Williams & Wilkins
Health

Philadelphia · Baltimore · New York · London
Buenos Aires · Hong Kong · Sydney · Tokyo

Publisher: Julie K. Stegman
Senior Product Manager: Heather Rybacki
Product Manager: Kristin Royer
Marketing Manager: Shauna Kelley
Design Coordinator: Joan Wendt
Art Director: Jennifer Clements
Manufacturing Coordinator: Margie Orzech
Production Services: Absolute Service, Inc.

351 West Camden Street
Baltimore, MD 21201

Two Commerce Square
2001 Market Street
Philadelphia, PA 19103

Third Edition

Printed in China.

Library of Congress Cataloging-in-Publication Data

Diagnostic medical sonography. The vascular system / edited by Ann Marie Kupinski.
    p. ; cm.
Vascular system
Includes bibliographical references and index.
ISBN 978-1-60831-350-1 (alk. paper)
I. Kupinski, Ann Marie. II. Title: Vascular system.
[DNLM: 1. Cardiovascular System--ultrasonography. 2. Vascular Diseases--ultrasonography. WG 141]

616.1'307543--dc23
                        2012002011

Care has been taken to confirm the accuracy of the information presented and to describe generally accepted practices. However, the authors, editors, and publisher are not responsible for errors or omissions or for any consequences from application of the information in this book and make no warranty, express or implied, with respect to the contents of the publication. Application of the information in a particular situation remains the professional responsibility of the practitioner.

The authors, editors, and publisher have exerted every effort to ensure that drug selection and dosage set forth in this text are in accordance with current recommendations and practice at the time of publication. However, in view of ongoing research, changes in government regulations, and the constant flow of information relating to drug therapy and drug reactions, the reader is urged to check the package insert for each drug for any change in indications and dosage and for added warnings and precautions. This is particularly important when the recommended agent is a new or infrequently employed drug.

Some drugs and medical devices presented in this publication have Food and Drug Administration (FDA) clearance for limited use in restricted research settings. It is the responsibility of the health care provider to ascertain the FDA status of each drug or device planned for use in their clinical practice.

To purchase additional copies of this book, call our customer service department at **(800) 638-3030** or fax orders to **(301) 223-2320**. International customers should call **(301) 223-2300**.
Visit Lippincott Williams & Wilkins on the Internet: **http://www.lww.com.** Lippincott Williams & Wilkins customer service representatives are available from 8:30 am to 6:00 pm, EST.

10 9 8 7 6 5 4

To my husband, Mitchell, and son, Justin,
for their continual encouragement and love.
They are the best part of my life. Sharing this
book with them makes it even more special.

And to those who will read this book,
remember that "Learning is not attained by
chance, it must be sought for with ardor and
diligence."—Abigail Adams
Hopefully this book will provide knowledge
beneficial to your education, helpful in your
careers, and valuable to your patients.
Never stop learning.

Contents

PART 4 • PERIPHERAL VENOUS

PART 5 • ABDOMINAL

PART 6 • MISCELLANEOUS

Acknowledgements

I would first like to thank editors Diane Kawamura (Abdomen and Superficial Structures) and Susan Stephenson (Obstetrics and Gynecology) for their support throughout the completion of the three volumes of *Diagnostic Medical Sonography*. It was great to work with these talented individuals and their ideas and knowledge were a tremendous help.

The team of individuals at Lippincott Williams and Wilkins deserves my sincerest gratitude for their support, encouragement, knowledge and patience. I'd like to especially thank Peter Sabatini, Acquisitions Editor and Kristin Royer, Product Manager as this textbook would not have been possible without them. In addition, I'd like to extend my appreciation to Kelly Horvath, Development Editor, Jennifer Clements, Art Director and all the others on our team who helped get this textbook completed. I would also like to thank Rachel Kendoll, Vascular Technology Program Director at Spokane Community College for her help with some of the online ancillary materials.

When I was first approached about this textbook, I knew it would only be as good as the authors I could get to contribute to it. I tried to gather a group from a broad range of backgrounds and experiences. Our authors include individuals from the Pacific Northwest to South Florida, New England to Southern California and multiple facilities in between as well as international contributors from Australia, Brazil and England. The strength and thoroughness of this textbook is due to the fantastic authors who contributed to this project. I am so thankful to have their expertise and their wonderful chapters.

Images are a key component to any textbook. I'd like to thank the various authors within the book who helped contribute additional images for other chapters. There are several other individuals I would like to thank who contributed images: Phillip J. Bendick, PhD, RVT, Royal Oak, MI; Karen Burns, RN, RVT, MBA, Chicago, IL; Michael Ciarmiello, Albany, NY; David Cosgrove, FRCR, London, England; Steven Feinstein, MD, Chicago, IL; Kimberly Gaydula, BS, RVT, Chicago, IL; Damaris Gonzalez, RVT, RDMS, Chicago IL; Kathleen Hannon, RN, MS, RVT, RDMS, Boston, MA; John Hobby, RVT, Pueblo, Co; Debra Joly, RVT, RDMS, RDCS, Houston, TX; Steve Knight, BSc, RVT, RDCS, Boston, MA; Kimberly Lopresti, RDCS, Philadelphia, PA; Daniel Matz, Frimley, Surrey, England; Antonio Sergio Marcelino, MD, Sao Paulo, Brazil; Patricia "Tish" Poe, BA, RVT, RDCS, FSVU, Cincinnati, OH; Jeff Powers, PhD, Bothell, WA; Besnike Ramadani, BS, RVT, Chicago IL; Robert Scissons, RVT, FSVU, Toledo OH; William B. Schroedter, BS, RVT, RPhS, FSVU, Venice Fl; Carlos Ventura, MD, Sao Paulo, Brazil; Hans-Peter Weskott, MD, Hannover, Germany; Jean White, RVT, RPhS, Venice, FL. A special thanks goes out to my friends at GE Healthcare: Mike Arbaugh, Cindy Owen, Jim Sitter and Billy Zang and Unetixs Vascular: Tony Castillo, Brewster Merrill and Don Tibbals for their assistance and contributions to image acquisitions.

Lastly, I'd like to thank those people in my life who have personally helped me get to this point to function as an editor of a textbook. Thanks to my coworkers for their support. Thanks to the numerous medical and scientific professionals at Albany Medical Center and my vascular friends across the country who have taught me so much. Special thanks goes to Sister Theresa Wysolmerski, CSJ, PhD of the College of Saint Rose for getting me started with exploring science and helping me in so many ways. A big thank you goes out to Mr. Peter Leopold, MB, BCh, MCh, FRCS Eng/Ed for having enough patience to teach me to scan and answer my countless questions on vascular disease. Finally to my family and friends, especially my parents, son and husband who have given me so much love and support through the years, thank you so very much!

Preface

This is the first edition of *Diagnostic Medical Sonography: The Vascular System*. Ultrasound educators and colleagues encouraged and supported the development of this textbook. It contains fundamental materials and advanced topics hoping to appeal to readers with diverse educational backgrounds and experiences. This textbook is intended to be used as either an introduction to the profession or as a comprehensive reference guide. The content provides groundwork for an essential understanding of anatomy, physiology, and pathophysiology. This material is expected to benefit sonographers, vascular technologists, students, practitioners, and physicians caring for patients with vascular disease.

The first section of this textbook presents basic vascular anatomy as well as arterial and venous physiology. The next four sections contain chapters that focus on specific components of the vascular system, namely the cerebrovascular, peripheral arterial, peripheral venous, and abdominal vascular systems. The sixth and final section contains additional chapters with topics relevant to vascular ultrasound, including the use of quality assurance statistics. Sonographic examination techniques, technical considerations, pitfalls, and diagnostic criteria are just some of the sections contained within the chapters. Within the peripheral arterial section, a chapter focuses on nonimaging physiologic arterial testing, which is often performed in conjunction with ultrasound testing. When appropriate, complementary testing procedures are also presented within several chapters.

Every attempt was made to compile an up-to-date and factual textbook. The reader should find the format of the chapters easy to follow, interesting, and comprehensive. Normal and abnormal sonographic findings are depicted in numerous illustrations throughout the chapters. Several case study examples are also provided throughout the chapters.

The goal of this textbook was to be as complete as possible while recognizing that augmentation with ongoing supplemental information from peer-reviewed journals will be required. Learning is a lifelong process that can be a challenge but should be looked upon as a welcome exercise. The essential information contained within this textbook should establish a basis for those seeking to build their knowledge of vascular ultrasound.

Contributors

Clifford T. Araki, PhD, RVS, RVT
Professor, Medical Imaging Sciences
Director, Vascular Sonography Program
School of Health Related Professions
University of Medicine and Dentistry of
    New Jersey
Scotch Plains, NJ

Enrico Ascher, MD
Professor of Surgery, Mount Sinai
    School of Medicine
Chairman, Vascular Institute of New York
New York, NY

Dennis F. Bandyk, MD, FACS, FSVU
Professor of Surgery
Division of Vascular and Endovascular
    Surgery
University of California—San Diego
    School of Medicine
La Jolla, CA

Kari A. Campbell, BS, RVT
D. E. Strandness Jr. Vascular Laboratory
University of Washington Medical
    Center, Seattle, WA

Cynthia Cannon, BA, BS, RVT
Instructor, Medical Imaging Sciences
Clinical Coordinator, Vascular
    Technology Program
School of Health Related Professions
University of Medicine and Dentistry of
    New Jersey
Scotch Plains, NJ

Gwendolyn Carmel, BS, RVT
Clinical Physiologist and Technical
    Director, Vascular Laboratory
East Orange VA Medical Center
East Orange, NJ

**Kathleen A. Carter, BSN, RN,
RVT, FSVU**
Vascular Laboratory Clinical
    Consultant/Educator
Norfolk, VA

Terrence D. Case, MEd, RVT, FSVU
Cardiovascular Program Consultant
Hollywood Beach, FL

Michael Costanza, MD, FACS
Division of Vascular Surgery and
    Endovascular Services
SUNY Upstate Medical University
VA Health Care Network Upstate
    New York
Syracuse, NY

**M. Robert De Jong, RDMS,
RVT, FSDMS**
Radiology Technical Manager,
    Ultrasound
Johns Hopkins Hospital
Baltimore, MD

Colleen Douville, BA, RVT
Director, Cerebrovascular Ultrasound
Program Manager, Clinical
    Neurophysiology
Swedish Neuroscience Institute,
    Swedish Medical Center
Seattle, WA

Eileen French-Sherry, MA, RVT, FSVU
Assistant Professor
Program Director and Acting Chair
Department of Vascular Ultrasound and
    Technology
Rush University—College of Health
    Sciences
Chicago, IL

Monica Fuller, RDMS, RVT
Johns Hopkins Hospital
Baltimore, MD

Anil Hingorani, MD
Associate Professor of Surgery, Mount
    Sinai School of Medicine
Cochairman, Vascular Institute of
    New York
New York, NY

Zafar Jamil, MD
Clinical Professor of Surgery
New Jersey Medical School
University of Medicine and Dentistry of
    New Jersey
Newark, NJ

Jenifer F. Kidd, RN, RVT, DMU, FSVU
Senior Vascular Sonographer
Gosford Vascular Laboratory
Gosford, NSW, Australia

Ann Marie Kupinski, PhD, RVT, RDMS, FSVU
North Country Vascular Diagnostics, Inc.
Glens Falls, NY
Clinical Associate Professor of Radiology
Albany Medical College
Albany, NY

Steven A. Leers, MD, RVT
Associate Professor of Surgery
Division of Vascular Surgery
Director, UPMC Vascular Laboratories
University of Pittsburgh Medical Center
Pittsburgh, PA

Wayne C. Leonhardt, BA, RT, RDMS, RVT, APS
Lead Sonographer, Technical Director, and Clinical Instructor
Department of Ultrasound
Alta Bates Summit Medical Center, Merritt Pavilion
Oakland, CA

Peter W. Leopold, MB, BCh, MCh, FRCS Eng/Ed
Chief of Vascular Surgery
Frimley Park Hospital
Camberley, Surrey, United Kingdom

Natalie Marks, MD, RVT
Vascular Institute of New York
Brooklyn, NY

Gregory L. Moneta, MD
Professor and Chief of Vascular Surgery
Oregon Health and Science University
Portland, OR

Daniel A. Merton, BS, RDMS, FSDMS, FAIUM
Clinical Instructor and Technical
    Coordinator of Research
The Jefferson Ultrasound Research and
    Education Institute
Department of Radiology
Thomas Jefferson University
Philadelphia, PA

Anne M. Musson, BS, RVT
Senior Vascular Associate
Noninvasive Vascular Laboratory
Dartmouth-Hitchcock Medical Center
Lebanon, NH

Terry Needham, RVT, FSVU
Needham Vascular Consulting
Chattanooga, TN

Diana L. Neuhardt, RVT, RPhS
CompuDiagnostics, Inc.
Phoenix, AZ

Marsha M. Neumyer, BS, RVT, FSVU, FSDMS, FAIUM
International Director
Vascular Diagnostic Educational
    Services
Harrisburg, PA

Mark Oliver, RVT, RPVI, FACP, FSVU
Codirector, Vascular Laboratory
Gagnon Cardiovascular Institute
Attending Physician
Morristown Memorial Hospital
Morristown, NJ

Aaron Partsafas, MD
Vascular Surgeon
Providence Health and Services
Medford, OR

Jesenia Pineda, BS, RVT
Chief Technologist
Vascular Laboratory
Saint Michael's Medical Center
Newark, NJ

Sergio X. Salles Cunha, PhD, RVT, FSVU
Consultant
Angiolab—Noninvasive Vascular
    Laboratories
Curitiba, PR and Vitoria, ES, Brazil

Gail Egan Sansivero, MS, ANP
Nurse Practitioner
Community Care Physicians
Instructor of Radiology
Albany Medical College
Albany, NY

Leslie Millar Scoutt, MD
Professor of Diagnostic Radiology and
    Surgery
Chief, Ultrasound Service
Medical Director, The Noninvasive
    Vascular Laboratory
Yale University School of Medicine
Yale—New Haven Hospital
New Haven, CT

Jack I. Siegel, RVT
Technical Director, Vascular Laboratory
Medical University of South Carolina
Charleston, SC

David Singh, MD
Interventional Radiologist
Holy Name Medical Center
Teaneck, NJ

Michael J. Singh, MD
Program Director, Vascular Surgery
    Integrated Residency and Fellowship
Director, University Vein Care Center
Associate Professor of Surgery
University of Rochester Medical Center
Rochester, NY

Gary Siskin, MD
Professor and Chairman
Department of Radiology
Albany Medical Center
Albany, NY

S. Wayne Smith, MD, FACP, FSVM, RVT, RPVI
Medical Director
Vascular Diagnostic Center
Rex Hospital
University of North Carolina Health Care
Raleigh, NC

Cheryl Sura, LPN, BS, RVT
Technical Director, Noninvasive
    Vascular Laboratory
University of Rochester Medical Center
Rochester, NY

Steven R. Talbot, RVT, FSVU
Technical Director, Vascular Laboratory
Research Associate, Division of Vascular
    Surgery
School of Medicine
University of Utah Medical Center
Salt Lake City, UT

Patrick A. Washko, BSRT, RDMS, RVT
Technical Director
Vascular Diagnostic Center
Rex Hospital
University of North Carolina Health Care
Raleigh, NC

R. Eugene Zierler, MD
Professor of Surgery
University of Washington School of
    Medicine
Medical Director, D. E. Strandness Jr.
    Vascular Laboratory
University of Washington Medical Center
    and Harborview Medical Center
Seattle, WA

Robert M. Zwolak, MD, PhD, FACS
Professor of Surgery
Section of Vascular Surgery
Dartmouth-Hitchcock Medical Center
Lebanon, NH
Chief of Surgery
White River Junction VA Medical Center
White River Junction, VT

Using This Series

The books in the *Diagnostic Medical Sonography* Series will help you develop an understanding of specialty sonography topics. Key learning resources and tools throughout the textbook aim to increase your understanding of the topics provided and better prepare you for your professional career. This User's Guide will help you familiarize yourself with these exciting features designed to enhance your learning experience.

18 Abnormalities of the Placenta and Umbilical Cord

Lisa M. Allen

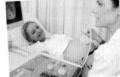

OBJECTIVES

Recognize the sonographic appearance of placental and umbilical cord anomalies

Discuss developmental variations in placental size, shape, and configuration

Identify placenta previa classifications

Explain placental abruption and the associated risk factors

List placenta accreta classifications and known risk factors

Name the various abnormalities of umbilical cord insertion into the placenta

Describe cystic and solid masses of the umbilical cord

KEY TERMS

succenturiate lobe | circummarginate placenta | circumvallate placenta | placenta previa | placental abruption | placenta accreta spectrum | chorioangioma | amniotic band syndrome | uterine synechiae | marginal insertion | battledore placenta | velamentous insertion | true knot | false knot | nuchal cord | cord prolapse | vasa previa | single umbilical artery | cord entanglement | umbilical cord hemangioma | umbilical cord coiling | umbilical coiling index

GLOSSARY

Aneurysm Focal dilatation of an artery

Bilobed placenta Placenta where the lobes are nearly equal in size and the cord inserts into the chorionic bridge of tissue that connects the two lobes

Body stalk anomaly Fatal condition associated with multiple congenital anomalies and absence of the umbilical cord

Breus' mole Very rare condition where there is massive subchorionic thrombosis of the placenta secondary to extreme venous obstruction

Extrachorial placenta Attachment of the placental membranes to the fetal surface of the placenta rather than to the underlying villous placental margin

False knot Bending, twisting, and bulging of the umbilical cord vessels mimicking a knot in the umbilical cord

Gastroschisis Periumbilical abdominal wall defect, typically to the right of normal cord insertion, that allows for free-floating bowel in the amniotic fluid

Limb–body wall complex Condition characterized by multiple complex fetal anomalies and a short umbilical cord

Marginal insertion (a.k.a. battledore placenta) Occurs when the umbilical cord inserts at the placental margin instead of centrally

Mickey Mouse sign Term used to describe the cross-section of the three-vessel umbilical cord or the portal triad (portal vein, hepatic artery, common bile duct)

Omphalocele Central anterior abdominal wall defect of the umbilicus where abdominal organs are contained by a covering membrane consisting of peritoneum, Wharton's jelly, and amnion

Placentomegaly Term that refers to a thickened placenta

Synechia (Asherman's syndrome) Linear, extra amniotic tissue that projects into the amniotic cavity with no restriction of fetal movement

Thrombosis Intraplacental area of hemorrhage and clot

True knot Result of the fetus actually passing through a loop or loops of umbilical cord creating one or more knots in the cord

425

CHAPTER OBJECTIVES

Measurable objectives listed at the beginning of each chapter help you understand the intended outcomes for the chapter, as well as recognize and study important concept within each chapter.

GLOSSARY

Key terms are listed at the beginning of each chapter and clearly defined, then highlighted in bold type throughout the chapter to help you to learn and recall important terminology.

PATHOLOGY BOXES

Each chapter includes tables of relevant pathologies, which you can use as a quick reference for reviewing the material.

CRITICAL THINKING QUESTIONS

Throughout the chapter are critical thinking questions to test your knowledge and help you develop analytical skills that you will need in your profession.

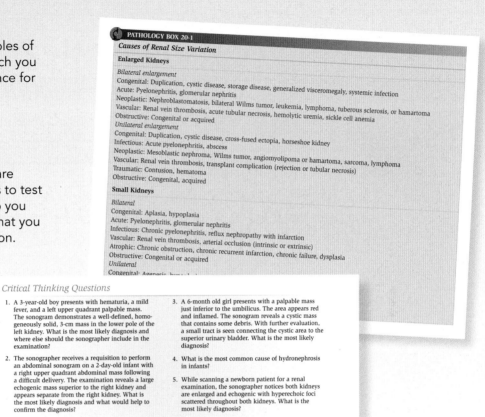

PATHOLOGY BOX 20-1

Causes of Renal Size Variation

Enlarged Kidneys

Bilateral enlargement
Congenital: Duplication, cystic disease, storage disease, generalized visceromegaly, systemic infection
Acute: Pyelonephritis, glomerular nephritis
Neoplastic: Nephroblastomatosis, bilateral Wilms tumor, leukemia, lymphoma, tuberous sclerosis, or hamartoma
Vascular: Renal vein thrombosis, acute tubular necrosis, hemolytic uremia, sickle cell anemia
Obstructive: Congenital or acquired
Unilateral enlargement
Congenital: Duplication, cystic disease, cross-fused ectopia, horseshoe kidney
Infectious: Acute pyelonephritis, abscess
Neoplastic: Mesoblastic nephroma, Wilms tumor, angiomyolipoma or hamartoma, sarcoma, lymphoma
Vascular: Renal vein thrombosis, transplant complication (rejection or tubular necrosis)
Traumatic: Contusion, hematoma
Obstructive: Congenital, acquired

Small Kidneys

Bilateral
Congenital: Aplasia, hypoplasia
Acute: Pyelonephritis, glomerular nephritis
Infectious: Chronic pyelonephritis, reflux nephropathy with infarction
Vascular: Renal vein thrombosis, arterial occlusion (intrinsic or extrinsic)
Atrophic: Chronic obstruction, chronic recurrent infarction, chronic failure, dysplasia
Obstructive: Congenital or acquired
Unilateral
Congenital: Agenesis, hypoplasia

Critical Thinking Questions

1. A 3-year-old boy presents with hematuria, a mild fever, and a left upper quadrant palpable mass. The sonogram demonstrates a well-defined, homogeneously solid, 3-cm mass in the lower pole of the left kidney. What is the most likely diagnosis and where else should the sonographer include in the examination?

2. The sonographer receives a requisition to perform an abdominal sonogram on a 2-day-old infant with a right upper quadrant abdominal mass following a difficult delivery. The examination reveals a large echogenic mass superior to the right kidney and appears separate from the right kidney. What is the most likely diagnosis and what would help to confirm the diagnosis?

3. A 6-month old girl presents with a palpable mass just inferior to the umbilicus. The area appears red and inflamed. The sonogram reveals a cystic mass that contains some debris. With further evaluation, a small tract is seen connecting the cystic area to the superior urinary bladder. What is the most likely diagnosis?

4. What is the most common cause of hydronephrosis in infants?

5. While scanning a newborn patient for a renal examination, the sonographer notices both kidneys are enlarged and echogenic with hyperechoic foci scattered throughout both kidneys. What is the most likely diagnosis?

RESOURCES

You will also find additional resources and exercises online, including a glossary with pronunciations, quiz bank, sonographic video clips, and weblinks. Use these interactive resources to test your knowledge, assess your progress, and review for quizzes and tests.

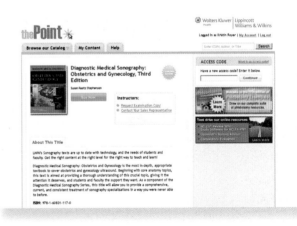

1 Vascular Anatomy

Ann Marie Kupinski

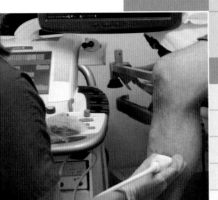

OBJECTIVES

Define the major components of the vascular system

Describe the arrangement of the blood vessel walls

Identify the major vessels of the arterial system

Identify the major vessels of the venous system

KEY TERMS

arteriole | artery | capillary | vein | venule

GLOSSARY

arteriole a small artery with a muscular wall; a terminal artery that continues into the capillary network

artery a blood vessel that carries blood away from the heart

capillary a small blood vessel with only an endothelium and a basement membrane through which the exchange of nutrients and waste occurs

vein a blood vessel that carries blood toward the heart

venule a small vein that is continuous with a capillary

Ultrasound is a medical imaging modality used to define various structures as well as any pathology within the body. Sonographers and vascular technologists control the ultrasound equipment and the acquisition of the images and thus are vital to obtaining accurate and adequate clinical information. In order to successfully perform an ultrasound examination, thorough knowledge of anatomy is essential. This chapter will present the basic anatomic components of the vascular system. Additional detailed anatomic information pertaining to specific organs, regions, pathology, or disorders is contained within several of the subsequent chapters.

VASCULAR ARCHITECTURE

Blood is circulated throughout the body by a network of arteries, veins, and capillaries. Arteries carry blood that is rich in nutrients and oxygen from the heart out to the various organs and tissue beds. Veins return the deoxygenated blood with waste materials back toward the heart. Capillaries are part of

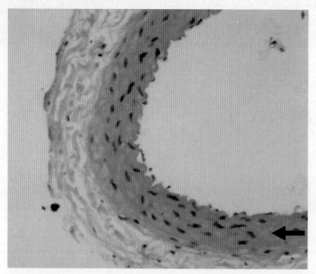

Figure 1-1 Cross section of an arterial wall. The *black arrow* is indicating the thick layer of smooth muscle cells within the tunica media.

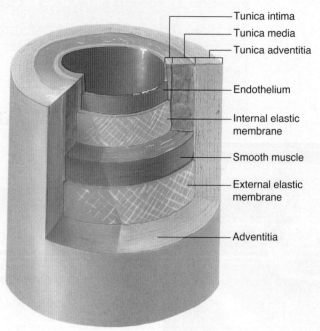

Tunica intima
Tunica media
Tunica adventitia
Endothelium
Internal elastic membrane
Smooth muscle
External elastic membrane
Adventitia

Figure 1-2 Schematic diagram of arterial and venous walls illustrating the tunica intima, tunica media, and tunica adventitia.

the microvasculature where the exchange of oxygen, nutrients, and waste occurs.

ARTERIES

Arteries and veins have three layers of cells within their vessel walls (Fig. 1-1). These layers are called the tunica intima, tunica media, and tunica adventitia, respectively (Fig. 1-2). The tunica intima is the innermost layer consisting of an endothelial cell lining with connective tissue components beneath it. This is the layer of cells in contact with the blood. The tunica media is the middle layer and is a strong muscular layer. It is the thickest component of an arterial wall. It is composed mainly of smooth muscle cells circularly arranged around the vessel. There are varying amounts of elastic fibers and collagen present. The tunica adventitia is the outmost layer of a blood vessel wall and is in contact with the tissue surrounding the vessel. The tunica adventitia is composed of connective tissue, nerve fibers, and small vessel capillaries.

Arteries are classified according to their size. Arterioles are about 100 μm or less in diameter. They have been called the "stopcocks" of the vascular system. They are the principal point of resistance to blood flow within the vascular system. Circular smooth muscle layers control the degree of contraction of these vessels and thus alter vessel resistance. Small- and medium-sized arteries average approximately 4 mm in diameter. This group of vessels includes all the arteries excluding the aorta and its largest branches. Small- and medium-sized arteries have well-developed smooth muscle layers. They also have more elastic and fibrous tissue than the arterioles. Large elastic arteries are the aorta and its

largest branches (the brachiocephalic, common carotid, subclavian, and common iliac arteries). They have a large amount of elastic fibers in their walls and less smooth muscle cells.

VEINS

Veins have the same laminar structures as the arteries, although they tend not to be as muscular as the arteries. In some veins, they have more elastic fibers and collagen than muscle fibers. Their walls are thinner in comparison to arteries of similar size. Wall thickness does vary depending on the region of the body, with lower extremity veins having thicker walls than upper extremity veins.

Venules are the smallest component of the venous system and measure approximately 20 μm in diameter. Their walls are mainly connective tissue. Some venules are as permeable to certain substances as the capillaries, and some exchange occurs across these vessels. Small- and medium-sized veins range in diameter from 1 to 10 mm. These include all the veins except the portal vein and the venae cavae and their main branches. The small- and medium-sized veins have a thin tunica adventitia. Large veins include the portal vein, inferior and superior venae cavae, and their main branches. The bulk of these large veins is an adventitial layer of fibrous and elastic tissue.

A unique feature of veins is the presence of valves (Fig. 1-3). Most veins have valves that prevent the retrograde movement of blood. Valves are formed

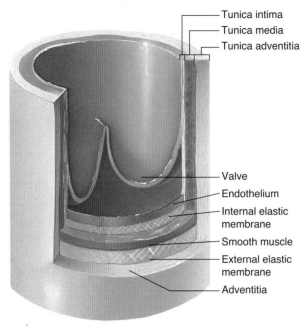

Figure 1-3 Schematic diagram of a venous valve.

CAPILLARIES

The capillaries are the smallest vessel in the body, measuring approximately 8 μm in diameter, just big enough to let a red blood cell pass through. Their walls are composed primarily of a layer of endothelial cells and a small amount of basement membrane. This layer of endothelial cells is typically referred to as the tunica intima. These thin walls are ideal for the diffusion of products across the capillaries. The capillaries are the primary place in the body where nutrient exchange occurs. Oxygen and nutrients pass across the capillaries into the tissue, while at the same time, carbon dioxide and waste products leave the tissues and enter the blood of the capillary. Capillary permeability does vary somewhat depending on the tissue bed with efficient barriers in place such as the diffusion of large molecules, particularly in the brain.

Blood enters into the capillary from the arterial side of the circulation via the arterioles. Blood leaves the capillary on the venous side of the circulation via the venules. There are different types of capillaries characterized by slightly different arrangements of the endothelial cells. There are also places in the body where an arteriole and venule are connected together without a true capillary between them.

by inward projections of the tunica intima and are strengthened by the presence of collagen and elastic fibers. The valves are covered by endothelial cells. Valves are bicuspid, which mean they have two leaflets that are shaped as semilunar cusps. They attach to the vein wall by their convex edges, and their free concave edges are oriented toward the heart. When blood flow reverses, the valves close and blood fills a slightly enlarged space between the wall of the vein and the valve, called the sinus. Valves are numerous in the legs where venous flow moves against the force of gravity. Valves are usually absent within the veins of the thorax and abdomen.

CEREBROVASCULAR ANATOMY

The principal arteries supplying the head and neck are the right and left common carotid arteries (CCAs). The left CCA is the second of three major vessels that arise from the aortic arch (Fig. 1-4). The right CCA

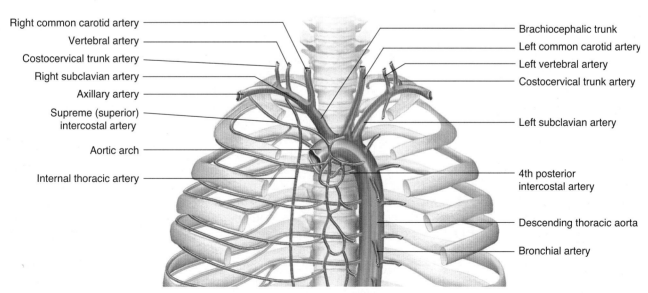

Figure 1-4 Illustration of the aortic arch and its major branches: the brachiocephalic, left common carotid, and left subclavian arteries.

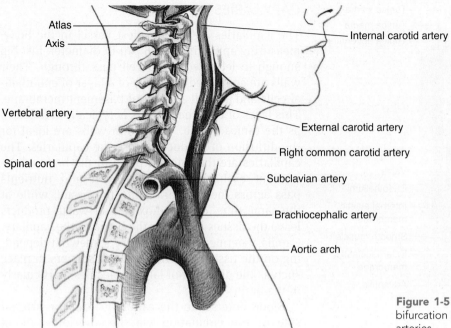

Atlas

Axis

Internal carotid artery

Vertebral artery

External carotid artery

Right common carotid artery

Spinal cord

Subclavian artery

Brachiocephalic artery

Aortic arch

Figure 1-5 View of the common carotid artery bifurcation into the internal and external carotid arteries.

originates from the brachiocephalic artery (formerly called the innominate artery). The CCA ascends the neck laterally and bifurcates into the internal carotid (ICA) and external carotid arteries (ECAs) in the mid cervical region at the upper border of the thyroid cartilage (Fig. 1-5). The right and left ICA supplies much of the blood to the brain and eyes. They usually lie laterally to the ECAs and have no extracranial branches. The intracranial segment of the ICA consists of three portions, namely, the petrous, the cavernous, and the cerebral. The ophthalmic artery is the first branch of the cerebral portion of the ICA. The ophthalmic artery has several branches, including the supraorbital, the frontal, and the nasal arteries. Terminal branches of the ophthalmic artery anastomose with the ECA and may provide sources of collateral flow. The cerebral portion of the ICA terminates into four branches: the anterior cerebral, the middle cerebral, the posterior communicating, and the anterior choroidal arteries.

The ECAs are usually medial to the ICAs and more superficial. Eight branches arise off the external ECA: the superior thyroid, the lingual, the facial, the occipital, the posterior auricular, the ascending pharyngeal, the maxillary, and the superficial temporal arteries (Fig. 1-6). The superficial thyroid is usually the first branch of the ECA. The ECA normally does not supply blood flow to the brain but can serve as an important collateral pathway.

The vertebral arteries arise off the subclavian arteries and ascend the neck (Fig. 1-7). The right and left vertebral arteries, along with the right and left ICA, are the four vessels that supply the brain with

blood. The vertebral artery enters the transverse process of the sixth cervical vertebra and runs superiorly. The vertebral artery continues coursing through the foramina in the transverse process of the other five cervical vertebrae. It then bends medially before entering the cranial cavity through the foramen magnum. After entering the skull, the two vertebral arteries join to form the basilar artery.

The circle of Willis is a unique arrangement of the branches of the ICAs and vertebral arteries. This arrangement of vessels provides a vital collateral network to maintain cerebral perfusion in the event of disease. The circle of Willis is formed anteriorly by the right and left anterior cerebral arteries, which are interconnected via the anterior communicating artery and posteriorly by the right and left posterior cerebral arteries, which are connected via the posterior communicating arteries (Fig. 1-8).

Venous drainage of the head and neck includes the external jugular, the internal jugular, and the vertebral veins (Fig. 1-9). The external jugular courses through the neck and returns blood from portions of the cranial cavity, the face, and the neck. The external jugular vein flows into the subclavian vein. The internal jugular vein collects blood from the brain and superficial parts of the face and neck. The internal jugular vein courses along the anterior–lateral edge of the ICA and CCA. The internal jugular vein unites with the subclavian vein to form the brachiocephalic (innominate) veins. The vertebral vein is formed from numerous small tributaries of the internal vertebral venous plexuses. These vessels join with small veins from the muscles of the neck

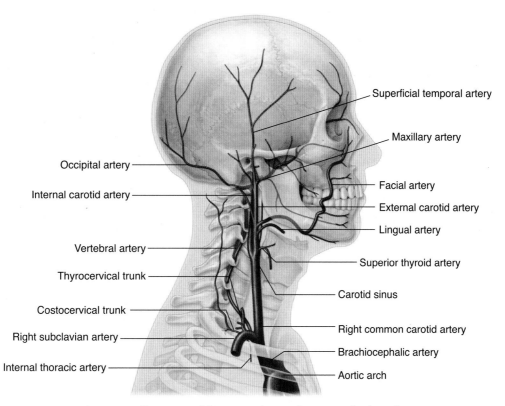

Figure 1-6 Illustration of the external carotid artery and its branches.

Superficial temporal artery

Maxillary artery

Occipital artery

Internal carotid artery

Facial artery

External carotid artery

Lingual artery

Vertebral artery

Superior thyroid artery

Thyrocervical trunk

Costocervical trunk

Carotid sinus

Right subclavian artery

Right common carotid artery

Internal thoracic artery

Brachiocephalic artery

Aortic arch

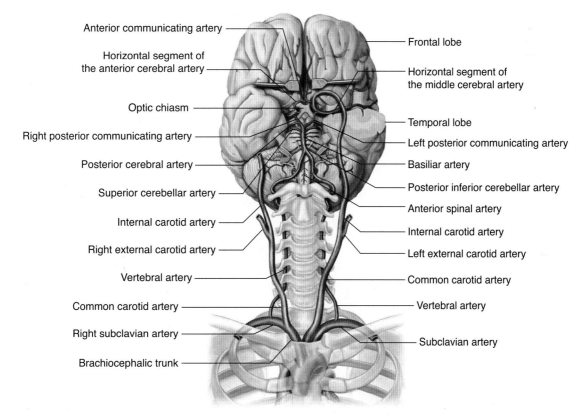

Figure 1-7 Diagram indicating the orientation of the vertebral arteries through the cervical vertebrae and into the cranial cavity.

Anterior communicating artery

Horizontal segment of
the anterior cerebral artery

Frontal lobe

Horizontal segment of
the middle cerebral artery

Optic chiasm

Right posterior communicating artery

Temporal lobe

Left posterior communicating artery

Posterior cerebral artery

Basiliar artery

Superior cerebellar artery

Posterior inferior cerebellar artery

Anterior spinal artery

Internal carotid artery

Internal carotid artery

Right external carotid artery

Left external carotid artery

Vertebral artery

Common carotid artery

Common carotid artery

Vertebral artery

Right subclavian artery

Subclavian artery

Brachiocephalic trunk

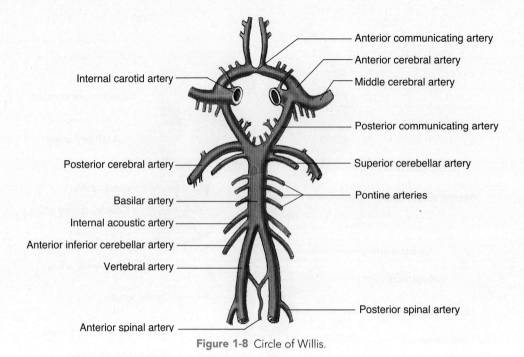

Internal carotid artery

Anterior communicating artery

Anterior cerebral artery

Middle cerebral artery

Posterior communicating artery

Posterior cerebral artery

Superior cerebellar artery

Basilar artery

Pontine arteries

Internal acoustic artery

Anterior inferior cerebellar artery

Vertebral artery

Posterior spinal artery

Anterior spinal artery

Figure 1-8 Circle of Willis.

and form a dense plexus around the vertebral artery. These veins descend in the transverse foramina of the cervical vertebrae. This plexus ends in a single trunk, the vertebral vein, which emerges from the sixth cervical vertebra and empties into the brachiocephalic vein.

THE AORTIC ARCH AND UPPER EXTREMITY ARTERIES

The ascending aorta begins at the aortic valve and runs upward, becoming the aortic arch. It continues upwards and backwards, crossing the trachea. It

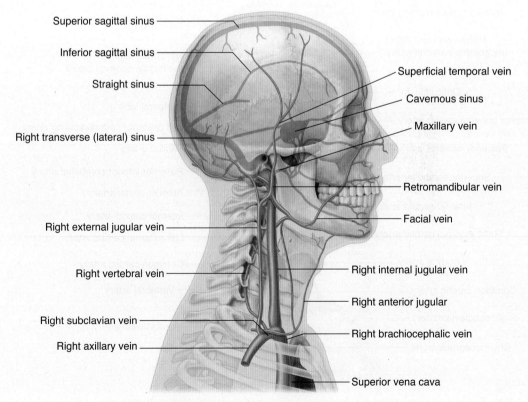

Superior sagittal sinus

Inferior sagittal sinus

Straight sinus

Right transverse (lateral) sinus

Superficial temporal vein

Cavernous sinus

Maxillary vein

Retromandibular vein

Facial vein

Right external jugular vein

Right vertebral vein

Right internal jugular vein

Right anterior jugular

Right subclavian vein

Right brachiocephalic vein

Right axillary vein

Superior vena cava

Figure 1-9 Venous drainage of the brain, head, and neck.

then continues posteriorly on the left side of the trachea and curves downward, becoming the descending aorta.

The first and largest branch of the aortic arch is the brachiocephalic artery (see Fig. 1-4). The brachiocephalic artery is typically 4 to 5 cm in length. At the sternoclavicular joint, the artery divides into the right CCA and the right subclavian artery. The second branch of the aortic arch is the left CCA. The last branch of the aortic arch is the left subclavian artery.

The subclavian arteries give rise to branches that supply the brain, the neck, thoracic wall, and the shoulder, including the vertebral and internal mammary arteries (Fig. 1-10). Beyond the outer border of the first rib, the subclavian artery becomes the axillary artery. From the axilla to approximately 1 cm below the elbow joint, the artery is known as the brachial artery. The largest branch of the brachial artery is the deep brachial artery, or profunda brachii. The brachial artery ends by dividing into the radial and ulnar arteries near the neck of the radius.

The ulnar artery is usually slightly larger than the radial artery. The ulnar artery continues distally and courses along the ulnar border of the wrist. Beyond this point, the artery becomes the superficial palmar arch (Fig. 1-11). Major branches of the ulnar artery include the ulnar recurrent and interosseous arteries in the forearm, the palmar and dorsal carpal branches at the wrist, and the deep palmar and superficial palmar arch of the hand. The radial artery passes along the radial aspect of the forearm to the wrist, and then winds around the lateral aspect of the wrist to the dorsum of the wrist. It continues distally to join the deep palmar branch of the ulnar artery to form the deep palmar arch (Fig. 1-12). Branches of the radial artery include the radial recurrent, muscular, palmar carpal, and superficial palmar arteries. The superficial and deep palmar arches of the hand are continuations of the ulnar and radial arteries, respectively. The superficial palmar arch is completed by a branch of the radial artery. The deep palmar arch is completed by a branch of the ulnar artery. Both systems supply the digital arteries.

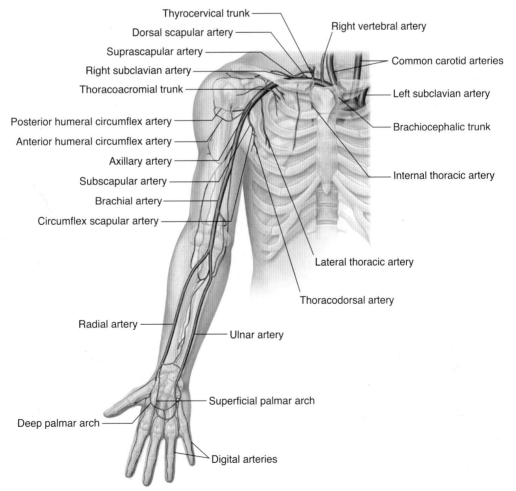

Figure 1-10 Diagram of the upper extremity arterial system.

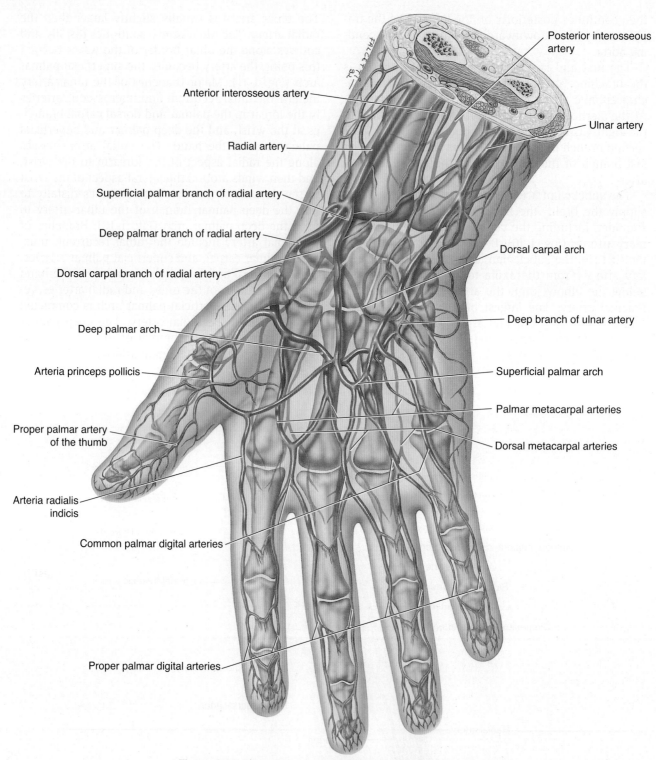

Figure 1-11 Ulnar artery terminating into the superficial palmar arch.

Labels on figure:

Posterior interosseous artery
Ulnar artery
Anterior interosseous artery
Radial artery
Superficial palmar branch of radial artery
Deep palmar branch of radial artery
Dorsal carpal branch of radial artery
Dorsal carpal arch
Deep branch of ulnar artery
Deep palmar arch
Superficial palmar arch
Arteria princeps pollicis
Palmar metacarpal arteries
Proper palmar artery of the thumb
Dorsal metacarpal arteries
Arteria radialis indicis
Common palmar digital arteries
Proper palmar digital arteries

THE SUPERIOR VENA CAVA AND UPPER EXTREMITY VENOUS SYSTEM

The dorsal digital veins unite to form the dorsal metacarpal veins, which end in a venous network on the back of the hand. The radial part of the network drains into the cephalic vein, and the ulnar part of the network drains into the basilic vein. The palmar digital veins flow over the palmar surface of the wrist and help form the medial antebrachial veins (Fig. 1-13).

The veins of the arm have both superficial and deep components similar to the lower extremities.

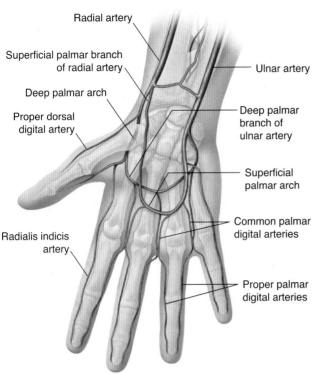

Radial artery

Superficial palmar branch of radial artery

Deep palmar arch

Proper dorsal digital artery

Ulnar artery

Deep palmar branch of ulnar artery

Superficial palmar arch

Radialis indicis artery

Common palmar digital arteries

Proper palmar digital arteries

Figure 1-12 Radial artery supplying the deep palmar arch.

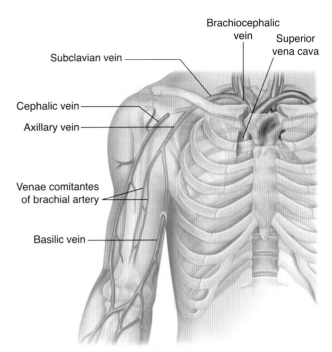

Brachiocephalic vein

Superior vena cava

Subclavian vein

Cephalic vein

Axillary vein

Venae comitantes of brachial artery

Basilic vein

Figure 1-14 View of the upper extremity veins crossing the axillary region.

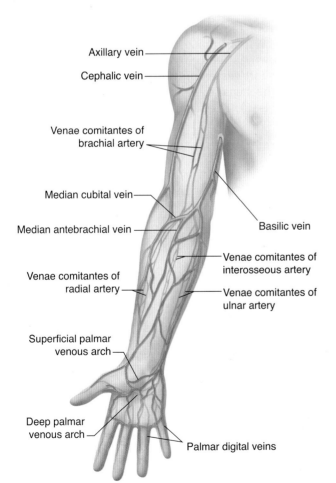

Axillary vein

Cephalic vein

Venae comitantes of brachial artery

Median cubital vein

Median antebrachial vein

Basilic vein

Venae comitantes of interosseous artery

Venae comitantes of radial artery

Venae comitantes of ulnar artery

Superficial palmar venous arch

Deep palmar venous arch

Palmar digital veins

Figure 1-13 Venous drainage of the hand and veins of the upper extremity.

The superficial veins of the arm include the cephalic, basilic, and medial antebrachial veins. The cephalic vein winds around the radial border of the forearm and continues along the lateral border of the biceps muscle. It then empties into the axillary vein just below the clavicle (Fig. 1-14). The basilic vein courses along the ulnar aspect of the forearm and continues proximally along the medial border of the biceps muscle. It joins the brachial vein to form the axillary vein. Both the cephalic and basilic veins communicate with the median cubital vein at the antecubital fossa. The median antebrachial vein courses the forearm slightly toward the ulnar side of the arm. It ends into either the median cubital vein or the basilic vein.

The deep venous branches of the forearm are the venae comitantes of the radial, ulnar, and interosseous arteries. They are paired veins, which follow the path of the arteries. These branches all unite at the elbow to form the brachial veins. There are usually two brachial veins, which course along each side of the brachial artery. The axillary vein begins at the junction of the brachial and basilic veins. It becomes the subclavian vein just past the outer border of the first rib. The axillary vein lies medial to the axillary artery, which it partially overlaps. The brachiocephalic veins are formed at the junction of the internal jugular and subclavian veins at each side of the base of the neck. The superior vena cava is formed by the junction of the two brachiocephalic veins just behind the right side of the sternum.

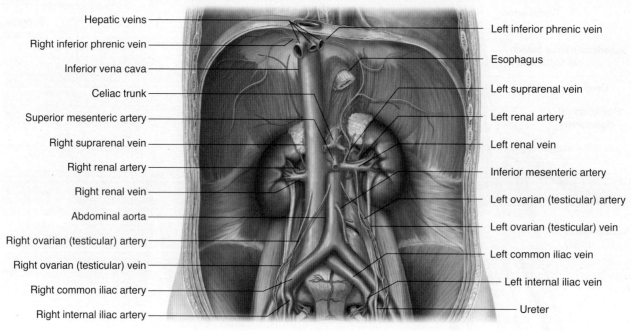

Hepatic veins
Right inferior phrenic vein
Inferior vena cava
Celiac trunk
Superior mesenteric artery
Right suprarenal vein
Right renal artery
Right renal vein
Abdominal aorta
Right ovarian (testicular) artery
Right ovarian (testicular) vein
Right common iliac artery
Right internal iliac artery

Left inferior phrenic vein
Esophagus
Left suprarenal vein
Left renal artery
Left renal vein
Inferior mesenteric artery
Left ovarian (testicular) artery
Left ovarian (testicular) vein
Left common iliac vein
Left internal iliac vein
Ureter

Figure 1-15 The abdominal aorta and its branches, as well as the inferior vena cava and its tributaries.

MAJOR VESSELS OF THE THORAX, ABDOMEN, AND PELVIS

The descending thoracic aorta is the continuation of the aorta beyond the aortic arch. Branches of the descending aorta include the bronchial, esophageal, phrenic, intercostal, and subcostal arteries. The abdominal aorta begins at the level of the 12th thoracic vertebra as it passes through the aortic hiatus of the diaphragm (Fig. 1-15). There are three major branches of the anterior aspect of the abdominal aorta. The first branch is the celiac artery. This is also known as the celiac trunk or celiac axis. It is a fairly short vessel, only 1–2 cm in length. It gives rise to the hepatic, splenic, and left gastric arteries (Fig. 1-16). The superior mesenteric artery is the

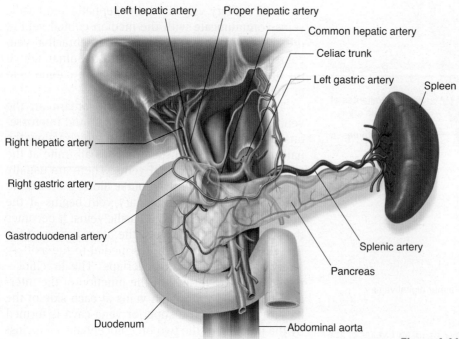

Left hepatic artery
Proper hepatic artery
Common hepatic artery
Celiac trunk
Left gastric artery
Spleen
Right hepatic artery
Right gastric artery
Gastroduodenal artery
Splenic artery
Pancreas
Duodenum
Abdominal aorta

Figure 1-16 The celiac artery and its branches.

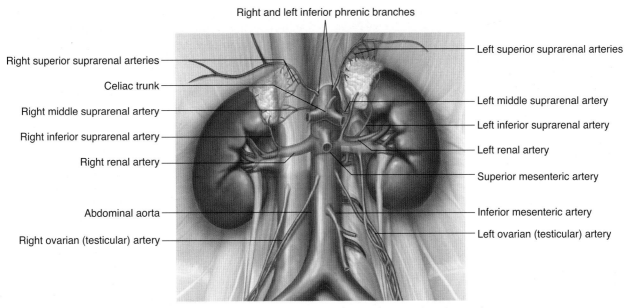

Figure 1-17 View of the branches of the abdominal aorta, including the renal arteries.

next branch of the aorta, just below the celiac artery (Fig. 1-17). It supplies most of the small intestine and some of the large intestine. It courses inferiorly, running parallel with and anterior to the aorta. The last anterior branch of the aorta is the inferior mesenteric artery. It arises about 3 or 4 cm above the aortic bifurcation. It mainly supplies the large intestine.

The renal arteries branch off the lateral aspect of the aorta just below the superior mesenteric artery (see Fig. 1-17). The right renal artery is longer and usually slightly higher than the left renal artery. The right renal artery courses posterior to the inferior vena cava as it continues to the right kidney. Both renal arteries approach the kidneys slightly posterior to the renal veins.

Just below the level of the renal arteries, two additional arteries branch off the anterior–lateral aspect of the aorta. These are the testicular arteries in the male and the ovarian arteries in the female. Posteriorly, off the aorta, there are four pairs of lumbar arteries. These course laterally and posteriorly along the lumbar vertebrae. Occasionally, there is a fifth smaller pair. A single middle sacral artery is a small posterior branch of the aorta. It arises just above the bifurcation of the iliac vessels.

The aorta terminates at the level of the fourth lumbar vertebra into the right and left common iliac arteries (Fig. 1-18). The common iliac arteries each bifurcate into the external and internal iliac arteries. The internal iliac arteries, which are also known as the hypogastric arteries, supply the pelvic organs. The external iliac arteries continue distally to supply the lower extremities. At the inguinal ligament,

these arteries are then known as the common femoral arteries.

The venous system of the pelvis is composed of the external iliac veins, which are the continuation of the common femoral veins above the inguinal

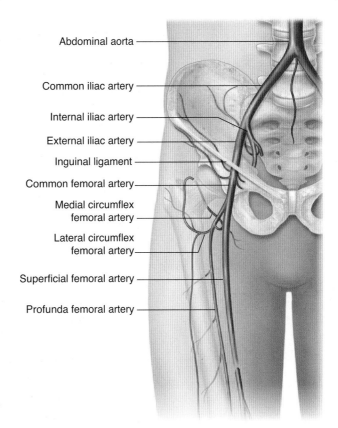

Figure 1-18 Diagram of the termination of the abdominal aorta into the iliac vessels.

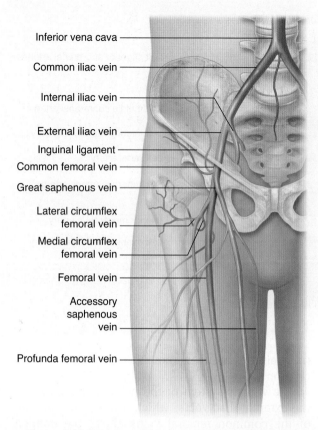

Inferior vena cava

Common iliac vein

Internal iliac vein

External iliac vein

Inguinal ligament

Common femoral vein

Great saphenous vein

Lateral circumflex
femoral vein

Medial circumflex
femoral vein

Femoral vein

Accessory
saphenous
vein

Profunda femoral vein

Figure 1-19 Diagram of the venous system of the pelvis.

ligament (Fig. 1-19). The internal iliac veins join the external iliac veins to form the common iliac veins. The left common iliac vein courses proximally, passing beneath the right common iliac artery at the level of the aortic bifurcation. The left and right common iliac veins join to form the inferior vena cava. The inferior vena cava travels through the abdomen along the right side of the aorta. The renal, hepatic, lumbar, ovarian, and testicular veins drain into the inferior vena cava.

The liver has a unique arrangement of vessels (Fig. 1-20). The hepatic artery (a branch of the celiac artery) carries fully oxygenated blood into the liver. It typically supplies 30% of the total blood flow into the liver. The liver receives the remaining 70% of its blood flow via the portal vein. The portal vein forms at the junction of the splenic and superior mesenteric veins posterior to the neck of the pancreas and anterior to the inferior vena cava. Drainage of the liver is accomplished by the hepatic venous system, which drains into three hepatic veins: the left, the right, and the middle hepatic veins. These three hepatic veins empty into the inferior vena cava. The middle and left hepatic veins join into a common trunk before entering the inferior vena cava in approximately 96% of individuals (Fig. 1-21).

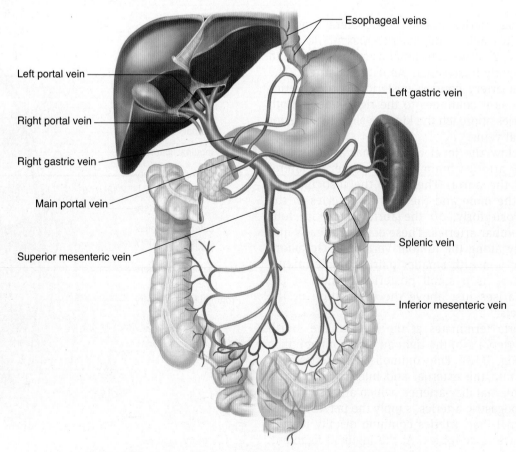

Esophageal veins

Left portal vein

Right portal vein

Right gastric vein

Main portal vein

Superior mesenteric vein

Left gastric vein

Splenic vein

Inferior mesenteric vein

Figure 1-20 Diagram illustrating the main portal vein and its tributaries.

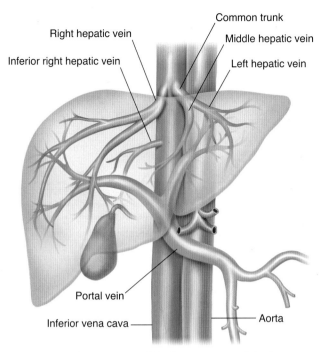

Figure 1-21 Diagram of the hepatic veins of the liver.

THE ARTERIES AND VEINS OF THE LOWER EXTREMITIES

The common femoral artery is the continuation of the external iliac artery below the inguinal ligament (Fig. 1-22). The common femoral artery divides into the superficial femoral and the profunda femoris arteries. The profunda femoris artery is also known as the deep femoral artery. The profunda femoris artery is posterior and lateral to the superficial femoral artery. Branches of the profunda femoris artery include numerous perforators and the medial and lateral circumflex arteries. The superficial femoral artery courses distally, passing through the adductor canal. The popliteal artery is the continuation of the superficial femoral artery and courses behind the knee in the popliteal fossa. Branches of the popliteal artery include the sural and genicular arteries. Terminal branches of the popliteal artery include the anterior tibial, posterior tibial, and peroneal arteries (Fig. 1-23). Initially, the popliteal artery bifurcates into the anterior tibial artery and the tibial–peroneal trunk. The tibial–peroneal trunk continues for a

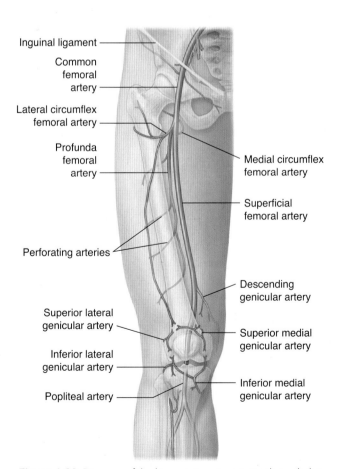

Figure 1-22 Diagram of the lower extremity arteries through the thigh.

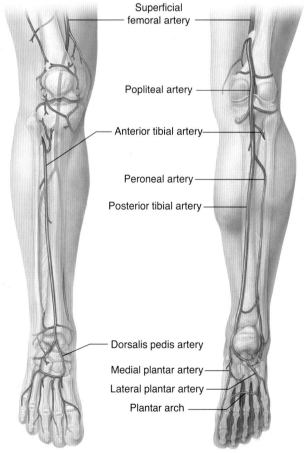

Figure 1-23 Diagram of the lower extremity arteries through the calf.

short distance and bifurcates again into the posterior tibial and peroneal arteries. The anterior tibial artery passes through an opening in the interosseous membrane, then proceeds distally in the anterior compartment of the leg. It continues anterior to the ankle joint and becomes the dorsalis pedis artery. The posterior tibial artery courses medially in the posterior compartment of the leg. It runs behind the medial malleolus and terminates into the medial and lateral plantar arteries. The peroneal artery is located deep within the leg and descends along the medial aspect of the fibula. It terminates into branches that communicate with the posterior and anterior tibial arteries. The arteries of the foot include the medial and lateral plantar and dorsalis pedis arteries, which all help to give rise to the plantar arch. Arising off the plantar arch are the metatarsal arteries, which divide into the digital arteries.

The veins of the leg have both deep and superficial systems. The dorsal venous arch of the foot joins into the great saphenous vein (GSV) just anterior to the medial malleolus. The GSV is

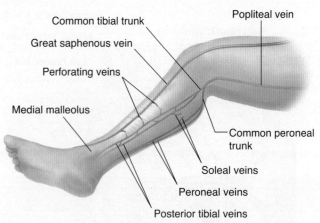

Figure 1-25 Diagram of the orientation of the peroneal and posterior tibial veins of the calf.

the longest vein in the body. It ascends the leg medially with several tributaries emptying into the GSV before it terminates into the common femoral vein at the saphenofemoral junction (Fig. 1-24). The small saphenous vein (SSV) begins as

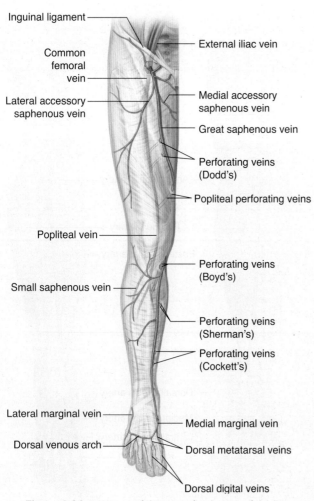

Figure 1-24 Diagram of the superficial veins of the leg.

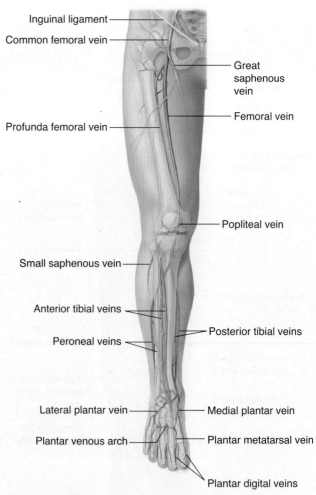

Figure 1-26 Diagram of the lower extremity deep venous system.

a continuation of the lateral segment of the dorsal venous arch of the foot. The SSV courses posteriorly up the calf, penetrating the deep fascia in the upper half of the calf. In approximately 70% of individuals, the SSV terminates into the popliteal vein at the saphenopopliteal junction. In the remainder of cases, the SSV continues above the knee as the vein of Giacomini.

The deep venous system begins with the deep plantar arch, which continues as the medial and lateral plantar veins. These veins then unite to form the posterior tibial veins (Fig. 1-25). The pared posterior tibial veins accompany the posterior tibial artery. The paired peroneal veins ascend the calf in the same plane as the peroneal artery. Approximately two-thirds of the way up the calf, the peroneal veins join the posterior tibial veins to form the tibio-peroneal trunk veins. The anterior tibial veins are the continuation of the vena comitantes of the dorsalis pedis artery. The anterior tibial veins pass between the tibia and fibula through the upper part of the interosseous membrane. The veins then unite with the tibio-peroneal trunk veins to form the popliteal vein. The popliteal vein is medial to the popliteal artery distally and moves lateral to the artery as it passes through the adductor canal. The femoral vein is the continuation of the popliteal vein and accompanies the superficial femoral artery to the groin (Fig. 1-26). The profunda femoral (deep femoral) vein courses the thigh along the profunda femoris artery. The profunda femoris and femoral veins unite to form the common femoral vein. The common femoral vein lies medial to the common femoral artery. The external iliac vein is the continuation of the common femoral vein above the inguinal ligament.

SUMMARY

In summary, the blood vessels of the body have the same basic microscopic arrangement. Varying combinations of muscle, collagen, elastic fibers, and connective tissue provide essential differences between the arteries and veins to allow for their specific functions. Arteries and veins of differing sizes are oriented to provide for the efficient delivery of nutrients to the organs and tissue beds as well as to return blood back to the heart to complete the cycle. The network of arteries and veins is complex but, if examined by region (arm, leg, abdomen, etc.), can be easier to understand. Proper knowledge of vascular anatomy will aid the vascular technologist or sonographer to achieve a technically adequate vascular ultrasound examination.

Critical Thinking Questions

1. When examining the carotid system, the physician asks you to be sure to document the origin of the superficial thyroid artery. Normally, in which direction should you focus your examination in order to visualize this vessel?

2. In your department, part of the documentation includes tapping over the superficial temporal artery and observing the ECA Doppler signal for oscillations in the waveform produced by the tapping. This is done to confirm the vessel being insonated is the ECA. Why are there no oscillations within the ICA?

3. If a patient presents with an abdominal aortic aneurysm that is present from just below the renal arteries to the bifurcation of the common iliac arteries, what branches of the aorta may be involved in the aneurysmal dilation?

4. You are asked to examine a patient with a penetrating injury to the medial aspect of the mid-thigh. What vessels may have sustained an injury and thus should be thoroughly examined?

SUGGESTED READINGS

1. Gilroy AM, MacPherson BR, Ross LM. *Atlas of Anatomy.* New York, NY: Thieme; 2008.
2. Kadir S, ed. *Diagnostic Angiography.* Philadelphia, PA: W.B. Saunders; 1986.
3. Krstić RV. *Human Microscopic Anatomy: An Atlas for Students of Medicine and Biology.* Berlin, Germany: Springer-Verlag; 1991.
4. Netter FH. *Atlas of Human Anatomy.* 4th ed. Philadelphia, PA: Saunders-Elsevier; 2006.
5. Standring S, ed. *Gray's Anatomy: The Anatomical Basis of Clinical Practice.* 40th ed. Edinburgh, Scotland: Churchill-Livingstone; 2008.

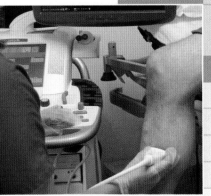

2 Arterial Physiology

Ann Marie Kupinski

OBJECTIVES

List the various hemodynamic forces acting upon the arterial system

Describe the relationship between pressure, flow, and resistance

Identify the factors that control peripheral blood flow

Define physiologic changes associated with arterial disease

KEY TERMS

inertia | kinetic energy | laminar flow | potential energy | pressure | resistance | turbulence | velocity | viscosity

GLOSSARY

inertia the tendency of a body at rest to stay at rest or a body in motion to stay in motion

kinetic energy the energy of work or motion; in the vascular system, it is in part represented by the velocity of blood flow

laminar flow flow of a liquid in which it travels smoothly in parallel layers

Poiseuille's law the law that states that the volume flow of a liquid flowing through a vessel is directly proportional to the pressure of the liquid, and the fourth power of the radius is inversely proportional to the viscosity of the liquid and the length of the vessel

potential energy the stored or resting energy; in the vascular system, it is the intravascular pressure

viscosity the property of a fluid that resists the force tending to cause fluid to flow

A general understanding of the physiology of the vascular system is important when performing ultrasounds on the circulatory system. Although anatomy provides information on the structures being scanned, one must understand function too. There are numerous factors that impact the arterial system. Relationships that govern blood flow result in spectral waveforms that can vary depending on the system being scanned. This chapter will review the basics of normal arterial physiology as well as pathophysiology.

FLUID ENERGY

Blood, like any other fluid, will move from one point to another in response to differences in total energy. The total energy of a system is made up of both potential and kinetic energy. Potential energy is also known as stored or resting energy. In the vascular system, it is represented primarily by the intravascular pressure, which distends the vessels. This pressure is supplied by the contraction of the heart. Kinetic energy is the energy of work or motion. The velocity of moving blood represents the kinetic energy component of the vascular system. Blood will move from an area of high energy (pressure) to an area of lower energy (pressure). The highest pressure in the vascular system occurs in the left ventricle of the heart where the pressure is approximately 120 mm Hg. The blood leaves the left ventricle, flowing down an energy (pressure) gradient until it returns to the right atrium. The lowest pressure is found at the right atrium where pressure is 2 to 6 mm Hg.

There is another component to the energy of the vascular system related to differences in the level of body parts. Gravitational potential energy is the potential for doing work related to the force of gravity. If blood is positioned above a reference point (which is usually the right atrium), it has the ability to do work because gravity will act on the blood to move it downward. The gravitational potential energy is reduced in dependent parts of the body (below the reference point). Hydrostatic pressure is also pressure within the vessels related to the reference point of the right atrium.

Hydrostatic pressure increases in lower portions of the body due to the weight of the column of blood within the vessels. The farther below the reference point, the greater the hydrostatic pressure. The formula for gravitational potential energy is the same as hydrostatic pressure but with an opposite sign. Thus, gravitational potential energy and hydrostatic pressure tend to cancel each other out. More information about hydrostatic pressure will be discussed in Chapter 3.

THE BERNOULLI PRINCIPLE

The Bernoulli principle states that when a fluid flows without a change in velocity from one point to another, the total energy content remains constant, providing no frictional losses. However, in reality, there is always some energy that is "lost." Of course, energy cannot be lost, but it is merely transferred to a different form. In the vascular system, energy is mostly dissipated in the form of heat due to friction.

The total energy in the vascular system is a balance between potential energy (pressure) and kinetic energy (velocity). If the velocity of blood goes up, there must be a pressure decrease. One can think of this as taking energy from one form (the blood pressure) in order to increase another form of energy (the blood velocity). This principle is used in cardiac imaging. By measuring the velocity at the stenotic valve, one can determine the pressure drop across a valve and thus the clinical significance (Fig. 2-1).

VISCOSITY AND INERTIA

In the vascular system, energy "losses" are the result of viscosity and inertia. Viscosity is the property of a fluid that resists the force tending to cause fluid to flow. It can be defined as the friction existing between bordering layers of fluid. Imagine two open containers, one filled with water and one filled with honey. If both containers were tilted to allow the liquids to pour out, the water would flow more quickly than the honey. The honey is more viscous than the water, and more viscous fluids flow more slowly. Blood viscosity increases with increases in hematocrit (the concentration of red blood cells). Hematocrit is the most important influence on blood viscosity.

Inertia is the tendency of a body at rest to stay at rest or a body in motion to stay in motion unless acted upon by an outside force. It is one of the fundamental principles of physics described by Sir Isaac Newton. A classic example of the force of inertia is, when riding in a car when the brakes are applied, an individual has the tendency to move forward. The seat belt is the outside force that stops this forward movement. Inertial losses in the vascular system occur whenever blood is forced to change direction or velocity. In order to change direction, a force needs to be applied and some energy is "lost." Inertial "losses" depend on the density and velocity of the blood flow. In blood vessels, energy "losses" due to viscosity effects are greater than those due to inertia.

VELOCITY AND FLOW

Often, the terms "blood velocity" and "blood flow" are used interchangeably, but they mean two different things. Velocity refers to the rate of movement (displacement) with respect to time. It has the units of distance per unit of time, such as centimeters per second or meters per second. Blood flow is also referred to as volume flow. It represents the volume of something moved per unit of time. It has the units of milliliters per second, liters per second, milliliters per minute, or liters per minute.

Velocity and flow are related by the equation:

$$V = \frac{Q}{A}$$

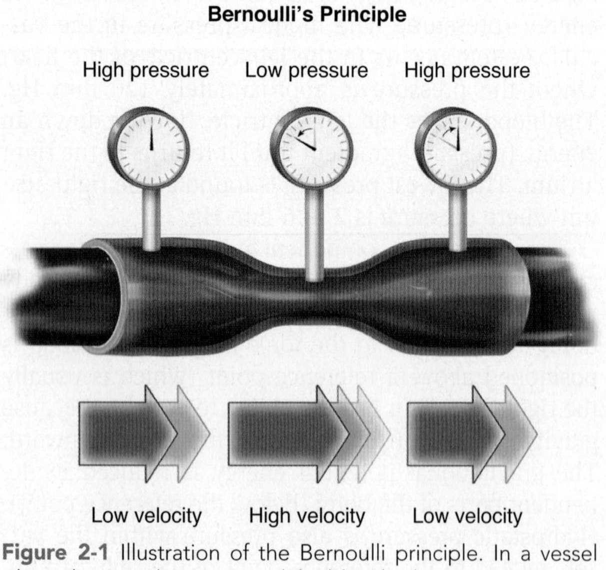

Bernoulli's Principle

High pressure   Low pressure   High pressure

Low velocity   High velocity   Low velocity

Figure 2-1 Illustration of the Bernoulli principle. In a vessel where the area decreases and the blood velocity increases, the pressure must decrease.

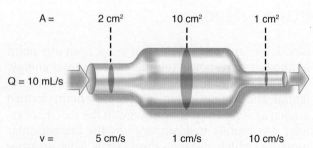

A =   2 cm²   10 cm²   1 cm²

Q = 10 mL/s

v =   5 cm/s   1 cm/s   10 cm/s

Figure 2-2 This illustrates the changes in velocity as a result of changes in diameter. Note there is a steady rate of flow throughout the conduit.

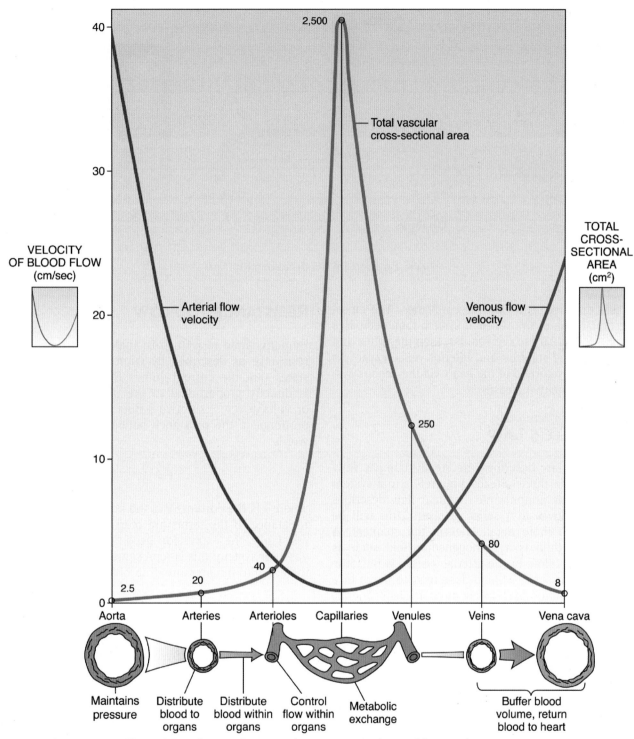

Figure 2-3 A diagram illustrating the cross-sectional area of the vascular system.

where V is velocity, Q is volume flow, and A is area. Given a constant flow, velocity will vary inversely related to the cross-sectional area. Thus, if the flow is the same, the velocity must increase if the area of a blood vessel decreases (Fig. 2-2). This change in velocity allows one to estimate the degree of cross-sectional stenosis within an individual vessel such as the internal carotid artery.

Throughout the entire circulatory system, the cross-sectional area increases from the aorta moving through the arteries, then arterioles, and finally into the capillaries (Fig. 2-3). Blood velocity thus decreases as blood travels from the aorta, through the arteries, then the arterioles, and finally through the capillaries. This slowing down of blood flow at the capillary level is important in the proper exchange of nutrients and

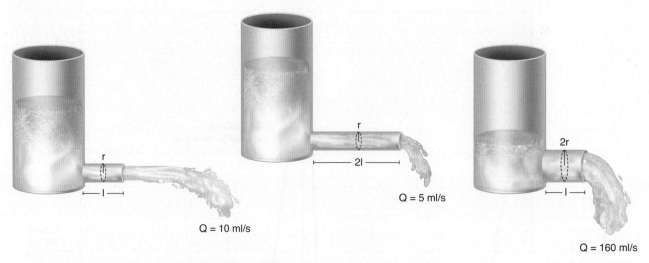

Figure 2-4 Effects of radius and length on flow.

waste that occurs within the capillaries. The cross-sectional area of the vascular system then decreases from the capillary to the venules, then the veins, and lastly into the superior and inferior venae cavae. As the blood is returned to the heart via the venous system, the velocity increases.

POISEUILLE'S LAW

Poiseuille's law describes the steady laminar flow of Newtonian fluids. Steady flow refers to a system where flow is nonpulsatile. Laminar flow describes flow that moves in a series of layers (this will be discussed in more detail later in the chapter). A Newtonian fluid is a homogeneous fluid such as air or water. Flow in the arterial system is pulsatile and thus not steady. Blood does tend to move in a laminar fashion, at least in some portions of the arterial system. Blood is definitely not homogeneous and thus is non-Newtonian. However, even with all these variations, Poiseuille's law is used to define pressure/flow relationships in the vascular system.

The full definition of Poiseuille's law states:

$$Q = \frac{\pi \, (P_1 - P_2) r^4}{8\eta l}$$

where Q is flow, r is the radius of the vessel, l is the length of the vessel, P_1–P_2 is the pressure difference, η is the viscosity of the blood, and $\pi/8$ is the constant of proportionality. Examining the terms of Poiseuille's law, a greater change in pressure will produce an increase in flow (providing the other components stay the same). If the viscosity of the blood increases, flow will decrease. If the radius of a vessel changes, this will have a significant impact on flow because it is the radius to the 4th power that is directly proportional to flow (Fig. 2-4).

RESISTANCE TO FLOW

Hemodynamic resistance is analogous to electrical resistance as described by Ohm's law. Ohm's law states that the current (flow) through two points is directly proportional to the potential difference or voltage across the two points and inversely proportional to the resistance between them. In other words:

$$I = \frac{V}{R}$$

where I is the current, V is the voltage, and R is the resistance. If the terms are rearranged to solve for resistance, the expression becomes R = V/I. In the vascular system, this is represented as resistance being equal to the pressure drop divided by the flow:

$$R = \frac{\Delta P}{Q}$$

Looking back to the components of Poiseuille's law, it can be determined that resistance can be expressed as:

$$R = \frac{8\eta l}{\pi r^4}$$

In the circulatory system, the length of a given vessel is virtually constant and the blood viscosity does not vary. Thus, changes in resistance are virtually all due to variations in the radius. It is the smooth muscle cell layer within the media of the wall of a vessel that varies resistance by altering vessel radius.

In the vascular system, various types of vessels lie in series with one another. In addition, individual members of each category of vessels are arranged in parallel with each other. The notable exceptions to this are the renal and splanchnic vasculatures where capillary systems are arranged in a series.

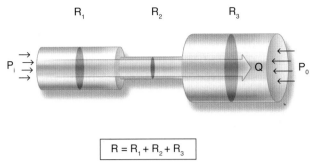

$$R = R_1 + R_2 + R_3$$

Figure 2-5 A diagram illustrating multiple resistances in series.

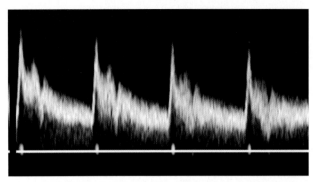

Figure 2-7 A low-resistance flow profile with antegrade flow throughout the cardiac cycle.

For resistances in series, the total resistance of the entire system equals the sum of the individual resistances (Fig. 2-5):

$$R_T = R_1 + R_2 + R_3$$

Thus, multiple stenoses along the same blood vessel will increase the total resistance.

For resistances in parallel, the reciprocal of the total resistance of the system equals the sum of the reciprocals of the individual resistances (Fig. 2-6):

$$\frac{1}{R_T} = \frac{1}{R_1} + \frac{1}{R_2} + \frac{1}{R_3}$$

The more parallel elements in a network, the lower the overall resistance of the network will be. An example of a resistance in parallel is a collateral artery. A collateral artery dilates in response to ischemia produced by a flow-limiting stenosis in a main artery, such as the superficial femoral artery. When adding a collateral pathway, around a stenosis, this will have the effect to lower the total resistance.

PERIPHERAL RESISTANCE

Most flow can be described as either high resistance or low-resistance flow. A low-resistance flow profile characteristically has antegrade flow throughout the cardiac cycle (Fig. 2-7). This is the result of dilation of the arteriolar bed. The internal carotid and the vertebral, celiac, splenic, hepatic, and renal arteries will display low-resistance flow.

A high-resistance flow profile displays both antegrade and retrograde flow (Fig. 2-8). In systole, flow is antegrade. In early diastole, flow reversal occurs. This is due to slight vasoconstriction of the distal arterioles. The radius of these vessels is decreased, thus increasing the resistance to flow. As the flow traveling down the vessel encounters the high-resistance arteriolar bed, some flow is reflected back up the vessel. This produces a "reflected wave," which is apparent on ultrasound spectral analysis as well as on continuous Doppler tracings and plethysmographic waveforms. Depending on the compliance of the more proximal vessels, a third antegrade flow component may be present. This feature of distensible vessels will be discussed later in this chapter. Vessels that normally display high-resistance flow patterns include the external carotid and the subclavian, distal aorta, iliac, fasting superior mesenteric, and resting peripheral arteries.

Some high-resistance tissue beds can change into low-resistance beds. This happens with extremity arteries after exercise. Exercise produces vasodilation, which decreases the resistance to flow. This

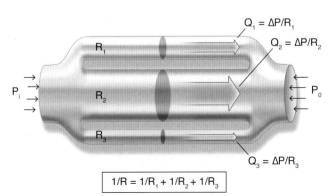

$$1/R = 1/R_1 + 1/R_2 + 1/R_3$$

Figure 2-6 A diagram illustrating multiple resistances in parallel.

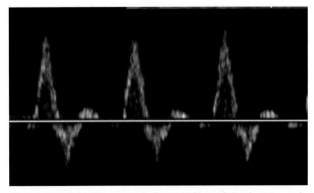

Figure 2-8 A high-resistance flow profile with both antegrade and retrograde flow.

results in changing the flow profile into a low-resistance pattern with antegrade flow throughout the cardiac cycle. The same change can occur within the superior mesenteric artery. After eating, this tissue bed also vasodilates, changing the flow profile into a low-resistance pattern. In both these circumstances, the low-resistance pattern results in an increase in blood flow to meet the increased metabolic demand.

LAMINAR AND TURBULENT FLOW

Under certain conditions, flow in a cylindrical tube (or blood vessel) will be laminar or streamlined. At the entrance to a vessel, all elements of the blood flow stream will have the same velocities (often referred to as plug flow). As the flow progresses in the vessel, a thin layer in contact with the wall will adhere to the wall and become motionless. The layer of fluid next to this layer must move against this motionless layer and therefore moves slowly due to friction between the layers. The adjacent more central layer travels a little more rapidly. The layers at the center of the tube move the fastest and their velocity is equal to twice the mean velocity across the entire cross section of the tube. At a distance equal to several tube diameters away from the entrance, laminar flow becomes fully developed. Thus, at the beginning of a vessel, the flow profile is rather blunted. The longitudinal velocity profile becomes parabolic at a point several diameters away from the entrance of a vessel (Fig. 2-9).

Turbulent flow is described as irregular motions of the fluid elements. Definite laminae are no longer present but rapid radial mixing occurs. A greater pressure is required to move a given flow of fluid through a tube under turbulent conditions as compared to those for laminar flow.

Turbulence is best defined in terms of a dimensionless quantity, the Reynolds number (Re). The Reynolds number is proportional to the inertial

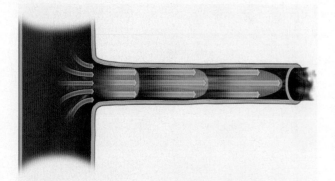

Figure 2-9 Flow through a tube illustrating plug flow at the entrance of the tube and parabolic flow distal to the entrance.

forces and to the viscous forces acting on a fluid. In the vascular system, Re is directly proportional to the velocity of the blood, the density of the blood, and the radius of the blood vessel. It is inversely proportional to the viscosity of the blood. Because blood density and viscosity are relatively constant, turbulence develops mainly due to changes in the velocity of blood and the size of the blood vessel. For Re below 2,000, flow will be laminar. For Re above 2,000, turbulence will develop. As blood flows through a stenosis, the vessel radius is reduced by the presence of atherosclerotic disease, and velocity increases. This results in turbulence, which is routinely documented as the flow exits the stenotic area.

THE ARTERIAL SYSTEM: A HYDRAULIC FILTER

The principal function of the arterial system is to distribute blood to the capillary beds throughout the body. The arterial system consists of various-sized vessels with varying volumes and distensibility. The arterial system, composed of elastic conduits and high-resistance terminals, constitutes a hydraulic filter analogous to resistance-capacitance filters of electrical circuits. Hydraulic filtering converts the intermittent (pulsatile) output of the heart to a steady flow through the capillaries. Steady flow in the capillaries ensures adequate exchange or nutrients and wastes.

The entire stroke volume is discharged from the heart during systole. Part of the energy of the cardiac contraction is dissipated as the kinetic energy of the forward blood flow. The remainder is stored as potential energy by the distensible arteries. During diastole, the elastic recoil of the arterial walls converts the potential energy into blood flow. This produces antegrade flow in late diastole (Fig. 2-10). If the arterial walls were rigid, no capillary flow would occur during diastole.

Arterial elasticity and capacitance are essential properties to allow for proper blood flow. The change in volume divided by the change in pressure represents capacitance or compliance. Normal capacitance of arteries is greatest over a median range of pressure variations. (Just like a balloon, which is hardest to inflate at the very beginning and again at just before it is completely full, but it is easiest to inflate at intermediate volumes.) Capacitance decreases with age as the vessel walls become rigid. As a vessel wall becomes stiffer with age, this results in an increase in systolic pressure as well as pulse pressure. Pulse pressure is the difference between the systolic and diastolic pressures.

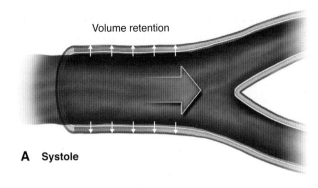

A   Systole

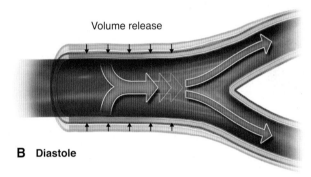

B   Diastole

Figure 2-10 A diagram illustrating the distensibility of the arterial walls, **(A)** systole expanding the vessel walls, **(B)** antegrade flow in diastole produced by the elastic recoil of the vessels.

Control of Peripheral Circulation

Peripheral circulation is controlled centrally by the nervous system and locally by conditions at the tissue bed. Vessels involved in regulating blood flow are called the resistance vessels, the arterioles. The vessel diameter is varied by contracting or relaxing the smooth muscle cells in the medial layer of the vessel wall. The constant contraction of these muscle cells provides a degree of vasomotor tone.

The arterioles that control blood flow to a particular region or organ lie within the area or within the organ tissue itself. These arterioles are exposed to various chemicals in that region, and changes in concentrations of many substances can impact the arterioles. For instance, if interstitial oxygen levels fall because the cells are using more oxygen, this results in the arterioles dilating. When this vasodilation occurs, blood flow to the area will increase and bring more oxygen. This is an example of a local feedback mechanism that controls blood flow. Not only will oxygen levels alter the vasomotor tone, but carbon dioxide, hydrogen ions, and potassium ions will also have an effect. These are

just a few of the substances that can locally impact blood flow.

There are nerve fibers of the sympathetic nervous system that innervate the arterioles. These nerve fibers release norepinephrine, which causes an increase in the tone of the arterioles. These vasoconstrictor nerves normally have a continual activity, resulting in a contractile tone of the arterioles.

At any given point in time, some arterioles are open and some are closed. If all arterioles were open at the same time, blood pressure would fall very low. Flow into many tissue beds appears to be autoregulated. This means a constant level of blood flow is maintained over a wide range of perfusion pressures. Resistance vessels dilate in response to high blood pressure and constrict in response to low blood pressure. These actions help maintain a constant flow of oxygen and nutrients to vital organs.

Hemodynamics of Arterial Disease

Atherosclerotic changes begin with a lipid streak that consists of subintimal deposits of fat. Lesions that are of concern include fibrous and complicated plaques. Fibrous plaque has a smooth surface and is composed of smooth muscle and fibrous tissue and lacks calcification. Complicated plaque has an irregular surface and loss of the normal endothelium and calcification is present. The exposure of the subendothelial collagen matrix is thrombogenic and may cause platelets to accumulate. Atherosclerosis typically develops at branch points and at bifurcations.

Most abnormal energy losses in the arterial system result from stenoses or obstruction of the vessel lumen (Fig. 2-11). According to Poiseuille's law, viscous energy losses within a stenosis are inversely proportional to the 4th power of the radius and directly proportional to its length. Thus, the radius of a stenosis is more important than its length. Even a small change in radius will result in large changes in flow. A doubling in the length of a stenosis will yield a doubling in the associated energy losses. A decrease in the radius of a vessel by half will increase the energy losses by a factor of 16 (because it is the radius to the 4th power in Poiseuille's law).

Inertial energy losses are encountered at the entrance and the exit of a stenosis. More energy is lost at an abrupt change rather than a gradual tapering. A great deal more inertial energy is lost when blood exits a stenosis because the kinetic energy may be dissipated in the turbulent jet.

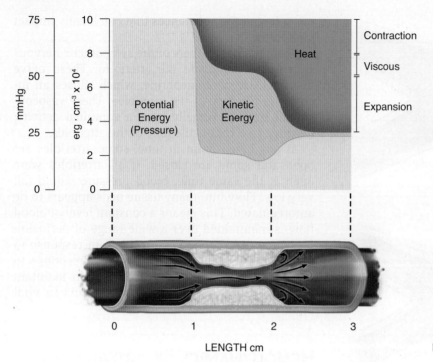

Figure 2-11 Energy losses across a stenosis.

A critical stenosis is defined as a degree of narrowing at which pressure and flow begin to be affected. Experimentally, changes in pressure and flow do not occur until the cross-sectional area has been reduced by 75% (or a 50% diameter reduction). Because energy losses also depend on the velocity of blood flow, in high-flow (low-resistance) systems, significant drops in pressures and flow occur with less severe narrowing than in low-flow systems. Therefore, a critical stenosis varies with the resistance of the run-off bed. In the carotid or coronary systems (low-resistance systems), a critical stenosis may be reached with less narrowing than in the resting lower extremity (high resistance). In the exercising leg, resistance drops, flow increases, and a stenosis may become critical or flow limiting.

Collateral vessels are preexisting pathways that enlarge with a stenosis or occlusion. They are one of the main mechanisms to compensate for a stenosis. Collateral arteries can be divided into (1) stem arteries, which are the large branches; (2) midzone collaterals, which are the small intramuscular branches; and (3) reentry arteries, which are the vessels that rejoin a major artery distal to the area of stenosis or occlusion (Fig. 2-12). The resistance of the collateral bed is almost fixed and will only slightly dilate gradually. Exercise, sympathectomy, and vasodilator drugs have little effect on collaterals unlike the peripheral run-off bed.

Blood flow increases with exercise to at least three to five times resting flow in normal limbs. In limbs with mild-to-moderate disease, blood flow is increased far less. In patients with multilevel disease,

flow after exercise may change very little. At rest, blood pressure distal to an arterial lesion will decrease with mild-to-moderate disease and even more with severe disease. Exercise will cause a further decrease in peripheral pressure.

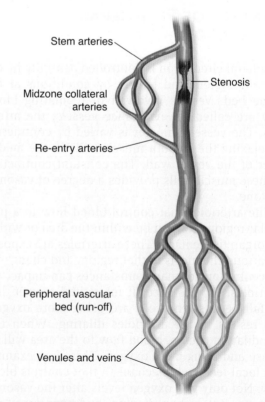

Figure 2-12 Collateral arteries including stem arteries, midzone collaterals, and reentry arteries.

SUMMARY

The hemodynamics of the arterial system includes unique relationships between pressure, resistance, and flow. Blood flow follows the same rules that govern the movement of other fluids. Understanding the factors that influence the movement of blood flow in the arterial system will make it easier to understand the velocities and waveforms encountered during ultrasound examinations.

Critical Thinking Questions

1. You are examining a patient with a lower extremity bypass graft from the common femoral artery to the popliteal artery. The flow is constant throughout the graft but, at one point, you detect a velocity increase on spectral analysis. What must be happening in this area?

2. Would increasing the viscosity of blood or increasing length of a conduit have a greater effect on decreasing blood flow?

3. You examine a popliteal artery that displays continuous forward (antegrade) flow throughout the entire cardiac cycle. In the absence of any disease or pathology, what is the most likely explanation of these findings?

SUGGESTED READINGS

1. Carter SA. Hemodynamic considerations in peripheral vascular and cerebrovascular disease. In: Zwiebel WJ, Pellerito JS, eds. *Introduction to Vascular Ultrasonography*. 5th ed. Philadelphia, PA: Elsevier Saunders; 2005:3–17.
2. Guyton AC, Hall JE. *Textbook of Medical Physiology*. 11th ed. Philadelphia, PA: Saunders; 2005.
3. Koeppen BM, Stanton BA. *Berne & Levy Physiology*. 6th ed. Philadelphia, PA: Mosby; 2009.
4. Mohrman DE, Heller LJ. *Cardiovascular Physiology*. New York, NY: McGraw-Hill; 1997.
5. Oates C, ed. *Cardiovascular Haemodynamics and Doppler Waveforms Explained*. Cambridge, MA: Cambridge University Press; 2001.
6. Zierler RE. Hemodynamics of normal and abnormal arteries. In: Zierler RE, ed. *Strandness's Duplex Scanning in Vascular Disorders*. 4th ed. Philadelphia, PA: Lippincott Williams & Wilkins; 2010:47–55.

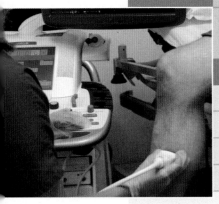

3 Venous Physiology

Ann Marie Kupinski

OBJECTIVES

List the hemodynamic factors which affect venous blood flow

Describe the components of hydrostatic pressure

Identify the forces that lead to edema formation

Define the changes that occur at rest and with exercise in the venous system

KEY TERMS

calf muscle pump | edema | hydrostatics | resistance | transmural pressure | venous insufficiency

GLOSSARY

edema excessive accumulation of fluid in cells, tissues, or cavities of the body

hydrostatic pressure the pressure within the vascular system due to the weight of a column of blood

transmural pressure the pressure on the walls of a vessel

venous insufficiency abnormal retrograde flow in veins

The venous system is usually perceived to be rather passive. It is generally believed that the arterial system does all the work and the veins just return the blood back to the heart. However, changes in venous blood flow can cause various complications from varicose veins to pulmonary emboli. Venous disease affects a significant portion of the population. Several factors affect the movement of blood throughout the venous system. This chapter will present the major features of venous physiology and pathophysiology.

VENOUS CAPACITANCE

Veins are known as the capacitance vessels of the body. They serve an important role acting as a reservoir. The venous side of the circulatory system holds approximately two-thirds of the total blood volume of the body (Fig. 3-1). The arterial side of the circulatory system typically holds about 30% of the blood volume with the remaining 3% to 4% within the capillaries. The cross-sectional area of a fully distended vein can be three to four times that of the corresponding companion artery. Often, the veins are paired structures and this adds to their ability to hold blood.

VENOUS RESISTANCE

By changing the cross-sectional area, veins can vary their resistance. When distended, they offer almost no resistance to blood flow. When partially empty, they assume an elliptical cross-sectional shape that offers a great deal of resistance to blood flow. When a vein is distended and takes on a more circular shape, it offers less resistance to blood flow. Remember the importance of the radius of a vessel to the resistance. Their ability to change shape permits veins to accommodate increases in blood flow without causing increases in the pressure gradient to the heart.

At several areas within the body, veins naturally offer resistance to flow. Veins tend to collapse as they enter the thorax. The subclavian veins are compressed by the first rib. The jugular veins collapse because of atmospheric pressure. Changes in resistance to blood flow within these upper extremity veins are usually minimal but can vary depending on the patient position and intravascular pressures. The inferior vena cava can be compressed by abdominal organs and intra-abdominal pressure, both of which will affect the venous return through the inferior vena cava. The effect of intra-abdominal pressure on resistance to venous flow will be discussed in more detail when describing resting venous dynamics later in this chapter.

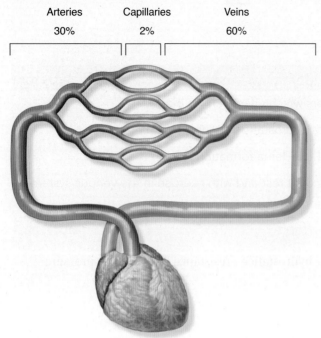

Figure 3-1 A schematic drawing of the distribution of blood volume through the circulatory system.

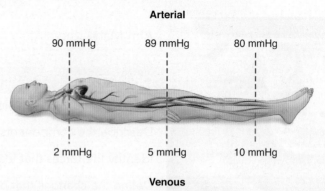

Figure 3-3 Pressures within the arteries and veins in a supine individual.

HYDROSTATICS

A major force affecting the venous system is hydrostatic pressure. Hydrostatic pressure is caused by the weight of a fluid as measured compared to a reference point. As stated in the preceding chapter, the reference point of the human body is the right atrium. Hydrostatic pressure is equal to $\rho \times g \times h$ where ρ is the density of blood, g is the acceleration due to gravity, and h is the height of the column of blood.

Pressure within a blood vessel is equal to the dynamic pressure supplied by the contraction of the heart plus the hydrostatic pressure (Fig. 3-2). Hydrostatic pressure affects both the arteries and the veins equally. Because the dynamic pressure is so low in the veins, the hydrostatic pressure plays a greater role in determining the overall venous pressure. When supine, all the arteries and veins are roughly the same level as the right atrium; therefore, the hydrostatic pressure is negligible (Fig. 3-3). Pressure throughout the vascular system is roughly equal to the dynamic pressure. In this position, the pressure in the veins at the ankle level is about 15 mm Hg.

When standing, an individual who is approximately 6 ft tall will add a hydrostatic pressure component of about 102 mm Hg at the ankle. This occurs in both the arteries and the veins so that the pressure gradient across the capillary bed is the same as it was in the supine position (about 80 mm Hg). During

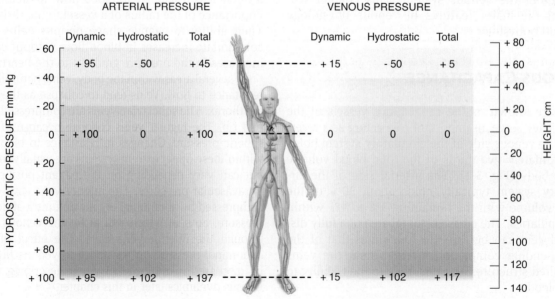

Figure 3-2 A drawing illustrating dynamic and hydrostatic pressure within the vascular system.

exercise, the pressure in the veins falls lower than 20 mm Hg. This has the result of increasing the pressure gradient (to about 177 mm Hg) across the capillaries. This increased pressure gradient will increase blood flow needed during exercise. Remember from the preceding chapter, blood will move down an energy (pressure) gradient; and the bigger the gradient, the more blood flow.

In an uplifted arm, the hydrostatic pressure is negative. The hydrostatic pressure at the wrist would be approximately −50 mm Hg. Combining the hydrostatic pressure with a dynamic pressure of 15 mm Hg would yield a total intravascular pressure of −35 mm Hg. However, pressure within the veins cannot fall lower than the tissue pressure of 5 mm Hg or the veins would collapse and no blood flow would occur. The pressure gradient across the capillary in this uplifted arm does decrease to 40 mm Hg as compared with 80 mm Hg in the supine position.

PRESSURE–VOLUME RELATIONSHIPS

Because veins are collapsible tubes, their shape is determined by transmural pressure. Transmural pressure equals the difference between the pressure within the vein and the tissue pressure. At low transmural pressure, a vein will assume a dumbbell shape. As the pressure within a vein increases, the vein will become elliptical. At high transmural pressures, the vein will become circular (Fig. 3-4).

Changes in vein shape are associated with large increases in venous volume (Fig. 3-5). As such, veins can accommodate large changes in volume with very little changes in pressure. The walls of a vein are rather elastic, but a very large change in pressure is needed to change the volume of the vein when it is circular as compared with partially collapsed and elliptical. When supine, the transmural pressure is low. However, upon standing, the pressure increases and the walls stiffen such that the

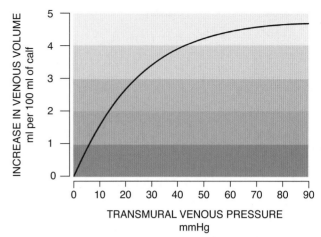

Figure 3-5 Venous pressure–volume curve.

venous volume will change little even with large changes in pressure.

Elastic compression stockings are available in varying degrees of pressure with some patients wearing stockings with 15 mm Hg pressure. This pressure is exerted on the limb producing an increase in the tissue pressure. Thus, with 15 mm Hg stockings, the tissue pressure increased from about 5 mm Hg to 15 mm Hg. This results in a net decrease in the transmural pressure of 10 mm Hg. When supine, this 10 mm Hg difference will greatly reduce venous volume. However, when standing, these low-pressure compression stockings will have little effect because of the increased pressure within the vein caused by the hydrostatic pressure. This is one reason why higher pressure compression stockings are often employed to aid individuals while sitting or standing.

EDEMA

Edema is a consistent sign of increased venous pressure. The Starling equilibrium describes the movement of fluid across the capillary (Fig. 3-6). Forces that act to move fluid out of the capillary are the intracapillary pressure and the interstitial osmotic pressure. Forces that tend to favor the reabsorption of fluid from the interstitium are the interstitial pressure and the capillary osmotic pressure. Osmotic pressure is the pressure exerted by fluid when there is a difference in the concentrations of solutes across a semipermeable membrane, in this case, the capillary endothelium. Normally, the forces are fairly balanced so that there is little overall fluid loss. What little fluid normally moves out into the interstitial space is picked up by the lymphatics. While standing, the increased capillary pressure is no longer balanced by the reabsorptive forces and fluid loss

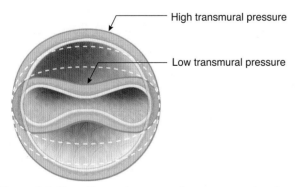

Figure 3-4 The effects of transmural pressure on the shape of a vein.

Arteriole   Capillary   Venule

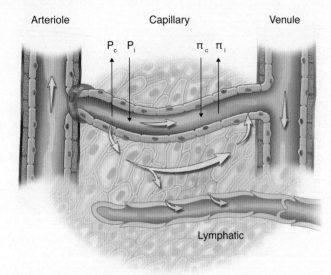

Figure 3-6 The Starling forces governing the movement of fluid across the capillary bed.

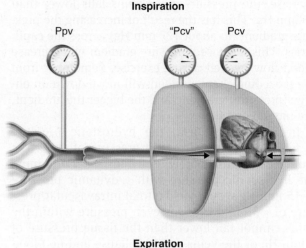

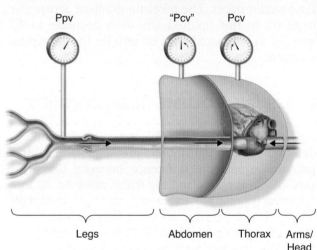

Figure 3-7 Resting venous flow and changes with respiration.

occurs. Edema formation is limited by the action of the calf muscle pump. The contraction of the calf muscles acts to empty the veins and decrease the venous pressure. With venous thrombosis, the venous pressure is increased. The increased venous pressure will be transmitted back through the venous system, into the smaller veins (venules) and finally, the capillaries. This increase in pressure at the capillary level will result in edema formation. As described earlier, the use of compression stockings will increase the interstitial pressure, which will increase fluid reabsorption thus decreasing edema. Elevating the legs will reduce the intracapillary pressure (by lowering the hydrostatic pressure), which also limits edema formation.

VENOUS DYNAMICS AT REST

Changes in intrathoracic and intra-abdominal pressure have a profound effect on the venous return to the heart. During inspiration, the diaphragm descends, which decreases the pressure with the chest cavity. This causes blood to pool into the pulmonary vascular bed as well as pulls air into the lungs. Also during inspiration, the descending movement of the diaphragm results in an increase in intra-abdominal pressure. This collapses the inferior vena cava, which impedes venous return from the legs. Upon expiration, the diaphragm moves upward, which decreases intra-abdominal pressures. This results in an increase in blood flow from the legs and a decrease in blood flow into the thorax (Fig. 3-7).

With a deep venous thrombosis, venous pressure is increased in the legs because of an increase in venous resistance caused by the occluded or partially

occluded veins (Fig. 3-8). Variations in abdominal pressure with respiration have little effect on the pressure gradient from the legs. Normal phasic venous flow from the lower extremity may be reduced or absent. Venous flow from the legs may become continuous as the venous pressures in the legs exceed the normal changes in intra-abdominal venous pressures.

VENOUS DYNAMICS WITH EXERCISE

The calf muscle pump aids in the return of blood from the legs against the force of gravity (hydrostatic pressure). The muscles act as the power source. The intramuscular sinusoids within the gastrocnemius and soleal muscles as well as the deep and superficial veins all play a part in this mechanism. The valves are necessary to ensure efficient action of the muscle pump (Fig. 3-9). Closure of the valves in the deep veins decreases the length of the column of blood, which helps reduce the venous pressure.

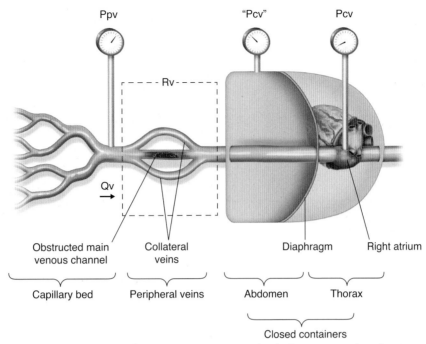

Figure 3-8 Venous pressure changes associated with deep venous thrombosis.

At rest, blood pools in the leg and is only propelled passively by the dynamic pressure gradient created by the contraction of the left ventricle. Contraction of the calf muscles can generate pressures greater than 200 mm Hg. This compresses the veins forcing blood upward (back to the heart) in both the deep and superficial veins. The valves are closed in the perforating veins and in the veins of the distal calf to prevent reflux of the blood. Upon relaxation, because these veins in the calf are empty, blood is drawn into the area from the superficial veins via perforators. More distal veins also help to fill the calf

veins upon relaxation (Fig. 3-10). In the more proximal segments of the leg, the valves close to prevent reflux of blood from these segments.

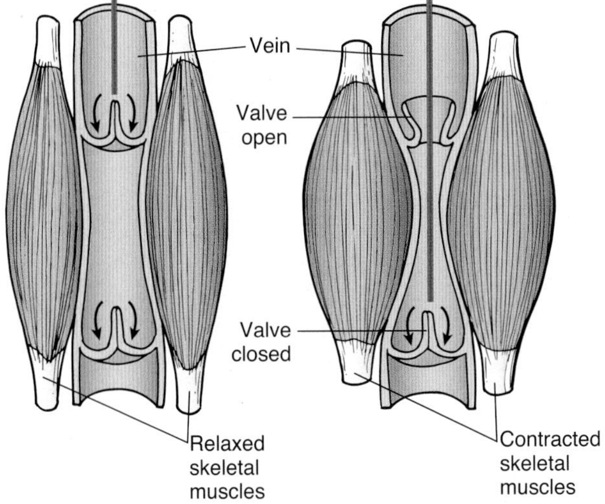

DISORDERS

PRIMARY VARICOSE VEINS

Varicose veins that develop in the absence of a deep venous thrombosis are referred to as primary varicose veins. With primary varicose veins, incompetent valves may be found in the common femoral and great saphenous vein. In some patients, valves may be congenitally absent from the common femoral and iliac veins. Only rarely are primary varicose veins associated with the small saphenous vein. With primary varicose veins, the calf muscle pump still works to propel blood upward during a contraction. However, during relaxation, blood falls back down the superficial veins because of valvular incompetence (Fig. 3-11). This blood then reenters the deep system through the perforators. This creates an inefficient circular motion of blood. Venous pressure is increased because of the presence of a long column of blood caused by the incompetent valves.

SECONDARY VARICOSE VEINS

Secondary varicose veins are mainly the result of deep venous thrombosis. The valves in the deep, superficial, and perforating veins are incompetent and

Figure 3-9 Structure of a venous valve.

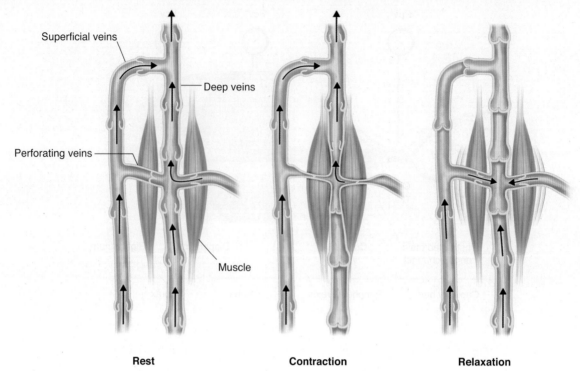

Superficial veins

Deep veins

Perforating veins

Muscle

Rest   **Contraction**   **Relaxation**

Figure 3-10 Patterns of normal venous flow at rest and with calf contraction.

there may be a degree of residual venous obstruction (Fig. 3-12). Because of the obstruction, the superficial veins may function as collaterals, and blood may flow out from the deep to the superficial veins even at rest. Venous flow patterns are completely disrupted in these patients. The flow through the perforators can be bidirectional, thus increasing pressure within the superficial system. More blood is forced distally because of the incompetent valves in both the deep and superficial systems resulting in

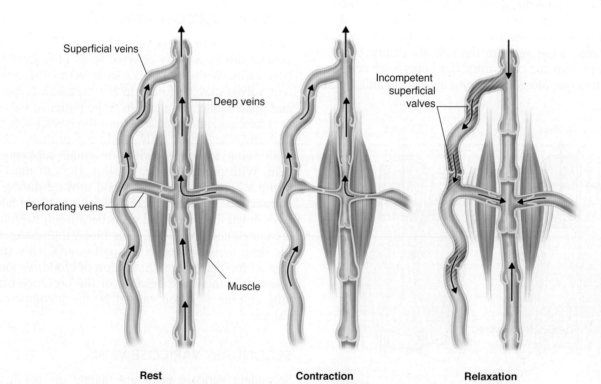

Superficial veins

Deep veins

Incompetent superficial valves

Perforating veins

Muscle

Rest   **Contraction**   **Relaxation**

Figure 3-11 Patterns of venous flow with primary varicose veins.

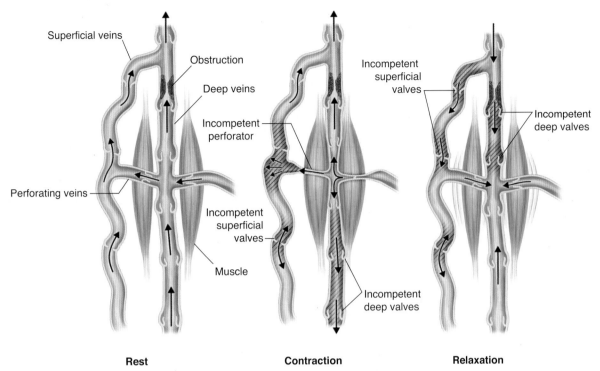

Figure 3-12 Patterns of venous flow with secondary varicose veins.

increased venous pressure. If residual thrombus is present, the proximal obstruction to blood flow will also add to increased venous pressure in the leg.

VENOUS STASIS ULCERS

The effect of persistent increased venous pressure or venous hypertension is distention of the capillaries and increased capillary pressure. This results in slightly opening the junctions between the endothelial cells. This will cause plasma proteins to move out of the vascular space and into the tissue. As a consequence to this protein movement, additional fluid will also enter the interstitial space. There are several theories about how the tissue damage occurs, leading to ulceration. One theory involves fibrin accumulating around the capillaries in the interstitial space. This collection of fibrin, termed a *fibrin cuff*, leads to limited oxygen transfer across the capillaries. Another theory involves the migration and trapping of white blood cells in the capillaries and venules. The plugging of the capillaries and venules by these white blood cells also results in limited oxygen transfer into the tissue bed. The decreased oxygen transfer produces tissue ischemia. As the ischemia progresses, ulceration occurs. Venous stasis ulcers are a serious end result of this extreme form of venous disease.

PREGNANCY AND VARICOSE VEINS

During pregnancy, the inferior vena cava and the iliac veins can be compressed by the enlarged uterus while lying supine, particularly in the third trimester. This can produce a continuous venous outflow signal from the legs that is no longer responsive to changes in pressure brought on by respiration. This change in lower extremity venous flow is a result of increased venous pressure due to compression of the pelvic veins. This can be alleviated somewhat by turning the patient on her side so that the weight of the gravid uterus no longer impinges on the venous structures.

Humoral factors circulating during pregnancy cause the veins to be more compliant. This factor plus the increased venous pressure, which occurs later in pregnancy due to the size of the uterus can cause significant venous distention. The final result is a decrease in the velocity of venous flow. This can contribute to the development of a deep venous thrombosis.

Pregnancy does not cause varicose veins. Increased venous pressure and venous distention can magnify predisposing factors. Thus, varicose veins often first appear during pregnancy. Typically, varicose veins become more severe with subsequent pregnancies.

SUMMARY

Understanding some of the factors that play a role in the movement of blood within the vein will be helpful when performing venous ultrasound. Venous capacitance, transmural pressure, hydrostatic pressure, as well as other anatomic and physiologic components help to govern venous flow. Venous physiology affects what is observed on the ultrasound image as well as the venous Doppler signals obtained during a duplex ultrasound examination.

Critical Thinking Questions

1. You are examining a patient's calf veins with ultrasound, and the veins appear small and difficult to visualize. The patient is lying supine, with their head slightly elevated. What is one simple change not involving the ultrasound system that can be done to make the veins easier to image?

2. Is the venous pressure higher or lower than normal in a common femoral vein that demonstrates a continuous venous Doppler signal with no respiratory phasicity?

3. A patient presents for a venous examination with clinically evident varicose veins and no history of a deep vein thrombosis or venous ulceration. Would venous insufficiency be more likely in the deep or superficial system or both?

SUGGESTED READINGS

1. Carter SA. Hemodynamic considerations in peripheral vascular and cerebrovascular disease. In: Zwiebel WJ, Pellerito JS, eds. *Introduction to Vascular Ultrasonography*. 5th ed. Philadelphia, PA: Elsevier Saunders; 2005:3–17.
2. Eberhardt RT, Raffetto JD. Chronic venous insufficiency. *Circulation*. 2005;111(18):2398–2409.
3. Guyton AC, Hall JE. *Textbook of Medical Physiology*. 11th ed. Philadelphia, PA: Saunders; 2005.
4. Koeppen BM, Stanton BA. *Berne & Levy Physiology*. 6th ed. St. Louis, MO: Mosby; 2009.
5. Kupinski AM. Dynamics of venous syndrome. *Vascular US Today*. 2006;11:1–20.
6. Meissner, MH. Venous anatomy and hemodynamics. In: Zierler RE, ed. *Strandness's Duplex Scanning in Vascular Disorders*. 4th ed. Philadelphia, PA: Lippincott Williams & Wilkins; 2010:56–60.
7. Mohrman DE, Heller LJ, eds. *Cardiovascular Physiology*. New York, NY: McGraw-Hill; 1997.
8. Oates C. *Cardiovascular Haemodynamics and Doppler Waveforms Explained*. Cambridge, NY: Cambridge University Press; 2001.

4 The Extracranial Duplex Ultrasound Examination

Kari A. Campbell and R. Eugene Zierler

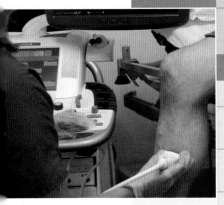

OBJECTIVES

List the essential components of a carotid duplex ultrasound examination

Describe the normal waveform characteristics of the extracranial carotid vessels

Define the common diagnostic criteria used to evaluate the extracranial carotid vessels

Describe common pathology observed during a carotid duplex ultrasound examination

KEY TERMS

carotid artery | carotid duplex | extracranial cerebrovascular disease | spectral analysis | stroke | vertebral artery

GLOSSARY

bruit an abnormal "blowing" or "swishing" sound heard with a stethoscope while auscultating over an artery such as the carotid; the sound results from vibrations that are transmitted through the tissues when blood flows through a stenotic artery; although the presence of a bruit is a sign of arterial disease, the absence of a bruit is less diagnostic because all stenoses are not associated with bruits

carotid bulb a slight dilation involving variable portions of the distal common and proximal internal carotid arteries, often including the origin of the external carotid artery; this is where the baroreceptors assisting in reflex blood pressure control are located; the carotid bulb tends to be most prominent in normal young individuals

Doppler angle most commonly defined as the angle between the line of the Doppler ultrasound beam and the arterial wall (also referred to as the "angle of insonation"); this is a key variable in the Doppler equation used to calculate flow velocity

spectral analysis spectral analysis is a signal processing technique that displays the complete frequency and amplitude content of the Doppler flow signal; the spectral information is usually presented as waveforms with frequency (converted to a velocity scale) on the vertical axis, time on the horizontal axis, and amplitude indicated by a gray scale

spectral broadening an increase in the "width" of the spectral waveform (frequency band) or "filling-in" of the normal clear area under the systolic peak; this represents turbulent blood flow associated with arterial lesions

transient ischemic attack (TIA) an episode of stroke-like neurologic symptoms that typically lasts for a few minutes to several hours and then resolves completely; this is caused by temporary interruption of the blood supply to the brain in the distribution of a cerebral artery

Evaluation of the extracranial cerebrovasculature was the first clinical application of the duplex ultrasound device that was developed at the University of Washington in the late 1970s.[1,2] Although B-mode imaging and Doppler flow detection had been used separately to characterize vascular disorders, the duplex concept combined real-time B-mode imaging and pulsed Doppler flow detection in a single instrument to obtain both anatomic and physiologic information on the status of blood vessels. In addition to the B-mode imaging and pulsed Doppler systems, the first duplex scanning instrument contained a spectrum analyzer for generating Doppler spectral waveforms. The position of the Doppler beam and the pulsed Doppler sample volume was indicated by a line and a cursor superimposed on the B-mode image. Ultrasound technology has advanced significantly since the introduction of the duplex scanner, with improved B-mode image resolution, a wider selection of transducers, and alternative approaches to displaying flow information such as color Doppler and power Doppler. Unlike catheter contrast arteriography, which can be interpreted in terms of a specific percentage of diameter reduction, duplex scanning classifies arterial lesions into categories that include ranges of stenosis severity.

The primary goal of noninvasive testing for extracranial cerebrovascular disease is to identify patients who are at risk for stroke due to atherosclerotic plaque and to facilitate treatment by either carotid endarterectomy or stenting. A secondary goal is to document progressive disease in patients already known to be at risk for recurrent stenosis after intervention. Duplex scanning can also detect a variety of nonatherosclerotic conditions that involve the extracranial carotid and vertebral arteries, such as dissection, fibromuscular dysplasia, trauma, arteritis, radiation effects, and aneurysms.

SONOGRAPHIC EXAMINATION TECHNIQUES

The major indications for a duplex scan of the carotid and vertebral arteries include an asymptomatic neck bruit; hemispheric cerebral or ocular transient ischemic attacks (TIAs); a history of stroke; screening prior to major cardiac, peripheral vascular, or other surgery; and a follow-up after carotid endarterectomy or stenting. Atherosclerotic lesions of the extracranial carotid arteries can be present without neurologic symptoms and some may produce a neck bruit. Experience has shown that only about one-third of bruits are related to high-grade (≥50% diameter reducing) internal carotid stenoses.[3,4] Symptoms of cerebrovascular disease can be produced by emboli from atherosclerotic plaques, reduction of flow due to high-grade stenoses, and arterial thrombosis. An important mechanism for both transient and permanent neurologic deficits appears to be small emboli consisting of platelet aggregates or atheromatous debris arising from ulcerated plaques in the extracranial carotid system. Hemorrhage or necrosis within a plaque may lead to ulceration and the appearance of symptoms. Although high-grade stenoses can reduce flow through the involved internal carotid artery, this is rarely a primary cause of symptoms because of the collateral circulation available through the circle of Willis.

Symptoms typically associated with extracranial carotid artery lesions include TIAs, amaurosis fugax, reversible ischemic neurologic deficits (RINDs), and strokes. A TIA is sometimes referred to as a "mini stroke" and is characterized by focal weakness (paralysis) or numbness (paresthesia) involving some combination of the face, arm, and leg on one side of the body. Difficulty speaking (aphasia) may also occur. These symptoms occur on the side of the body opposite to the affected carotid artery and cerebral hemisphere. Symptoms of a TIA typically last from several minutes to a few hours, but not longer than 24 hours. Amaurosis fugax is a TIA of the eye that produces transient monocular blindness on the same side as the responsible carotid artery lesion. A RIND is similar to a TIA but with symptoms lasting between about 24 and 72 hours. A stroke, also known as a cerebrovascular accident (CVA), results in fixed or permanent neurologic deficits. The symptoms of vertebrobasilar arterial insufficiency are less specific than those related to the carotid circulation and include dizziness, diplopia, and ataxia. In general, patients with transient neurologic symptoms in the distribution of an internal carotid artery (TIAs, RINDs, amaurosis fugax) are considered to be at risk for stroke.[5] For patients with TIAs, the overall stroke risk is about 6% per year, with a 12% risk of stroke during the first year after onset of symptoms. Patients who survive their initial stroke have a continuing stroke risk in the range of 6% to 11% per year.[6]

PATIENT PREPARATION

In preparation for the carotid artery duplex evaluation, the patient should remove jewelry and tight clothing from the neck area, allowing unobstructed access to the cervical carotid artery segments. Interview the patient to obtain the pertinent past medical history and current signs or symptoms that prompted the request for a carotid duplex evaluation (Table 4-1). A brief physical examination can be performed, which includes palpation of pulses for strength and symmetry (carotid, axillary, brachial, radial) and auscultation

TABLE	4-1

Patient Interview for Pertinent Medical History

- Are you being treated for high blood pressure (hypertension)?
- Are you being treated for high cholesterol (hypercholesterolemia)?
- Do you have diabetes? If so, for how long? Is it treated with diet control, oral medication, or insulin?
- Have you had a heart attack (myocardial infarction) or chest pains?
- Have you ever had surgery or other interventions on any of your blood vessels (coronary artery bypass graft or stent placement, carotid endarterectomy or stent placement, peripheral arterial revascularization)?
- Have you had a stroke or "mini stroke" (CVA, TIA) in the past?
- Have you recently or are you currently experiencing stroke-like symptoms that include:
  - Weakness or numbness down one side of your body
  - Difficulty with balance or walking
  - Slurred speech or difficulty forming words
  - Dizziness, nausea, or vomiting
  - Severe headache
  - Vision disturbances such as "cloudiness" or perhaps like a "shade" coming down over one eye

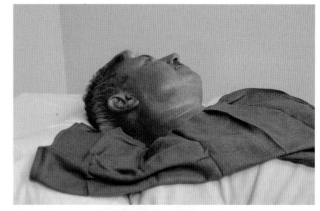

Figure 4-1 The correct patient position for performing a carotid artery duplex evaluation. The patient's chin is elevated and the head is turned 45° away from the side being examined.

with a stethoscope for bruits (high, middle, and low neck, and in the region of the clavicle).

PATIENT POSITIONING

Place the patient in a supine position on the stretcher. The head of the bed may be elevated and a pillow placed beneath the patient's knees for comfort. In rare instances when the patient cannot tolerate lying supine, this examination may be performed with the patient sitting in a chair, although it is not an ideal position due to potential patient movement and poor ergonomics for the sonographer or vascular technologist. Position a pillow equally beneath the patient's head and shoulders and adjust to have the patient's chin tilted up, rather than down toward the chest. If this cannot be accomplished, forego the pillow and provide a towel underneath the patient's neck for support. The patient's head should be turned away from the side examined, approximately 45° from midline (Fig. 4-1).

Avoiding Repetitive Stress Injury

Career longevity depends greatly on proper sonographer/technologist positioning by helping to avoid repetitive stress injuries (RSIs). Being ambidextrous,

practicing flexibility, and properly positioning equipment can help lessen the severity of RSI symptoms. Being ambidextrous can be particularly helpful. A sonographer or technologist should develop the ability to scan with either hand. Alternating scanning hands will extend the life of hands, arms, and shoulders by taking stress off of one set of muscles at various times throughout the day. Practice flexibility by keeping muscles limber and stretched while keeping hydrated throughout the day. Taking the time to stretch the hands, arms, shoulders, and back before and after each examination is imperative to prevent RSI. There are many written, diagrammatic, and video resources available demonstrating these techniques. Maintaining proper hydration allows muscles to be less vulnerable to injury and promotes healing. Position the equipment properly by taking time to arrange the stretcher or bed and the ultrasound machine, getting as close to the patient as possible. Particularly on an inpatient floor, this involves moving equipment and furniture around the room to allow access close to the patient. Develop the ability to scan from the right and left sides as well as from the head of the bed. In order to decrease strain on the neck and shoulder muscles, the scanning arm should be maintained as close to the technologist's body as possible. Rolled towels or the bed can be used to rest the scanning arm.

EQUIPMENT

Proper transducer selection is essential to successfully completing the carotid artery duplex evaluation. The two key factors to consider when selecting a transducer are transmit frequency for image quality and transducer "footprint" for access and visualization (Fig. 4-2). A transducer such as a linear array with a 7-4 MHz frequency will generally provide the best

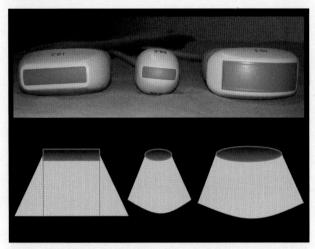

Figure 4-2 Suitable transducers for performing a carotid artery duplex evaluation: linear 9-3 MHz (for average size necks), curvilinear 8-5 MHz (for short necks and small spaces), and curvilinear 5-2 MHz (for deeper depths).

image resolution and most options for Doppler angle correction. The midrange transmit frequencies provide high resolution at depths of 2 to 10 cm. The transducer footprint is rectangular, approximately 4 cm long, and narrow (approximately 1 cm wide).

An alternative transducer selection may be warranted in certain circumstances. A curvilinear array with a frequency range of 8-5 MHz is preferred when access to the neck is limited, as is the case with a short neck, internal jugular intravenous lines, or tracheotomy ties. This transducer provides similar image quality to a 7-4 MHz linear array due to similar midrange transmit frequency. The face of the transducer is slightly curved, with a small rectangular footprint, which is approximately 2.5 cm in length and narrow (approximately 0.5 cm wide). This is an excellent type of transducer to access areas around lines and bony structures. Use of a phased array, sector 4-1 MHz or curvilinear 5-2 MHz transducer may be necessary when vessels are located more deeply than usual in the neck.

SCANNING TECHNIQUE

The carotid artery duplex evaluation generally includes bilateral examination of the common carotid artery (CCA), internal carotid artery (ICA), and external carotid artery (ECA), as well as the vertebral artery at the mid-neck and proximal subclavian artery. In special circumstances, a unilateral or limited evaluation may be performed. The carotid arteries are interrogated in both transverse and long-axis orientations using grayscale B-mode imaging, color Doppler ultrasound (CDU), and pulsed wave (PW) spectral Doppler.

Beginning with B-mode imaging, place the transducer on the anterior-lateral neck midway between the clavicle and the angle of the mandible to locate the vessels. Sweep along the carotid arteries in transverse orientation from the clavicle to the angle of the mandible. Move the transducer to the more anterior and posterior aspects of the neck to locate the clearest image path, and observe the location of the arteries and veins relative to one another. Turn the transducer into the long-axis plane and image the length of the CCA, ICA, and ECA from clavicle to above the angle of the mandible. Document intraluminal echoes such as plaque or other intimal defects, as well as any other areas of interest throughout the carotid arteries and surrounding tissues. Minimal B-mode image documentation should include long-axis views of the CCA, ICA, and the bifurcation region.

Next, use the color Doppler modality to image the carotid segments in transverse orientation and sweep once again from the clavicle to the angle of the mandible. The color Doppler scale is a representation of the mean flow velocity, and the scale should generally be set in the range of 20 to 40 cm/s. Document the distal CCA and the proximal ICA and ECA at the bifurcation in both transverse and long-axis or longitudinal orientations. Additionally, document any color Doppler disturbance, areas of aliasing or mosaic flow patterns, and observe any color Doppler speckling in the tissues that may indicate a color Doppler bruit.

The pulsed wave spectral Doppler modality is then selected, beginning low in the neck on the right and insonating the brachiocephalic (innominate) artery if possible. As previously stated, use of a smaller footprint transducer is often ideal for insonating behind the clavicle or sternum. Evaluation of the distal segment of the brachiocephalic artery and origins of the right and left CCA are considered optional. However, when turbulent Doppler flow is found in the proximal and mid-segments of either CCA, this step becomes imperative. With the left CCA originating directly off the aortic arch, this portion of the vessel is unable to be imaged with a standard linear array transducer and additional transducers and approaches are necessary. Sweep the Doppler sample volume throughout the proximal, mid-, and distal segments of the CCA, documenting representative peak systolic Doppler flow velocities (PSVs). It is not always necessary to document the end-diastolic Doppler flow velocities (EDVs) throughout the CCA. However, measure the EDV when the flow appears more resistive and compare it to the contralateral segment.

Clearly differentiate the ICA from the ECA using one or both of the following methods. The ECA can be identified by finding the artery with multiple branches beyond the carotid bifurcation. Of note, there are normal anatomical variants in which a branch may arise from the proximal ICA or the distal CCA (this is

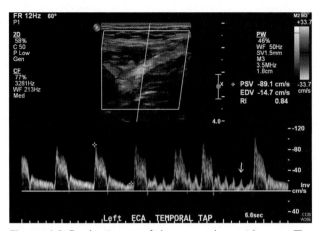

Figure 4-3 Duplex image of the external carotid artery. The Doppler flow signal is affected by oscillations on the ipsilateral temporal artery.

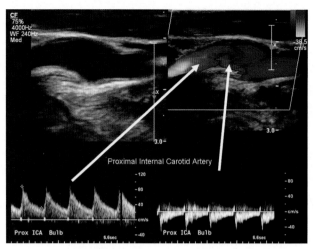

Figure 4-4 Duplex image of normal Doppler flow separation in the proximal internal carotid artery (carotid bulb).

generally the superior thyroid artery). A second technique involves the palpation of the pulse of the superficial temporal artery just anterior to the ear, then oscillating the flow by "tapping" on the artery (the "temporal tap" maneuver) while insonating flow in the proximal segment of the ECA (Fig. 4-3). An artifact from the tapping (oscillations) should be visible in the spectral waveform from the ECA but not from the ICA. The temporal tap technique is not always accurate, particularly in patients with an ICA occlusion and an ECA collateralization. In some patients, the temporal tap may also produce oscillations within the ICA if the temporal artery is tapped too strongly. In addition, if the temporal artery is inadequately tapped, oscillations will not be generated within the ECA Doppler spectrum. Therefore, the temporal tap can be helpful in many patients but should be used with caution.

Sweep the Doppler sample volume from the distal CCA into the ECA, continuously insonating to document the highest peak systolic velocity in the proximal ECA segment. Continue to move the Doppler sample volume through the proximal and mid-segments to determine whether any waveform changes are present. When elevated flow velocities are obtained in the ECA, document the presence or absence of poststenotic turbulence to help determine hemodynamic significance.

Return to the distal CCA and sweep the Doppler sample volume into the proximal ICA to detect the presence of stenosis at the origin of the ICA. Document flow separation in the carotid bulb, if present, which appears as a small area of flow reversal. This typically is located along the outer wall of the bulb on the side opposite to the flow divider, as shown in Figure 4-4. As plaque formation progresses and fills in the carotid bulb, the area of flow separation

disappears. It is not necessary to measure the flow velocity of this reversal component. Laminar flow may actually be difficult to demonstrate in patients with large carotid bulbs. Move the sample volume throughout the carotid bulb to detect the highest PSV and EDV with the most laminar waveform obtainable. Continue to insonate through the carotid bulb and the proximal, mid-, and distal segments of the ICA. Often, the distal segment of the ICA is difficult to visualize or insonate beyond the angle of the mandible. It is particularly important to evaluate these segments of the ICA in patients who are at risk for fibromuscular dysplasia (young- to middle-aged females). For this application, curved or phased array transducers are ideal.

The next vessel evaluated is the vertebral artery. Place the transducer at the anterior-medial aspect of the mid-neck in the long-axis position. Once the CCA has been identified, slowly slide or angle the transducer posteriorly, focusing deep to the CCA to view the vertebral artery between the transverse processes of the cervical vertebrae. Take care to properly identify flow direction and document waveform contour at the level of the mid-neck. An abnormal waveform contour or flow direction indicates hemodynamically significant stenosis of the ipsilateral proximal subclavian artery, which will be discussed later. When turbulent Doppler flow is detected in the vertebral artery at low-to-mid neck, evaluate the origin and proximal segments to identify a stenosis.

Finally, place the transducer in transverse orientation at the base of the neck to insonate the supraclavicular subclavian artery. Set the Doppler sample volume as far proximally in the vessel as possible, then sweep distally to obtain the highest PSV and the most laminar Doppler spectral waveform. If elevated velocities are detected, determine

PATHOLOGY BOX 4-1

Carotid Artery Pathology

Pathology	Sonographic Appearance		
	B-Mode Image	Color Flow Doppler	Doppler Spectral Waveform
Normal Internal carotid artery	No plaque or wall thickening	Complete filling of the lumen Flow separation zone along the outer wall of the bulb	PSV<125 cm/s Narrow frequency band with a "window" under the systolic peak Flow (or boundary layer) separation along the outer wall of the bulb
Severe (80%–99%) Internal carotid stenosis	Extensive plaque, often with acoustic shadowing due to calcification	Narrowing of the lumen Aliasing in the color flow image	PSV ≥125 cm/s and EDV ≥140 cm/s Spectral broadening throughout the cardiac cycle
Internal carotid string sign	Extensive plaque, often with acoustic shadowing due to calcification	Severely narrowed lumen Power Doppler may show a small lumen	Variable velocity (high, low, or undetectable flow) May be decreased diastolic flow in the ipsilateral common carotid artery
Internal carotid occlusion	Extensive plaque filling the lumen, often with acoustic shadowing due to calcification	No filling of the lumen beyond the bulb by color flow or power Doppler	No flow in the internal carotid artery Decreased diastolic flow in the ipsilateral common carotid artery
Subclavian steal (brachial systolic pressure gradient >15 mm Hg)	May be plaque in the subclavian artery on the side of the decreased pressure	Retrograde flow in the ipsilateral vertebral artery	Increased PSV in the subclavian artery on the side of the decreased pressure Retrograde or "hesitant" flow in the ipsilateral vertebral artery May be increased PSV in the contralateral vertebral artery

hemodynamic significance by sampling distally in the infraclavicular segments of the subclavian artery, documenting the presence or absence of post-stenotic turbulence.

PITFALLS

The majority of patients' carotid arteries are difficult to visualize high in the neck (distal ICA) and very low in the neck (proximal CCA or brachiocephalic artery). Patients with short and thick necks will likely have difficult visualization due to vessel depths and difficult access. The low-range transmit frequencies allow for better Doppler penetration and image

capability at deeper depths. A 4-1 MHz phased array transducer has a flat, small footprint, which is approximately 3 cm in square. A 5-2 MHz curvilinear transducer also has low-to-mid range transmit frequencies and smoother image resolution than the phased array transducer. The curvilinear transducer has a curved and rectangular footprint, approximately 6 cm in length and 1.5 cm wide, which is a larger footprint than the phased array. The primary challenge when using these alternative transducers is the limited options for angle correction and beam steering. The sector, wedge-shaped imaging format does not allow for Doppler beam steering as does a linear array transducer.

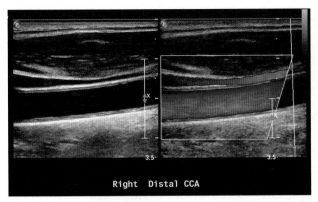

Figure 4-5 B-mode image of the common carotid artery, with the intimal–medial layer clearly visible.

DIAGNOSIS

Ultrasound image quality using modern technology is vastly improved compared to early ultrasound systems. In the early days of duplex scanning, the B-mode image was primarily used for locating the vessels of interest, and spectral Doppler waveforms provided nearly all the information on vessel patency. Today, Doppler continues to provide the most reliable data on the degree of stenosis. However, due to the higher resolution of B-mode images generated by modern instruments and the use of harmonic imaging techniques, great amounts of data are being gleaned by researchers on plaque composition, intimal–medial thickness, and overall vessel wall condition.[7,8] Common findings are summarized in Pathology Box 4-1.

B-MODE CHARACTERISTICS

A normal carotid artery has smooth vessel walls with no appreciable plaque in the vessel lumen. The intimal–medial layer is clearly visible as a thin grey-white line on the innermost part of the wall and is uniform throughout the length of the vessel (Fig. 4-5). The adventitial layer is visible outside of the intimal–medial layer, appearing as brighter white than the adjacent tissues. The lumen of the vessel is anechoic. It is not unusual for a mobile-appearing echo to be present within the lumen of the carotid artery in both planes; this represents a normally occurring reverberation artifact of the wall of the adjacent internal jugular vein.

Most abnormalities of the carotid artery are easily detectable on B-mode imaging. These include plaque formation, intraluminal defects (such as intimal dissection or thrombus), and iatrogenic injuries (such as pseudoaneurysm or arteriovenous fistula involving the adjacent internal jugular vein).

Plaque

Modern B-mode imaging can provide detailed information on both the surface and the internal composition of atherosclerotic plaque. Plaque formation can occur along any segment of the common, internal, or external carotid arteries; however, plaque most commonly forms at the common carotid bifurcation (in the distal common carotid and the proximal internal and proximal external carotid arteries). In the early stages, plaque appears as a thickening of the intimal–medial layers, and a fibrous cap may form between the bulk of the plaque and the lumen (Fig. 4-6A,B).

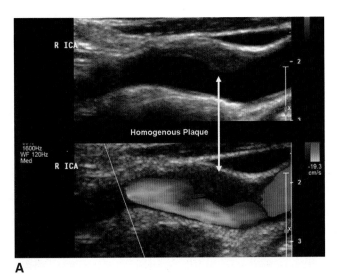

A

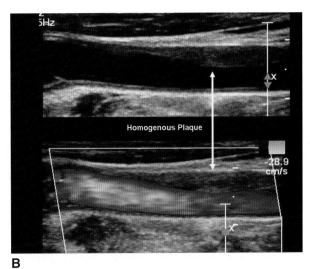

B

Figure 4-6 B-mode and color Doppler images demonstrating smooth homogenous plaque in the carotid arteries. **A:** Homogenous plaque internal carotid artery. **B:** Homogenous plaque in the common carotid artery. The fibrous cap is visible as a brighter line along the intraluminal aspect of the plaque.

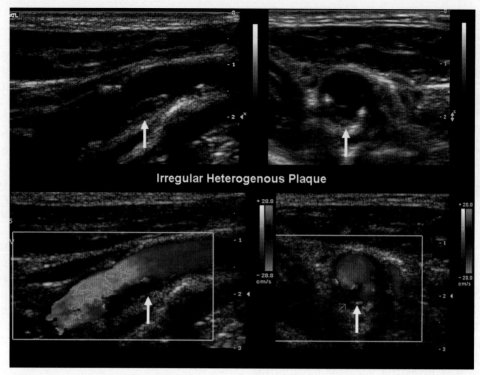

Figure 4-7 B-mode and color images of heterogeneous irregular plaque in the proximal internal carotid artery. Note the color-Doppler flow eddy at the area of apparent plaque compromise, which indicates possible ulceration *(arrows)*.

The surface of the plaque can be described as smooth or irregular, but use of the term "ulcerated" is generally discouraged. Strictly speaking, an ulcer refers to an area where there is loss of the vascular endothelium, and although some irregular plaques may be ulcerated, this is not a finding that is reliably documented by ultrasound (Fig. 4-7). Ulceration is best documented by a pathologic specimen at the time of surgery. The internal features of atherosclerotic plaque are often described qualitatively according to their echogenicity as either homogenous or heterogeneous.

Homogenous plaque is uniform in appearance and is often of relatively low echogenicity. In general, low echogenicity correlates with a high lipid content and the presence of fibrofatty tissue. A smooth appearing fibrous cap may also be present. Heterogeneous plaque, also described as mixed-echogenicity plaque, may be comprised of fatty material as well as areas of calcium, which tend to cause brighter echoes and acoustic shadowing (Fig. 4-8). Acoustic shadowing occurs when calcium attenuates the transmission of ultrasound and creates a "shadow" deep to the calcified area. An echolucent region in a heterogeneous plaque may represent either lipid or hemorrhage (Fig. 4-9).

A plaque has the potential to rupture, exposing the plaque contents to the arterial lumen and to flowing blood. Bleeding within the plaque beneath an intact fibrous cap is referred to as intraplaque

hemorrhage and can cause the plaque to become "unstable." These unstable plaques can expand, increasing both the degree of stenosis and the potential to produce emboli to the brain. Ulceration or rupture of the fibrous cap is a feature of unstable plaque that also increases the risk of thrombus formation and subsequent embolization. The clinical value of characterizing plaque surface features and internal composition by B-mode imaging is

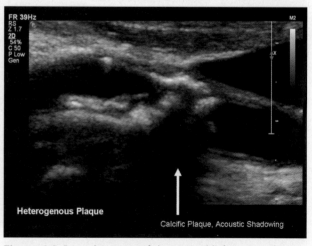

Figure 4-8 B-mode image of the carotid bifurcation demonstrating heterogeneous plaque with mixed echogenicity, calcification, and acoustic shadowing.

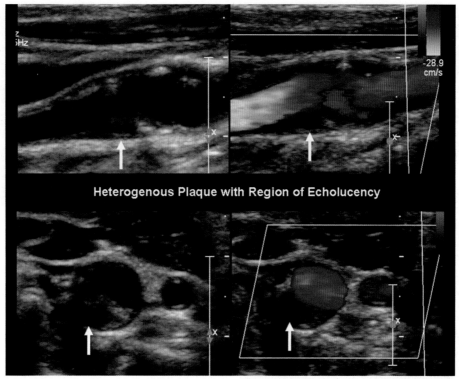

Heterogenous Plaque with Region of Echolucency

Figure 4-9 B-mode and color image of the proximal internal carotid artery demonstrating plaque with echolucency *(arrows)*. These findings may represent lipid core versus intraplaque hemorrhage.

controversial. Retrospective analyses suggest that plaques that are predominately echolucent or irregular are more likely to be associated with neurologic symptoms than are predominately echodense or smooth plaques.[8–10]

Intraluminal Defects

Intraluminal defects in the carotid arteries include disruption of the intima with blood from the true lumen flowing between the layers of the vessel wall. This separation of the layers is referred to as an arterial dissection and creates a second (false) flow lumen within the vessel. (Chapter 5 will present additional examples of dissections.) Dissections tend to occur in a spiral pattern along the vessel, narrowing the true lumen and creating a generally ineffectual false lumen, which may go on to thrombose. Intimal dissections occur either spontaneously or due to trauma. It is crucial to differentiate a carotid artery dissection from an internal jugular vein wall artifact. Multiple views should be used to confirm the dissection. Interrogate with color Doppler for disturbed flow patterns that usually display opposite directions of flow within the two lumens (Fig. 4-10A–C). It is usually possible to identify distinctly different flow patterns within the separate true and false lumens with spectral Doppler waveforms. Flow patterns may reveal normal or stenotic

characteristics in one lumen and delayed backfilling into the second lumen.

Spontaneous dissections commonly begin at the aortic root and may be associated with thoracic aortic aneurysm formation. Once the dissection process has begun, the vessel walls continue to separate along the length of the artery with the force of blood through each cardiac cycle. Traumatic dissections can begin at any point along the vessel wall following blunt trauma or torsion. Examples include injury by the cross-chest component of a seat belt during a motor vehicle accident, blunt force from sports activities or equipment, and chiropractic manipulation of the neck. Smaller intimal defects can occur, presenting as short intimal flaps that do not extend along a great length of the vessel. Although some of these defects resolve spontaneously, some may extend and be associated with thrombosis and or embolization.

Carotid artery thrombosis is rare, and differentiation of a thrombus from softly echogenic homogeneous plaque can be challenging. The soft uniform echoes are similar in both acute thrombus and some homogeneous plaques (Fig. 4-11A,B). The etiology of carotid artery thrombosis is most often related to progressive atherosclerotic plaque with eventual obliteration of the remaining vessel lumen by thrombus. Other possible contributing factors include cardiogenic embolus, trauma, and dissection.

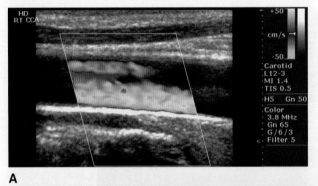

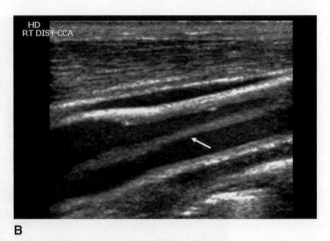

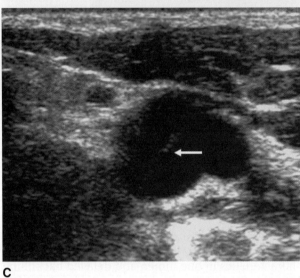

Figure 4-10 A: A common carotid artery dissection illustrating color flow variations within both the true and false lumens. **B:** Sagittal B-mode image of the distal common carotid artery illustrating an intraluminal defect (arrow). **C:** Transverse B-mode image across the carotid bifurcation with the dissected lumen (arrow) visible within the internal carotid artery.

Iatrogenic Injury

Iatrogenic injury is defined as any adverse patient condition that is induced inadvertently by a health care provider in the course of a diagnostic procedure or therapeutic intervention. Iatrogenic injury to the carotid artery can occur during catheter interventions or venous line placement. An inadvertent puncture of the carotid artery has the potential to cause a pseudoaneurysm at the puncture site, an arteriovenous fistula between the CCA and the internal jugular or external jugular veins, or intimal dissection (Fig. 4-12A,B). Intraluminal arterial injury can be caused by instrumentation with catheters and

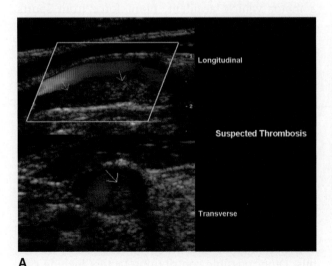

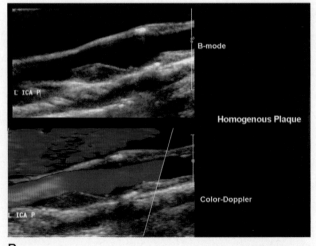

Figure 4-11 B-mode and color Doppler images of softly echogenic material within the lumen of the carotid artery. **A:** Duplex ultrasound findings in conjunction with patient history indicate carotid artery partial thrombosis. **B:** Findings indicate soft homogenous plaque.

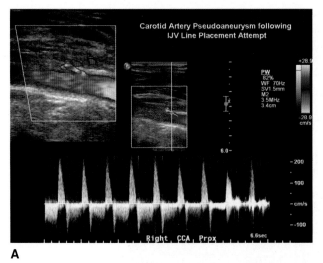
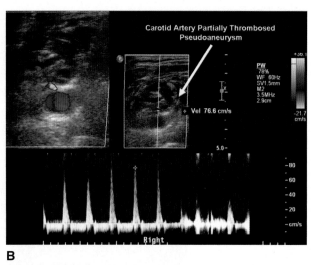

A   **B**

Figure 4-12 Common carotid artery pseudoaneurysm following internal jugular vein line placement attempt. **A:** Duplex ultrasound demonstration of to-and-fro flow in the neck of the pseudoaneurysm, arising from the common carotid artery. **B:** Duplex image of the pseudoaneurysm, which is mostly thrombosed.

wires during procedures on the carotid or intracranial arterial segments, including balloon angioplasty and stent deployment.

SPECTRAL DOPPLER CHARACTERISTICS

In addition to the information the B-mode image reveals about the carotid arteries, each segment must be insonated and the flow velocity and waveform contour should be carefully evaluated with spectral Doppler waveform analysis. Duplex ultrasound is unique in that the information collected is both anatomic and physiologic, as compared to the purely anatomic information provided by standard intra-arterial contrast arteriography and computed tomography arteriography (CTA). The physiologic data provides hemodynamic information for interpretation of flow changes proximal and distal to any given insonated location. The spectral Doppler component provides the most reliable means for assessing vessel patency and classifying the degree of stenosis.

Doppler Waveform Contour

Doppler waveform contour is directly related to cardiac output, vessel compliance, and the status of the distal vascular bed (peripheral resistance). The Doppler waveform contour in a normal CCA, ICA, or ECA has a brisk systolic acceleration, sharp systolic peak, and a clear spectral window (Fig. 4-13). Because the ICA supplies the brain directly, it has the lowest peripheral resistance and shows the highest diastolic flow velocities with forward flow throughout the cardiac cycle. The ECA normally supplies a relatively high resistance vascular bed, which includes the muscles of the face and mouth. This

produces lower diastolic flow velocities and often results in a multiphasic waveform similar to that of a peripheral artery. The Doppler waveform from the CCA takes on the characteristics of both the internal and external carotid arteries, as it supplies both branches; however, about 70% of the normal CCA flow volume passes through the ICA, so the CCA usually has a low resistance flow pattern with forward flow throughout the cardiac cycle (Fig. 4-14). The brachiocephalic artery has a higher resistance flow pattern that reflects the status of the multiple vascular beds that it supplies: arm (high resistance), face (high resistance), and brain (low resistance).

The carotid sinus or carotid bulb is a slight focal dilation in the artery where baroreceptors assisting in reflex blood pressure control are located. The carotid bodies, which are chemoreceptors involved in the control of respiratory rate, are also nearby. The carotid bulb typically involves the proximal ICA, but the dilated segment may also include the distal CCA or the origin of the ECA. How to classify the severity of an ICA stenosis within the carotid bulb has been the subject of much research. The normal carotid bulb will have an area of "flow separation" along the outer wall on the side opposite to the flow divider, as discussed previously. This area of flow separation is created when flow from the CCA enters the widened bulb segment. This change in vessel geometry creates a helical flow pattern that includes a zone of reversed, lower velocity flow (Fig. 4-15). The appearance of flow separation in this situation is considered to be normal and usually correlates with minimal or no plaque in the bulb. A more characteristic low resistance ICA flow pattern is present in the bulb along the flow divider and in the distal ICA beyond the bulb. As plaque develops it can fill

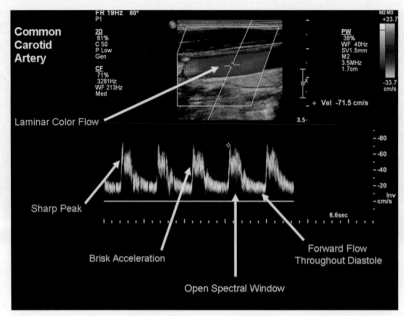

Figure 4-13 Normal Doppler arterial flow through the common carotid artery.

in the bulb, leaving a residual segment of vessel that is more uniform in diameter, and the area of flow separation disappears. Therefore, even though the Doppler arterial waveform contour may be normal, the absence of flow reversal in the bulb can be considered abnormal.

Changes in the contour of the Doppler waveform associated with arterial disease depend greatly on the location of the site of insonation relative to the stenosis or obstruction. In addition, collateral pathways can influence waveform contour depending on the location of the stenosis relative to proximal and distal arterial branches. Standard Doppler principles dictate that the Doppler arterial waveform within a significant stenosis will be characterized by a high-velocity jet. The waveform contour

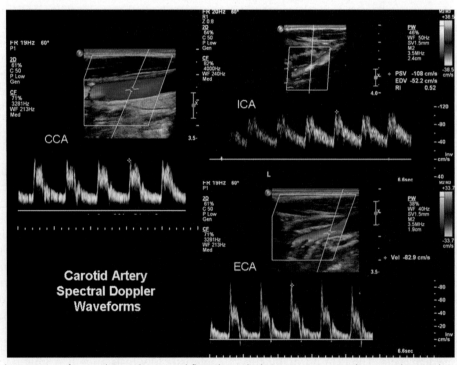

Figure 4-14 Duplex images of normal Doppler arterial flow through the common carotid, external carotid, and internal carotid arteries.

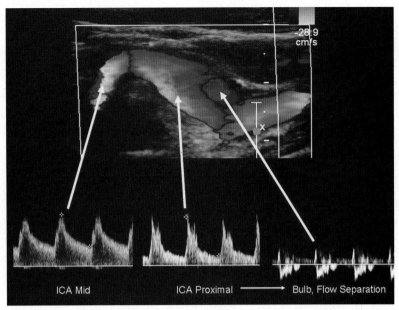

Figure 4-15 Duplex image of normal Doppler arterial flow characteristics through the carotid bulb and internal carotid artery.

distal to a significant stenosis will be dampened, with decreased flow velocity, delayed acceleration, and a rounded peak. This is sometimes referred to as a "tardus-parvus" pattern (Fig. 4-16). When the site of insonation is immediately distal to the stenotic lesion, poststenotic turbulence will be present, resulting in spectral broadening. The high-velocity jet and the maximal spectral broadening may only be evident for a few vessel diameters distal to the stenosis, so it is important to sample flow with the PW Doppler relatively close to the lesion. As the severity of stenosis increases, the downstream extent

of the high-velocity jet and dampened poststenotic flow tends to increase. The features of Doppler waveforms obtained proximal to a stenosis depend on the severity of the lesion and the intervening collateral vessels. If there are abundant collateral vessels, the waveform may appear essentially normal. If collateral flow is limited and the stenosis is severe, the waveform will have a "high resistance" pattern with low velocity or absent diastolic flow (Fig. 4-17). The most severe stenoses, which are nearly occlusive, will produce the most abnormal, preocclusive waveform contour known as "string-sign" flow.

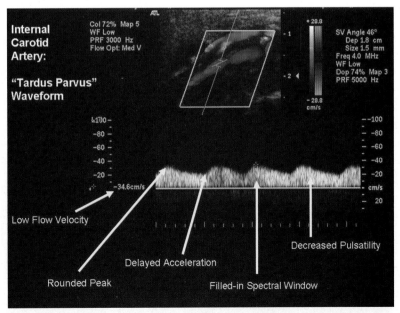

Figure 4-16 Abnormal dampened Doppler arterial waveform contour in the internal carotid artery described as "tardus and parvus."

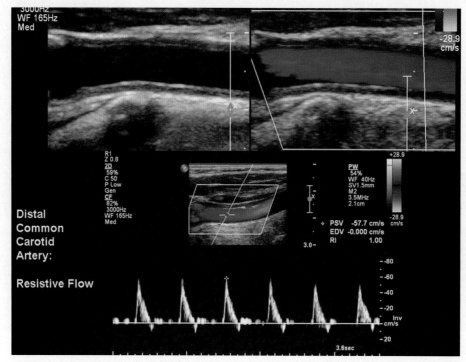

Figure 4-17 Abnormal, resistive Doppler arterial flow through the common carotid artery in the setting of an internal carotid artery occlusion.

"Steal" Waveform Contours

Another spectral waveform abnormality is the "steal" phenomenon. This describes the situation where one vascular bed draws blood away or steals from another, which tends to occur when two runoff beds with different resistances are supplied by a limited source of inflow. The degree of arterial steal depends on the severity of the stenosis and the resistance offered by the various downstream vascular beds.

A "latent" steal describes flow that is beginning to show signs of reversal, but is not yet completely retrograde. There are progressing stages of abnormal flow, which indicate an impending steal. "Hesitant" waveforms possess a deep flow reversal notch when flow pauses before progressing cephalad (Fig. 4-18). When the deep notch in the Doppler waveform extends below the baseline, with a portion of the flow fully retrograde during part of the cardiac cycle, these waveforms are described as "alternating" or bidirectional. In the case

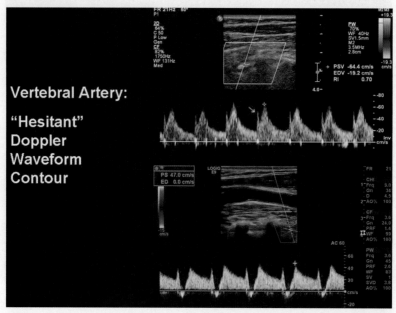

Figure 4-18 Duplex images of abnormal "hesitant" Doppler vertebral artery flow, indicating latent subclavian steal phenomenon.

of a progressive proximal subclavian artery stenosis, changing pressure gradients at the origin of the ipsilateral vertebral artery can change the ratio of antegrade to retrograde flow in the vertebra to the point where flow is entirely in the retrograde direction—a "complete" steal. In this setting, it is important to determine

the flow direction based on the color Doppler and spectral Doppler settings. Abnormal steal patterns can also develop in the presence of a brachiocephalic artery stenosis or occlusion. Blood flow can be affected in the carotid distribution (Fig. 4-19A) as well as within the subclavian and vertebral arteries (Fig. 4-19B).

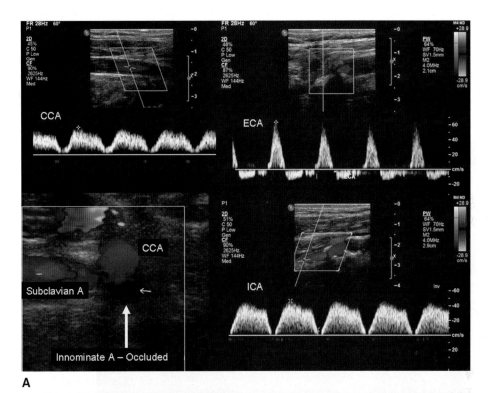

A

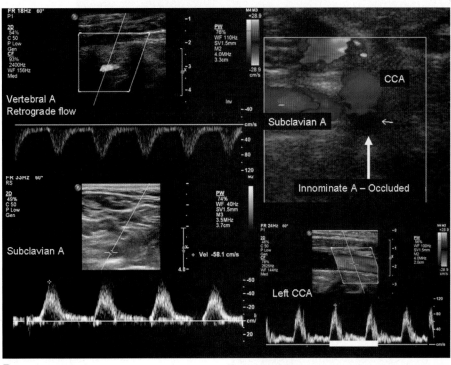

B

Figure 4-19 Duplex images demonstrating brachiocephalic artery occlusion. **A:** Abnormal Doppler arterial flow through the carotid distribution. **B:** Abnormal Doppler flow through the subclavian and vertebral distribution.

Vessel-Specific Abnormal Waveform Contours

"String sign" flow is characterized by blunted, somewhat resistive waveforms and is the pattern that precedes complete occlusion of the vessel (Fig. 4-20A,B). This is most likely to be found in a severely diseased ICA. It is important to differentiate string sign flow from complete vessel occlusion. With a string sign, the patient may still undergo an endarterectomy, whereas the patient with a completely occluded vessel will not be a surgical candidate. To aid in this differentiation, the vessels should be imaged along both the long axis and the transverse planes using color Doppler (with settings of low scale and high gain)

and power Doppler to detect the presence of any flow. Careful interrogation of the most distal extracranial ICA segment is important to avoid overlooking a patent but small lumen in that location.

A markedly decreased diastolic flow or resistive component and overall "blunted" appearing waveform in the extracranial ICA indicates a severe stenosis or occlusion in the more distal or intracranial segments (Fig. 4-21). This may be associated with severe distal extracranial ICA stenosis due to fibromuscular dysplasia or segmental dissection. These changes will be observed even when there is a stenosis in the proximal ICA. Resistive and blunted flow

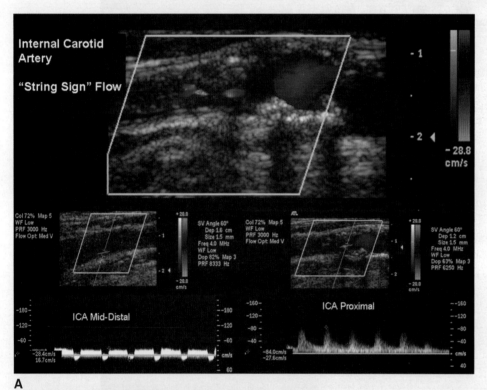

A

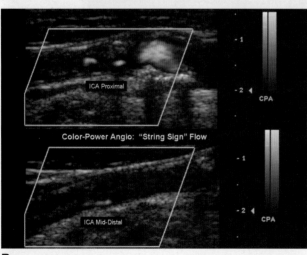

B

Figure 4-20 Duplex images of a functionally occluded internal carotid artery with "string sign" Doppler flow. **A:** Use of color Doppler and spectral Doppler modalities. **B:** Use of color power angio modality.

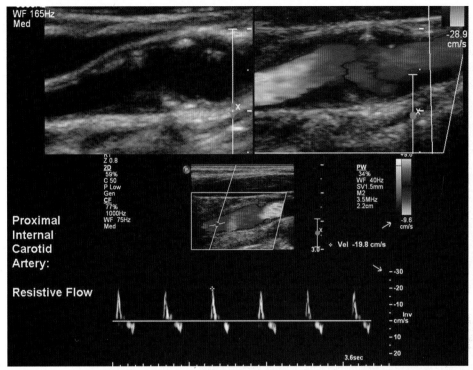

Figure 4-21 Duplex images of a patent proximal internal carotid artery and abnormal, blunted, and resistive Doppler arterial flow. Findings indicate distal extracranial versus intracranial severe stenosis or occlusion of the internal carotid artery.

in the ICA will also be reflected in the CCA. This is similar to the setting of extracranial internal carotid artery occlusion, where the flow pattern in the CCA takes on the features of the patent ECA. Careful comparison of the bilateral ICA end-diastolic velocities is imperative to verify hemodynamic significance of a unilateral distal stenosis.

Recognition of a severe ECA stenosis is generally straightforward. Atherosclerotic lesions of this vessel tend to involve the origin and proximal segments and are associated with a focal velocity increase, poststenotic turbulence (spectral broadening), and a dampened waveform distally. Diffuse increases in ECA velocity due to intracranial collateralization and compensatory flow may be found when the ipsilateral ICA is occluded.

Aortic valve or root stenosis will generate a symmetrically abnormal Doppler arterial waveform contour in the right and left carotid systems (Fig. 4-22A–C). Brachial systolic pressures may also be symmetrically low depending on the severity of the stenosis. Severe stenosis or occlusion of the brachiocephalic artery creates decreased pressure and waveform changes in the right CCA and subclavian artery and their distal branches. Therefore, when the brachiocephalic artery bifurcation is patent, there is the potential for a steal from the subclavian and the vertebral arteries to supply the common carotid circulation.

Severe stenosis or occlusion of the proximal, mid-, or distal CCA will affect the Doppler arterial waveform in the remaining peripheral segments of the CCA, as well as the ICA, and ECA. A severe distal CCA obstruction with continued patency of the carotid bifurcation is often referred to as a "choke lesion" (Fig. 4-23). Flow direction distal to a choke lesion depends on the local pressure gradients and can result in varying degrees of steal. In this situation, flow will typically reverse in the ECA to supply the ICA (Fig. 4-24). Rarely, flow will reverse in the ICA to supply the ECA in response to unusual intracranial collateral pathways. In these cases, it is important to make sure that the vessels have been correctly identified. When the internal carotid artery is occluded, Doppler arterial waveforms throughout the common carotid artery will be more resistive and more identical to the external carotid artery (Fig. 4-25A,B). Complete external carotid artery occlusion is uncommon due to multiple branches and abundant collateral pathways.

Special Considerations

Low cardiac output and a poor ejection fraction can affect systemic arterial pressure and Doppler arterial waveform contour throughout the carotid system. Doppler waveforms will be dampened with delayed acceleration in every artery evaluated, yet no stenosis or poststenotic turbulence will be identified.

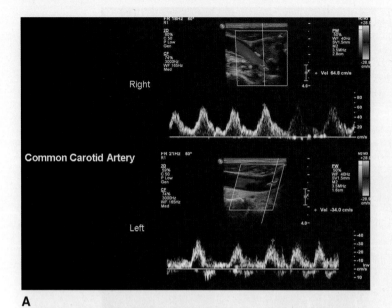

A

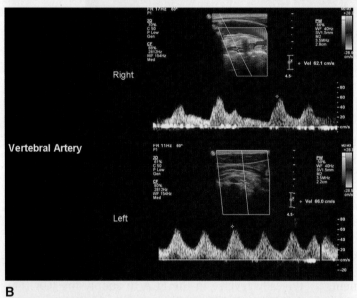

B

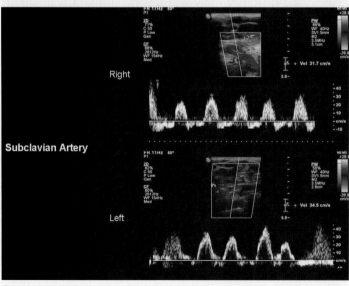

C

Figure 4-22 Duplex images demonstrating symmetrically abnormal Doppler arterial flow in the presence of known aortic stenosis, demonstrated in the right and left: **(A)** carotid arteries, **(B)** vertebral arteries, and **(C)** subclavian arteries.

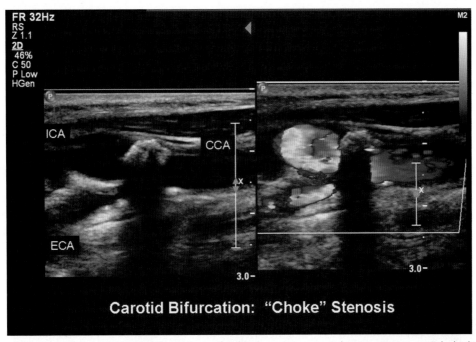

Figure 4-23 B-mode and color Doppler images of a distal common carotid artery stenosis or "choke lesion."

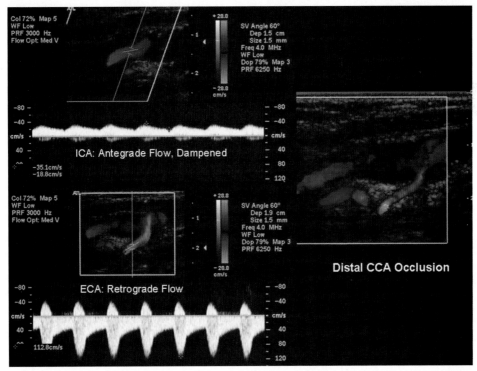

Figure 4-24 Duplex images demonstrating distal common carotid artery occlusion with retrograde Doppler flow through the external carotid artery and dampened antegrade flow through the proximal internal carotid artery.

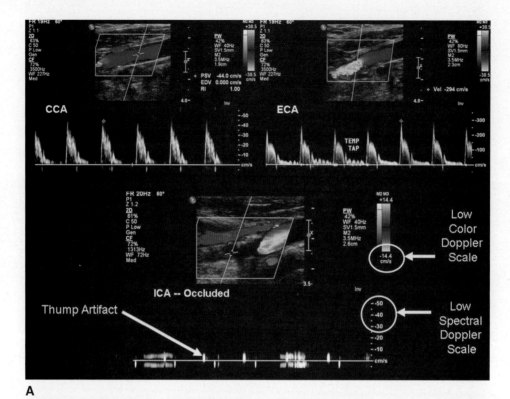

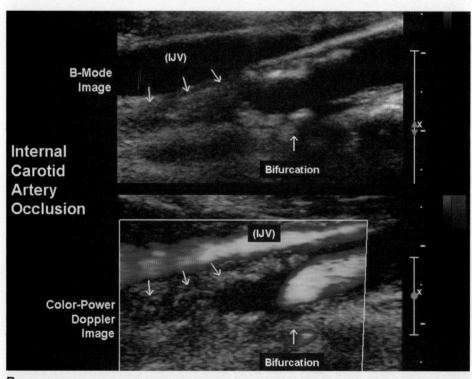

Figure 4-25 Duplex images of an internal carotid artery occlusion, no obtainable Doppler flow. **A:** Use of color Doppler and spectral Doppler modalities. **B:** Use of color power angio modality.

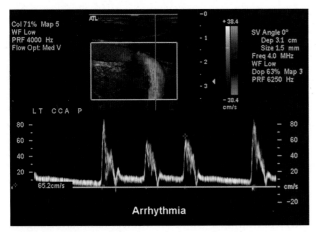

Figure 4-26 Doppler flow signal obtained in the common carotid artery, with arrhythmia.

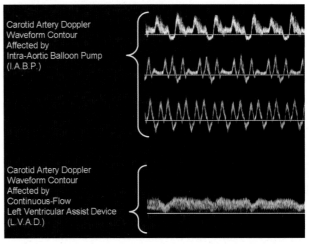

Figure 4-27 Carotid artery Doppler flow affected by cardiac assist devices: intra-aortic balloon pump (IABP) and left ventricular assist device (LVAD).

Differentiating low cardiac output from aortic stenosis can be difficult with duplex ultrasound. However, an unusual waveform with two prominent systolic peaks separated by a systolic retraction called "pulsus bisferiens" has been described in the carotid arteries of patient with aortic valvular disease and hypertrophic obstructive cardiomyopathy.[11] Cardiac arrhythmias (abnormal heart rhythms or rates) can also make interpreting Doppler waveforms difficult because standard velocity criteria may not apply and the waveform contour may be altered (Fig. 4-26).

Cardiac assist devices are used in patients with heart failure to support cardiac function, often while they are recovering from myocardial infarction or heart surgery. Some cardiac assist devices are intended for short-term use, whereas others may be in place for longer periods as a bridge to cardiac transplantation. A ventricular assist device (VAD) and an intra-aortic balloon pump (IABP) are two examples of cardiac assist devices. The effects of cardiac assist devices on Doppler arterial waveform contour is profound, creating patterns that may be unrecognizable as arterial flow. An example of a carotid artery Doppler waveform in a patient with an IABP is shown in Figure 4-27. Therefore, a "disclaimer" is necessary in the vascular laboratory report stating that waveform contour cannot be interpreted according to standard criteria. Hospital-based vascular laboratories are most likely to encounter these patients, as they are almost always inpatients. However, some of these devices are portable, so occasionally an outpatient may present to the vascular laboratory with one of these devices in place.

Measurement of Doppler Flow Velocity

Flow velocity obtained from Doppler waveforms serves as the primary criterion for classification of stenosis severity with duplex ultrasound. Obtaining

accurate Doppler information is highly dependent on proper examination technique, particularly using the correct angle of insonation. The Doppler angle of insonation is traditionally defined as the angle between the line of the ultrasound beam and the arterial wall at the site of the PW Doppler sample volume. This assumes that the direction of flow is parallel to the wall of the artery and requires that the angle cursor be aligned parallel to the vessel wall. However, "off-axis" flow (flow not parallel to the wall) is common in diseased arteries. When the direction of an off-axis flow jet can be determined based on the color Doppler image, some laboratories set the angle cursor parallel to the flow jet, but it has not been established that this is more accurate than setting the angle cursor parallel to the vessel wall.

All arterial velocity measurements should be obtained using an angle of insonation of 60° or less. This is accomplished by either adjusting the steering of the Doppler beam or by a transducer maneuver called "toe-heel." This maneuver involves slight transducer pressure at either end of the transducer (the toe or the heel) to push a vessel into a slight angle. This moves the vessel enough to create an angle of 60° or less. Although an in-depth discussion of Doppler physics is beyond the scope of this chapter, this recommendation is based on the concept that errors related to Doppler angles are more critical at large angles because the cosine changes more rapidly at angles approaching 90°.[12] Doppler shift frequencies also become very small at larger angles, which further reduces the accuracy of velocity measurements. For carotid duplex scanning, a Doppler angle of 60° or less results in clinically valid velocity information for the classification of stenosis severity.

Obtaining the most complete and accurate representation of flow velocity changes throughout the carotid arteries requires that the PW Doppler sample volume be moved slowly and continuously ("swept") along the vessel. Simply "spot checking" the flow pattern may overlook very focal or localized flow disturbances. In a segment where stenosis is suspected, sweep the sample volume cursor through the area, proximal to distal, evaluating flow at closely spaced intervals and moving the sample volume across the lumen to identify the highest velocity flow jet. As this is being done, the Doppler angle must be continually evaluated and adjusted to maintain proper alignment through each segment.

The carotid and vertebral artery systems are connected by the circle of Willis at the base of brain. The branches of the circle of Willis are variable and provide numerous collateral pathways to compensate for extracranial cerebrovascular disease. Potential collateral routes include posterior-to-anterior, side-to-side, and extracranial-to-intracranial. When there is a severe stenosis or complete occlusion of one ICA, velocities may be increased in the contralateral carotid system due to compensatory collateral flow. It is important to recognize this situation to avoid overestimating the extent of disease on the contralateral side. Compensatory flow is generally associated with a diffuse increase in flow velocity throughout the contralateral CCA and ICA, without a focal high-velocity jet or other localized flow disturbance. Even when a hemodynamically significant ICA stenosis is identified contralateral to a severe stenosis or occlusion, it is appropriate to comment that the Doppler flow velocity elevation may be due, in part, to the contralateral disease. More detailed information on specific intracranial collateral pathways can be obtained by a transcranial Doppler examination, as discussed in Chapter 7.

CRITERIA FOR CLASSIFICATION OF DISEASE

The B-mode imaging and Doppler waveform parameters for classification of carotid artery disease have been developed by comparing the results of duplex scanning with "gold standard" imaging modalities or surgical findings. These alternative standard imaging approaches include catheter contrast arteriography, CTA, and magnetic resonance arteriography (MRA). The majority of duplex ultrasound carotid criteria have been validated for the ICA. Therefore, it must be emphasized that such criteria cannot be applied to the CCA or ECA.

One of the most widely applied classification schemes for ICA stenosis was developed at the University of Washington under the direction of Dr. D. Eugene Strandness, Jr. These criteria classify ICA lesions into the following ranges of stenosis: normal, 1% to 15%, 16% to 49%, 50% to 79%, 80% to 99%, and occlusion (Table 4-2). Prospective validation of these criteria has demonstrated a 99% sensitivity for the detection of carotid disease and an 84% specificity for the identification of normal arteries.[13] The carotid duplex criteria have undergone periodic updating to remain relevant to current clinical practice.

TABLE 4-2

University of Washington Criteria for Classification of Internal Carotid Artery Disease

Arteriographic Diameter Reduction	Peak Systolic Velocity (PSV)	End Diastolic Velocity (EDV)	Spectral Waveform Characteristics
0% (Normal)	<125 cm/s	—	Minimal or no spectral broadening; boundary layer separation present in the carotid bulb
1%–15%	<125 cm/s	—	Spectral broadening during deceleration phase of systole only
16%–49%	<125 cm/s	—	Spectral broadening throughout systole
50%–79%	≥125 cm/s	<140 cm/s	Marked spectral broadening
80%–99%	≥125 cm/s	≥140 cm/s	Marked spectral broadening
100% (Occlusion)	—	—	No flow signal in the internal carotid artery; decreased diastolic flow in the ipsilateral common carotid artery

Diameter reduction is based on arteriographic methods that compared the residual internal carotid artery lumen diameter to the estimated diameter of the carotid bulb.
Velocity criteria are based on the angle-adjusted velocity using a Doppler angle of 60° or less.

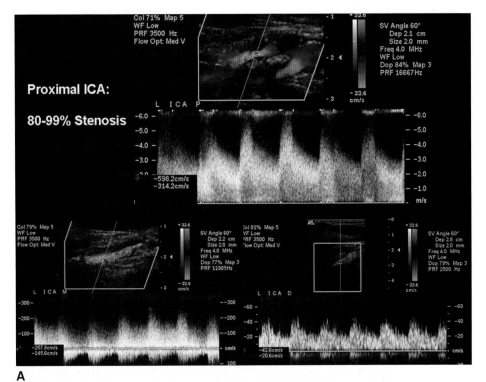

A

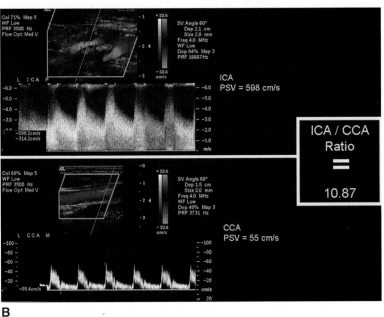

B

Figure 4-28 Duplex images demonstrating high-grade stenosis of the internal carotid artery. **A:** A stenosis of 80% to 99% of the proximal internal carotid artery with poststenotic turbulence. **B:** Calculation of the internal carotid artery (ICA) to the common carotid artery (CCA) ratio.

For example, the randomized trials that evaluated the efficacy of carotid endarterectomy (CEA) in the 1990s prompted the development of some new interpretation criteria.[14-16] In the North American Symptomatic Carotid Endarterectomy Trial (NASCET), patients with symptomatic internal carotid stenosis of 70% to 99% had dramatic benefit from an endarterectomy. Based on a detailed review of multiple Doppler waveform parameters, the best criteria for identifying a 70% or greater internal carotid stenosis, as defined in the NASCET, was a PSV of 230 cm/s or greater, or an internal carotid to common carotid PSV ratio (ICA/CCA ratio) of 4.0 or greater.[17] When calculating the ICA/CCA ratio, it is important to use the highest PSV from the stenotic site for the ICA value and the PSV in a normal mid-to-distal common carotid artery segment (where the imaged arterial walls are parallel) for the CCA value (Fig. 4-28). The ICA/CCA ratio is not valid in the presence of significant common carotid artery disease.

In the major North American CEA, trials the severity of internal carotid stenosis was calculated from arteriograms by comparing the diameter of the minimal residual lumen at the stenotic site to the diameter of the normal distal cervical internal carotid.[14] This approach to measuring the stenosis is now often referred to as the NASCET method. The categories of carotid stenosis in the University of Washington criteria were developed long before the CEA trials by comparing the diameter at the stenotic site to an estimate of the diameter of the normal carotid bulb. However, because the bulb often has a larger diameter than the distal internal carotid, the two methods of measuring stenosis do not give the same percentage of angiographic stenosis for the same lesion. Calculations of angiographic stenosis using the distal internal carotid as the reference vessel result in lower stenosis percentages than calculations using the bulb as the reference site. This effect is particularly striking for lesions in the middle of the stenosis range, and the differences decrease with increasing stenosis severity.

Recognizing the wide variability in the performance and interpretation of carotid duplex scans, a panel of authorities from a variety of medical specialties met in 2002 to develop a consensus regarding the key components of the carotid ultrasound examination and the most appropriate criteria for classification of disease.[18] The panelists recommended the consistent use of relatively broad categories to classify the degree of internal carotid stenosis. The panel also concluded that Doppler parameters are relatively inaccurate for subcategorizing stenoses of less than 50% diameter reduction and recommended that these lesions be reported under a single stenosis category. They noted that although PSV is a primary parameter for interpretation, its measurement is subject to significant variability. In order to minimize this variability, it was recommended that Doppler waveforms be obtained with an insonation angle as close to 60° as possible, but not exceeding 60°, and the sample volume should be placed within the area of maximal stenosis. Additional parameters such as the ICA/CCA ratio and EDV were regarded as secondary parameters. A summary of the consensus panel criteria is given in Table 4-3. It is important to emphasize that these criteria have not been subjected to retrospective or prospective evaluation and do not represent the results of any one laboratory or study. However, they can serve as a reference for those laboratories that have not been able to internally validate their own criteria.

As previously stated, criteria used for classifying ICA disease cannot be applied for lesions in the CCA or ECA. However, sites of significant stenosis in these vessels can still be identified by the presence of plaque on B-mode imaging and associated focal increases in velocity in Doppler waveforms. A stenosis of more than 50% can be inferred by the presence of a focally increased PSV followed by poststenotic turbulence.

COLOR AND POWER DOPPLER FINDINGS

The ability to display flow information using color Doppler and power Doppler has improved remarkably

---

TABLE 4-3

Consensus Panel Recommendations for Classification of Internal Carotid Artery Stenosis[18]

Normal: The ICA PSV is less than 125 cm/s and there is no visible plaque or intimal thickening. Normal arteries should also have an ICA/CCA ratio of less than 2.0 and ICA EDV of less than 40 cm/s.

ICA stenosis <50% is present when the ICA PSV is less than 125 cm/s and there is visible plaque or intimal thickening. Such arteries should also have an ICA/CCA ratio of less than 2.0 and an ICA EDV of less than 40 cm/s.

ICA stenosis of 50% to 69% is present when the ICA PSV is 125 to 230 cm/s and there is visible plaque. Such arteries should also have an ICA/CCA ratio of 2.0 to 4.0 and an ICA EDV of 40 to 100 cm/s.

ICA stenosis ≥70% to 99% but less than near occlusion is present when the ICA PSV is more than 230 cm/s and there is visible plaque with lumen narrowing on grayscale and color Doppler imaging. The higher the PSV, the more likely (higher positive predictive value) that there is severe disease. Such stenoses should also have an ICA/CCA ratio of more than 4.0 and an ICA EDV of more than 100 cm/s.

Near occlusion of the ICA: The velocity parameters may not apply. "Preocclusive" lesions may be associated with high, low, or undetectable velocity measurements. The diagnosis of near occlusion is therefore established primarily by demonstration of a markedly narrowed lumen with color Doppler. In some near occlusive lesions, color or power Doppler can distinguish between near occlusion and occlusion by demonstrating a thin wisp of flow traversing the lesion.

Occlusion: There is no detectable patent lumen on grayscale imaging and no flow with pulsed Doppler, color Doppler, or power Doppler. Near occlusive lesions may be misdiagnosed as occlusions when only grayscale ultrasound and pulsed Doppler spectral waveforms are used.

ICA, internal carotid artery; PSV, peak systolic velocity; CCA, common carotid artery; EDV, end diastolic velocity; ICA/CCA ratio, maximal ICA PSV divided by the maximal CCA PSV.

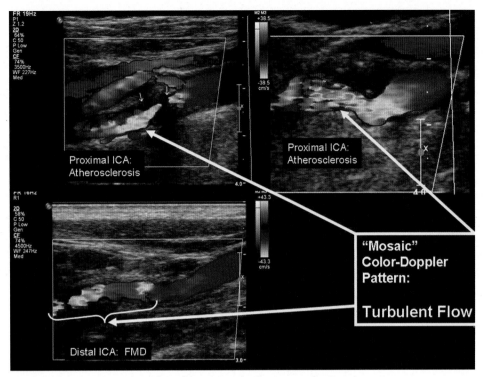

Figure 4-29 Turbulent arterial flow demonstrated with mosaic color Doppler pattern.

in recent generations of ultrasound machines. However, the diagnostic relevance of these methods for the carotid duplex evaluation remains secondary to Doppler velocities. The main benefit from using the color Doppler and power Doppler modalities is the rapid identification of flow disturbances and determining the location and direction of high velocity jets. When set with appropriate sensitivity, the flow disturbances associated with poststenotic turbulence are readily demonstrated with color Doppler imaging (Fig. 4-29). Power Doppler is particularly helpful in detecting extremely low flow velocities, including "string sign" flow.

There are several adjustments that can be made to optimize the color Doppler image and maintain proper sensitivity. Whenever possible, the color Doppler scale should be set high enough so that no color aliasing is present during any phase of the cardiac cycle and low enough so that color fills the patent lumen with even the lowest velocities (Fig. 4-30). This may not be feasible when a wide range of velocities is present, and in this setting, color aliasing can be used to identify the sites of high velocity flow. The color Doppler transmit frequency can be adjusted to provide better resolution or penetration, depending on vessel depth.

Smooth, single color in the low-to-medium tone range indicates laminar flow. When the flow velocity exceeds the color Doppler scale, aliasing occurs with brighter tones of color progressing to the opposite

color (e.g., red to blue). Turbulent flow produces a typical "mosaic" color Doppler pattern (Fig. 4-31). Regardless of the color-flow characteristics, Doppler spectral waveforms must always be used to classify the severity of disease.

The power Doppler modality displays flow based on the amplitude of the Doppler signal rather than the frequency shift and thus does not give any information on flow direction. This representation of blood flow is relatively independent of the angle of insonation. The main advantage of power Doppler is its ability to detect low-flow states.

VERTEBRAL ARTERY STENOSIS

Although the vertebral artery cannot be visualized in its entirety due to acoustic shadowing as the vessel courses through the transverse processes of the cervical vertebrae, the proximal vertebral artery is usually evaluated during a routine carotid duplex scan. Normal vertebral artery flow has the same pattern as the ICA, with a low resistance pattern and antegrade (toward the brain) flow throughout the cardiac cycle. Waveform characteristics include a brisk systolic acceleration, sharp peak, and relatively high diastolic flow (Fig. 4-32). A proximal vertebral artery stenosis will produce abnormal dampened waveforms distally with delayed acceleration, a rounded peak, and possibly poststenotic turbulence. Vertebral artery stenoses generally occur at the origin of the vessel

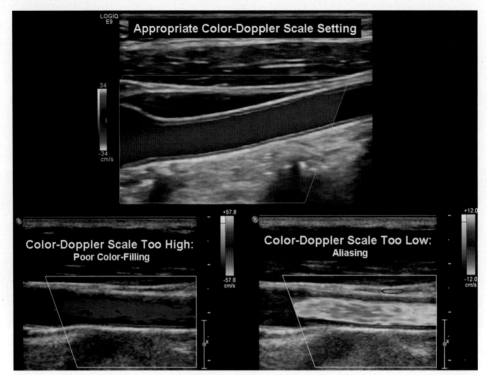

Figure 4-30 Color Doppler scale settings: appropriate, too high, and too low.

from the subclavian artery. There are no specific velocity criteria for grading of vertebral artery stenoses, but a stenosis may be suspected if there is a focal increase in PSV at the origin of greater than 150 cm/s.

Stenosis or occlusion in the more distal segments of the vertebral artery (extracranial or intracranial vertebral) will be apparent in waveforms from the cervical segments. In this situation, Doppler waveforms will have brisk systolic acceleration and a sharp peak, but there will be a high resistance pattern with minimal or no forward flow in diastole (Fig. 4-33). This waveform characteristic is referred to as resistive or blunted. When these findings are present, evaluate flow in the contralateral vertebral artery to help determine if the distal lesion is in the ipsilateral vertebral or the basilar artery. When clinically indicated, transcranial Doppler may be used to insonate the intracranial vertebral arteries and basilar artery directly.

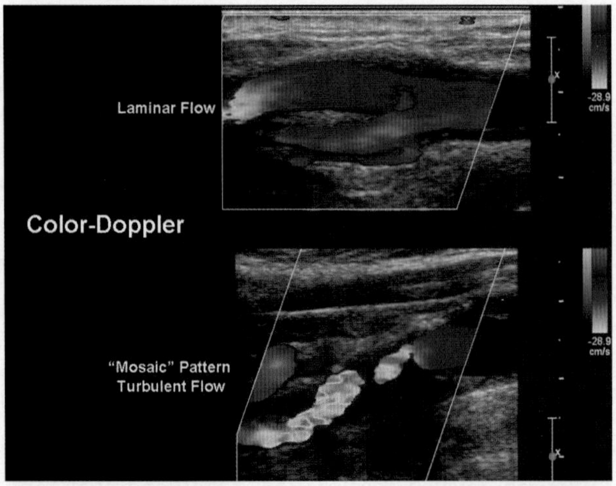

SUBCLAVIAN STEAL

The general features of a vascular steal have been discussed previously. A hemodynamically significant stenosis in the proximal subclavian artery will result in a brachial systolic pressure gradient of more than 15 to 20 mm Hg. Whenever a brachial pressure gradient is present, the vertebral arteries should be evaluated for a possible steal phenomenon. Subclavian steal occurs with severe stenosis or occlusion of the subclavian artery (or brachiocephalic artery on the right) proximal to the origin of the vertebral artery. This causes decreased pressure at the origin of the ipsilateral vertebral that can lead to reversed flow in that artery as the abnormal pressure gradient "steals" blood from the vertebral circulation to supply the arm.

As upper extremity arterial inflow obstruction progresses, so do the different stages of abnormal vertebral artery flow. Doppler arterial waveform contour will progress from normal antegrade to antegrade with a deep notch at the mid-cardiac cycle.

Figure 4-31 Color Doppler images comparing laminar color Doppler flow and abnormal turbulent color Doppler flow (mosaic pattern).

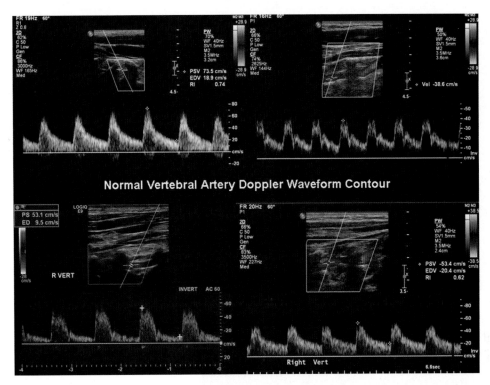

Figure 4-32 Duplex images demonstrating various normal vertebral artery Doppler waveform contours.

In the next phase toward a complete steal, this notch extends below the baseline progressing toward alternating (to-and-fro) flow. Vertebral artery flow direction will be fully retrograde in the case of a complete subclavian steal (Fig. 4-34).

Reactive Hyperemia

Reactive hyperemia is a provocative noninvasive test that can be used to augment a subclavian steal from the "latent" stage to the "complete" stage. Reactive hyperemia testing begins with a blood pressure cuff on the upper arm. The cuff is inflated to a pressure that is more than systolic pressure for 3 to 5 minutes, and duplex scanning is performed to continuously monitor the vertebral artery. At the end of the inflation period, the cuff is rapidly deflated while the ipsilateral vertebral artery flow is observed. The test is considered positive when flow in the vertebral artery completely reverses direction.

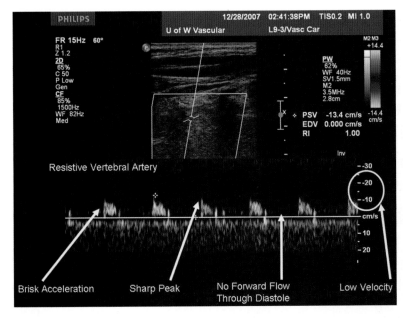

Figure 4-33 Abnormal, resistive, and blunted vertebral artery Doppler waveform contour, which indicates distal (versus intracranial) severe stenosis or occlusion.

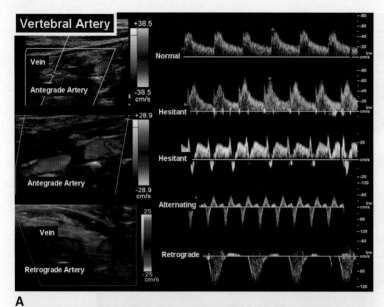

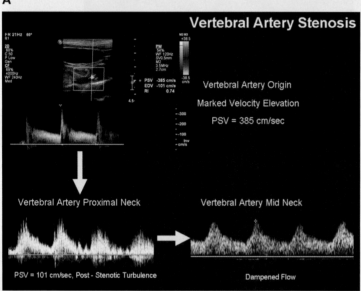

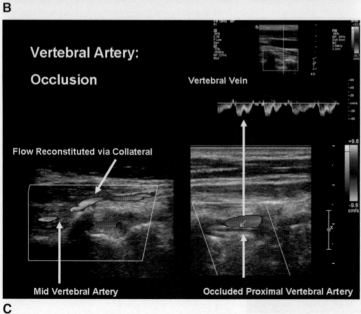

Figure 4-34 Abnormal vertebral artery Doppler flow signals. **A:** Progression from normal waveform contour to reversed vertebral artery flow. **B:** Vertebral artery stenosis. **C:** Proximal extracranial vertebral artery occlusion with collateral artery reconstitution.

In cases where one vertebral artery is congenitally or pathologically small in caliber, the contralateral vertebral artery will often dilate and carry increased flow to compensate. In the case of severe ipsilateral subclavian steal, the contralateral vertebral artery flow may be elevated. In complex cases where one or both of the carotid arteries (particularly the ICA) are compromised, Doppler flow velocities will be elevated through the vertebral arteries to compensate through collateral pathways involving the circle of Willis.

SUMMARY

The use of ultrasound in the diagnosis of extracranial carotid disease has become a standard tool used by clinicians. The combination of real-time B-mode imaging, spectral Doppler analysis and color Doppler imaging has proven to be highly accurate and reproducible. Multiple studies have lead to reliable criteria by which to grade stenosis. Atherosclerotic disease can be easily detected and monitored with ultrasound techniques in order to prevent serious consequences such as stroke.

Critical Thinking Questions

1. Your initial B-mode and Doppler evaluation of the left carotid system suggests that there may be occlusion of the internal carotid artery. What key features will help to confirm an occlusion of this vessel?

2. A carotid–vertebral artery duplex examination has been requested on a patient who is in the cardiac intensive care unit awaiting a cardiac transplantation. The patient has an intra-aortic balloon pump (IABP). Doppler waveform contour is markedly altered, and there is an arrhythmia. What is the best way to approach this duplex examination in terms of interpreting the Doppler velocities and flow patterns and application of other diagnostic criteria?

3. During a carotid–vertebral artery duplex examination, you document high-grade, 80% to 99% stenosis of the left proximal internal carotid artery. There is minimal plaque visible in the right proximal internal carotid artery (and through the carotid bifurcation), yet the peak systolic velocity is diffusely increased at 165 cm/s. Is this a 50% to 79% stenosis? What may account for the elevated Doppler flow velocities contralateral to the 80% to 99% stenosis? How would you describe this in the vascular laboratory report?

4. Brachial systolic pressures are asymmetrical: right = 86 mm Hg, left = 138 mm Hg. As you begin the carotid–vertebral artery duplex, you find an abnormal, dampened, and hesitant Doppler waveform contour through the right proximal common carotid artery. What do you expect the remainder of the carotid–vertebral artery duplex examination to reveal?

REFERENCES

1. Barber FE, Baker DW, Nation AWC, et al. Ultrasonic duplex echo-Doppler scanner. *IEEE Trans Biomed Eng.* 1974;21(2):109–113.
2. Beach KW. D. Eugene Strandness, Jr., MD, and the revolution in noninvasive vascular diagnosis. Part 1: foundations. *J Ultrasound Med.* 2005;24(3):259–272.
3. Fell G, Breslau P, Knox RA, et al. Importance of noninvasive ultrasonic Doppler testing in the evaluation of patients with asymptomatic carotid bruits. *Am Heart J.* 1981;102(2): 221–226.
4. Fell G, Phillips DJ, Chikos PM, et al. Ultrasonic duplex scanning for disease of the carotid artery. *Circulation.* 1981;64:1191–1195.

5. Johnston SC, Gress DR, Browner WS, et al. Short-term prognosis after emergency department diagnosis of TIA. *JAMA*. 2000;284(22):2901–2906.

6. Whisnant JP. The role of the neurologist in the decline of stroke. *Ann Neurol*. 1983;14(1): 1–7.

7. Santos RD, Nasir K. Insights into atherosclerosis from invasive and non-invasive imaging studies: should we treat subclinical atherosclerosis? *Atherosclerosis*. 2009;205(2):349–356.

8. Grogan JK, Shaalan WE, Cheng H, et al. B-mode ultrasonographic characterization of carotid atherosclerotic plaques in symptomatic and asymptomatic patients. *J Vasc Surg*. 2005;42(3):435–441.

9. El-Barghouty N, Geroulakos G, Nicolaides A, et al. Computer assisted carotid plaque characterization. *Eur J Vasc Endovasc Surg*. 1995;9(4):389–393.

10. Takiuchi S, Rakugi H, Honda K, et al. Quantitative ultrasonic tissue characterization can identify high-risk atherosclerotic alteration in human carotid arteries. *Circulation*. 2000;102:776–770.

11. Rohren EM, Kliewer MA, Carroll BA, et al. A spectrum of Doppler waveforms in the carotid and vertebral arteries. *AJR Am J Roentgenol*. 2001;181(6):1695–1704.

12. Kremkau FW. *Diagnostic Ultrasound Principles and Instruments*. St. Louis, MO: Saunders Elsevier; 2006.

13. Moneta GL, Mitchell EL, Esmonde N, et al. Extracranial carotid and vertebral arteries. In: Zierler RE, ed. *Strandness's Duplex Scanning in Vascular Disorders*. 4th ed. Philadelphia, PA: Lippincott Williams & Wilkins; 2010:87–100.

14. North American Symptomatic Carotid Endarterectomy Trial Collaborators. Beneficial effect of carotid endarterectomy in symptomatic patients with high-grade carotid stenosis. *N Engl J Med*. 1991;325(7):445–453.

15. European Carotid Surgery Trialists' Collaborative Group (ECST). MRC European Carotid surgery Trial: interim results for symptomatic patients with severe (70–99%) or with mild (0–29%) carotid stenosis. *Lancet*. 1996;347:1591–1593.

16. Executive Committee for Asymptomatic Carotid Atherosclerosis Study: endarterectomy for asymptomatic carotid artery stenosis. *JAMA*. 1995;273:1421–1428.

17. Moneta GL, Edwards JM, Papanicolaou G, et al. Screening for asymptomatic internal carotid artery stenosis: duplex criteria for discriminating 60% to 99% stenosis. *J Vasc Surg*. 1995;21:989–994.

18. Grant EG, Benson CB, Moneta GL, et al. Carotid artery stenosis: gray-scale and Doppler US diagnosis—Society of Radiologists in Ultrasound Consensus Conference. *Radiology*. 2003;229:340–346.

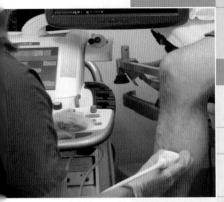

5 Uncommon Pathology of the Carotid System

Eileen French-Sherry

OBJECTIVES

Recognize patient signs and symptoms of carotid artery pathology beyond atherosclerosis

Identify uncommon pathology in the carotid arteries

Plan an appropriate duplex exam to assist in the diagnosis of unusual pathology in the carotid arteries

Create interpretable images of unusual carotid pathology using B-mode, Doppler, and color duplex ultrasound techniques

Avoid pitfalls in scanning and documenting unusual pathology in the carotid arteries

KEY TERMS

aneurysm | arteritis | carotid body tumor | dissection | fibromuscular dysplasia | intimal flap | pseudoaneurysm | radiation injury | tortuosity

GLOSSARY

aneurysm a localized dilatation of the wall of an artery

arteritis inflammation of an artery

carotid body tumor a benign mass (also called paraganglioma or chemodectoma) of the carotid body, which is a small round mass at the carotid bifurcation

dissection a tear along the inner layer of an artery that results in the splitting or separation of the walls of a blood vessel

fibromuscular dysplasia abnormal growth and development of the muscular layer of an artery

wall with fibrosis and collagen deposition causing stenosis

intimal flap a small tear in the wall of a blood vessel resulting in a portion of the intima and part of the media protruding into the lumen of the vessel; this free portion of the blood vessel wall may appear to move with pulsations in flow

pseudoaneurysm a dilation of an artery with disruption of one or more layers of the vessel wall causing an expanding hematoma; also called false aneurysm

tortuosity the quality of being tortuous, winding, twisting

Atherosclerosis is clearly the most common pathology that is encountered during a carotid ultrasound examination. However, the vascular sonographer will be faced with other forms of disease and abnormalities while scanning the carotid arteries. Some of these abnormalities will be observed more frequently, such as tortuosity, whereas others are fairly rare, such as a carotid artery aneurysm. It is important to know the ultrasound presentation and scanning requirements when presented with nonatherosclerotic

carotid disease. This chapter will review several of these less common findings observed during carotid duplex scans.

TORTUOSITY AND KINKING

Sonographers frequently encounter tortuous carotid arteries with varying degrees of winding and bending. Some of these vessels will be kinked with a very sharp angulation of the artery. As many as one-quarter of adults will have some degree of angulation within their internal carotid artery (ICA). Often, this is a bilateral finding.

SIGNS AND SYMPTOMS

Tortuous carotid arteries are usually asymptomatic, but a kinked artery may cause symptoms of stroke or transient ischemic attack (TIA), particularly upon turning the head. Tortuous carotid arteries may be congenital, affecting more women than men, but most patients with symptoms are of the older adult population.[1] Frequently, a referring physician will mistake a very tortuous proximal common carotid (CCA) or brachiocephalic (innominate) artery for a carotid aneurysm because a large tortuous vessel that courses superficially may appear to be a very pulsatile mass upon palpation and/or upon being seen pulsing in the proximal neck. A duplex ultrasound scan can easily differentiate the two.

SONOGRAPHIC EXAMINATION TECHNIQUES

Although tortuosity is not uncommon in the CCA, the ICA is actually more likely to be redundant. It is a challenge to follow these vessels in long and transverse views and takes considerable skill and experience to identify the course of the vessel as it changes planes and while it curves, loops, and sometimes kinks (Fig. 5-1). Color is nearly essential to follow tortuous arteries and care must be taken not to accidentally move on to a branch that the tortuous artery may be crossing. Moving slowly up the neck

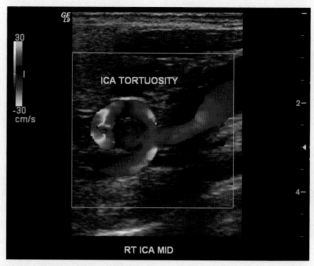

Figure 5-2 Color clearly demonstrates a looped internal carotid artery with higher velocities (aliasing) along the outer walls of the vessel as the flow courses upward on the left side of the image and as it moves downward in the red segment in the middle of the image. (Image courtesy of Damaris Gonzalez, RVT, RDMS, Rush University, Vascular Laboratory.)

while concentrating only on the next 0.5 cm at a time will enable the sonographer to move the transducer along the plane needed to follow the vessel. The sonographer will be forced to move the transducer along unusual oblique angles and planes and, in transverse view, even move it proximally at times while the vessel turns upon itself. It is often not possible to obtain a picture of the entire tortuous segment in one image, but if it can be done, it creates a beautifully complex color picture (Fig. 5-2). Although Doppler angles close to zero degrees may occur causing color aliasing in the vertical segments of the artery, flow also naturally increases along the outer edges of a curve and may also cause aliasing in the color display.

The next challenge is to obtain interpretable Doppler waveforms and velocities on a tortuous carotid artery.[2] If there is no atherosclerotic disease or tight kink, Doppler waveforms should preferentially be taken on a straighter portion of the vessel, just before and after a curve, rather than directly at the point of the tightest curve. If you must measure the velocity on a curved segment of artery (perhaps in those cases where plaque is noted or a tight kink is suspected), the angle cursor is set so that the very middle of the angle-correct cursor is parallel to the walls of the artery (perhaps in those cases where plaque is noted or a tight kink is suspected), even though one or both ends of the cursor may not appear to be aligned correctly (Fig. 5-3)

As in any carotid duplex examination, the sample volume should be kept center stream and small despite the fact that velocities are higher along the outside of the curve. The inside of a curve may have

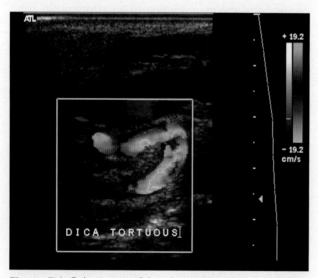

Figure 5-1 Color is a useful tool to appreciate the tortuous course of this distal ICA. (Image courtesy of Kimberly Gaydula, BS, RVT, University of Chicago, Vascular Laboratory.)

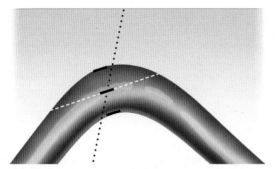

Figure 5-3 Appropriate angle correction techniques when sampling along a curved portion of the vessel.

lower velocities and demonstrate flow separation at or just distal to the curve. Some laboratories may choose to place the sample volume at the highest point of velocity whether or not it is along the wall. Although this process will ensure that no high velocities will be missed, in the case of the curved vessel, a sample volume placed along the outer wall will possibly make the interpretation even more difficult as velocities measured here will be more likely to enter the abnormal range even in a normal artery.

Technical Considerations

A standard carotid duplex examination, as described in the preceding chapter, should be completed first. Additional transverse and longitudinal color images of the tortuous carotid segments should be obtained. Scroll the sample volume through the tortuous segment or kink and document Doppler velocities pre- and post-curve or kink, setting the middle of the angle-correct cursor parallel to the walls of the vessel, as described previously. Transverse and longitudinal B-mode images should be used to identify any plaque along the curved segment. A transverse B-mode image may be helpful in identifying the diameter of the artery at a tight kink. Some laboratories may document flow changes past a kink and/or symptoms while the patient turns his or her head.

DIAGNOSIS

High velocities naturally occur past a curve, making it difficult to apply strict velocity criteria on tortuous vessels. However, recognizing this normal flow phenomenon should be helpful to identify false-positive velocity increases when the arterial lumen appears normal. Unfortunately, there is no specific velocity criterion to apply to tortuous vessels due to the variety of angulations that may occur. Careful analysis of B-mode images with and without color in multiple planes can be helpful as adjunct data to confirm that velocity changes around the curve are due to plaque formation or a significant kink rather than just a normal flow response to a curve in the vessel. In the case of a significant stenosis, poststenotic turbulence will be present and will persist beyond the area in question.

DISSECTIONS/INTIMAL FLAPS

An arterial dissection is simply a separation of the layers of an artery, typically the intima from the media, caused by a tear in the intima. The dissected intima, which may include some of the media, typically flaps or flutters freely in the arterial lumen, although some may appear stable. Some dissections may result in a pseudoaneurysm, which forms because of a weakening in the arterial wall caused by the splitting of the layers of the vessel wall.

The intimal tear creates a false lumen, where blood can flow and/or a thrombus can form. Blood can exit the false lumen in either of two ways. It can enter and exit the false lumen through the same tear, or it can exit via a secondary tear either distal or proximal to the original tear (Fig. 5-4A,B). Either configuration will result in differing flow patterns in the false lumen compared to the true lumen. A false lumen may (1) demonstrate antegrade flow due to the blood continuing through a secondary tear into the true lumen, (2) have blood flow into and out of the false lumen in a to-and-fro pattern, (3) thrombose to form a stenosis or occlude the entire artery as it stretches across the true lumen of the artery, or (4) demonstrate reversed flow direction.

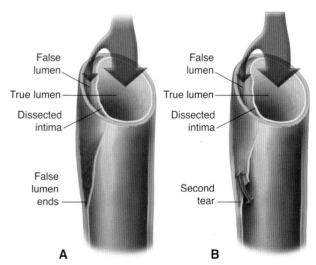

Figure 5-4 A: Diagram of a blind-ended dissection. **B:** Diagram of a dissection with a secondary tear.

SIGNS AND SYMPTOMS

A carotid artery dissection usually originates in the aorta and extends into the CCA. Some of these dissections that originate within the aortic arch may be associated with diseases such as Marfan's syndrome or Ehlers-Danlos syndrome. However, it may also originate in the distal ICA and extend proximally or it may appear at the distal end of the carotid bifurcation during a duplex scan. These dissections can be either spontaneous or traumatic. Following carotid endarterectomy, an intimal flap may also form in the area of the endarterectomized segment.

A carotid dissection may be an unexpected finding in those patients where the dissection extends from the aorta because these dissections may cause no cerebral symptoms or pain. Although pain is not a typical symptom of patients with atherosclerosis, the patient with a dissection, particularly one that begins in the internal carotid artery, may present with pain in the head, face, or neck, or with or without hemispheric symptoms. Dissection is usually suspected when a young patient (typically 35 to 50 years old) presents with symptoms of stroke despite having no risk factors for atherosclerosis and particularly with a history of trauma. The trauma that may cause a dissection may not be evident at first because it could be as subtle as a cough or turning the head or it could be a more obvious blunt trauma to the head or neck. Stretching of the artery may have occurred during these events, causing a tear in the arterial wall, or there may be an intimal weakness predisposing the individual to this consequence. With dissections that appear to be spontaneous, the primary risk factor is often hypertension.[3–6]

SONOGRAPHIC EXAMINATION TECHNIQUES

The first duplex ultrasound finding indicating that a dissection may be present is either an unusual color pattern in a section of an artery that otherwise shows no signs of atherosclerosis or the presence of a thin white line in the lumen that appears to flutter with each pulse. In B-mode, it is important to investigate the continued presence of the white line in both longitudinal and transverse views and to be sure that it is not a refraction artifact from a nearby venous valve (Figs. 5-5 and 5-6). If the white structure can be visualized in multiple views, including anterior–posterior (AP) and lateral planes, it is much more likely to be a dissection rather than an artifact. If the media is also involved, the white structure may appear thicker and may move less.

The flow patterns on each side of the dissected intima need to be investigated with Doppler, and each will be quite different (Fig. 5-7A–C). In the case where there is only one tear in the intima, blood

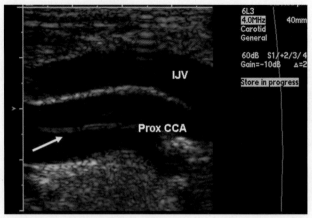

Figure 5-5 A longitudinal view of the thin, bright structure *(arrow)* in the lumen of this proximal common carotid artery (prox CCA) clearly documents a dissection. The internal jugular vein (IJV) is shown anterior to the CCA. (Image courtesy of Damaris Gonzalez, RVT, RDMS, Rush University, Vascular Laboratory.)

flow in the true lumen may continue to show a low-resistance Doppler signal. It may also demonstrate a stenotic velocity pattern if the false lumen has enough thrombus within it to block a significant portion of the artery and form a stenosis. The stenosis formed by a thrombosed false lumen is typically very smooth and tapered and may be longer than the stenosis formed by atherosclerotic plaque. If the thrombosed false lumen causes a tight stenosis or occlusion of the distal ICA, the proximal and mid-ICA may have a high resistance flow pattern typical of a distal ICA occlusion with little or no diastolic flow.

If there is still flow in the false lumen with a blind end, the flow pattern will be highly resistant. There may be portions of the false lumen with reversed flow direction because the blood has nowhere else to go but back into the true lumen through the original hole in the intima. In the case where there is both an

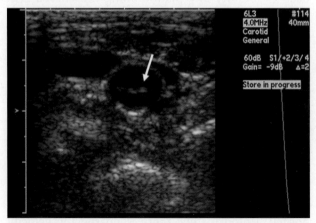

Figure 5-6 A transverse view of the thin, bright structure in the lumen of this common carotid artery clearly documents the dissection *(arrow)*. (Image courtesy of Damaris Gonzalez, RVT, RDMS, Rush University, Vascular Laboratory.)

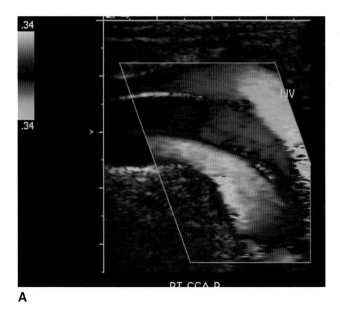

A

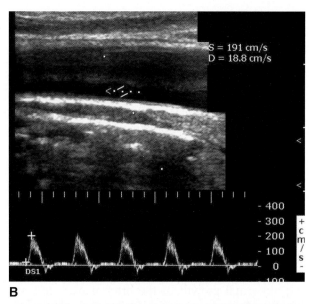

B

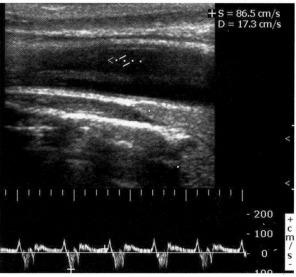

C

Figure 5-7 **A:** Color filling of the true and false lumens of this dissected artery document different directions of flow in each. The two lower flow channels are the true and false lumens of the CCA. The uppermost blue lumen is the IJV. (Image courtesy of Damaris Gonzalez, RVT, RDMS, Rush University, Vascular Laboratory.) **B:** Spectral Doppler waveforms taken from the true lumen of a CCA dissection. Note the increased resistance to flow. **C:** Spectral Doppler waveforms taken from the false lumen of a CCA dissection. Note the to-and-fro flow pattern.

inflow and outflow tear in the intima, the flow patterns within each lumen can be forward but different or one may demonstrate a reversed flow direction. Do not confuse an apparent change in direction of flow from the helical or corkscrew flow pattern that is sometimes seen in the CCA with a true dissection. The true dissection will typically reveal a white line between the differing flow patterns, which will be absent in a corkscrew pattern of flow in the normal CCA seen in transverse view.

Technical Considerations

Following the completion of a standard carotid duplex examination, additional images are required. B-mode images of the dissection should be documented using longitudinal, transverse, and multiple planes if possible. Obtain Doppler waveforms and velocities in both

the false and true lumen for a dissection, and pre- and post-flap for a short intimal flap. Color images can be used to demonstrate location, proximal and distal ends of dissection, open or thrombosed lumen, tapering of stenosis, length of stenosis, and dissection.

DIAGNOSIS

In the presence of a carotid dissection, the carotid duplex examination may not show any evidence of atherosclerotic disease, particularly in a young patient. Careful evaluation of the B-mode image will reveal a thin white structure in the arterial lumen. This represents the dissected intimal layer as well as some connective tissue and may to be fluttering or still, depending on if the medial layer is included in the dissected segment, making it thicker, or if the false lumen is completely or partially thrombosed. The stenosis in this case is typically smooth and tapered in nature, in the proximal/mid-CCA or mid-/distal ICA beyond the bifurcation. It is difficult to completely differentiate between this situation and a long smooth atherosclerotic plaque; however, there will likely be more evidence of atherosclerosis in adjacent arteries in the latter case. Color changes are likely to be noticed in either the proximal and mid-CCA, or in the mid-/distal ICA beyond the bifurcation. An important characteristic to identify the dissected artery is the distinctly different flow patterns in the true and false lumens by analysis of the Doppler waveforms.

FIBROMUSCULAR DYSPLASIA

Fibromuscular dysplasia (FMD) is a disease involving abnormal growth of the arterial wall and may involve the intima, media, and/or adventitia. The media is the most common location for the abnormal growth of smooth muscle cells and fibrous tissue. The abnormal growth will sometimes cause narrowing of the arterial lumen in multiple sections with normal walls or slight aneurysmal dilatation in between the stenotic segments. This essentially causes a "string of beads" appearance of the artery on arteriography with larger and smaller diameters in sequence.

SIGNS AND SYMPTOMS

Fibromuscular dysplasia is primarily seen in young (25 to 50 years old) Caucasians, occurring in females three times more commonly than men.[4-7] The most common location of disease is the renal arteries, and hypertension is frequently seen with renal involvement. The second most common vessel impacted is the internal carotid artery. Patients with carotid FMD often have no symptoms and can present with a cervical bruit. Embolization may occur and cause TIAs. In addition, approximately 30% of patients' carotid FMDs may have cerebral aneurysms.

SONOGRAPHIC EXAMINATION TECHNIQUES

A young person who is referred to the vascular laboratory for a carotid duplex examination should be evaluated for evidence of FMD. Bilateral disease is typical. The typical "string of beads" appearance of the artery may not be clearly appreciated at first because this disease primarily involves the distal ICA, where the vessel often courses deeply into the tissue, making detailed images difficult. The first sign of FMD during a duplex exam is most likely to be a sudden turbulence with high velocities in the distal

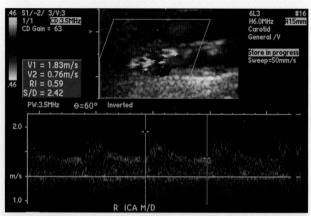

Figure 5-8 An internal carotid artery with FMD. In the area of FMD in the mid-/distal ICA, the Doppler spectral waveform demonstrates marked turbulence with spectral broadening that is clearly different than the normal waveform seen in the proximal ICA. (Image courtesy of Besnike Ramadani, BS, RVT, University of Chicago, Vascular Laboratory.)

ICA after the proximal arteries have shown no sign of atherosclerosis (Fig. 5-8). The sonographer may need to change to a lower frequency probe to visualize more distally in the internal carotid artery (Fig. 5-9). Power Doppler may be helpful in visualizing the characteristic beading in the artery, avoiding the distraction of aliasing from the marked turbulence (Fig. 5-10).

Technical Considerations

The distal ICA should be carefully examined with color, Doppler, and B-mode looking for a sudden turbulence distally after a normal appearing common

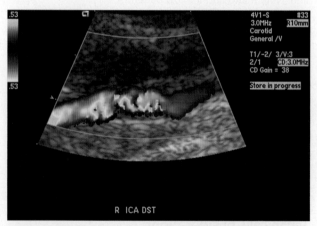

Figure 5-9 FMD. This is an image obtained from the same patient illustrated in Figure 5-8. A 3-MHz transducer was used and positioned posterior to the ear to obtain this view of FMD in the distal ICA. The image clearly depicts the turbulence and suggests a beading appearance of the artery. (Image courtesy of Besnike Ramadani, BS, RVT, University of Chicago, Vascular Laboratory.)

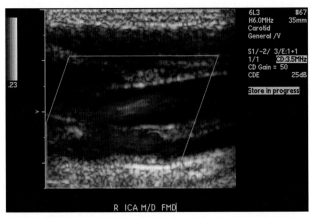

Figure 5-10 Power color is helpful in documenting the dilatations and narrowing, which are characteristic of FMD. (Image courtesy of Besnike Ramadani, BS, RVT, University of Chicago, Vascular Laboratory.)

carotid and proximal ICA. A lower frequency probe may be needed to visualize the very distal ICA behind the ear.

Additional images are required when faced with the FMD patient. There should be an image of distal ICA in longitudinal view with color demonstrating turbulence or lack of it. A velocity waveform must be taken in the distal ICA at the point of highest velocity, confirming stenosis if present, and turbulent waveform configuration. Power Doppler imaging should be used within the distal ICA if turbulence is noted to attempt to demonstrate changes in diameter or a "string of beads" appearance. In this same area, a B-mode image should be used to further demonstrate changes in diameter, especially if color bleeding is difficult to control. If evidence of FMD is noted in the carotids, the referring physician may order a renal artery exam because FMD is often found in multiple vessels.

DIAGNOSIS

A young patient with no evidence of carotid atherosclerotic disease in the bifurcation who demonstrates marked turbulence in the distal ICA with increased velocities should be considered as having ultrasound characteristics consistent with FMD. A "string of beads" appearance of the distal ICA on B-mode, color, or power Doppler imaging aids in the confirmation of FMD. However, the gold standard for the diagnosis of FMD is angiography.

CAROTID BODY TUMOR

The carotid body is a 1- to 1.5-mm structure located in the adventitia of the carotid bifurcation. It has a role in control of blood pressure, arterial pH, and blood gases. A tumor of the carotid body may form, which is easily seen with duplex ultrasound. These tumors are classified as paragangliomas and are usually not malignant.

SIGNS AND SYMPTOMS

Carotid body tumors (CBTs) are usually asymptomatic. Typically, patients notice a small lump in the anterior neck that has been growing slowly over a period of years. There may be a slight discomfort in the area and some patients may notice dysphagia, headaches, or a change in their voice.[4,8]

SONOGRAPHIC EXAMINATION TECHNIQUES

Carotid body tumors are easily seen on duplex ultrasound as a well-defined mass located between the ICA and external carotid artery (ECA) at the bifurcation, splaying the two vessels apart (Fig. 5-11). These tumors are highly vascular in nature, being fed by the ECA and its branches, which can often be seen entering the mass with color flow. The color scale may need to be decreased to identify these small vessels (Fig. 5-12). Doppler will typically demonstrate low resistance waveforms within the tumor.

Technical Considerations

When scanning a patient with a carotid body tumor, a color image of the mass is recorded to document it's vascularity. Color imaging should also be used to determine the proximity of the ICA and ECA to the mass.[4] Multiple B-mode images in various planes are used to determine the overall dimensions.

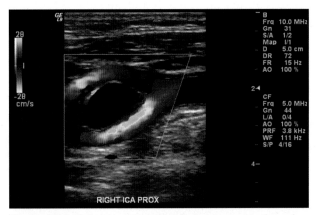

Figure 5-11 This color image clearly demonstrates the splaying of the ECA (near field) and ICA (far field) by the mass of a CBT. (Image courtesy of Damaris Gonzalez, RVT, RDMS, Rush University, Vascular Laboratory.)

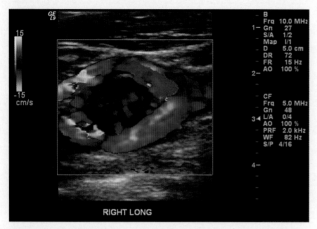

RIGHT LONG

Figure 5-12 The color scale was decreased in order to appreciate color within the mass of a CBT. (Image courtesy of Damaris Gonzalez, RVT, RDMS, Rush University, Vascular Laboratory.)

DIAGNOSIS

Location of a highly vascularized mass most clearly identifies a carotid body tumor on duplex ultrasound. The CBT is clearly located at the carotid bifurcation, splaying the ICA and the ECA. It is typically highly vascular and fed by ECA branches. Doppler waveforms within the tumor are typically low resistant. It is important to the surgeon to note the length of the tumor and if the tumor just touches the carotid vessels, partially surrounds them, or completely encases the ICA, ECA, and/or CCA.

CAROTID ANEURYSM

An aneurysm is a dilatation of the artery that involves all three layers of the arterial wall. True carotid aneurysms are very rare. The most common location for carotid artery aneurysms is within the CCA and often occurs at the bifurcation. Atherosclerosis appears to be the cause in the majority of cases. Some carotid aneurysms are the result of infection and are termed mycotic aneurysms.[9]

SIGNS AND SYMPTOMS

Usually, the patient with suspicion of a carotid aneurysm presents with a nontender, pulsatile mass in the neck. The patient may be asymptomatic or may have symptoms of a TIA or stroke. Rupture is also rare, but there may be cranial nerve dysfunction such as hoarseness of the patient's voice.[10]

SONOGRAPHIC EXAMINATION TECHNIQUES

True carotid aneurysms are rare. Be sure to take multiple B-mode images in longitudinal and transverse planes to give a complete picture of the suspected

aneurysm. Also compare the diameters of the CCA, ICA, and contralateral carotid system.

Technical Considerations

Longitudinal and transverse B-mode and color images of the widest area of the vessels should be documented. Measure the widest diameter in the transverse view in both AP and lateral. To avoid overestimating the diameter, measure the widest diameter in longitudinal view *along the axis of flow*. This is a helpful confirmation of vessel diameter particularly in a slightly tortuous vessel. Lastly, the diameter of the normal segments of the CCA and ICA bilaterally should be measured in longitudinal and transverse views for comparison to the dilated area.

DIAGNOSIS

True carotid aneurysms are rare. It is difficult to differentiate a large carotid bulb from a medium or small aneurysm. Some authors have described the true aneurysm at the bulbous portion of the ICA or CCA as having a diameter >200% of the ICA or >150% of the CCA (Fig. 5-13).[9]

PSEUDOANEURYSM

A pseudoaneurysm (PA), also known as a false aneurysm, is also very uncommon in the carotid arteries. Pseudoaneurysms are typically caused by penetrating trauma or iatrogenic injury, creating a perforation

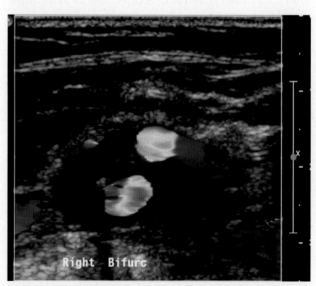

Right Bifurc

Figure 5-13 This image depicts a transverse view of a mycotic aneurysm at the carotid bifurcation. (Reprinted with permission from Journal for Vascular Ultrasound 2010;34:81.)

in the artery wall, whereby blood can extravasate out the arterial wall into the surrounding tissue.[4] Pseudoaneurysms may also form at an endarterectomy site or the anastomosis of a carotid bypass graft. The blood flow outside of the artery wall forms a spherical or ovoid mass bordered by the surrounding tissues. There may or may not be a thrombus formed within the mass or sac. The channel connecting the pseudoaneurysm mass to the artery is called the pseudoaneurysm "neck," and may be short or long, wide or thin. Characteristically, blood flow within the neck has a to-and-fro appearance as blood flows out of the artery, to the mass, and back into the artery again.

SIGNS AND SYMPTOMS

Patients will usually present with a palpable, pulsatile mass in the neck associated with a history of trauma, whether iatrogenic or otherwise. The presence of a carotid bypass graft with a pulsatile mass is also an appropriate indication for a duplex ultrasound examination. A TIA or stroke is also possible, but rupture rarely occurs.

SONOGRAPHIC EXAMINATION TECHNIQUES

A transverse overview of the carotid arteries in color will typically be the easiest and fastest way to determine the area of interest for further examination. A mass, either partially or completely filled with color, will be noted adjacent to the artery. Typically, the color flow within the pseudoaneurysm in transverse view will demonstrate a "yin-yang" appearance, with a red color on half of the mass and a blue color on the other half, demonstrating flow into and out of the mass. Upon further investigation with careful color control of gain and scale, a point will be noted in the artery wall as a defect, which allows blood flow extending beyond the arterial wall into the color-filled "neck" of the pseudoaneurysm. The neck may be short with flow going directly into the mass, or long and winding. The diameter of the disruption in the wall and the neck of the pseudoaneurysm are variable. However, the key feature of the neck is a to-and-fro Doppler flow pattern, usually with high velocities. Velocities in the pseudoaneurysm mass itself are typically much lower due to the larger diameter. Pseudoaneurysms may thrombose spontaneously, so a variable amount of thrombus may be present. The color scale may be decreased to obtain adequate color filling. Steering angles and planes of view may need to be varied to estimate the percentage of mass that is thrombosed.

A sonographer must be careful not to confuse a pseudoaneurysm with an enlarged lymph node or a tumor. A lymph node or tumor may also appear to be a mass with color flow within it, but the flow patterns in a lymph node or a branch feeding the node will have either a typical arterial waveform, not to-and-fro, or demonstrate a venous waveform pattern. A tumor will also be missing the pendulum flow pattern in the branches feeding it, which are characteristic of a true pseudoaneurysm.

TECHNICAL CONSIDERATIONS

A transverse overview of carotid artery from clavicle to mandible is performed first to identify a mass adjacent to the artery. Color is very helpful in identifying a pseudoaneurysm, especially if it is not completely filled with a thrombus. Document the PA in color demonstrating the red and blue color pattern associated with these structures. The largest diameter of the PA should be measured in both longitudinal and transverse views. Some laboratories choose to estimate the amount of thrombus in the PA (i.e., 30%, 50%, nearly completely thrombosed) as this will help the clinician to decide on a treatment. Many PAs thrombose spontaneously, and those with long necks that are nearly thrombosed are most likely to completely thrombose without intervention. B-mode images may document this estimate in multiple planes of view.

To identify the location of the source of the PA, color is used to follow the neck from the PA to the artery. In addition, there will be a color change along the wall of the native artery at the perforation (i.e., color aliasing) and possibly a color bruit. Spectral Doppler is used to identify the to-and-fro flow pattern associated with the neck of a true PA. If possible, try to measure the perforation in the artery wall using B-mode. This is not always possible and the measurement should be taken very carefully. It can be used as an estimate of the size of the wall injury. Lastly, demonstrate Doppler flow patterns pre-PA and post-PA in the native artery.

DIAGNOSIS

Pulsatile color flow in the mass with a yin-yang, red and blue appearance is the classic presentation of a PA. The most important characteristic to demonstrate for the diagnosis of PA is the to-and-fro Doppler flow pattern in the neck of the PA. As mentioned in the preceding section, a thrombus may or may not be noted in the mass and an estimate of the percentage of the thrombus may be helpful to the physician.

RADIATION-INDUCED ARTERIAL INJURY

Radiation-induced arterial injury (RIAI) is caused by the use of therapeutic irradiation during treatment for various tumors. The treatment with radiation preferentially injures cancer cells with less injury to other tissues. However, there is a potential effect on blood vessels due to the presence of endothelial cells, which are sensitive to the radiation. Capillaries, arterioles, and venules are primarily involved, but it may also affect the carotid arteries in some patients. Injury to the vasa vasorum in the medial layer of the artery causes fibrosis. This and the repopulation of the endothelium may result in a narrowing of the lumen. Other risk factors, such as hypercholesterolemia and hypertension, may add to the effect of the radiation, but not all patients develop these lesions.[11]

SIGNS AND SYMPTOMS

Patients will present with a history of radiation often several years prior to their examination. Often, these patients lack the typical risk factors for atherosclerosis. An atypical location of an atherosclerotic stenosis may tip the examiner to RIAI. In many patients, there is an absence of other atherosclerotic plaque in the carotids, which makes a single unusually located stenosis suspicious. TIA or CVA may be the effects of these lesions.

SONOGRAPHIC SCANNING TECHNIQUES

The distribution, extent of stenosis, and sonographic characteristics of radiation-induced disease are different from the commonly encountered atherosclerotic disease. The ultrasound examination must include thorough B-mode imaging of the common carotid arteries as there is a higher incidence of common carotid artery radiation-induced stenosis as compared to bifurcation and ICA disease. Transverse and longitudinal B-mode images should be taken to document the echogenicity of these lesions. As with all carotid examinations, spectral Doppler and color-flow imaging are used to assess the areas of stenosis.

Technical Considerations

A standard carotid duplex ultrasound examination is performed, although imaging may be difficult in some patients due to the changes in the tissue from the radiation. Poor echogenicity and hard, rather than supple neck tissue is common in postradiated patients. Any surgery that may have altered the

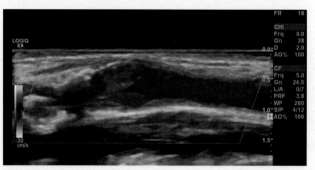

Figure 5-14 RIAI. This image depicts an occlusion of the ICA in a 51-year-old man following radiation. There is no color filling of the ICA, only filling of the CCA. Note the several hypoechoic areas within the lesion. (Image courtesy of Kathleen Hannon, RN, MS, RVT, RDMS, Massachusetts General Hospital, Vascular Laboratory.)

neck anatomy may also make the scan difficult, but rarely impossible, to obtain pertinent information. A careful history should be taken of the patient's past medical history in terms of any radiation treatment in the past, and the exact location of the treatment can alert the interpreting physician to this phenomenon.

DIAGNOSIS

An atypical location of the carotid lesion with a history of radiation treatment in the past makes RIAI suspicious of the cause of the lesion. Stenotic lesions, which are radiation-induced, are significantly longer than the nonradiation-induced lesions. The area of maximum stenosis in the radiation-induced lesions also tends to be located at the distal end of the stenotic area. The stenotic lesions do not typically contain calcifications and may have hypoechoic foci (Figs. 5-14 and 5-15).

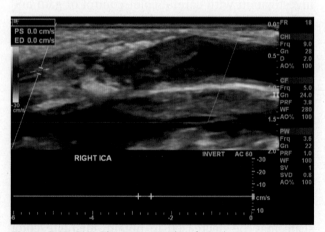

Figure 5-15 RIAI. This image is taken from the same patient as shown in Figure 5-14. Spectral Doppler confirms the occlusion in the ICA. (Image courtesy of Kathleen Hannon, RN, MS, RVT, RDMS, Massachusetts General Hospital, Vascular Laboratory.)

ARTERITIS

Arteritis is an inflammation of the artery wall that results in breakdown of parts of the wall structure and may conclude in occlusion and sometimes distal ischemia. In the vascular laboratory, two forms of arteritis may be seen in a carotid artery examination, Takayasu's disease, or temporal arteritis, a form of giant cell arteritis.

Takayasu's arteritis affects the aortic arch and great vessels, including the brachiocephalic, carotid, and subclavian arteries. Giant cell arteritis affects medium and larger sized arteries, so it may also affect the aortic arch and carotid arteries, but the vascular laboratory is usually asked to look specifically at the superficial temporal artery to assist in the diagnosis. There are no definitive ultrasound criteria for arteritis, and it is diagnosed through a series of blood tests and clinical presentations.

SIGNS AND SYMPTOMS

There is a wide variety of clinical presentations for arteritis and no known etiology. However, autoimmune deficiencies are thought to be the suspect in these diseases, and women outnumber men 2:1. Although both young and old can be afflicted with arteritis, young people generally present with Takayasu's disease, and temporal arteritis generally affects the elderly. In Takayasu's disease, there may be claudication of the arms with no radial pulses if the subclavian arteries are affected. TIA, visual changes, stroke, and multiple bruits may also be encountered.[12] Temporal arteritis is likely to cause headaches, low-grade fever, jaw claudication, tenderness in the temporal region, and visual problems, including blindness.

SONOGRAPHIC EXAMINATION TECHNIQUES

Takayasu's arteritis will generally be suspected in young people, especially young women. It may result in a vascular laboratory request for a carotid and renal examination because the obstruction of the arch and great vessels are most commonly seen in this order: subclavian, common carotid, aorta, and renal arteries. If lesions are seen in the carotid arteries, they are likely to appear as long, smooth, homogeneous narrowings in the artery, and appear to be more of a general wall thickening as opposed to typical atherosclerotic plaque within the lumen.

Giant cell arteritis may affect branches of the ECA including the facial, occipital, and internal maxillary, but the most accessible branch is the superficial temporal artery (STA). The STA can be scanned as it progresses up the temporal side of the head above the ear and across the forehead. If an echolucent or lightly echogenic "halo" surrounds the artery at any point, it is a positive sign of arteritis. The inflammation in this disease may be spotty, affecting segments of the artery and may include stenosis or occlusion. It is best to use the highest frequency transducer, such as a 12-MHz or 15-MHz transducer. The STA is best located anterior to the ear, and if normal in that area, a pulse can be palpated. The course of the artery should be followed transversely along the side of the head and across the forehead where there are branches. Look for the characteristic "halo" to identify areas of inflammation and avoid "spot checking" because the inflamed areas are intermittent and may be missed without a complete scan of the temporal artery. Look for areas of stenosis or occlusion, if possible with color. It is best to obtain a Doppler waveform if any areas of aliasing are found in color. Otherwise, a sample Doppler signal with a high-resistance waveform can be documented and is considered normal.

Technical Considerations

When performing an ultrasound on a patient with Takayasu's arteritis, pay special attention to obtain Doppler waveforms in the most proximal areas possible (i.e., the brachiocephalic artery on the right and as proximal as possible on the left). Be sure to obtain bilateral brachial pressures and subclavian artery waveforms to assess the involvement of the subclavian arteries in the disease and/or the proximal or distal aorta. Take multiple B-mode images in longitudinal and transverse views and closely examine these for any arterial thickening or stenoses, especially in the common carotid arteries.

With temporal arteritis, the entire course of the STA should be examined with transverse B-mode imaging. This approach is used to identify any areas with a halo or document no evidence of a halo with at least three representative images in transverse view. Use color-flow imaging to get an overview representation of flow within the temporal artery. Obtain a Doppler sample of a normal segment and any areas suspected of stenosis or occlusion.

DIAGNOSIS

Although there is no definitive test for these inflammatory diseases, duplex ultrasound can assist with information used to affirm the diagnosis. Takayasu's patients will typically have an unusual appearance of thickened artery walls with some patients demonstrating long, narrowed stenoses of the common carotid arteries. Often, the disease appears to be concentric and evenly distributed when imaged in transverse view. This is in contrast to atherosclerotic disease, which is often eccentric and irregular. These patients will have abnormalities primarily related to the proximal common carotid arteries and subclavian arteries, sometimes with abnormal waveforms indicating proximal disease in the aorta or the origins of the great vessels. If the aortic arch is affected proximally, bilateral changes in the common carotid waveforms will be noted, such as slow upstroke and lower than typical velocities bilaterally. If the aorta is stenosed in the area between the brachiocephalic and the left common carotid, the left CCA and left subclavian artery waveforms may be turbulent, dampened, and display lower velocities than the right CCA and subclavian arteries.

An echolucent halo around the temporal artery is a strong indicator of temporal arteritis. Recent studies on the diagnostic value of the halo report sensitivity of 75% to 86% and specificity of 83% to 92% in patients with temporal arteritis.[13,14] Again, intermittent areas of focal velocity increases will be observed.

PATHOLOGY BOX 5-1

Uncommon Carotid System Pathology

Pathology	B-Mode	Color	Doppler
Dissection or intimal flap	White line within lumen; may be moving. Seen in transverse and longitudinal views. An occluded or thrombosed segment may cause smooth and tapered stenosis.	May be two colors on each side, aliasing if high velocities present.	Two clearly different flow patterns on each side of white line. May be occluded, high resistance, or reversed flow direction in one lumen.
Aneurysm	Section of artery at least 200% of normal ICA or 150% of normal CCA by some authors. Very rare.	Widened area of artery with flow separation and/or partial thrombosis.	Low velocities due to large diameter.
Pseudoaneurysm	Mass adjacent to artery postpenetrating or iatrogenic injury. May have various levels of thrombosis or no evidence of thrombosis.	Color within mass has yin-yang (red/blue) pattern of color flow.	Distinct to-and-fro flow pattern in neck of pseudoaneurysm.
Fibromuscular dysplasia (FMD)	Difficult to see "string of beads" widening and narrowing in distal ICA.	Velocity and/or power color may demonstrate "string of beads."	Doppler waveforms typically show a sudden change from normal bulb and mid-ICA to markedly turbulent flow pattern with high velocities in distal ICA.
Temporal arteritis	Echolucent "halo" around sections of STA.	Color may show aliasing if stenoses occur.	Doppler pattern demonstrates high velocities if stenosis is present but not likely.
Carotid body tumors (CBTs)	Mass between ICA and ECA splays arteries apart.	Color demonstrates highly vascular mass. ECA feeds mass.	Doppler demonstrates low resistant waveforms within mass.
Tortuosity	Difficult to follow tortuous vessels with B-mode alone.	Color highly useful to follow tortuous vessels. Color aliasing seen frequently due to sharp angulation (closer to zero degrees) and/or higher velocities past curve. Flow separation inside curve.	Velocities naturally increase as blood flows around a curve. Center of angle cursor (angle correct) set parallel to walls for velocity measurements. Edges of angle cursor may be off-parallel as long as center is parallel to walls.

SUMMARY

Sonographers expect to observe atherosclerotic plaque during carotid ultrasound examinations. There are several other well-characterized diseases that may present within the extracranial portion of the carotid vessels. Understanding the various pathologies and the associated ultrasound findings will aid in the proper diagnosis of these less commonly encountered carotid abnormalities.

Critical Thinking Questions

1. While examining a tortuous internal carotid artery, you observe an area of color aliasing. What can you can do in order to determine if there is a stenosis?

2. When obtaining a Doppler waveform from the false lumen of a dissection, what direction would you expect the flow to be going?

3. A patient presents with a pulsatile neck mass. What would be helpful to differentiate the mass?

REFERENCES

1. Lin PH, Lumsden AB. Carotid kinks and coils. In Ernst CB, Stanley JC, ed. *Current Therapy in Vascular Surgery.* 4th ed. St. Louis, MO: Mosby; 2001:114–117.
2. Polak JF, Dobkin GR, O'Leary DH, et al. Internal carotid artery stenosis: Accuracy and reproducibility of color Doppler-assisted duplex imaging. *Radiology* 1989;173:793-798.
3. Treiman RL, Treiman GS. Carotid artery dissection. In: Ernst CB, Stanley JC, ed. *Current Therapy in Vascular Surgery.* 4th ed. St. Louis, MO: Mosby; 2001:108–111.
4. Zweibel WJ, Pellerito JS. Carotid occlusion, uncommon carotid pathology and tricky carotid cases. In: Zweibel WJ, Pellerito JS, ed. *Introduction to Vascular Ultrasonography.* 5th ed. Philadelphia, PA: Elsevier; 2005:191–210.
5. Morasch R, Pearce WH. Extracranial cerebrovascular disease. In: Fahey VA, ed. *Vascular Nursing.* 4th ed. Philadelphia, PA: Elsevier; 2004:290–291.
6. Daigle R. Carotid color duplex imaging. In: Daigle RJ, ed. *Techniques in Noninvasive Vascular Diagnosis.* 2nd ed. Littleton, CO: Summer Publishing; 2002:23–48.
7. Kulbaski MJ, Smith RB. Surgical treatment of fibromuscular dysplasia of the carotid artery. In: Ernst CB, Stanley JC, ed. *Current Therapy in Vascular Surgery.* 4th ed. St. Louis, MO: Mosby; 2001:112–114.
8. Hallett JW. Carotid body tumors. In: Ernst CB, Stanley JC, ed. *Current Therapy in Vascular Surgery.* 4th ed. St. Louis, MO: Mosby; 2001:118–122.
9. Bekker D, Hannon K, Jaff MR, et al. Carotid artery mycotic aneurysm identified by duplex imaging. *J Vasc Ultrasound.* 2010;34(2):80–81.
10. Stanley JC. Extracranial carotid artery aneurysms. In: Ernst CB, Stanley JC, ed. *Current Therapy in Vascular Surgery.* 4th ed. St. Louis, MO: Mosby; 2001:104–107.
11. Modrall JG, Rosen SF, McIntyre KE. Radiation-induced arterial injury. In: Ernst CB, Stanley JC, ed. *Current Therapy in Vascular Surgery.* 4th ed. St. Louis, MO: Mosby; 2001:131–134
12. Webb TH, Perler BA. Takayasu arteritis. In: Ernst CB, Stanley JC, ed. *Current Therapy in Vascular Surgery.* 4th ed. St. Louis, MO: Mosby; 2001:122–127.
13. LeSar CJ, Meier GH, DeMasi RJ, et al. The utility of color duplex ultrasonography in the diagnosis of temporal arteritis. *J Vasc Surg.* 2002;36(6):1154–1160.
14. Ball EL, Walsh SR, Yang TY, et al. Role of ultrasonography in the diagnosis of temporal arteritis. *Brit J Surg.* 2010;97(12):1765–1771.

6 Ultrasound Following Surgery and Intervention

Clifford T. Araki, Cynthia Cannon, Gwendolyn Carmel, Jesenia Pineda, and Zafar Jamil

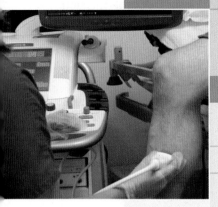

OBJECTIVES

Describe the ultrasound protocols unique for carotid scanning in postendarterectomy and poststent patients

Define normal and abnormal criteria associated with carotid stents

List the pathology encountered in a postoperative or postinterventional carotid ultrasound

KEY TERMS

carotid artery stenting | carotid endarterectomy | eversion carotid endarterectomy | restenosis | supra-aortic endovascular treatment

GLOSSARY

arteriotomy a surgical incision through the wall of an artery into the lumen

carotid artery stenting a catheter-based procedure in which a metal mesh tube is deployed into an artery to keep it open following balloon angioplasty to dilate a stenosis

carotid endarterectomy a surgical procedure during which the carotid artery is opened and

plaque is removed in order to restore normal luminal diameter

in-stent restenosis a narrowing of the lumen of a stent, which causes a stenosis

polytetrafluoroethylene (PTFE) a synthetic graft material used to create grafts and blood vessel patches; a common brand name is Gore-Tex

The concept of a vascular laboratory has, since its inception, revolved around the care of patients who may be candidates for surgery or who have had surgery. The duplex ultrasound evaluation that is conducted on patients who have had a carotid endarterectomy (CEA) should be performed by someone who knows the complications of surgery. Now with carotid artery stenting (CAS) becoming mainstream, vascular sonographers must be cognizant of the issues associated with both surgical and endovascular interventions. Differences exist in the procedure and complications that impact the interpretation of duplex testing whether it is performed in preprocedure planning, in the immediate postprocedure period, or in long-term follow-up.

This chapter is intended for the vascular sonographer but also presents issues that are important to the vascular surgeon or interventionalist. The clinician's concerns are different for CEA and CAS. It is important for sonographers to recognize that the duplex data collected post-CAS will not be interpreted

in the same fashion as for CEA and that the documentation will be different. It is also important to recognize that although CEA procedures are relatively stable, CAS is in the midst of its technological refinement. Developments could further impact how the sonographer will perform the duplex examination for either type of patient follow-up.

CAROTID ENDARTERECTOMY

To evaluate the CEA patient either within the first 30 days or in a long-term follow-up, the sonographer needs to be familiar with the operation and the complications that can arise during and after the procedure. Most surgical procedures have been standard over the years but new modifications are relevant to the practicing vascular sonographer.

The traditional CEA is an open operation that is performed through an arteriotomy made longitudinally from the normalized internal carotid artery (ICA), through the bulb, and into the common carotid artery (CCA). The external carotid artery (ECA) is not normally involved with significant disease, and therefore is typically not part of the procedure. Exposure is made sufficient to allow for the complete removal of the atheromatous material, which may extend from the distal CCA into the distal taper of the proximal ICA. Once the plaque is removed, the arteriotomy may be closed primarily by suturing together the cut edges of the arterial wall. In smaller diameter vessels, primary closure may narrow the lumen to the point of stenosis, particularly if the sutures are made deep to the incision.

Problems of stenosis associated with the CEA are more common at the distal border of the arteriotomy, where the ICA normalizes. At that point, common potential problems that may lead to a stenosis include (1) narrowing as a result of closure; (2) plaque retained from an incomplete excision; and (3) a neointimal hyperplastic response to the operation, which occurs within subsequent months of follow-up. Of the three, only the latter can truly be characterized as a restenosis. Other forms of stenosis are caused by technical errors of the operation.

Because stenotic narrowing can result from closing the arteriotomy primarily, surgeons will often reduce the potential for stenosis by suturing in a patch to widen the lumen. The patch also reduces the potential intrusion a hyperplastic response that may develop a restenosis.[1]

SURGICAL PATCHES

The sonographer evaluating patients in follow-up to a CEA should expect to see patients with patches, particularly in female patients, whose arteries tend to be narrower than that of males. Patches for CEA may be either an autogenous vein or synthetic. The latter are constructed of either Dacron or polytetrafluoroethylene (PTFE). Veins used for the patch may be a cervical vein that is exposed and harvested from the incision site or a segment that is taken from the great saphenous vein at the ankle. Veins are often everted to create a patch with double wall thickness that will be stronger than the vein that is incised and flattened for a single wall patch. The vein is everted to allow the vein intima to face the lumen of the artery.[1]

EVERSION VERSUS TRADITIONAL CEA

In recent years, vascular surgeons are performing the operation using a technique called eversion CEA. The procedure, popular in Europe but less common in the United States, is receiving attention. Instead of using a long axis arteriotomy and patch, eversion CEA is performed with a complete transection of the

ICA at the bifurcation or of both the ICA and the ECA. An endarterectomy is performed by everting the cut ends of the arteries away from the incision and peeling the arterial wall away from the plaque as it is everted. The ends of the arteries are reverted to their normal position for subsequent reattachment. The procedure does not require a patch because the sutures are placed on the widened bulb of the ICA.[2]

To the vascular sonographer, the eversion CEA will be less obvious in its presentation than the traditional CEA with patch. It will appear more like the traditional revascularization that was closed primarily (without a patch). Sutures, if visible, will surround the ICA circumferentially. In the standard CEA, the suture line will have an orientation along the long axis of the ICA, on its superficial wall. The eversion technique has the advantage of not requiring a patch because the full diameter of the distal taper of the ICA is retained and possibly enlarged in the process of feathering the plaque beyond the bulb. The sonographer should expect to see less restenosis in the eversion CEA than in the CEA with a primary closure, but eversion appears to have equivalent restenosis to the traditional CEA with a patch.[2]

SONOGRAPHIC EXAMINATION TECHNIQUES

Most follow-up evaluations arise as scheduled outpatient appointments. Emergent testing is infrequently requested in an immediate postoperative patient.

Patient Preparation

The CEA evaluation may be particularly difficult in the immediate postoperative period. Sutures, staples, and dressings all compromise access for the sonographer. Sterile techniques including sterile imaging pads, gel, transducer covers, or bio-occlusive dressings should be used to minimize the risk of infection when scanning a patient in the first 48 hours following surgery. Once the skin has healed, there is little impedance to the ultrasound examination. No specific preparation is typically required other than to remove jewelry or clothing that may limit access to the neck.

In the long term, patients with CEA should be followed with duplex ultrasound testing. For any follow-up protocol, it is important that the first duplex exam be performed within 1 month of the CEA. This serves as the baseline study that will provide the velocity data to which all subsequent follow-ups should be compared.

Patient Positioning

The patient should be positioned supine with a small pillow placed under the head and shoulders. The patient's chin should be tilted up and the head turned away from the side being examined. Occasionally, if the patient cannot lie supine, the examination can be performed with the patient in a sitting position. Conducting an examination with the patient sitting upright is not ideal because, in this position, the patient often does not remain still and it adds strain to the sonographer.

Scanning Techniques

A standard carotid duplex ultrasound examination is performed for the CEA patient. The CCA, ICA, and ECA are examined using B-mode and color-flow imaging techniques. Spectral Doppler is taken throughout the vessels at the typical levels specified in Chapter 4. There are particular areas to be closely examined, and these are described in the following section.

Technical Considerations

Primary concerns for the evaluation of the CEA patient include stenosis from residual plaque or intimal flap, suture narrowing, or thrombotic narrowing/occlusion. The ultrasound findings along the endarterectomy site as well as at the ends of the endarterectomy site must be carefully examined for any of these primary concerns. In the immediate postoperative period, the information obtainable may be restricted to knowing whether there is flow in the distal cervical ICA. The quality of flow then also becomes important to determine whether poststenotic turbulence exists.

The sonographer will, in all likelihood, not have any information on how the CEA was performed. It would be best to assume that a traditional CEA was performed and a patch was used. If a patch is identified, it should be determined whether the patch is synthetic or autogenous. A synthetic patch may appear to have a woven appearance to the walls (in the case of a Dacron patch) or demonstrate two brightly echogenic lines (in the case of a PTFE, which is double layered). Vein patches will more closely resemble the native vessel.

Any patient with neck swelling on the side of a CEA should be evaluated for the possibility of hematoma, infection, or pseudoaneurysm. All are associated with a synthetic patch. A vein patch may be associated with patch rupture. The objectives for a duplex evaluation should be to identify the presence of a fluid collection or encapsulated mass in the soft tissue that surrounds the patch, remembering that the patch and swelling associated with the CEA will typically lie superficial to the endarterectomy. An encapsulated mass is associated with a hematoma or pseudoaneurysm but may also suggest the presence of inflammatory tissue associated with infection. The appearance of a perivascular fluid collection above an irregular buckling of the Dacron patch has also been described as an indication of a pending or active infection (Fig. 6-1).[3]

An extravascular leak or pseudoaneurysm is not common but, if detected in a synthetic patch, its most likely source is a suture disruption. Extravasation in a vein patch is associated with a rupture of the patch. A hematoma can also occur as synthetic patches can have problems with suture hole bleeding that tends not to be seen in vein patches. Fibrin sealants or hemostatic agents are used to reduce bleeding but may lead to hematomas if ineffective. A hematoma may also be the result of blood extravasated from surrounding tissue. Early infection may present as a wound complication and hematoma. Late infection may be evident as neck swelling. According to Knight and Tait,[3] most cases of synthetic patch infections are painless, with no local or systemic signs of infection. Infection is typically not associated with vein patches and is rare with synthetic patches with at an occurrence rate of 0.18% in the latter.[1] Given

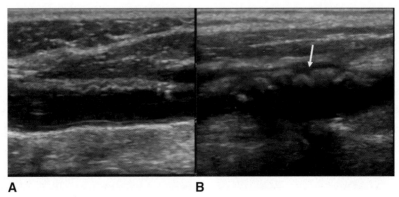

A   **B**

Figure 6-1 Endarterectomy Dacron patch. **A:** Normal Dacron patch along the superficial wall of endarterectomy site. **B:** Abnormal Dacron patch with buckling of the patch and hypoechoic mass *(arrow)* suggestive of extraluminal fluid collection providing evidence of infection.

this, sonographers may not consider this a problem of concern. Still, a duplex evaluation is often the first diagnostic step and the sonographer must know of these abnormalities in order to perform an adequate assessment when evaluating a swollen neck.

Pitfalls

In the early postoperative period within the first few days after surgery, ultrasound visualization should be expected to be complicated by air entrapped in the matrix of a synthetic patch or introduced in the hemostatic agents applied prior to closure or by wound hematomas. Because entrapped air often obliterates the ultrasound image directly above the CEA site, the sonographer is often required to visualize the carotid bifurcation from the most posterior approach possible.

By the time of a first postoperative follow-up, the image is no longer compromised by entrapped air. Wound hematomas should have been substantially reduced. Nonreduction and tenderness should be considered particularly problematic in the presence of a swollen neck.

DIAGNOSIS

Intravascular problems associated with the CEA may include both stenotic or nonstenotic pathology. One type of nonstenotic issue associated with the CEA includes an oversized or irregular patch that gives the vessel an aneurysmal appearance. Diameters are important measurements in these cases. It should be remembered that a patch identified as synthetic is more thrombogenic than an autogenous patch. Slower flows in an aneurysmal patch are more likely to laminate thrombus in a synthetic patch. Evaluating an oversized patch for mural thrombi can be significant to the patient. Another nonstenotic problem is loosely mobilized material may be detected within the lumen at the site of CEA. The material may be an intimal flap or loose strands of suture material. The intimal flap is of considerable concern to the surgeon. Either may embolize material, but the intimal flap has the greater potential for occlusion. Intimal flaps will appear on the B-mode image as a small disruption along the wall with a short piece of material (the intimal and some additional wall material) protruding into the vessel lumen. Intimal flaps will produce disturbed color flow patterns and, depending on the extent, cause elevated velocities (Fig. 6-2).

Stenotic problems can be differentiated as technical problems of surgery or restenosis. Stenoses identified within the first postoperative month should be considered technical problems of surgery. They could be the result of narrowing in primary closure or of remnant plaque that was not properly resected during the procedure. The latter is often called a "shelf lesion." The cut edge of the plaque is left, which creates an abrupt, stepped edge in the arterial wall. A shelf lesion may be located at the proximal or distal edges of the CEA. It is more commonly associated with the distal edge, particularly when a "high bifurcation" limits surgical access and prevents an adequate feathering or tapering of the plaque. On a B-mode image, the edge of the residual plaque will be easy to visualize adjacent to the endarterectomized segment of the vessel wall. A stenosis may also be caused by a nonocclusive thrombus adherent to the wall that developed from the manipulations of surgery. This thrombus can be associated with the

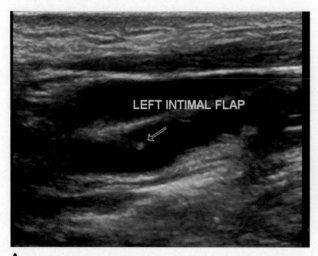

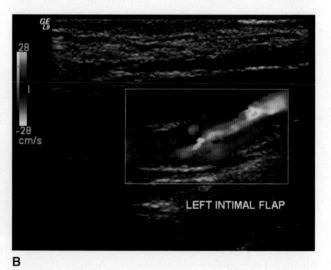

A

B

Figure 6-2 Post-CEA carotid intimal flap. **A:** Grayscale image with defect (*at arrow*) projecting into lumen along the anterior wall of the ICA. **B:** Color flow imaging noting turbulence along the area of the flap.

CEA site and patch.[4] Lastly, although the post-CEA exam is targeted at the operative site, there is still the possibility of missed lesions in the proximal CCA or the innominate artery (on the right) that had been overlooked in the presurgical workup.

Restenosis

Although a stenosis seen 1 month postsurgery is typically associated with surgery in the form of retained plaque or thrombus, narrowing in the first 24 months after a CEA is considered a result of neointimal hyperplasia. The hyperplastic lesion is considered relatively benign with the low thromboembolic potential of a fibrotic plaque. After 2 years, a stenosis is considered atherosclerotic and potentially more problematic, with risks approaching that of the asymptomatic lesion. Restenosis rates vary widely in the literature, but Rosenborough and Perler estimate the incidence of restenosis as 6% to 14% after a CEA.[5]

When evaluating the patient in follow-up, some laboratories may adjust velocity criteria post-CEA. Most will use the preprocedural velocity criteria established by the lab to identify the presence of a stenosis. Sonographers may question the need for postoperative surveillance if the restenosis rate is relatively low and the lesion is relatively benign. In some respects, it matches the surveillance of the asymptomatic lesion. Unlike the primary asymptomatic lesion, however, the hyperplastic response to surgery has the potential to become virulent with a rapid progression to occlusion. The primary aims of the surgeon are to identify the restenosis early and, when the disease is found to progress in follow-up, to intervene before it reaches occlusion. Follow-up is also important for the contralateral bifurcation. Atherogenesis has a degree of symmetry. Patients treated for disease in one carotid bifurcation are at risk of aggressive disease in the contralateral bifurcation. Postoperative surveillance should always be performed bilaterally (Pathology Box 6-1).

CAROTID ARTERY STENTING

In 2005, carotid artery stenting (CAS) accounted for only 9.6% of patients treated for extracranial cerebrovascular disease.[6] Held back by concerns of high complication rates and low reimbursements, CAS has not benefitted from wide use. Complication rates for CAS continue to decrease with the increased use of cerebral protective devices and retrograde flow flushing of the ICA during stenting.

The rapid evolution of CAS since 2005 can be demonstrated in three publications. In 2008, the Society for Vascular Surgery (SVS) published guidelines for

PATHOLOGY BOX 6-1

Common Pathology Associated with CEA

Pathology	Ultrasound Characteristics
Residual plaque	Plaque observed at end of CEA site, may have abrupt stepped edge (shelf lesion); color and spectral Doppler may display turbulence or elevated PSV depending on severity
Intimal flap	Disruption along vessel wall with moving material observed within lumen; disturbed color flow patterns and elevated PSV often present
Occlusion	No color filling, no lumen detected, no spectral Doppler signal
Infected patch	Irregular buckling of patch material along vessel wall; perivascular fluid accumulation
Hematoma	Nonvascular mass adjacent to vessel; may appear cystic or contain various levels of echogenicity
Pseudoaneurysm	Dilated area attached to vessel with flow demonstrated on color and spectral Doppler; to-and-fro pattern flow may be detected in connection between dilated sac and native vessel; color swirling (yin-yang appearance) present within dilated sac
Restenosis	Focal area of elevated velocities with poststenotic turbulence; homogeneous material present along the wall in cases of restenosis due to hyperplasia

CEA, carotid endarterectomy; PSV, peak systolic velocity.

the management of carotid stenosis.[7] It was recommended that CEA be used for the moderate-to-severe symptomatic carotid stenoses and asymptomatic lesions. CAS was only recommended for symptomatic patients with high perioperative risk and not for asymptomatic stenoses.

In 2010, the Carotid Revascularization Endarterectomy vs. Stenting Trial (CREST) reported its long awaited results.[8] Although preliminary results demonstrated that CAS patients suffered more strokes than CEA patients in the 30 days postprocedure, this finding was balanced by the number of heart attacks in the CEA group. Within the immediate postoperative period, there was no statistical difference between CAS and CEA in heart attacks and strokes. This equivalence was found to continue over the trial's median follow-up of 2.5 years. Also significant was the study's finding that the outcomes were similar between CAS and CEA in asymptomatic patients.

Participating interventionalists in CREST were well vetted and the devices used for CAS were well controlled. In early 2010, an interim report from the International Carotid Stenting Study (ICSS) group was released at the same time as CREST. The European ICSS trial compared CAS with CEA in symptomatic patients and demonstrated that CAS resulted in a greater statistical risk of stroke, myocardial infarction, or death than CEA (8.5% vs. 5.2%). ICSS investigators recommended CEA as the treatment of choice over CAS.

This result may be interpreted to suggest that, in actual practice, CAS may have a more mixed outcome.[9] Major differences between ICSS and CREST were the lesser experience required of ICSS interventionalists performing CAS and in the ICSS use of all devices approved. When CREST placed stricter limits on interventionalists and devices, results improved. General CAS use in the United States is not as restrictive, and the results could be better reflected in the ICSS trial than in CREST and may result in an increased risk of stroke.

Still, the demonstration of equivalence between CEA and CAS in rigorously controlled applications speaks to increased use. Should reimbursement for CAS relax, the vascular laboratory will see greater numbers of patients treated with CAS, and sonographers must be prepared for duplex-related issues associated with CAS.

Pre- and postprocedure ultrasound testing for CAS is performed as it relates to technical issues associated with the CAS procedure and the stent that is implanted "for life." There are aspects of the procedure that are important for the sonographer and should be described. These not only relate to the carotid bifurcation but also to the path that the catheter follows toward the stenosis. The latter is important because the vascular sonographer may be involved in defining the status of that path before or after CAS is performed.

STENTING TECHNIQUES

Catheter manipulations for CAS are typically performed after accessing the common femoral artery at the groin. Postprocedural complications are not limited to the carotid bifurcation but may include dissection, thrombosis, or perforations within the path where devices encounter difficulty.

Once at the carotid bifurcation, the guide wire must be passed across the lesion. The guide wire will usually first be used to position an embolic protection device (EPD), then to position the balloon, and stent catheters that are used subsequently. All catheters must gain access to the ICA segment that lies distal to the stenosis. After the EPD is placed, a balloon catheter is typically used to predilate the lesion. Following this, a stent catheter is then positioned over the lesion and deployment starts from beyond the distal border of the stenosis. The stent is unsheathed by retracting the stent catheter over the lesion. This deploys a self-expanding stent that should cover the entire lesion from its distal through proximal borders. A second balloon catheter is usually positioned and inflated to ensure full expansion of the stent. For full coverage, a stent length should be selected that will extend 5 mm beyond the lesion proximally and distally once it is deployed. The stent may extend from the CCA into the bulb, and coverage of the ECA is not considered a contraindication for the procedure.

SONOGRAPHIC EXAMINATION TECHNIQUES

Sonographic evaluation of the post-CAS patient should be approached using the same basic patient positions and techniques as the routine scanning of native carotid arteries. In the normal mid-cervical level bifurcation, the stent should be fully visible by ultrasound. Its proximal and distal borders should be easily identifiable.

There are important additional images required for complete documentation of a stented vessel. B-mode image, color, and spectral Doppler waveforms should be recorded proximal to the stent, at the proximal attachment site, within the midportion of the stent, at the distal attachment site, and distal to the stent. Because stent border stenosis is most common, documentation of the highest velocities in these locations (Fig. 6-3) can be particularly useful in serial comparisons. Sonographers should evaluate stents by color or power Doppler for narrowing (Fig. 6-4). Any evidence of diffuse narrowing within a stent even without velocity changes should be flagged for increased vigilance. Some laboratories choose to use color or power Doppler to aid in the measurement of the minimum stent and flow channel diameters to assist in the categorization of any disease. Any diameter measurement made from the ultrasound image should be used with caution as diagnostic accuracy of these is limited and highly dependent on technique. The B-mode image along the entire stent as well as proximal and distal stent attachment sites must be carefully examined for hyperplastic growth across the stent itself or for progression of the disease at the attachment sites. In addition, the B-mode image should be examined for any evidence of stent compression, incomplete deployment, or other deformation.

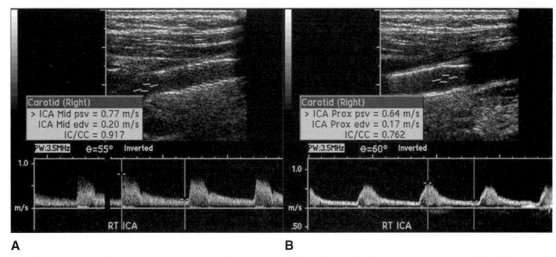

Figure 6-3 Carotid stent velocities representative of proximal and distal stent borders. Documentation should represent highest velocities detected within these segments—near distal **(A)** and proximal **(B)** borders of the stent.

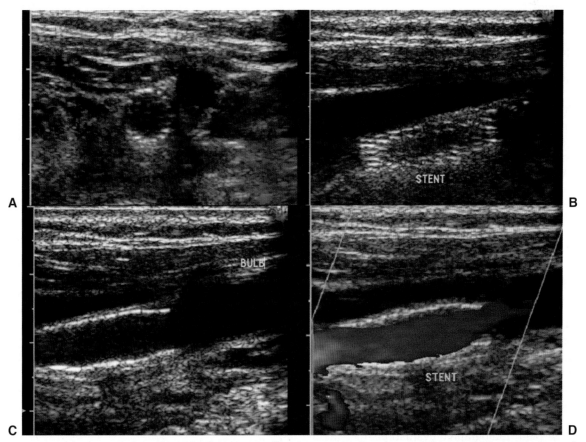

Figure 6-4 Carotid stent with B-mode and color imaging illustrating minimal evidence of disease. **A:** Transverse view of stent. **B:** Longitudinal view of stent slightly offset to demonstrate stent walls. **C:** Longitudinal view of stent at proximal attachment site. **D:** Longitudinal view of stent with color flow imaging. Color does not completely fill the lumen along the superficial wall of the stent. This image serves as evidence of a mild Type III lesion.

Pitfalls

Dense calcification that produced shadows in the preprocedural scan will be present in the follow-up evaluation and will compromise the B-mode image and Doppler interrogation of the stented vessel. Multiple views should be used to avoid areas of acoustic shadowing. In some vessels, this is not possible; therefore, signals distal to the calcific areas will be important in determining the presence of disease. Turbulence distal to these areas likely indicates that a stenosis is present.

Dense circumferential calcification is problematic during the stent placement as well. It restricts balloon expansion of the lesion during stenting, which in turn increases procedural manipulation and adds the risk of an inadequate expansion. Both are reasons for sonographers to pay particular attention to velocity changes with the area of calcification. Added manipulation may increase the hyperplastic response, and inadequate expansion may lead to residual stenosis.

DIAGNOSIS

The normal ultrasound appearance of a carotid stent should reveal the walls of the stent apposed to the walls of the vessel. These walls should be relatively uniform and color filling should be observed out to the edges of the stent. The velocity spectra through the stent should not demonstrate any focal increases. The CAS patient can present with some unique pathology. For the vascular sonographer, the forms of concern include stent fracture, stent migration, thrombus formation, dissection, intimal flap, intimal hyperplasia, and in-stent restenosis (Pathology Box 6-2).

Stent Fracture and Migration

To date, migration and fracture have not been seen as significant problems. Stent fractures are generally considered rare (1.9% in 78 patients).[10,11] Still, biomechanical forces associated with head tilting, neck rotations, and swallowing have been found to distort stents in carotid bifurcation. Temporary lengthening, twisting, and crushing deformations were demonstrated in cinefluoroscopy.[12] Long-term effects were evident in plain radiographic evaluations of patients followed for an average of 18 months. Stent fractures, most of which were benign, were found in 29% of 48 stents.[13] Only 3 of 14 stent fractures were associated with flow velocity changes. Fractures were strongly associated with calcification and it was suggested that torsional motions of a stent that repeatedly rubbed against a hard, calcified surface during rotations of the neck may have been at fault. Compromises to the

PATHOLOGY BOX 6-2

Common Pathology Associated with CAS

Pathology	Ultrasound Characteristics
Restenosis	Focal area of elevated velocities with poststenotic turbulence; homogeneous material present along the stent wall
Stent fracture	Irregular border of stent with abrupt edge apparent; color and spectral Doppler turbulence noted
Stent deformation	Border of stent appears to protrude into vessel lumen; color flow channel is reduced; elevated PSV may be present depending on degree of deformation
Thrombus	Homogeneous, smooth bordered material present within stent or native vessel; reduced color flow lumen; elevated PSV
Dissection	White line seen within vessel lumen using multiple views, may be seen moving; disturbed color flow and spectral Doppler will be present on both sides of dissection
Occlusion	No color filling, no lumen detected, no spectral Doppler signal

PSV, peak systolic velocity; CAS, carotid artery stenting.

architectural integrity of the stent should be considered as time dependent. Sonographers may need to be alert to the possibility that biomechanical distortion with repeated neck flexion could create a fracture and stimulate a late hyperplastic response. The natural history of a stent is still unknown and the wearing of the device over the long term may lead to late occurrences. In the case of a stent deformation, the border of the stent may appear to protrude into the vessel lumen (Fig. 6-5). A stent fracture will produce an abrupt edge within the stented portion with associated changes in the color flow signals.

In-Stent Restenosis

When evaluating a patient in follow-up to CAS, restenosis will be the greatest concern to the sonographer. Restenosis rates following CAS, reported in the literature and tabulated by Sullivan, were highly variable among investigators and ranged from 2% to 75%.[14] A number of studies indicate that restenosis following CAS (at 20% to 25%) is higher than

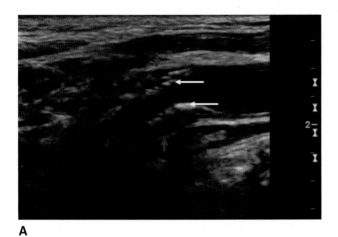
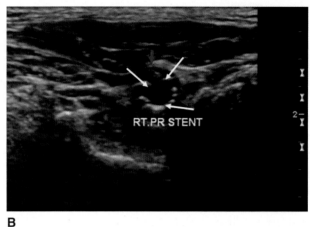

A   **B**

Figure 6-5 B-mode images of a deformed stent. Stent walls *(white arrows)* are not apposed to vessel walls *(red arrows)*. Extensive plaque is observed between vessels walls and stent. **A:** Longitudinal view. **B:** Transverse view.

following CEA. As with CEA, restenosis is considered to be a low-risk neointimal hyperplastic lesion with an occurrence within the first 2 years of stenting. A difference in the hyperplastic response may, however, lie in the type of insult. Hyperplasia with CEA is considered an early occurrence in response to a single insult. De Borst et al. suggests that the hyperplasia following CAS may be an ongoing response to the presence of an implanted foreign object.[15] Given these findings, follow-up surveillance may appear more significant for CAS than for CEA.

Lal et al. characterized the in-stent restenosis (ISR) in five sonographic distribution patterns (Table 6-1).[16] All ISRs are described as intimal hyperplasia with its typical homogeneously hypoechoic appearance. The most common form of ISR (Type I) developed at the stent border and comprised 40% of the restenosis that were identified by B-mode and color/power Doppler. The most severe was occlusion (Type V), which was rare at 1.2%. The second most severe form of ISR, Type IV, was diffuse proliferative narrowing of the stent lumen. Type IV lesions were found in 20% of ISRs and was most predictive of the

need for reintervention. On an interesting note, Lal et al. found that Type IV ISR tend to be associated with diabetes and concurred with other investigators that diabetes is a predictor of aggressive intimal hyperplasia.[16]

Changes in Velocity Criteria

Although increased ISR rates were reported with stents over CEA, other concurrent studies have documented that flow velocity elevations occur in post-CAS patients without the presence of stenosis. It was considered that the stent may impose a rigid matrix that reduces arterial compliance and decreases the elastic expansion of the stented segment. The result may be an elevation in velocities within the stent that could be misinterpreted as a restenosis.

Flow velocity elevations have lead investigators to propose a number of new velocity criteria to use when evaluating the post-CAS patient.[17–24] Table 6-2 compares the proposed criteria. All elevate the velocity thresholds for the moderate and high-grade stenosis.

TABLE 6-1		
Classification of In-stent Restenosis (ISR)[16]		
Class	**Type**	**Description**
Type I	Focal end-stent ISR	Hyperplastic stenosis associated with one or both stent borders; lesions are ≤10 mm in length
Type II	Focal intrastent ISR	Central hyperplastic stenosis or incomplete stent expansion (mid-stent wasting); lesions are ≤10 mm in length
Type III	Diffuse intrastent ISR	Hyperplastic accumulation throughout the stent; lesions are >10 mm long
Type IV	Diffuse proliferative	Hyperplasia that diffusely narrows the stent toward occlusion and extends beyond the margins of the stent; lesions are >10 mm long
Type V	Occlusion	No flow or lumen is identified

TABLE	6-2

Post-CAS Duplex Ultrasound Criteria

STENOSIS THRESHOLD	ABURAHMA[17]		SETACCI[18]			CHI[23]		CHAHWAN[22]		LAL[20]		ZHOU[19]			ARMSTRONG[24]	
	PSV	EDV	PSV	EDV	I/C	PSV	I/C	PSV	EDV	PSV	I/C	PSV	EDV	I/C	PSV	EDV
20%								137	20	150	2.15					
30%	154	42	105													
50%	224	88	175			240	2.45	195	62	220	2.7					
70%			300	140	3.8	450	4.3					300	90	4.0		
75%															300	125
80%	325	119						300	96	340	4.15					

PSV, peak systolic velocity; EDV, end-diastolic velocity; I/C, ICA/CCA PSV ratio.

In Table 6-2, the primary discriminator for a significant stenosis is the peak systolic velocity (PSV). End-diastolic velocity (EDV) did not appear as discriminating,[20,23] with the exception of one study.[24] The ICA/CCA PSV ratio, although reported, did not appear to substantially add to the determination of restenosis.

The PSV threshold for the 50% stenosis varied from 175 to 240 cm/s among criteria, suggesting it may not be a good discriminator for moderate stenosis. It was noted in the literature and verified by this range of velocities that velocity was not uniformly elevated among all patients. This suggests that PSV may not provide a reliable estimate for moderate stenosis.

High-grade stenosis was defined differently among investigators as a diameter reduction of 70%, 75%, or 80% but its PSV threshold was relatively consistent at 300 to 340 cm/s, with one outlier at 450 cm/s.[24] The EDV threshold for high-grade stenosis varied slightly more at 96 to 140 cm/s and, when used, the ICA/CCA ratio varied from 3.8 to 4.15. These results suggest that a PSV of 300 to 325 cm/s could serve as a relatively good predictor of a high-grade restenosis (Fig. 6-6).

Post-CAS Surveillance

Early poststenting surveillance is as important for CAS patients as it is for CEA patients. The first ultrasound generally occurs within 1 month of the procedure to detect any technical problems associated with retained stenosis, thrombus, or stent deployment and to set baseline velocity data. Velocity elevations associated with changes in arterial compliance should be evident at this stage. Any subsequent velocity elevations should be considered potential evidence of restenosis.

After the 1-month evaluation, follow-up surveillance will typically address the development of restenosis in the hyperplastic lesion. As with CEA,

restenosis develops asymptomatically and duplex surveillance is intended to detect the aggressive disease. The goal of surveillance is to identify the restenosis that could advance to occlusion, and the rate of progression is as important as the identification of the high-grade lesion. More frequent follow-up is indicated if significant changes in velocity are detected between surveillance scans.

As noted, a duplex may not reliably detect moderate stenosis following CAS. This softening of the velocity criteria post-CAS should not significantly compromise surveillance. An individual patient can still be followed serially over multiple scans through the development of a moderate stenosis if the angle correction is appropriately maintained. A PSV of 175 cm/s found in a stent at baseline should not raise concerns if it remained unchanged in serial testing. If, on subsequent testing, PSV rose to 200 cm/s then 250 cm/s, these data are consistent with the rapid progression of a moderate stenosis. Intervention may

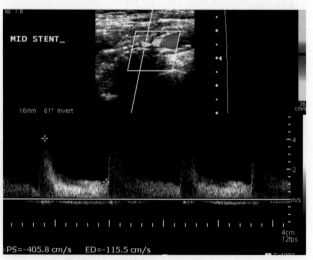

Figure 6-6 Carotid stent with elevated PSV at 405 cm/s. Note the narrowed color filling in the stent as well as color aliasing. These findings are consistent with a >70% restenosis.

be indicated with further workup before velocities reach the PSV threshold for a high-grade stenosis.

For CAS, Armstrong et al. uses a schedule similar to CEA with 6-month surveillance for the first 18 months.[24] Patients are then monitored annually if, by velocity criteria, they have less than a 50% stenosis. Patients will remain on a 6-month interval if they have lesions greater than 50% on the CAS side or on the contralateral side. Should the lesions become symptomatic on either side or the disease on either side progress asymptomatically to the high-grade lesion, they are considered for intervention.

SUMMARY

Issues associated with CEA and CAS remain in flux. CEA remains the traditional approach toward treating the bifurcation lesion and, although new techniques are evolving, its issues are relatively stable. Issues in CAS are poorly defined but given recent findings in CAS, the vascular sonographer should anticipate the volume of CAS to increase, possibly at the expense of CEA. It is important for vascular sonographers to recognize that significant differences exist in the duplex evaluation of CEA and CAS patients seen in follow-up. They should also recognize that the results of diligent post-CAS surveillance will determine the future of CAS. Duplex ultrasound will be the most important way of characterizing the behavior of this implanted device over time.

Critical Thinking Questions

1. You are asked to do a carotid ultrasound in the recovery room on a patient who just underwent a CEA. What approach would you use to image the CEA site and why?

2. You perform an ultrasound examination on a patient who is 2 weeks post-CEA. You observe echogenic material along the wall of the vessel with color aliasing and elevated velocities. What is the most likely cause of the stenosis?

3. When scanning patients who have had a CAS or CEA, will either patient group present a problem with acoustic shadowing and why?

REFERENCES

1. Muto A, Nishibe T, Dardik H, et al. Patches for carotid artery endarterectomy: current materials and prospects. *J Vasc Surg.* 2009;50(1):206–213.
2. AbuRahma AF. Processes of care for carotid endarterectomy: surgical and anesthesia considerations. *J Vasc Surg.* 2009;50(4):921–933.
3. Knight BC, Tait WF. Dacron patch infection following carotid endarterectomy: a systematic review of the literature. *Eur J Vascular Endovasc Surg.* 2009;37(2):140–148.
4. Flanigan DP, Flanigan ME, Dorne AL, et al. Long-term results of 442 consecutive, standardized carotid endarterectomy procedures in standard-risk and high-risk patients. *J Vasc Surg.* 2007;46(5):876–882.
5. Roseborough GS, Perler BA. Carotid artery disease: endarterectomy. In: Cronenwett JL, Johnston KW, eds. *Rutherford's Vascular Surgery.* 7th ed. Philadelphia, PA: Saunders/Elsevier; 2010:1443–1468.
6. Timaran CH, Veith FJ, Rosero EB, et al. Intracranial hemorrhage after carotid endarterectomy and carotid stenting in the United States in 2005. *J Vasc Surg.* 2009;49(3):623–628.
7. Hobson RW II, Mackey WC, Ascher E, et al. Management of atherosclerotic carotid artery disease: clinical practice guidelines of the Society for Vascular Surgery. *J Vasc Surg.* 2008; 48(2):480–486.
8. Brott TG, Roubin G, Howard G, et al. The Randomized Carotid Revascularization Endarterectomy vs Stenting Trial (CREST): primary results. Paper presented at: International Stroke Conference; February 24–28, 2010; San Antonio, TX.

9. ICSS Investigators. Carotid artery stenting compared with endarterectomy in patients with symptomatic carotid stenosis (International Carotid Stenting Study): an interim analysis of a randomized controlled trial. *Lancet.* 2010;375(9719):985–997.

10. Varcoe RL, Mah J, Young N, et al. Relevance of carotid stent fractures in a single-center experience. *J Endovasc Ther.* 2008;15:485–489.

11. Surdell D, Shaibani A, Bendok B, et al. Fracture of a Nitinol carotid artery stent that caused restenosis. *J Vasc Interv Radiol.* 2007;18(10):1297–1299.

12. Robertson SW, Cheng CP, Razavi MK. Biomechanical response of stented carotid arteries to swallowing and neck motion. *J Endovasc Ther.* 2008;15(6):663–671.

13. Ling AJ, Mwipatayi P, Gandhi T, et al. Stenting for carotid artery stenosis: fractures, proposed etiology and the need for surveillance. *J Vasc Surg.* 2008;47(6):1220–1226.

14. Sullivan TM. Surveillance and follow-up after carotid angioplasty and stenting. In: Mansour MA, Labropoulos N, eds. *Vascular Diagnosis.* Philadelphia, PA: Elsevier Saunders; 2005:183–191.

15. de Borst GJ, Vos JA, Reichmann B, et al. The fate of the external carotid artery after carotid artery stenting. A follow-up study with duplex ultrasonography. *Eur J Vasc Endovasc Surg.* 2007;33(6):657–663.

16. Lal BK, Kaperonis EA, Cuadra S, et al. Patterns of in-stent restenosis after carotid artery stenting: classification and implications for long-term outcome. *J Vasc Surg.* 2007;46(5):833–840.

17. AbuRahma AF, Abu-Halimah S, Bensenhaver J, et al. Optimal carotid duplex velocity criteria for defining the severity of carotid in-stent restenosis. *J Vasc Surg.* 2008;48(3):589–594.

18. Setacci C, Chisci E, Setacci F, et al. Grading carotid intrastent restenosis: a 6-year follow-up study. *Stroke.* 2008;39(4):1189–1196.

19. Zhou W, Felkai DD, Evans M, et al. Ultrasound criteria for severe in-stent restenosis following carotid artery stenting. *J Vasc Surg.* 2008;47(1):74–80.

20. Lal BK, Hobson RW II, Tofighi B, et al. Duplex ultrasound velocity criteria for the stented carotid artery. *J Vasc Surg.* 2008;47(1):63–73.

21. Chauvapun JP, Armstrong PA, Johnson BL. The application of duplex surveillance after carotid intervention. *Perspect Vasc Surg Endovasc Ther.* 2007;19(4):362–367.

22. Chahwan S, Miller MT, Pigott JP, et al. Carotid artery velocity characteristics after carotid artery angioplasty and stenting. *J Vasc Surg.* 2007;45(3):523–526.

23. Chi YW, White CJ, Woods TC, et al. Ultrasound velocity criteria for carotid in-stent restenosis. *Catheter Cardiovasc Interv.* 2007;69(3):349–354.

24. Armstrong PA, Bandyk DF, Johnson BL, et al. Duplex scan surveillance after carotid angioplasty and stenting: a rational definition of stent stenosis. *J Vasc Surg.* 2007;46(3):460–465.w

7 Intracranial Cerebrovascular Examination

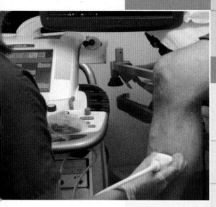

Colleen Douville

OBJECTIVES

Describe the arterial segments of the intracranial cerebral circulation that are standard to examine with transcranial Doppler (TCD) and transcranial duplex imaging (TCDI) techniques

Describe the anatomical approaches used to insonate the intracranial vessels in adults

List the current clinical applications for transcranial Doppler examinations

Describe normal velocities for each intracranial arterial segment examined with TCD and TCDI

Define the diagnostic criteria used to make the interpretation of collateral flow

List the values used for interpretation of >50% stenosis of the middle cerebral and intracranial internal carotid arteries

List criteria for vasospasm of the middle cerebral artery

Define the use of extracranial to intracranial ratios in vasospasm

KEY TERMS

anterior cerebral artery | anterior communicating artery | basilar artery | collateral flow | intracranial stenosis | middle cerebral artery | posterior cerebral artery | posterior communicating artery | transcranial Doppler | transcranial duplex imaging | vasospasm | vertebral artery

GLOSSARY

circle of Willis a roughly circular anastomosis of arteries located at the base of the brain

collateral a vessel that parallels another vessel; a vessel that is important to maintain blood flow around another stenotic or occluded vessel

Lindegaard ratio middle cerebral artery (MCA) mean velocity divided by the submandibular internal carotid artery (ICA) mean velocity; this ratio is useful in differentiating increased volume flow from decreased diameter when high velocities are encountered in the MCA or intracranial ICA

pulsatility expressed as Gosling's pulsatility index (peak systolic velocity minus end-diastolic velocity divided by the time averaged peak velocity)

Sviri ratio ratio calculation used to determine vasospasm from hyperdynamic flow in the posterior circulation; the bilateral vertebral artery velocities taken at the atlas loop are added together and averaged; this averaged velocity is then divided into the highest basilar mean velocity

transcranial Doppler (TCD) a noninvasive test that uses ultrasound to measure the velocity of blood flow through the intracranial cerebral vessels

transcranial duplex imaging (TCDI) a noninvasive test on the intracranial cerebral blood vessels that uses ultrasound and provides both an image of the blood vessels as well as a graphical display of the velocities within the vessels

vasospasm a sudden constriction in a blood vessel causing a restriction in blood flow

Originally introduced by Rune Aaslid in 1982 and applied to patients with vasospasm secondary to subarachnoid hemorrhage (SAH), transcranial Doppler (TCD) and transcranial duplex imaging (TCDI) provide diagnostic information in patients with a variety of cerebrovascular diseases.[1] This ultrasound technology complements the neuroimaging techniques of computed tomography with contrast (CTA), magnetic resonance imaging with contrast (MRA), and cerebral angiography by providing physiological data in real time that can be repeated, which is a valuable tool when considering the complex dynamics of cerebral blood flow.

ANATOMY

TCD examinations directly study the intracranial conducting arteries that lie at the base of the brain, including the arterial anatomists called the circle of Willis and the major anterior and posterior arteries that supply the circle. To put things in perspective, it is useful to understand that these are small targets; the center of the circle of Willis is about the size of a thumbnail and, on average, the diameter of the basal cerebral arteries range from approximately 2 to 4 mm.[2,3]

Most cerebral arteries have a numerical classification system that describes each arterial segment by name and number with the number referring to either the anatomical course or a branch point. Variations in the circle of Willis are frequent in 18% to 54% of individuals and result from anomalies in vessel caliber, course, and origin of branches.[4,5]

The anterior circulation is formed by the intracranial continuation of the internal carotid artery (ICA), which first becomes accessible by TCD exam in the cavernous portion, which is usually referred to as the carotid "siphon" because of its tortuous course (Fig. 7-1). The siphon is broken down into three segments: the parasellar (C_4), the genu (C_3), and the supraclinoid (C_2). The ICA pierces the dura, then enters the subarachnoid space, and terminates (C_1) by dividing into the middle cerebral (MCA) and anterior cerebral (ACA) arteries. Significant branches to a TCD study that arise from the distal ICA are the ophthalmic artery (OA) and posterior communicating arteries (PCOAs).

The MCA branches and courses laterally from the ICA as the main trunk or M_1 segment and bifurcates or trifurcates into M_2 branches that quickly angle upward into the insular area. There is very little asymmetry between the left and right middle cerebral arteries. The ACA (A_1 or precommunicating segment) begins and courses medially from the ICA for a short distance before passing forward as the

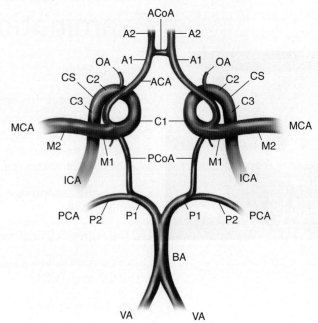

Figure 7-1 Circle of Willis and branches with abbreviations used for each arterial segment.

A_2 or postcommunicating segment. The two ACAs are connected above the optic chiasm by the anterior communicating artery (ACOA). There are frequent variations between the two ACAs, mainly consisting of differences in diameter or curvature.[4–6]

The intracranial posterior circulation is a continuation of the vertebral arteries (VAs) that pass through the foramen magnum and enter the subarachnoid space (V_4 segment) and course beneath the brain stem. Major branches, the posterior inferior cerebellar arteries (PICAs), usually arise from the distal part of the vertebral (V_4) and supply the brain stem and cerebellum. The VAs may have a tortuous course and often are of unequal size.[6] The basilar artery (BA) is created by the joining together of the two VAs and ends by terminating into the right and left posterior cerebral arteries (PCAs). It gives rise to two paired sets of branches, the anterior inferior cerebellar (AICA) and superior cerebellar (SCA) arteries along with numerous, small penetrating branches.[7]

The initial short segment of the PCA arising from the BA and prior to the PCOA is called the P_1 or precommunicating segment. Beyond this point it becomes the P_2, postcommunicating segment, which winds around the cerebral peduncle. The PCOA anatomically connects the anterior and posterior circulations but may be hypoplastic. The PCA normally arises from the BA but can have a "fetal origin" in 18% to 27% of the population, meaning it is dependent on the ICA for flow, either exclusively or in combination with the BA.[7]

SONOGRAPHIC EXAMINATION TECHNIQUES

PATIENT PREPARATION

Using simple language explain the test to the patient, instruct the patient to be quiet, and, unless necessary, not to speak during the exam. Take a relevant history from the patient or refer to medical records and make note of relevant indications for the test. When working in the intensive care unit (ICU) setting, check with the nurse before changing the level of the head. Take and record the blood pressure.

PATIENT POSITION

The patient is examined supine with the head slightly elevated during examination of the anterior circulation when using the transtemporal, transorbital, and submandibular approaches. It is advisable to use a rolled hand towel or a very small pillow to allow maximum access to the head and neck. The patient should be made as comfortable as possible as his or her cooperation and stillness is important to obtaining a good study. A semidark room facilitates relaxation as well as better image visualization on the ultrasound screen. To minimize variations in the spectral waveforms caused by fluctuating physiological variables, allow time for the heart, respiratory rate, and blood pressure to reach a steady state before beginning the study.

The VAs and BA require insonation through the foramen magnum. Place the patient in the lateral decubitus position supporting the face and head with a small pillow or towel with the neck aligned centrally. Palpate at midline about 1.25 in down from the skull base and flex the neck slightly. If the patient cannot be turned onto his or her side, the examination can be performed with the patient supine with the head rotated to the opposite side of insonation and the transducer placed just to the left or right side of the foramen magnum. For ambulatory patients, the upright sitting position is a feasible alternative with the neck flexed slightly and the head supported by the patient's arms and hands for stabilization. For ICU or other hospital inpatients that cannot be turned or optimally positioned, the head can be propped up using a rolled towel and turned away from the side of insonation. This will create a space large enough for the transducer to be placed at either midline or just lateral to the foramen magnum and will usually provide adequate access to the VAs and BA.

TECHNOLOGIST POSITION

The position of the sonographer may vary according to the setting. Outpatients are studied from the head or the side of the examination table, but for inpatients the equipment and the sonographer will usually be placed at the side of the bed. Dedicated TCD instruments often have remote controls, allowing for the manipulation of the instrument at a distance from the machine. Duplex ultrasound systems are more limited and require closer proximity of the machine and the sonographer.

A nonimaging TCD transducer is smaller than most imaging probes and unique ergonomic injuries can result from gripping the transducer too tightly and bending the thumbs and wrists backward. To avoid tendonitis and other injuries of the hands, grip the transducer with minimal pressure, rest when the hand becomes tired, and seek out preventative exercises from an ergonomics specialist.

EQUIPMENT

A dedicated nonimaging TCD instrument uses a 1 to 2 MHz pulsed wave transducer, spectral analysis, and additionally, may have M-mode capabilities. Software allows for the computation of peak systolic velocity (PSV), end-diastolic velocity (EDV), time averaged peak velocity (TAP-V), and Goslings pulsatility index (PI) at a minimum. Cursors and spectral outline tracers are available to compute values when automatic computations are erroneous. Additional software will function for specific applications such as monitoring for emboli, trending velocities, and displaying temporal changes in velocity.

The addition of power M-mode in 2002 uses simultaneous signal acquisition from 32 gates to create a display that demonstrates flow intensity and direction in bands of color (red is flow directed toward the transducer and blue is flow directed away from the transducer). The display ranges from 25 to 85 mm and corresponds to the course and depth of the arteries. Information in the power M-mode display helps the user find signals by creating a kind of visual road map much in the way color flow facilitates duplex imaging.

Standard duplex ultrasound technology allows for TCDI exams through the use of a broadband phased-array transducer with a Doppler frequency range usually of 2 to 3 MHz and imaging frequencies in the range of 4 MHz software provides computational packages similar to those found on dedicated TCD systems; however, TCDI is not routinely used for monitoring applications because the transducer size is too large to attach to the head and most companies have not developed instruments, hardware, or software for these applications.

REQUIRED DOCUMENTATION

In general, documentation for both techniques (TCD and TCDI) will be based on spectral waveforms. The B-mode and color Doppler information yielded in TCDI studies primarily facilitates acquisition of spectral

Doppler signals by providing a kind of color road map. Exceptions to this are color or power Doppler signals supporting identification of anomalous vessels and B-mode providing evidence of brain midline shifts and the visualization of masses. M-mode captures high intensity transient signals representing emboli. Documentation will vary according to the type of study being performed and will be discussed for each application later in the chapter.

The intracranial arteries are a continuation of the cervical internal and vertebral arteries and, as such, examining them in a proximal to distal order will facilitate interpretation. Spectral Doppler waveforms from each of the listed arterial segments from the right and left cerebral hemispheres and posterior circulation constitute a complete study.[7] When pathology is present, additional waveforms may be required to demonstrate abnormal flow characteristics.

Limited TCDs may be done for a number of reasons, such as repeat exams of affected vessels only, in acute stroke when using a fast protocol to determine single vessel patency,[8] when monitoring for microemboli, or when monitoring during an intervention. Required documentation will depend on the specifics of the study, why it was ordered, and which arteries are of interest. At a minimum, one spectral waveform from each artery or arterial segment studied is documented in normal exams or multiple waveforms to demonstrate the pathologies that are required for an adequate interpretation to be made.

Spectral Doppler Characteristics

Acquisition of a good spectral Doppler waveform from each required segment is essential as interpretation depends almost entirely on these signals. In TCD studies, the sample volume size is relatively large in comparison to the size of the arteries, which are on average only 2 to 4 mm in diameter and therefore even normal waveforms have the appearance of spectral broadening. The biggest difference between TCD and extracranial velocity calculations is the common use of a TAP-V obtained from the entire cardiac cycle, which is used for interpretation rather than the single point PSV and EDV used in extracranial carotid studies. This value is described differently by various manufacturers and for simplification is often referred to as the *mean* velocity (this term will also be used in this chapter). Quantitative values of mean velocity and PI are used along with waveform morphology and specific signatures seen in the amplitude of the waveform to make the formal interpretation in adults. Very high velocities and turbulent flow can be simultaneously displayed in signals detected in severe stenosis, vasospasm, collateral, and hyperdynamic flow creating complex waveforms. Instruments generally use an envelope trace that allows for real-time calculations of appropriate values; however, when the velocities become too complicated, these envelope tracers frequently fail to follow the true waveform outline and manual calculations become necessary. Depending on the equipment, different calculation methods are employed; one requires setting two cursors at the PSV and EDV and the second allows the user to trace the waveform contour with a cursor (Fig. 7-2).

With the exception of the OA, all of the arteries examined during a TCD exam supply the brain—a low resistance organ—with relatively high flow during diastole, similar to the extracranial ICA.

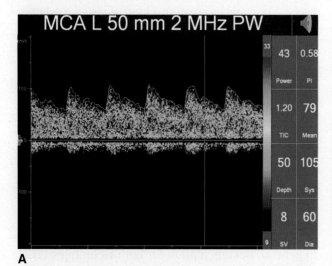
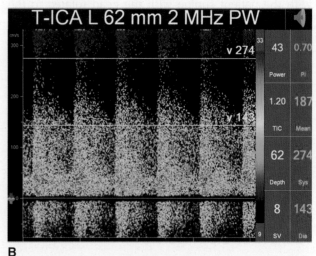

Figure 7-2 A: Spectral waveform from the MCA; envelope tracer calculates the time averaged peak velocity (mean). **B:** Nonoptimal spectral waveform from the MCA with the envelope tracer turned off and manual cursors set to peak systole and end diastole, resulting in a rough calculation of the mean velocity.

There are a wide range of normal values that vary primarily due to age, gender, cardiac effects, and by other intrinsic and extrinsic physiologic variables. Waveforms are evaluated for both quantitative and qualitative characteristics and with knowledge of physiological variables that can significantly influence flow findings.

Audio Signals

Doppler signals are audible as well as visible in the spectral waveform. With the increased sophistication of ultrasound instrumentation, there has been a trend toward diminishing the importance of hearing Doppler sounds. The human ear and brain are exquisitely designed to perceive subtle audio nuances and, when used for vascular studies, provide a feedback loop that informs the hand how to move to acquire a stronger signal and to increase gain to visualize the low amplitude, high velocity (pitch) signals that are otherwise drowned out by the high amplitude, low velocity turbulent signals. Developing good listening skills is especially important during nonimaging TCD and drives the acquisition of good signals but should not be minimized during TCDI examinations.

ANATOMICAL APPROACHES

Both TCD and TCDI use the same regions of the cranium to gain access into the basal cerebral arteries. Four approaches—also referred to as acoustic windows—are used to gain access into the cerebral vasculature; they are the transtemporal,[1] transorbital,[9] suboccipital,[10,11] and submandibular (Fig. 7-3).[12,13] A fifth approach involves obtaining the vertebral artery signals at the atlas loop and is used to facilitate calculation of a ratio specific to basilar artery vasospasm.[14,15]

Transtemporal Approach

The transtemporal approach is located over the temporal bone, superior to the zygomatic arch, and anterior and slightly superior to the tragus of the ear conch. Despite the relative thinness of the temporal bone, there is significant attenuation of the ultrasound at this interface. Early experiments measuring ultrasound energy transmission through the temporal bone showed that a large range of energy losses occurred between different skull samples and depended on the thickness of the bone.[16] There are individual variations in location of the temporal window, which is subdivided into posterior, middle, anterior, and frontal locations (Fig. 7-4). To find the site of optimal ultrasound penetration, all areas should be thoroughly explored. Window location determines the orientation of the transducer to the initial target, the MCA. Each area will require a somewhat different transducer angulation in order to be on axis with the arterial flow. From the posterior window, the beam is aimed slightly anterior and from an anterior or frontal window, it is aimed more posterior. Generally, the middle window requires a direct, neutral orientation (Fig. 7-5A).

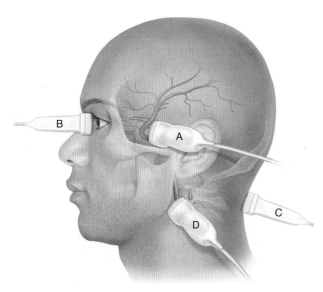

Figure 7-3 Four approaches used for intracranial exams: (*A*) transtemporal, (*B*) transorbital, (*C*) transoccipital, and (*D*) submandibular.

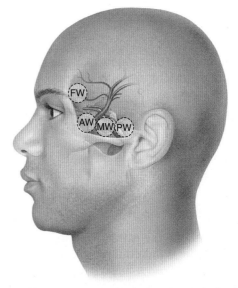

Figure 7-4 The transtemporal window located above the zygomatic arch with four possibilities for obtaining access through the temporal bone. *FW*, frontal window; *AW*, anterior window; *MW*, middle window; *PW*, posterior window.

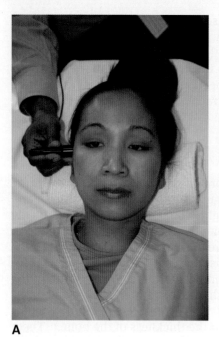 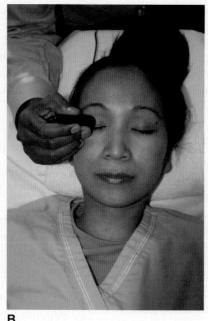 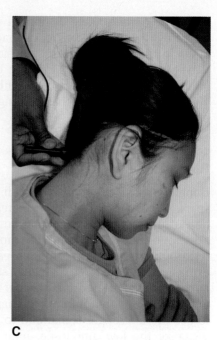

A   **B**   **C**

Figure 7-5 A: The most common position used for transtemporal access is the posterior window with the ultrasound beam oriented anteriorly. **B:** Transducer position for the orbit showing placement over the center of the eyelid with the beam aimed 15° to 20° medially. **C:** Midline transducer placement for the foramen magnum approach below the skull base and aimed toward the nasion.

Transorbital Approach

The orbital approach relies on the transmission of the ultrasound beam through the thin orbital plate of the frontal bone, optic canal, and superior orbital fissure; and signal attenuation is lower than for the temporal bone[10] (Fig. 7-5B). The power intensity is reduced to limit direct exposure to the eye and is guided by manufacturers' recommendations and the ALARA (as low as reasonably achievable) principle.

Foramen Magnum Approach

The foramen magnum approach takes advantage of the natural opening in the skull through which the spinal cord passes. The transducer is placed approximately 1.25 inches below the base of the skull, and the sound beam is aimed toward the nasion. The amount of soft tissue in this area varies considerably between individuals and will influence the depths at which the vertebral and basilar arteries are identified (Fig. 7-5C).

Submandibular Approach

This approach to the extracranial ICA is notably different than the standard technique used to study the carotid arteries with a linear probe and a 60° angle. The power can be quite low because the sound is not penetrating bone. The retromandibular ICA signal is obtained by using the TCD transducer and a zero degree angle of insonation. The transducer is placed at the angle of the jaw with the beam-directed cephalad. Signals obtained are usually used to calculate a Lindegaard ratio in patients with vasospasm secondary to SAH or for documenting distal ICA stenosis arising from fibromuscular dysplasia and dissections[11] (Fig. 7-6A).

Atlas Loop Approach

Originally described by von Reutern to study the extracranial VA using continuous wave Doppler,[2] obtaining VA signals at this location is used to calculate the BA/VA ratio, which, similar to the Lindegaard ratio, is useful to categorize a vasospasm or to confirm disease in routine examinations.[16] The transducer is placed approximately 1.25 inches below the mastoid process and behind the sternocleidomastoid muscle. Again, the power can be lowered as this is an extracranial signal and does not require penetration of bone (Fig. 7-6B).

STANDARD TRANSCRANIAL DOPPLER EXAMINATION TECHNIQUE

TCD studies are a diagnostic tool in the clinical management of patients with a variety of intracranial vascular abnormalities. The study provides physiologic information that complements anatomic imaging studies. The results may provide rationales for the treatment of brain ischemia and stroke.

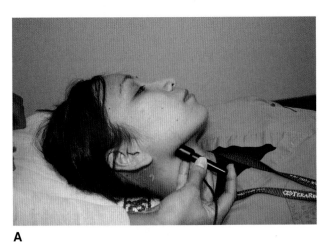

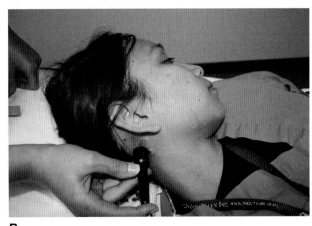

A   **B**

Figure 7-6 A: Obtaining the submandibular ICA at the angle of the jaw. **B:** Insonation of the vertebral artery in the region of the atlas loop.

Standard TCD exams are performed on inpatients and outpatients when ordered. A complete standard TCD exam consists of pulsed wave Doppler insonation of the basal cerebral arteries including the bilateral cavernous and terminal segments of the ICAs, OAs, MCAs, ACAs, PCAs, VAs, and the BA.[8] Additionally, in some populations, the extracranial retromandibular ICAs and VAs at the atlas loop will be examined to calculate vasospasm ratios (Table 7-1).

Doppler spectral waveforms are acquired in a blind fashion without the aid of B-mode or color Doppler, requiring a good understanding of the anatomy and physiology of the intracranial vessels and a precise, systematic approach to the exam performance.

TABLE 7-1

Basal Cerebral Arteries Insonated during Intracranial Exam, Their Abbreviations, and the Minimum Documentation for a Complete, Normal TCD or TCDI Study

Artery	Abbreviations	Number of Waveforms	Comments
Ophthalmic	OA	1	
Carotid siphon	CS	3	C2 (supraclinoid), C3 (genu), C4 (parasellar) if accessible
Terminal internal carotid	TICA	1	C1
Middle cerebral	MCA and MCA2	3	Proximal, mid, and distal, including MCA2 branches
Anterior cerebral (precommunicating segment)	ACA	1	
Anterior cerebral (postcommunicating segment)	ACA2	1	Only applies to TCDI
Anterior communicating artery	ACOA	1	When functioning as collateral
Posterior cerebral (precommunicating segment)	PCA1	1	
Posterior cerebral (postcommunicating segment)	PCA2	1	
Posterior communicating artery	PCOA	1	When functioning as collateral
Submandibular internal carotid artery	SM-ICA	1	When calculating Lindegaard index or documenting distal narrowing
Vertebral	VA4	3	Proximal, mid, and distal
Vertebral at the atlas loop (V3)	VA3		When calculating Sviri ratio for vasospasm
Basilar	BA	3	Proximal, mid, and distal

There are five primary criteria used to identify each vessel segment:

1. Approach: Each cranial window provides access to specific arteries only.
2. Sample volume depth: Each artery has a specific range of depths over which it courses.
3. Direction of blood flow relative to the ultrasound transducer.
4. The spatial relationship of one artery to another. For the anterior circulation, the reference vessel used to identify other arteries is the bifurcation of the terminal ICA.
5. Flow velocity: In general, the MCA > ACA > PCA = BA = VA. These relationships assist vessel identification and, when reversed, can be helpful in identifying pathological flow states.

See Table 7-2.[17,18]

Orbital Approach

Arteries identified through the orbital window include the OA and cavernous carotid (siphon). The acoustic intensity is lowered to the manufacturer's recommendations and close observation of the ALARA principle is used. The patient is asked to close his or her eyes gently and keep them shut until the end of the orbital exam to avoid getting ultrasound gel into the eye. A small amount of ultrasound gel is placed on the transducer and or closed eyelid, and the transducer is placed gently over the center of the closed eyelid and aimed 15° to 20°, toward the midline, and without applying any pressure to the eye.

At sample volume depths ranging from 40 to 60 mm, the OA can be identified isolated away from the carotid siphon. The unique waveform of the OA has low velocities and, due to the higher resistance bed of the eye compared with the brain, typically have low diastolic flow. The OA is studied to determine if flow is antegrade or retrograde, the latter being indicative of an external carotid artery (ECA) to ICA collateral flow.[10,11]

By increasing the sample volume to 60 to 70 mm, flow can be detected in the carotid siphon, so named because of its tortuous course at this location resulting in flow directionality that may be toward, away, or bidirectional depending on the orientation of the vessel segment to the transducer (although normally, the physiological direction of flow is antegrade) (Fig. 7-7).[10,11]

Temporal Approach

The arteries identified through the transtemporal approach include the MCA (M_1 and proximal M_2 segments), the ACA (A_1 segment), the terminal internal carotid artery (TICA), and the PCA (P_1 and proximal P_2 segments). The ACOA and PCOA are usually only identified when they are carrying an increased volume flow because they function as collaterals. Ample gel is applied to the transducer and to the patient's skin to create a good interface for the transmission of the ultrasound.[11]

Finding the exact location on the temporal bone that allows the best ultrasound penetration can be challenging and will be facilitated by being systematic in the exploration of this area and using small hand movements. To facilitate finding the temporal window, power is set at maximum and the sample volume is placed at a depth of 50 mm with the intention of finding the MCA.

The exam is begun by placing the transducer in the posterior window, aiming the beam slightly anterior and superior, and using a circular motion scanning for an audible Doppler signal and visual spectral display. If using M-mode, employ the same manual technique while also observing the M-mode display for a red color band at depths ranging from 30 to 65 mm.[19] If no or weak signals are obtained, the transducer is systematically moved to the middle and anterior or frontal locations and scanning is repeated until signal acquisition is accomplished.

Once a suitable acoustic window is identified, emphasis changes to identifying each arterial segment. Initial signals directed toward the transducer at a depth of 50 mm most often arise from the MCA. The sample volume depth is then reduced in a stepwise manner, tracing the MCA distally in 2 to 5 mm increments. Distally, the main trunk of the MCA divides into the M_2 segment and the branches course superior over the insula, have lower velocities, and flow direction may change to away from the transducer (Fig. 7-8).

The sample volume is then increased to trace the MCA proximally to its origin at 55 to 65 mm depth. The bifurcation of the terminal ICA into the MCA and ACA serves as a reference landmark for the remainder of the study. When using a large sample volume size (5 to 10 mm), the ACA and MCA are frequently seen simultaneously as a bidirectional signal as long as they are oriented on the same axis. The M-mode display will also show bands of color—red at shallower depths and, past the TICA bifurcation, a blue band will appear indicating flow away from the transducer, usually the ACA. A word of caution is in order because, at this depth, flow away from the transducer is not necessarily the ACA. If the beam is pointing slightly inferiorly, the tortuous TICA may also reveal flow away from the transducer, making it important to always know how the beam is being aimed relative to the landmark bifurcation signal (Fig. 7-9).

TABLE 7-2

Criteria Used to Identify Each Arterial Segment for a Full Diagnostic TCD Examination[18,19]

Cranial Approach	Arterial Segment	Flow Direction Relative to Transducer	Sample Volume Depth Ranges (mm)	Spatial Relationship to Landmark MCA/ACA Bifurcation	TCD Normal Mean Velocity Range and SD (cm/s)	TCDI (angle corrected) Normal Mean Velocity Range Age 20–39 (cm/s)	TCDI (angle corrected) Normal Mean Velocity Range Age 40–59 (cm/s)	TCDI (angle corrected) Normal Mean Velocity Range Age > 60 (cm/s)
Temporal	MCA (M1 and proximal M2)	M1 – Toward M2 – Away	30–60	Identical	55 +/–12	71–76	69–76	55–61
Temporal	TICA	Toward and/or away	60–70	Inferior	39 +/–9			
Temporal	ACA (A1)	Away	60–75	Anterior and superior	50 +/–11	57–62	57–64	48–54
Temporal	PCA (P1)	Toward	60–75	Posterior and inferior	39 +/–10	51–55	48–51	40–45
Temporal	PCA (P2)	Away	60–65	Posterior and inferior	40 +/–10	45–49	46–51	39–45
Orbital	OA	Toward	35–55		21 +/–5			
Orbital	Carotid siphon (C4, C3, C2)	Toward, bidirectional, away	65–80		C2 41 +/–11 C4 47 +/–14			
Submandibular	ICA	Away	35–80		30 +/–9			
Atlas loop	VA (V3)		40–50					
Foramen magnum	VA	Away	60–90		38 +/–10	42–47	38–43	30–36
Foramen magnum	BA	Away	70–120		41 +/–10	47–53	39–48	31–40

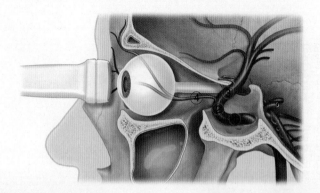

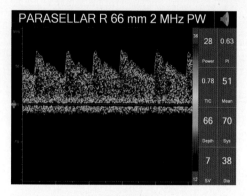

1 Parasellar

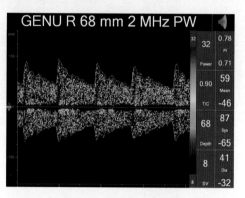

2 Genu

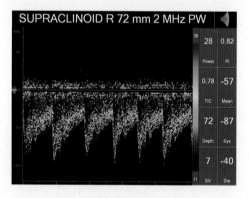

3 Supraclinoid

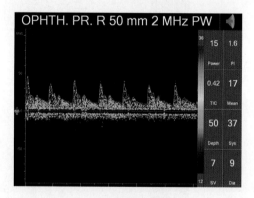

4 Ophthalmic

Figure 7-7 Orbital approach showing a lateral view of the carotid siphon and ophthalmic arteries. **1:** Low resistance waveform in parasellar segment of the intracranial ICA. **2:** Bidirectional signal seen at the genu. **3:** ICA siphon flow directed away from the transducer. **4:** Ophthalmic artery with high resistant, low velocity waveform.

From the bifurcation, the ACA is identified by increasing the sample volume depth and usually aiming the transducer slightly anterior and superior. The precommunicating segment of the ACA does exhibit variations in caliber with lower velocities found in hypoplastic segments. It can also vary its course and sometimes curves downward rather than upward in patients between the ages of 50 and 70 years.[2] The ACA can be traced to the midline of the brain, where bidirectional signals may again be detected related to insonation of the bilateral ACAs. The spectral waveform is normally directed away

from the transducer, although it can reverse direction when acting as collateral. The M-mode display will show a narrow band of blue color at the depth appropriate to the ACA. The ACOA is not identified until it acts as a collateral channel due to its diminutive size (Fig. 7-10).

To identify the TICA, the sample volume depth is returned to the landmark bifurcation and, at the same depth, aimed directly inferior. Velocities may appear low due to the anatomical course of the TICA relative to the sound beam, which tends to be perpendicular to the vessel, creating a larger

Middle Cerebral Artery

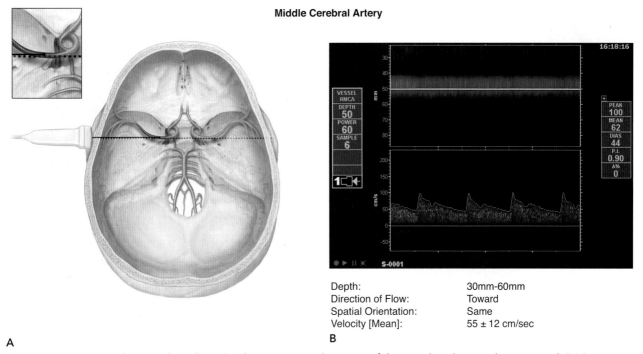

Depth: 30mm-60mm
Direction of Flow: Toward
Spatial Orientation: Same
Velocity [Mean]:   55 ± 12 cm/sec

A   B

Figure 7-8 A: Temporal approach to the MCA demonstrating placement of the sample volume in the main trunk (M1) segment and normal spectral waveform. **B:** M-mode display illustrating band of flow toward the transducer at depths of 30 to 60 mm, consistent with flow in the MCA.

angle of insonation and lower calculated velocities (Fig. 7-11).

Lastly, the PCA is located by again returning the sample volume to the ACA/MCA bifurcation, increasing the depth by 5 mm, and moving the transducer slightly posterior and inferior. Only very small movements are required because it is easy to overshoot

the amount of rotation used. The direction of flow in the P_1 segment and proximal P_2 segment is toward the transducer. The M-mode display will show a narrow red band representative of the P_1 and proximal P_2 at the appropriate depth, and the contralateral P_1 will appear blue at a greater depth. By increasing the depth to 70 to 80 mm, signals from both the right and

ACA/MCA Bifurcation

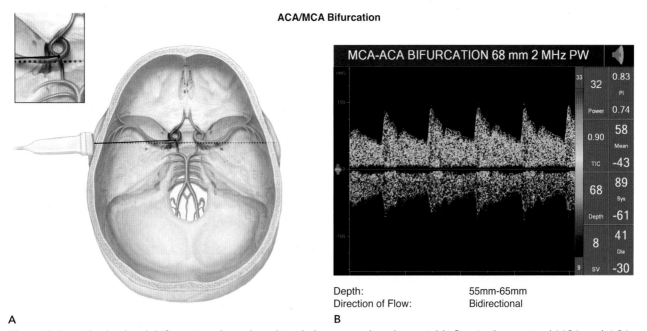

Depth: 55mm-65mm
Direction of Flow: Bidirectional

A   B

Figure 7-9 A: The landmark bifurcation where the relatively large sample volume yields flow in the proximal MCA and ACA. **B:** Bidirectional spectral waveform simultaneously demonstrating flow from the proximal MCA and ACA

Anterior Cerebral Artery

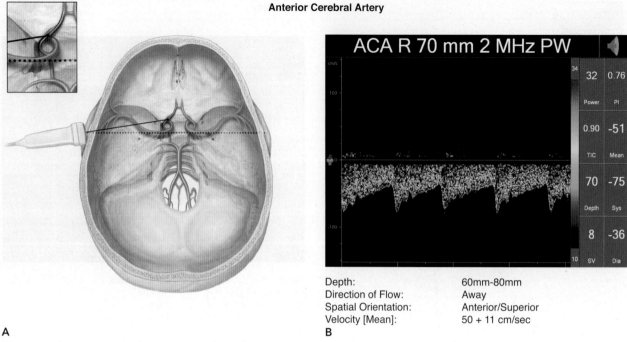

Depth: 60mm-80mm
Direction of Flow: Away
Spatial Orientation: Anterior/Superior
Velocity [Mean]:   50 + 11 cm/sec

A
B

Figure 7-10 A: Frequently, the ACA is located by further aiming the transducer in an anterior and superior manner. **B:** The spectral waveform demonstrates the ACA flowing away from the transducer.

left PCA are seen as they bifurcate from the tip of the BA, resulting in a bidirectional spectral waveform.

Once the P_1 segment is identified, continuing with further rotation in the same posterior–inferior direction, the P_2 segment flowing away from the transducer will be intersected. The PCOAs are usually not appreciated unless they are functioning as collateral pathways carrying an increased volume of blood with subsequent high velocities and turbulence (Fig. 7-12).

Terminal Internal Carotid Artery

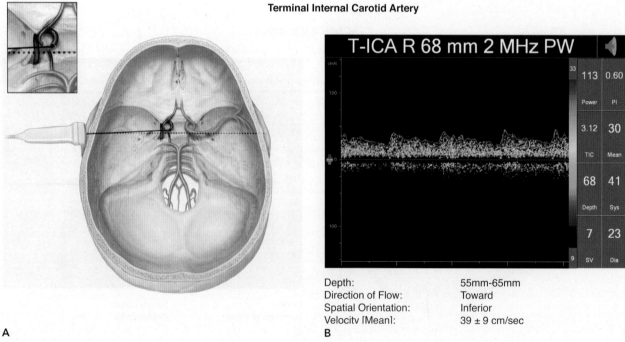

Depth: 55mm-65mm
Direction of Flow: Toward
Spatial Orientation: Inferior
Velocity [Mean]:   39 ± 9 cm/sec

A
B

Figure 7-11 A: With the sample volume depth located at the landmark bifurcation and aimed inferiorly, the terminal ICA is insonated. **B:** The spectral waveform from the TICA demonstrates relatively low velocities due to the poor angle of insonation.

Posterior Cerebral Artery (P1)

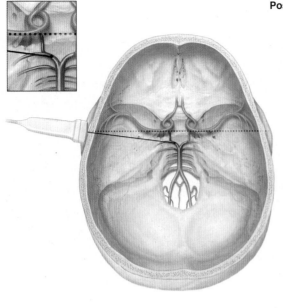

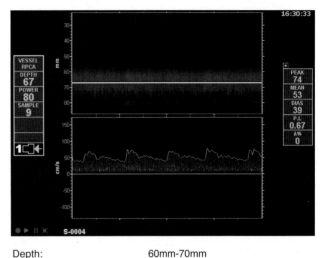

Depth:	60mm-70mm
Direction of Flow:	Toward
Spatial Orientation:	Posterior/Inferior
Velocity [Mean]:	39 ± 10 cm/sec

A

B

Figure 7-12 A: The PCA is identified by aiming the beam posterior and inferior from the depth of the very proximal ACA. The flow direction from the P1 and proximal P2 segments is toward the transducer. **B:** M-mode color bands showing the bilateral P1 segments as the beam crosses midline. Spectral waveform taken from the ipsilateral PCA.

Foramen Magnum Approach

The VAs and BA are studied using the suboccipital window with the transducer placed midline below the foramen magnum, the patient's head slightly flexed, and the ultrasound beam oriented upward toward the center of the patient's eyebrows. Normal direction of flow is away from the transducer but can reverse in any segment secondary to subclavian or innominate artery steals. Initially to find the window, the sample volume depth is set at 60 mm and by aiming minimally to the right and left toward the orbit of the eye signals are found. The right and left VAs are differentiated by having the signal drop out as one moves from side to side and because the waveforms frequently have a different shape. It is common to have a dominant and nondominant VA, and the flow velocities will be lower in the smaller vessel and the morphology of the waveform will have a different contour. Once the right and left vessels are differentiated, follow each from proximal to distal. In the near field around a depth of 55 mm, the signal becomes bidirectional as it begins to course extracranially and does so again at a depth of 65 mm, where the PICA branch arises. A more lateral orientation of the transducer to the foramen magnum can also be used to identify the VAs. However, from this approach it is possible to have the beam focused on the contralateral VA while thinking the ipsilateral VA is being insonated. This is usually only problematic if the left and right VA waveforms are very similar in shape and velocity, which occurs

about one-third of the time. The exact confluence of the two VAs into the BA may be difficult to determine with nonimaging TCD. In some cases, as the sample volume depth increases it begins to encompass both VAs simultaneously and the resultant spectral waveform will show them superimposed. The depth of the VA confluence varies with body habitus and has a range from approximately 69 +/− 7 mm.[20]

The BA curves below the brain stem and courses forward and superiorly; so to identify this segment, the transducer is slid slightly further down the neck and oriented somewhat higher than for the VAs. This artery is relatively long (33 +/− 6 mm) and may need to be traced for 3 to 4 cm in order to capture the distal segment.[19] Both the VAs and BA give off cerebellar branches, and when these are intersected, the signal becomes temporarily bidirectional (Fig. 7-13).

TRANSCRANIAL DOPPLER DUPLEX IMAGING SCANNING TECHNIQUE

The use of duplex ultrasound instrumentation to examine the intracranial circulation has both advantages and limitations. Accurate vessel identification and decreasing the learning curve time are two significant contributions of the TCDI technique. Disadvantages include a larger transducer footprint, which may limit access to small or difficult windows, and an inability to apply this technology to monitoring applications where the transducer is attached to a head frame

Vertebral Artery

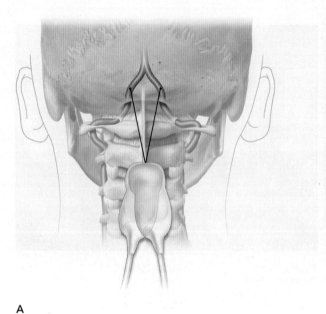

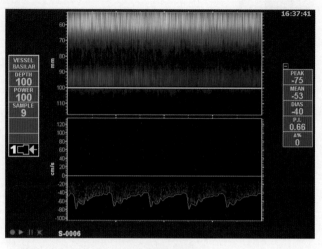

Depth:	60mm-90mm
Direction of Flow:	Away
Velocity [Mean]:	38 ± 10 cm/sec

A   **B**

Figure 7-13 A: Using the foramen magnum window to identify the intracranial vertebral arteries from a midline approach with spectral waveforms. **B:** M-mode display and spectral waveform from the basilar artery; notice the distance over which the BA travels.

and arteries are continually monitored over time. TCDI uses low frequency broadband phased-array transducers with Doppler frequencies in a range of 2 to 3 MHz and imaging frequencies up to 5 MHz.

Orbital Approach

Ultrasound energy passes through the orbit of the eye prior to penetrating the skull when using the trans-orbital window, and the U.S. Food and Drug Administration has lowered the maximum acoustic output allowable for this approach. This is in concern for potential bioeffects to the eye and most instruments have an orbital power setting that automatically limits the output.

The patient is placed in a supine position with both eyes gently closed. Instruct the patient to keep eyes shut until the orbital exam is complete and the acoustic gel has been removed. The transducer orientation marker is pointed medial for both the right and left side, and the probe is gently set on the center of the closed eyelid. The hand that holds the transducer can be stabilized by placing it on the patient's cheek for support. Do not apply any pressure to the eye.

B-mode image orientation will show medial to the left of the screen and lateral to the right. The globe of the eye will appear in the near field as a round echolu-cent structure. With the transducer in a true anterior/posterior orientation, the optic nerve shadow will extend from the distal rim at the center of the globe. With the color box set at the back of the globe and extending to include the proximal optic nerve shadow, the central retinal artery and vein, the lacrimal artery, as

well as the long and short posterior ciliary arteries can frequently be observed. These are all branches of the OA and supply blood flow to various parts of the eye.

Ophthalmic Artery

To locate the main branch of the OA, angle the transducer 15% to 20% and aim medially. This will distort the round shape of the globe, and the optic nerve shadow may disappear. Place the color box at a depth of 40 to 60 mm and lower the color scale (normal velocities are 21 +/− 5 cm/s). Normal flow direction is toward the transducer (red), and the path of the artery should be from lateral to medial as it courses across the optic nerve. Signals taken too shallow or too lateral may represent flow in the lachrymal artery branch. Place the spectral Doppler sample volume in the color box. The waveform will have a low velocity with high resistance similar to the extracranial ECA. Flow direction may reverse, velocity may increase, and pulsatility may decrease when the OA functions as a collateral channel in severe stenosis or occlusion proximally in the ICA (Fig. 7-14).

Carotid Siphon

There are no specific B-mode landmarks surrounding the cavernous carotid artery. Using the same transducer orientation as for the OA, the color box is placed at a depth of 60 to 75 mm and the color scale is increased (normal velocity is 47 +/− 14 cm/s). This tortuous section of the ICA may present as flow toward, away, or both. Spectral Doppler waveforms are obtained from each segment (Fig. 7-15).

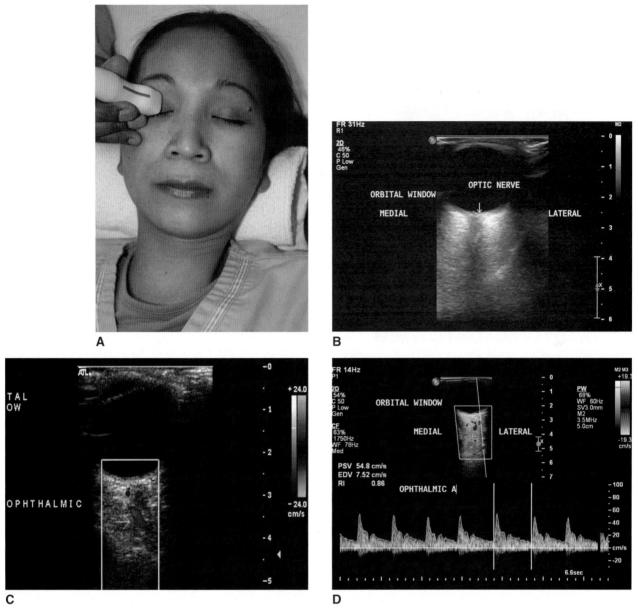

Figure 7-14 **A:** TCDI through using the orbital approach with the transducer orientation marker toward the patient's nose (medial). **B:** B-mode image of the globe and optic nerve *(arrow)* with the transducer in a true anterior–posterior position. **C:** Color Doppler of the ophthalmic artery *(arrow)*. **D:** Spectral Doppler waveform from the OA.

Temporal Approach

Begin the exam at maximum power to facilitate finding the acoustic window. Once the window is established, power can be adjusted following the ALARA principle, especially if the patient has a hemicraniectomy and the bone is absent.

The temporal window provides access to multiple arteries that, along with their branches, supply all lobes of the cerebrum. It is conventional to study the left and right hemispheres from the left and right temporal windows, respectively, even in patients with good windows so that spectral Doppler strength and angles of insonation are optimal.

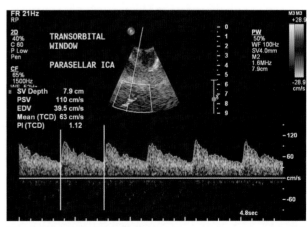

Figure 7-15 Color Doppler signals seen at depths corresponding to the carotid siphon.

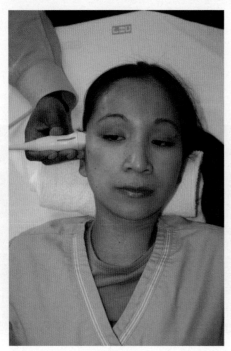

Figure 7-16 Temporal approach with transducer oriented in a cross-sectional plane and the orientation marker oriented toward the nose.

The transducer is positioned in cross section with the orientation marker oriented anteriorly or toward the patient's nose (Fig. 7-16). The grayscale image presents a cross-sectional view of the brain. The superficial portion of the image shows the ipsilateral cerebral hemisphere, and the deep portion of the image shows the contralateral cerebral hemisphere. Anterior is to the left of the screen, and posterior is to the right.

Identifying the Window Using B-Mode Landmarks

Apply a generous amount of gel over the temporal region of the head. Place the transducer just superior and parallel to the zygomatic arch. Set the field of view to at least 15 cm. If there is an adequate window, bright reflections are seen, forming a crescent shape at a depth of around 5 cm. This bright landmark arises from the lesser wing of the sphenoid bone (anterior) and the petrous ridge of the temporal bone (posterior). Tilt the transducer slightly caudad; directly below the tip of the sphenoid wing is the anterior clinoid process. If these reflections are absent, slide or tilt the transducer forward, backward, up, and/or down, using very slow, small motions until they appear. If all B-mode reflections are homogenous, there is no ultrasonic bone window (Fig. 7-17).

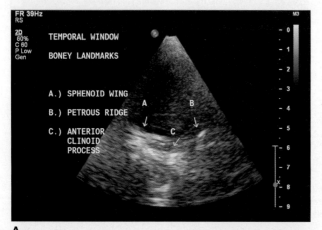

A

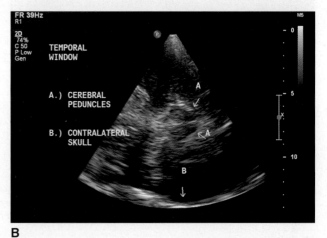

B

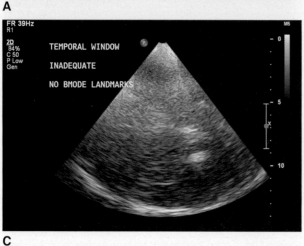

C

Figure 7-17 Temporal approach grayscale landmarks. **A:** Bright reflections returning from the sphenoid wing and petrous ridge and anterior clinoid process bone landmarks in the near field. **B:** Parenchymal landmarks including the cerebral peduncle and falx cerebri. **C:** Homogenous B-mode image with no landmarks consistent with mainly or totally absent temporal window.

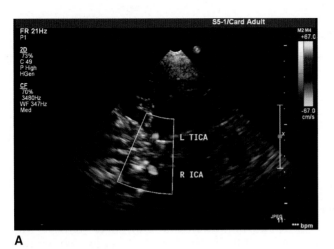

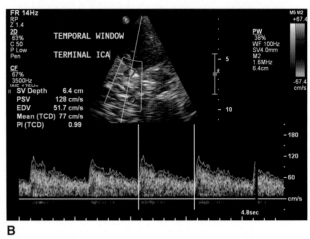

Figure 7-18 A: Color box placed over the anterior clinoid process bilateral TICAs. **B:** Spectral waveform from the TICA.

Tilt or slide the transducer slightly cephalad from bright reflections coming from the boney structures identified at the base of the brain and identify the following structures: (1) contralateral skull (note the depth of the inner table), midline of the brain will be at one-half this depth; (2) falx cerebri, seen as a bright, thin line produced by the reflection from the double layer of dura in the interhemispheric fissure at midline; and the (3) midbrain seen at midline and slightly posterior to the center of the screen image, which appears as an echolucent butterfly or heart-shaped structure.

Terminal Internal Carotid Artery

Decrease the field of view to 8 cm if the window is suboptimal. Relocate the boney landmarks and place the color box on the anterior clinoid process, around which the ICA courses. A small circle of color will appear; change the transducer orientation obliquely toward coronal and the color image will take on an "S" shape. This is the TICA, which is tortuous at this location and will appear both blue and red even though flow is normally antegrade. Sample with spectral Doppler and save the highest velocity. The angle of insonation for this segment of the ICA is not optimal and velocities will be lower than if sampled at zero degrees (Fig. 7-18).

Middle Cerebral Artery

The MCA is slightly above and parallel to the lesser wing of the sphenoid bone. From the TICA, move the transducer cephalad using deliberate, small, and slow motions. The main trunk of the MCA, flowing toward the transducer, is red. Branches coming off the distal MCA are often seen curving upward, toward the sylvian fissure, and are blue. To see MCA branches better, aim the beam upward. Sample the branches with spectral Doppler, then sample the main trunk sequentially in at least 5-mm increments, obtaining flow velocities distal, mid, and proximal. Turn the color scale up if there is color aliasing or down if there is poor color visualization (Fig. 7-19).

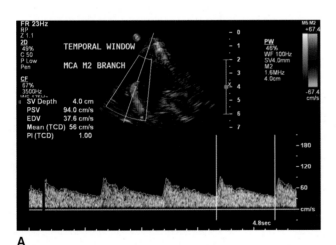

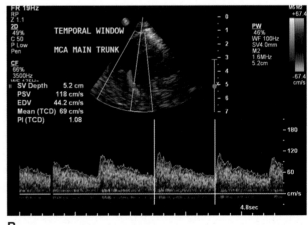

Figure 7-19 Color and spectral Doppler signals from **(A)** the M2 branches of the MCA and **(B)** the main trunk of the MCA.

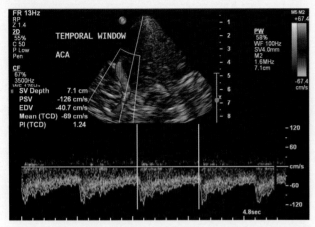

Figure 7-20 Color and spectral Doppler signals from the ACA (A1 segment); notice the surrounding B-mode image is usually not bright because the ACA usually courses above the boney processes.

Anterior Cerebral Artery

The short segment of the ACA can be challenging to identify with color flow, especially when the vessel is not oriented axially to the MCA. If not seen in tandem with the MCA, the following transducer adjustments are helpful: (1) twist the front end of the probe upward, (2) slide the probe upward, and (3) tilt the probe upward. The ACA does not lie in proximity to bone, and the surrounding B-mode image will not display the bright boney reflections seen surrounding the TICA. The precommunicating segment of the ACA is short and ends at midline. The proximal postcommunicating segment can often be seen coursing toward the left of the screen (anterior). The ACA is blue on color Doppler but can change direction when acting as collateral. Take spectral Doppler waveforms in 5-mm increments. If the color box does not fill, try using the spectral Doppler at the anticipated location for the ACA (Fig. 7-20).

The ACA has a high incidence of anatomical variation and may be hypoplastic or atretic, and most often exhibits asymmetries in the caliber between the right and left sides. When functionally absent, the crossover collateral ability (from one hemisphere to the other via the ACAs and ACOA) can be severely limited or absent.

Posterior Cerebral Artery

Locate the hypoechoic, butterfly-shaped midbrain using B-mode and place the color box around the midbrain, which is encircled by the PCAs. The P_1 will be flowing toward the transducer (red) as will the proximal P_2. Twist the transducer to open up the curving vessel. As the PCA curves around the midbrain, the flow orientation is away from the transducer (blue); this represents the postcommunicating or P_2 segment.

To differentiate between the P_1 and P_2 segments, set the color box to include the TICA simultaneously with the PCA. Draw an imaginary line between these two vessels and it will represent the PCOA. This artery can frequently be seen with color flow if the scale setting is low enough, even when it is not functioning as collateral. Flow in the ipsilateral PCA deeper than the imaginary line is the P_1 segment, and superficial to it is the P_2 segment. Obtain spectral Doppler signals along the PCA and document the highest velocity in the P_1 and P_2 segments (Fig. 7-21).

In normal anatomy the PCA originates from the BA, but in 18% to 27% of patients, it originates from the TICA either exclusively or in combination with the BA.[6] This is referred to as a fetal origin and can frequently be seen with TCDI. Fetal origin is highly suggested when there is no communication between the BA and the PCA, which is evidenced by no color or spectral Doppler signals that can be obtained from the short P_1 segment and a large vessel, originating

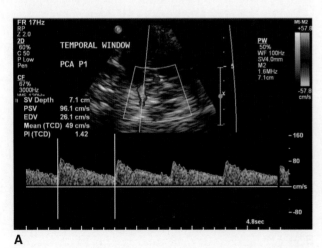

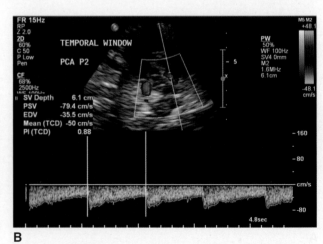

A   **B**

Figure 7-21 **A:** Hypoechoic cerebral peduncle and P1 segment of the PCA. **B:** P2 segment of the PCA.

from the TICA, and coursing posteriorly, which can be seen with color Doppler. A fetal origin PCA can have a significant clinical impact on patients with ICA stenosis and/or vertebrobasilar disease and should be noted in the comments and on the interpretation.

Foramen Magnum Approach

The foramen magnum is a large median opening penetrating the occipital bone. Place the transducer 1.25 inches below the skull base, aiming the beam toward the nasion. The bright bone reflections around this opening appear as a circle in the near field of the image (at a depth of about 5 cm). In order to find the best acoustic window, the transducer may be moved from one side or the other of the foramen magnum and twisted into an oblique or sagittal orientation. Turn the color Doppler on. Place the color box at a depth of 55 to 65 mm. The VAs appear as flow away from the transducer (blue) and may exhibit a high degree of tortuosity. In the near field, at around a 50- to 55-mm depth, the flow will be bidirectional, which is caused by the vessel changing course as it

travels from the atlas through the foramen magnum and into the V_4 segment.

Follow the two VAs to their confluence where they join to form the basilar artery. Sample each VA at 5-mm increments and obtain spectral waveforms. Document the highest velocity from each vessel. The VAs are often of unequal size, with one or the other dominant in 74% of the population.[7] The PICA arises from each distal VA and will appear as a branch, usually directed toward the transducers. At their confluence between 70 and 90 mm, the two VAs will join to form the BA that looks like a Y shape on the screen. Narrow the color box for a better frame rate and increase the depth of its placement.

The BA is 3 to 4 mm long and, in some patients, may extend to depths as great as 120 mm. Using TCDI, the mid and distal parts of the artery may be difficult to visualize with color flow, but the spectral Doppler sample volume can be placed to follow the trajectory of the BA, thus enhancing signal acquisition at greater depths. Obtain spectral Doppler waveforms at 5-mm increments and document the proximal, mid, and distal BA (Fig. 7-22).

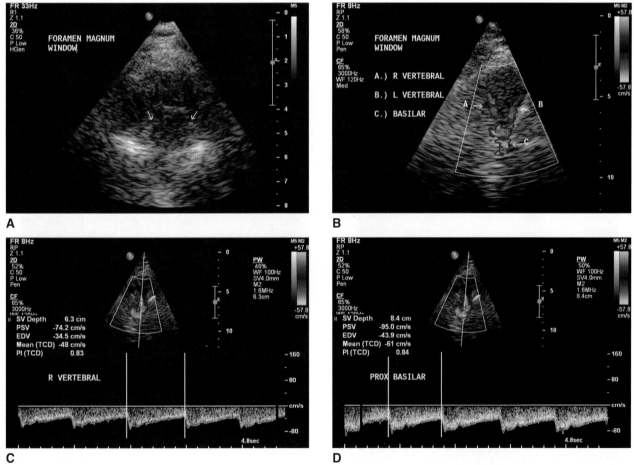

Figure 7-22 A: Grayscale showing the foramen magnum (*arrow*) surrounded by bright reflections from occipital bone. **B:** Bilateral VAs entering the cranium and coursing medially to form the basilar artery. **C:** Spectral waveform taken from the VA. **D:** Spectral waveform taken from the BA.

Submandibular Approach

The retromandibular extradural ICA is routinely obtained in patients with abnormalities, requiring calculation of the Lindegaard ratio including SAH, head trauma, intracranial stenosis, and arteriovenous malformations. This ratio, defined as MCA/SM-ICA, is important for differentiating vasospasm and stenosis of the MCA from hyperdynamic flow.[13,21] If the patient has >50% extracranial stenosis, the ratio calculation may be invalid and should not be used. Locating the ICA using this technique is also useful in determining distal arterial narrowing, which is often associated with carotid dissection or fibromuscular dysplasia.

Set the power to low and place the transducer at the angle of the jaw with the orientation marker facing up and aim slightly medial and posterior. The ICA will appear on the screen moving from right (more superficial) to left (deeper) and flowing away (blue) from the transducer. Place the sample volume at the depth providing the best zero degree angle, usually around 4 to 5 cm, and obtain a single spectral waveform with the highest obtainable velocity (Fig. 7-23).

TECHNICAL CONSIDERATIONS

About 10% of geriatric patients will have hyperostosis of the temporal bone and, due to high attenuation of

the ultrasound, no signals will be obtained through the temporal bone window. Hyperostosis occurs both unilaterally and bilaterally. Suboptimal windows provide some degree of penetration, but the numbers of arteries that can be identified are often limited. In patients without temporal access, a limited study using the transorbital and foramen magnum windows is performed.

Although a very light touch is used when the transducer is placed over the eye and care is taken to avoid applying any pressure, in order to avoid any unintentional abrasion do not perform the transorbital approach sooner than 6 weeks postoperative for a recent eye surgery.

There are significant anatomical variations of the circle of Willis causing challenges for accurate vessel identification, especially using nonimaging TCD. Anatomic anomalies include differences in the origin, caliber, and course of arteries. Problem areas include confusing the TICA with the PCA$_1$, and differentiating the right from the left VAs and the level of their exact confluence. Accuracy is low in the distal third of the BA because of the great depths required for its insonation and tortuosity.

PITFALLS

The accuracy of TCD findings is operator dependent. The learning curve is significant, requiring a minimum

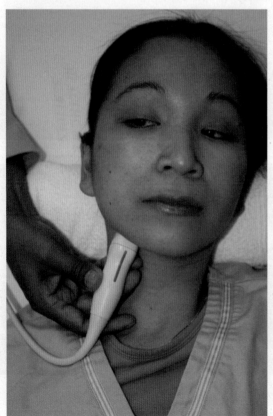

A

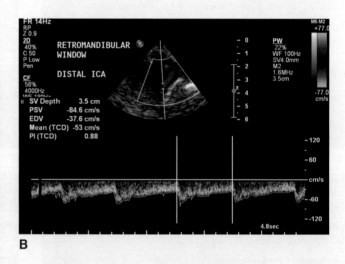

B

Figure 7-23 **A:** Transducer placement for the submandibular approach to the ICA. **B:** Color and spectral Doppler taken from the submandibular ICA.

of 6 months' testing experience and at least 100 abnormal studies with correlations for proficiency.

The calculation of velocity from the Doppler-shifted frequencies depends on the angle of insonation. Using a nonimaging technique, the angle is not measured and is operator dependent, requiring skill in obtaining the signal with the highest audible pitch and therefore the highest velocity.

Patient cooperation is required to obtain an accurate study; some patients may be agitated and unable to remain still and quiet.

In the setting of severe stenosis, vasospasm, collateral flow, and hyperemia, there can be very high velocities. Aliasing of the pulsed wave Doppler can occur and should be recognized.

DIAGNOSIS

Both TCD and TCDI rely on the Doppler spectral waveforms for interpretation of normal and abnormal exams. Normal Doppler spectral values have been established for each arterial segment. TCD interpretation requires a solid understanding of flow dynamics, systemic physiological variables that impact the cerebral circulation, and strong pattern recognition skills (see Table 7-2). The primary diagnostic features of the signals include (1) alteration in velocity, (2) deviations from laminar flow, (3) changes in pulsatility, and (4) changes in the direction of flow. Adjacent artery ratios, side-to-side, and extracranial-to-intracranial indices have been developed to help differentiate various findings.

The spectral waveform parameters include:
- Velocity: This is usually expressed in centimeters per second. Spectral analysis allows the quantification of the PSV, EDV, and TAP-V (commonly referred to as simply "mean velocity"). The mean velocity is the primary diagnostic feature used in TCD and TCDI.
- Pulsatility: In adults this is expressed as Gosling's pulsatility index (PI), which is calculated as:

$$PI = \frac{(PSV - EDV)}{TAP\text{-}V}$$

- Disturbed or turbulent flow: This is represented in the spectral waveform as high-amplitude, low-velocity signals and flow velocities below the zero baseline. It is also apparent as a disruption of the smooth contour of the waveform outer envelope.
- Systolic upstroke: This is the initial slope of the peak velocity envelope during the acceleration phase of systole.

- Lindegaard ratio: This is calculated as the MCA mean velocity divided by the submandibular ICA mean velocity. This ratio is useful in differentiating increased volume flow from a decreased diameter when high velocities are encountered in the MCA or intracranial ICA.
- Sviri ratio: This ratio is similar to the Lindegaard ratio for determining vasospasm from hyperdynamic flow in the posterior circulation. The bilateral VA mean velocities taken at the atlas loop are added together and averaged. This averaged velocity is then divided into the highest BA mean velocity (Fig. 7-24).

APPLICATIONS FOR INTRACRANIAL CEREBROVASCULAR EXAMINATIONS

There are multiple applications for intracranial cerebrovascular examinations. These applications have expanded over the years. As the technology has continued to advance, this has lead to further applicability for intracranial cerebrovascular evaluations. Pathology Box 7-1 lists some of the common abnormalities observed during TCD or TCDI examination.

TCD FINDINGS IN EXTRACRANIAL CAROTID ARTERY DISEASE—COLLATERAL FLOW

When an extracranial carotid artery stenosis reaches hemodynamic significance, the brain will compensate through the mechanisms of collateral flow and autoregulation. TCD is useful in identifying and assessing the presence and adequacy of collateral circulation and improving the understanding of the individual cerebral circulatory function and status. TCD assessment of cerebral collateralization also helps predict hemodynamic consequences of cross-clamping during carotid endarterectomy. There are three primary collateral patterns that can be accurately determined using TCD, and the diagnostic criteria for each collateral type are listed in the following sections (Fig. 7-25).

External Carotid to Internal Carotid through a Reversed Ophthalmic Artery[22,23]

- Direct evidence of carotid artery disease
- Retrograde flow in the OA
- Decreased pulsatility and increased velocity in the OA
- Obliteration, diminishment, or reversal of flow in the OA with compression of the branches of the ECA (superficial temporal, facial, or angular arteries)

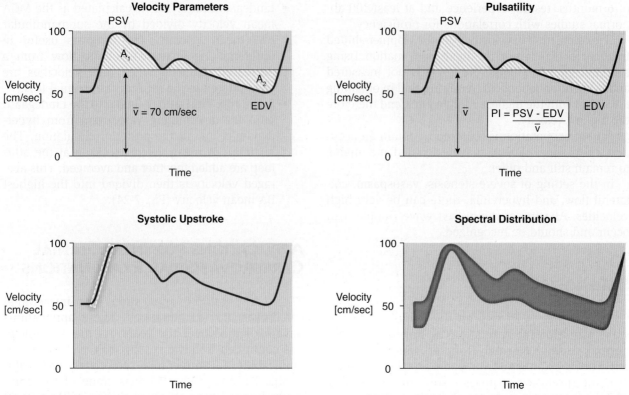

Figure 7-24 Diagnostic features of spectral waveforms for interpretation of TCD studies: mean velocity, pulsatility index, systolic upstroke, and distribution of the amplitude within the waveform.

Crossover Collateral through the Anterior Communicating Artery

- Direct evidence of carotid artery disease.
- Retrograde flow in the ACA, A_1 segment ipsilateral to the carotid disease.
- Increased flow velocities in the contralateral ACA (ACA mean velocity/ipsilateral MCA mean velocity >150%). The increase in velocity is related to the increase in volume flow as well as the diameter of the vessel carrying that increased volume. In individual cases, there can be crossover collateral with normal ACA velocities due to the large diameter of the ACA.
- There are usually very high velocities detected at midline in the small ACOA.

The accuracy of TCD in the identification of intracranial crossover collateralization through the ACOA in experienced laboratories has a sensitivity of 93%, a specificity of 100%, and an accuracy of 98%.[23,24]

PATHOLOGY BOX 7-1

Common Pathology Observed on TCD or TCDI Examinations

Pathology	Examination Findings
Stenosis	• Focal increase in velocity • Poststenotic turbulence • Greater than 30 cm/s hemispheric difference • Refer to Table 7-3 for complete criteria
Occlusion (acute, total)	• Absent flow on color imaging and Doppler • High resistance signal proximal to occlusion
Vasospasm (severe)	• MCA velocity >200 cm/s • Can be present in more than one artery • Temporal changes
Emboli	• Brief signal lasting <300 ms • Amplitude at least 3 dB above background • Unidirectional signal • Signal has snap, chirp, or moan sound

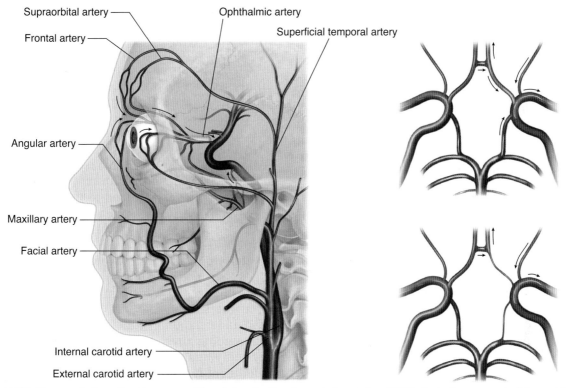

Supraorbital artery

Ophthalmic artery

Frontal artery

Superficial temporal artery

Angular artery

Maxillary artery

Facial artery

Internal carotid artery

External carotid artery

Figure 7-25 Changes in flow direction seen with collateralization through the circle of Willis, including reversal of the ophthalmic artery and reversal of the ACA ipsilateral to the stenosis/occlusion in the ICA.

Posterior to Anterior Collateral through the Posterior Communicating Artery

- Direct evidence of carotid artery disease
- Increased flow velocities in the ipsilateral PCA, P1 segment (PCA mean velocity/ipsilateral MCA mean velocity >125%)
- In individual cases, there can be PCOA collateral with lower velocities due to the large diameter and capacity of the collateral vessel
- Velocities in the PCOA, when detected, are usually quite high

The accuracy of TCD in the identification of posterior to anterior collateralization through the PCOA have been shown to have a sensitivity of 87%, a specificity of 96%, and an accuracy of 92%.[23,24]

Leptomeningeal Collateralization

Ipsilateral to a hemodynamically significant stenosis or occlusion of the main trunk of the MCA, high velocities may be observed in the ACA and PCA due to leptomeningeal collateralization.

INTRACRANIAL STENOSIS AND OCCLUSION

Intracranial arterial narrowing is a complicated subject with multiple causative factors and resultant complex pathophysiology. In general, stenoses and occlusions can be caused by intrinsic conditions and thromboembolic phenomena. TCD is useful for detection of >50% intracranial stenoses and occlusions.[24] It is a reliable diagnostic tool for finding disease if limitations and sources of error are carefully considered.

There are multiple conditions that produce intrinsic narrowing of the cerebral arteries, the most common being atherosclerotic disease. Additional uncommon noninflammatory conditions include dissection, fibromuscular dysplasia, radiation-induced vasculopathy, and Moyamoya disease. There are also a host of inflammatory vasculopathies and hematologic causes of stroke that may affect the basal cerebral vessels including temporal arteritis, meningitis, toxin-related vasculitis, and sickle cell disease.

Atherosclerosis

Approximately 9% or between 70,000 and 90,000 strokes in the United States every year result from intracranial atherosclerosis (ASO).[25] The effect of this disease is more significant for African Americans, Asians, and Hispanics[25-27] and the incidence of recurrent stroke in this population is high—reported to be up to 15% per year.[28,29]

ASO of the intracranial arteries involves the cavernous ICA, MCA, ACA, VA, BA, and PCAs. The four known factors that increase the risk of large artery atherosclerotic stenosis are hyperlipidemia, arterial hypertension, cigarette smoking, and diabetes mellitus.[30] Intracranial lesions may cause microemboli, which migrate into distal vascular territories causing ischemia and/or progress to significant severity or occlusion, which may result in perfusion failure, most notably in the absence of adequate collateral capacity. This latter may be a function of the site of the lesion, especially if it is located distal to the circle of Willis or due to anatomic anomalies.

Posterior Circulation

In the past, anterior circulation disease was better understood than posterior circulation. Caplan et al. developed a Posterior Circulation Registry (PCR) of patients with posterior circulation transient ischemic attacks (TIAs) or stroke. In their analysis, the incidence of intracranial VA stenosis was equal to that of the extracranial segments.

In the PCR, intracranial VA stenosis was present in 32% of patients, some bilaterally, and 2% had BA disease. Embolism was the most common mechanism of posterior circulation stroke with a preponderance of cardiac-origin embolism versus artery to artery. Additionally, poor outcomes were associated with cardiogenic embolism.[31]

Criteria for Intracranial Stenosis

As early as 1990, TCD criteria for stenosis and occlusion of the carotid siphon and MCA were reported in a large group of patients with TIA and stroke. In this seminal report by Ley-Poso and Ringelstein, 133 patients had TCD studies and conventional angiograms. Using multiple criteria, including focal velocity increases the site of stenosis, side-to-side velocity differences in analogous arteries, downstream hemodynamic effects in the spectral waveforms, and total lack of signal with positive identification of neighboring vessels, good results were achieved. The overall diagnostic accuracy for any lesion was 95.7%, with a sensitivity of 91.7%, and a specificity of 96.5%.[32]

Interpreting spectral waveforms requires knowledge of normal and abnormal values; appreciation of the changes in waveform morphology proximal to, at the site of, and distal to a stenosis; and a good understanding of the complex and sometimes confounding physiological variables that coexist in any individual patient at any point in time. The criteria put forth in Table 7-3 are useful as preliminary measurements. There are multiple systemic factors that significantly influence velocities and need to be factored in including age, heart rate, blood pressure, hematocrit, fever, and CO_2 levels (Table 7-3).[33]

TABLE 7-3					
Stenosis Criteria for the MCA (Middle Cerebral), ICA (Carotid Siphon), ACA/A1 (Anterior Cerebral), PCA/P1 (Posterior Cerebral), and Vertebral and Basilar Arteries					
Segment	Depth (mm)	Mean Velocity (cm/s)	Hemispheric Difference (cm/s)	Ratio to Adjacent Artery	Waveform Characteristics (Poststenotic)
MCA proximal	50–65	80–100	>30	>2 ≥50% >3 ≥70%	Turbulence, slow systolic upstroke, covibrations
MCA distal	40–50	80–100	>30	>2 ≥50% >3 ≥70%	Turbulence, slow systolic upstroke, covibrations
ICA (siphon)	55–65	70–90	>30	N/A	Turbulence, slow systolic upstroke, covibrations
ACA (A1)	65–75	>70	>30	ACA > MCA	Turbulence, slow systolic upstroke, covibrations
PCA	56–65	>50	N/A	PCA > ACA/ICA	Turbulence, slow systolic upstroke, covibrations
Basilar	75–110	>60	N/A	>30 cm/s	Turbulence, slow systolic upstroke, covibrations
Vertebral	40–75	>50	N/A	>30 cm/s	Turbulence, slow systolic upstroke, covibrations

Velocities represent mean values. The hemispheric difference compares the same artery on the contralateral side of disease. Ratio to an adjacent artery compares the diseased artery with a normal proximal segment of the same vessel or a homologous vessel.

Embolic Stenosis and Occlusion

The most common cause of occlusion beyond the circle of Willis is embolism, accounting for 15% to 30% of strokes, most of which occur in the territory of the MCA.[34] Several types of cardiac disease lead to cerebral embolism causing stenosis and occlusion including cardiac arrhythmias, ischemic heart disease, valvular disease, dilated cardiomyopathies, atrial septal abnormalities, and intracardiac tumors. Other sources of emboli include aortic arch atheroma, extracranial carotid and VA plaque, and crossing of a venous thrombus into the arterial tree in patients with patent foramen ovale.[31]

The use of cerebrovascular ultrasound in acute stroke requires a modified protocol that allows rapid insonation of the affected territory, supply arteries, and quick interpretation of the data. TCD can provide significant information regarding a thrombus in acute intracranial arterial occlusion, often a dynamic process that can involve recanalization. A TCD flow grading system was developed by Demchuk to predict the success of intracranial clot lysis and short-term improvement after ischemic stroke. Thrombolysis in brain ischemia (TIBI) measures residual flow around the clot and, in general, a larger amount of residual flow predicts the success of the thrombolysis.[35] For acute thrombosis, the TIBI scale is used to classify changes that can occur rapidly with recanalization and reocclusion in acute stroke (Table 7-4).

VASOSPASM

SAH, one of the most devastating types of stroke, accounts for 5% to 15% of all strokes and is fatal or disabling in about 60% of patients.[36,37] These patients suffer the initial effect of an intracranial bleed, the risks and complications associated with surgical or interventional treatments, and the sequelae of a host of medical complications. One of the most significant causes of delayed ischemic neurological deficits (DINDS) is the development of cerebral vasospasm during the first 2-week period following the initial bleed. The pathophysiology, diagnosis, prevention, and treatment of vasospasm continue to be topics of intense investigation aimed at improving clinical outcomes for these patients.

Cerebral vasospasm is the transient and delayed narrowing of the basal cerebral arteries following SAH, and the exact cause remains the subject of intense study. It is mainly seen in the large skull base arteries and, less frequently, in the distal branches of these vessels, and it is responsible for the significant morbidity and mortality seen in this population. The onset of arterial contraction, as demonstrated by angiography, begins 3 to 4 days following the initial bleed; peak narrowing develops at 6 to 8 days; and resolution occurs at 2 to 4 weeks post-SAH.[38] The incidence of angiographic vasospasm after SAH is greater than 50%, with symptomatic vasospasm affecting one-third of all aneurysmal SAH patients.[39] Neurological deficits caused by cerebral vasospasm may resolve or progress to infarction or death in spite of maximal therapy.

The medical management of cerebral vasospasm relies on hemodynamic therapy to improve cerebral blood flow. Calcium channel antagonists are widely used and have been shown to reduce poor outcomes. In patients with a clinically significant vasospasm that does not respond to maximal medical therapy, balloon angioplasty has been shown to be effective, improving neurological deficits. The timing of angioplasty is significant and patients need to be treated before cerebral infarction occurs.

In 2004, the American Academy of Neurology (AAN) published a special article addressing the use of TCD and TCDI for the diagnosis of multiple intracranial vascular abnormalities according to a rating

TABLE 7-4		
TIBI Scale for TCD Detection of MCA Recanalization during and following Thrombolytic Therapy		
TIBI Score	**MCA Flow (DSA)**	**TCD Signal Description**
0	Occluded with no residual flow	Absent, no flow signal
1	No antegrade residual flow	Low systolic only velocity signal
2	Subtotal occlusion with sluggish antegrade flow	Low velocity, damped systolic and diastolic signal, with slow systolic acceleration, with a PI <1.2
3	Subtotal occlusion with sluggish antegrade flow	High PI >1.2, systolic dominant signal with >30% decrease in velocity compared with contralateral MCA
4	Stenotic with recanalization	Increased velocity of >80 cm/s or >30% higher than contralateral MCA
5	Normal flow with total recanalization	Velocity comparable to contralateral MCA with <30% difference and similar PI

system. They gave TCD the highest rating (type A, class I to II evidence) when used for the detection and monitoring of angiographic vasospasm in the basal segments of the intracranial arteries, especially the MCA and BA.[40]

The goals of TCD in the setting of SAH are to detect elevated blood velocities that indicate cerebral vasospasm and identify patients at risk for DINDS. These patients are studied daily for detection of the onset, location, degree, and resolution of vasospasm for approximately 2 weeks following their initial bleed.

Accuracy of TCD is dependent on the expertise of the sonographer doing the studies. Interpretation is complicated in this setting by a set of potentially changing factors such as intracranial pressure, blood pressure, hematocrit, arterial CO_2, collateral flow, autoregulation, and responses to therapeutic interventions. TCD results in the anterior circulation are most reliable in the MCA. Mean flow velocities in the MCA ≥ 200 cm/s, a rapid daily rise in flow velocities, and a hemispheric ratio ≥ 6.0 predicts the presence of significant ($>50\%$ diameter reduction) angiographic MCA vasospasm.[41,42]

TCD is used in combination with cerebral blood flow (CBF) studies to facilitate treatment decisions. CBF studies measure perfusion to the brain territory affected by vasospasm. Often, the clinical exam on SAH patients is imprecise due to the severity of their condition. Complimentary TCD and CBF data inform the clinician in determining the appropriate treatments and their timing during the 2-week period when patients are at risk for a secondary ischemic insult from vasospasm.

More research is needed to better define exact velocity criteria for each arterial segment and by far the MCA has the highest correlative accuracy against cerebral angiography. More prospective studies are warranted to determine the predictive value for the posterior circulation (Table 7-5).[46]

EMBOLI MONITORING

TCD can be used to monitor for emboli during various procedures including carotid endarterectomy, carotid stenting, cardiopulmonary bypass surgery, and neurological procedures. A headband is used to secure the TCD transducer in place for continuous monitoring. Typically, the MCA is the vessel monitored for emboli. Most manufacturers have software within the TCD systems that will automatically count the number of microemboli. Microembolic signals (MESs) have also been referred to as high-intensity transient signals (HITSs) (Fig. 7-26). They have four characteristic components: (1) the signal is very short or brief, usually lasting for less than 300 ms; (2) the amplitude of the TCD signal must be at least 3 dB above the

TABLE 7-5

Vasospasm Criteria for Each Arterial Segment

Vasospasm Criteria	Velocity (cm/s)	Lindegaard or Sviri Ratio
MCA and ICA		
Mild	120–149	>3.0
Moderate	150–199	>3.0
Severe	>200	>6.0
Hyperdynamic flow	>80	<3.0
ACA		
Vasospasm (not graded)	>130	
Vasospasm versus collateral flow	>130	With the presence of MCA and/or ICA vasospasm
PCA		
Vasospasm (not graded)	>110	
Vasospasm versus collateral flow	>110	With the presence of MCA and/or ICA vasospasm
VA		
Vasospasm	>80	
BA		
Possible vasospasm	70–84	>2.0
Moderate/severe vasospasm	>85	>2.5
Severe vasospasm	>85	>3.0

background signals; (3) the signal is mainly unidirectional within the spectral waveform; and (4) the signal will produce a characteristic audible sound, which has been described as a "snap," "chirp," or "moan."[43]

The information gathered during the monitoring for emboli can be used to modify surgical techniques in order to reduce the risk of stroke. Pharmacologic interventions may also be used based on microembolic monitoring. The specific alterations during a procedure based on microemboli detection will vary depending on the surgeon, the patient, the number of microemboli, and the procedure being performed.

DETECTION OF CARDIAC SHUNTS

TCD can be used to detect the presence of a patent foramen ovale (PFO) or other right to left cardiac shunts.[44] The technique, often referred to as a bubble study, involves the intravenous injection of agitated

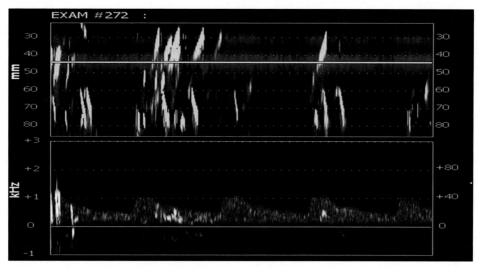

Figure 7-26 Example of a TCD signal illustrating the presence of microemboli. The bright white areas within the spectral waveform and within the m-mode tracing indicate microemboli.

saline mixed with air. A cardiac shunt is confirmed when there are HITS detected while monitoring the MCA using TCD. The more HITS detected, the more severe the cardiac shunt.

BRAIN DEATH

There are clinical criteria used in the determination of brain death. In addition, there are electroencephalographic criteria that must be met. Another parameter that is evaluated is the absence of intracranial circulation. TCD can be used to document cerebral circulatory arrest, which produces a characteristic to-and-fro TCD waveform. The waveforms have also been described as oscillatory or as reverberating signals. The waveform consists of a short systolic spike followed by either a small retrograde deflection in diastole or no flow in diastole. It should be mentioned that TCD is not used alone to make a diagnosis of brain death. TCD waveforms are used to correlate with other diagnostic tests as well as clinical criteria of brain death.[45]

SICKLE CELL DISEASE

TCD and TCDI play a vital role in evaluating children with sickle cell disease. These patients are prone to stroke involving the MCA and ACA. The Stroke Prevention Trial in Sickle Cell Anemia (STOP) study demonstrated that early detection of abnormal MCA velocities by TCD and subsequent initiation of a blood transfusion program was successful in reducing the rate of the first stroke.[46] The STOP trial also set the criteria for MCA velocities. If the MCA

mean velocity is less than 170 cm/s, it is considered normal in this patient group. A velocity of at least 170 cm/s but less than 200 cm/s is considered conditional or borderline. An MCA mean velocity ≥200 cm/s is considered abnormal. It is the current clinical practice to have all children with sickle cell disease undergo routine annual TCD screening. If the MCA velocities are found to be abnormal, then transfusion is recommended.

THE USE OF TCD WITH ACUTE STROKE

There has been increasing use of thrombolytic agents in patients with acute stroke. TCD plays an important role in patient selection as well as monitoring of these patients during and following these procedures. With constant TCD monitoring during the infusion of a thrombolytic agent, changes in MCA velocities can be immediately observed and provides an accurate and noninvasive tool to assess the recanalization procedure.[47]

A more recent expansion for the role of TCD includes its use to enhance the effect of thrombolytic agents. The success of a thrombolytic agent relies on the ability of the agent to come in contact with the thrombus. The more the agent can permeate a thrombus, the faster the lysis will occur. Ultrasound can provide mechanical energy to the thrombus interfaces and stagnant flow areas. Ultrasound can disaggregate portions of the fibrin stands, moving them slightly, which will promote flow through the area and aid in the delivery of the lytic agent.[48] Extensive research continues in this application for TCD.

SUMMARY

Intracranial cerebrovascular examinations with transcranial Doppler techniques can provide a vast amount of anatomic and physiologic data. The examination of the intracranial vessels requires extensive knowledge of anatomy and meticulous attention to technique. Various disease states can be evaluated with transcranial Doppler or transcranial imaging. A thorough understanding of the intracranial vessels will aid in the successful evaluation of patients presenting with suspected intracranial vascular disease.

Critical Thinking Questions

1. A TCD needs to be performed on a hospital inpatient that cannot be placed in a lateral decubitus position. Can the VAs and BA still be insonated and, if so, how?

2. While reviewing images from a TCD exam, should one expect to observe low resistance or high resistance signals?

3. When scanning via the transtemporal approach, two vessels are observed that appear to have branches. In order to determine which vessels are in view, what additional information needs to be taken into consideration?

4. A patient will require continued monitoring of MCA velocities. Which type of ultrasound probe would be best for this application and why?

REFERENCES

1. Aaslid R, Markwalder TM, Nornes H. Noninvasive transcranial Doppler ultrasound recording of flow velocity in cerebral arteries. *J Neurosurg.* 1982;57:769–774.
2. von Reutern GM, von Budingen HJ. *Ultrasound Diagnosis of Cerebrovascular Disease.* New York, NY: Thieme Medical Publishers; 1993.
3. Gabrielsen TO, Greitz T. Normal size of the internal carotid, middle cerebral and anterior cerebral arteries. *Acta Radiol Diagnosis.* 1970;101:68–87.
4. Lang J. Neurokranium, orbita, kraniozervikaler ubergang [Neurocranium, orbit, craniocervical transition]. *Klinische Anatomie des Kopfes.* [Clinical anatomy of the head]. Berlin, Germany: Springer; 1981.
5. Hodes PJ, Campy F, Riggs HE, et al. Cerebral angiography: fundamentals in anatomy and physiology. *Am J Roentgenol.* 1953;70:61–82.
6. Taveras JM, Wood EH. *Diagnostic Neuroradiology.* Baltimore, MD: Williams and Wilkins; 1976.
7. Alexandrov AV, Sloan MA, Wong LKS. Practice standards for transcranial Doppler ultrasound: part I—test performance. *J Neuroimaging.* 2006;17:11–18.
8. Alexandrov AV, Demchuk AM, Wein TH, et al. The yield of transcranial Doppler in acute cerebral ischemia. *Stroke.* 1999;30:1605–1609.
9. Spencer MP, Whisler D. Transorbital Doppler diagnosis of intracranial arterial stenosis. *Stroke.* 1986;17:916–921.
10. Aaslid R, ed. *Transcranial Doppler Sonography.* New York, NY: Springer-Verlag; 1986.
11. Arnolds BJ, von Reutern MG. Transcranial Doppler sonography. Examination techniques and normal reference values. *Ultrasound Med Biol.* 1986;12:115–123.
12. Lindegaard KF, Nornes H, Bakke SJ, et al. Cerebral vasospasm diagnosis by means of angiography and blood velocity measurements. *Acta Neurochir.* 1989;100:12–24.
13. Lindegaard KF. The role of transcranial Doppler in the management of patients with subarachnoid haemorrhage: a review. *Acta Neurochir.* 1999;72:59–71.
14. Soustiel JF, Shik V, Shreiber R, et al. Basilar vasospasm diagnosis: investigation of a modified "Lindegaard Index" based on imaging studies and blood velocity measurements of the basilar artery. *Stroke.* 2002;33:72–77.

15. Sviri GE, Ghodke B, Britz GW. Transcranial Doppler grading criteria for basilar artery vasospasm. *Neurosurg.* 2006;59:360–366.

16. Grolimund P. Transmission of ultrasound through the temporal bone. In: Aaslid A, ed. *Transcranial Doppler Sonography.* New York, NY: Springer-Verlag; 1986:10–21.

17. Ringelstein EB. A practical guide to transcranial Doppler sonography. In: Weinberger J, ed. *Noninvasive Imaging of Cerebrovascular Disease.* New York, NY: Alan R. Liss; 1989:75–121.

18. Martin PJ, Evans DH, Naylor AR. Transcranial color-coded sonography of the basal cerebral circulation reference data from 115 volunteers. *Stroke.* 1994;25:390–396.

19. Alexandrov AV, Demchuk AM, Burgin WS. Insonation method and diagnostic flow signatures for transcranial power motion (M-mode) Doppler. *J Neuroimaging.* 2002;12:236–244.

20. Schulte-Altedorneburg G, Droste DW, Popa V, et al. Visualization of the basilar artery by transcranial color-coded duplex sonography: comparison with postmortem results. *Stroke.* 2000;31:1123–1127.

21. Newell DW, Winn HR. Transcranial Doppler in cerebral vasospasm. *Neurosurg Clin N Am.* 1990;1:1–28.

22. Lindegaard K, Bakke S, Grolimund P. Assessment of intracranial hemodynamics in carotid artery disease by transcranial Doppler ultrasound. *J Neurosurg.* 1985;63:890–898.

23. Fujioka KA, Nonoshita-Karr L. The effects of extracranial arterial occlusive disease. *J Vasc Tech.* 2000;24(1):27–32.

24. Felberg RA, Christou I, Demchuk Am, et al. Screening for intracranial stenosis with transcranial Doppler: the accuracy of mean flow velocity thresholds. *J Neuroimaging.* 2002;12(1):9–14.

25. Sacco RL, Kargman DE, Gu Q, et al. Race–ethnicity and determinants of intracranial atherosclerotic cerebral infarction. The Northern Manhattan Stroke Study. *Stroke.* 1995;26:14–20.

26. Wityk RJ, Lehman D, Klag M, et al. Race and sex differences in the distribution of cerebral atherosclerosis. *Stroke.* 1996;27:1974–1980.

27. Feldmann E, Daneault N, Kwan E, et al. Chinese-white differences in the distribution of occlusive cerebrovascular disease. *Neurology.* 1990;40:1541–1545.

28. Jiang WJ, Wang YJ, Du B, et al. Stenting of symptomatic M1 stenosis of middle cerebral artery: an initial experience of 40 patients. *Stroke.* 2004;35:1375–1380.

29. The Warfarin-Aspirin Symptomatic Intracranial disease (WASID) Study Group. Prognosis of patients with symptomatic vertebral or basilar artery stenosis. *Stroke.* 1998;29:1389–1392.

30. Chaves CJ, Jones HR. Ischemic stroke. In: Jones HR, ed. *Netter's Neurology.* Teterboro, NJ: Icon Learning Systems; 2005:195–199.

31. Caplan LR, Wityk RJ, Glass TA, et al. New England Medical Center Posterior Circulation Registry. *Ann Neurol.* 2004;56:389–398.

32. Ley-Pozo J, Ringelstein EB. Noninvasive detection of occlusive disease of the carotid siphon and middle cerebral artery. *Ann Neurol.* 1990;28:640–647.

33. Alexandrov A, Neumyer M. Diagnostic criteria for cerebrovascular ultrasound. In: Alexandrov A, ed. *Cerebrovascular Ultrasound in Stroke Prevention and Treatment.* New York, NY: Futura–Blackwell, 2004:99–102.

34. Mohr JP, Lazar RM, Marshall RS, et al. Middle cerebral artery disease. In: Mohr JR, Choi DW, Grotta JC, et al., eds. *Stroke Pathophysiology, Diagnosis, and Management.* 4th ed. Philadelphia, PA: Churchill Livingstone; 2004:125–126.

35. Demchuk AM, Burgin WS, Christou I, et al. Thrombolysis in brain ischemia (TIBI) transcranial Doppler flow grades predict clinical severity, early recovery, and mortality in patients treated with tissue plasminogen activator. *Stroke.* 2001;32:89–93.

36. Bederson J, Awad IA, Wiebers DO, et al. Recommendations for the management of patients with unruptured intracranial aneurysms. *Circulation.* 2000;102:2300–2308.

37. Bederson JB, Awad IA, Wiebers DO. Recommendations for the management of patients with unruptured intracranial aneurysms: a statement for healthcare professionals from the Stroke Council of the American Heart Association. *Stroke.* 2000;31:2742–2750.

38. Weir B, Grace M, Hansen J, et al. Time course of vasospasm in man. *J Neurosurg.* 1978;48(2):173–178.

39. Dorsch NWC, King MT. A review of cerebral vasospasm in aneurismal subarachnoid haemorrhage: I. Incidence and effects. *J Clin Neurosci.* 1994;1(1):19–24.

40. Sloan MA, Alexandrov AV, Tegeler CH, et al. Assessment: transcranial Doppler ultrasonography: report of the therapeutics and technology assessment subcommittee of the American Academy of Neurology. *Neurology.* 2004;62:1468–1481.

41. Aaslid R, Huber R, Nornes H. Evaluation of cerebrovascular spasm with transcranial Doppler ultrasound. *J Neurosurg.* 1984;60(1):37–41.

42. Kincaid MS, Souter MF, Treggiari MM. Accuracy of transcranial Doppler ultrasonography and single-photon emission computed tomography in the diagnosis of angiographically demonstrated cerebral vasospasm. *J Neurosurg.* 2009;110(1):67–72.

43. Consensus Committee of the Ninth International Cerebral Hemodynamic Symposium. Basic identification criteria of Doppler microembolic signals. *Stroke.* 1995;26(6):1123.

44. Blersch WK, Draganski BM, Holmer SR, et al. Transcranial duplex sonography in the detection of patent foramen ovale. *Radiology.* 2002;225:693–699.

45. Wijdicks EFM. The diagnosis of brain death. *N Engl J Med.* 2001;344:1215–1221.

46. Adams RJ, McKie VC, Hsu L, et al. Prevention of a first stroke by transfusions in children with sickle cell anemia and abnormal results on transcranial Doppler ultrasonography. *N Engl J Med.* 1998;339:5–11.

47. Rubiera M, Cava L, Tsivgoulis G, et al. Diagnostic criteria and yield of real-time transcranial Doppler monitoring of intra-arterial reperfusion procedures. *Stroke.* 2010;41:695–699.

48. Alexandrov AV. Ultrasound enhancement of fibrinolysis. *Stroke.* 2009;40:S107–S110.

8 Indirect Assessment of Arterial Disease

Terry Needham

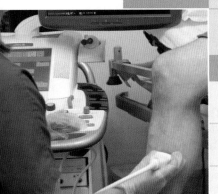

OBJECTIVES

Describe the types of indirect testing including systolic pressure measurements, Doppler waveforms, and plethysmography

Identify normal and abnormal continuous wave and plethysmographic waveforms

Define the various signs and symptoms associated with peripheral arterial occlusive disease

List the indirect testing techniques employed in an upper extremity evaluation

KEY TERMS

ankle-brachial index | claudication | photoplethysmography | plethysmography | rest pain

GLOSSARY

Allen test a series of maneuvers testing the digital perfusion of the hand while compressing and releasing the radial and ulnar arteries

ankle–brachial index the ratio of ankle systolic pressure to brachial systolic pressure

claudication pain in muscle groups brought on by exercise or activity that recedes with cessation of activity; can occur in the calf, thigh, and buttock

photoplethysmography an indirect physiologic test that detects changes in back-scattered infrared light as an indicator of tissue perfusion

plethysmography an indirect physiologic test that measures the change in volume or impedance in a whole body, organ, or limb

Raynaud's disease vasospasm of the digital arteries brought on by exposure to cold; can be caused by numerous etiologies

rest pain pain in the extremity without exercise or activity, thus "at rest"; can occur in the toes, feet, or ankle area

thoracic outlet syndrome compression of the brachial nerve plexus, subclavian artery, or subclavian vein at the region where these structures exit the thoracic cavity and course peripherally toward the arm

Indirect (nonimaging) testing modalities can be reliable for detecting the presence of peripheral arterial occlusive disease (PAOD) affecting the extremities and for categorizing its overall severity. The most common symptom of PAOD affecting the lower extremities is leg discomfort caused by activity, but which abates with cessation of the activity. This is termed intermittent claudication. Patients may describe the sensation of intermittent claudication as fatigue, or as a cramping, aching, or tiredness sensation, usually starting in the calf and perhaps progressing to the thigh and/or buttocks, according

TABLE 8-1

Variations in Leg Pain

Condition	Location	Associated with Exercise?	Relieved by?
Intermittent claudication	Buttock, thigh, hip, calf	Always	Stopping
Spinal stenosis	As previous	Yes, but also with standing	Sitting; flexing and moving spine
Herniated disc	Radiates down leg	Variable	Varies; aspirin or anti-inflammatories
Osteoarthritis	Hips, knees, ankles	Variable, not always produced	Varies; aspirin or anti-inflammatories

to the site and severity of the disease. The amount of activity that produces the symptoms can remain fairly reproducible for long periods unless there is accelerated progression of the PAOD. The site of the symptoms indicate the site(s) of the disease because they occur distal to the disease process, so claudication limited to the calf is associated with superficial femoral/popliteal or tibial artery disease, thigh symptoms with iliofemoral artery disease, and buttock claudication with either ipsilateral iliofemoral (if unilateral) or aortoiliac disease when bilateral.

It is important to distinguish between the causes of leg discomfort resulting from activity, especially for the mechanism(s) that result in the loss of postactivity symptoms.[1] Cessation of symptoms with quiet standing corresponds to true ischemic intermittent claudication, whereas correction requiring sitting and/or spinal flexure is more associated with spinal stenosis (Table 8-1). Claudication distances will decrease and symptom recovery time will increase as PAOD progresses, sometimes being accompanied by the signs of thickening of toenails and loss of toe hair. At the most severe levels of PAOD, the skin may become discolored and scaly and forefoot pain may be constant with claudication distance less than 50 ft. At these severe levels, raising the leg a foot or so above heart level will usually cause blanching of the skin on the foot, but which becomes red with dependency—elevation pallor/dependent rubor. Blueness of the toes, perhaps unilateral, can be the first indication of aneurysmal disease. This happens with embolization of aneurysm contents into distal segments of the limb and can progress to gangrene. The most common site for a peripheral aneurysm is at popliteal level, although these are associated more with sudden occlusion rather than with embolization.

PAOD in the upper extremity is encountered in <5% of all cases.[2] Typically, it is restricted to numbness, aching or tiredness associated with positional extrinsic compression in the shoulder girdle, or to cold-related vasospasm. Approximately 95% of all extrinsic compression-related symptoms have neurovascular origins, with only 3% to 4% from venous compression and arterial in only 1% to 2%.[3] This spectrum of symptoms are grouped as thoracic outlet syndrome (TOS).

Cold sensitivity is an intense episodic vasospasm related to cold exposure or to emotional stress.[4] It is generally referred to as Raynaud's phenomenon. It comprises both Raynaud's disease (also known as primary Raynaud's phenomenon) and Raynaud's syndrome (or secondary Raynaud's). The cause of primary Raynaud's is idiopathic. Secondary Raynaud's is associated with an underlying process such as scleroderma or trauma. The primary condition is usually bilateral, involving most of the digits (although the thumbs may be spared), whereas secondary causes may be unilateral, perhaps even affecting a single digit.

The various types of nonimaging tests that are commonly used to detect the presence of PAOD include systolic pressure determinations, Doppler waveforms, plethysmography, and photoplethysmography. These tests help determine overall limb perfusion and, thus, serve as an indicator of the functional status of a limb. However, they are less dependable when PAOD occurs at multiple levels because moderate-to-severe disease proximally can reduce flow energy distally, masking the presence of distal PAOD. This chapter will describe these indirect testing modalities, applications for such testing, and diagnostic criteria.

EXAMINATION PREPARATION

Although there are various types of indirect vascular tests, all have similar preparations that are needed prior to the start of testing. Proper patient preparation and positioning are required for adequate results.

PATIENT PREPARATION

The study starts with confirming the identity of the patient and verifying that the study ordered is appropriate to the patient's signs and/or symptoms.

The nature of the study should be explained to the patient and/or to an accompanying adult and an understanding of the explanation should be documented as part of a departmental quality assurance plan.

A relevant PAOD history for lower extremities should include:

- The clinical problem, signs/symptoms, onset/duration, and whether they are stable, improving, or deteriorating
- The site and extent of intermittent claudication and the time for the symptoms to abate following the symptom-producing activity
- Coexisting clinical conditions: stroke/transient ischemic attack, carotid artery disease, heart attack, coronary artery disease, hypertension, diabetes, lipid disorder(s)
- Smoking history
- Family's cardiac/peripheral vascular history
- Exercise activity

For the upper extremities, a similar history to that for the lower extremity should be obtained, excluding intermittent claudication but including the following:

- Symptoms related to positional causes of arm fatigue/numbness/aching
- Symptoms related to cold sensitivity

PATIENT POSITIONING

The examination table should be low enough for the patient to access safely, preferably without using a step stool. The ideal height for this is 22 inches to 24 inches, although this will then be too low for the comfort of the technologist (if standing throughout the test), so the exam table should be able to be elevated. Table width should be sufficient to avoid danger of the patient falling if rolled to a lateral decubitus position (which facilitates access at groin level, according to body habitus). For lower extremity testing, the patient should be supine and the head should be raised slightly on a pillow so that the patient is comfortable, but not so high that heart level is elevated. Legs should be rotated outward slightly, with the knees flexed, allowing access for the Doppler transducer to the popliteal artery.

When using volume plethysmography, the legs should be supported by placing a pillow under the heel to prevent the cuffs from being compressed by the bed, while being careful not to elevate it above heart level. To avoid artifacts from the effect of hydrostatic pressure, systolic pressures should be measured with the point of measurement at the same (horizontal) level as the heart.

For upper extremity testing, the patient position is similar to that for a lower extremity exam, but a pillow behind the knees will reduce back strain and enhance patient comfort. The arm should be abducted *slightly*, supported on a pillow to ensure muscle relaxation, but maintained at heart level—this is particularly important when measuring systolic pressures.

Once the patient has been appropriately positioned, the working height of the exam table should be adjusted (usually, between 28 inches and 32 inches) in accordance with the height of the technologist. Table height can be lower when the exam is carried out with the technologist or sonographer in a sitting position, and this is an acceptable way of reducing back strain for the technical staff. To avoid positional injury to the staff when sitting throughout the study, the equipment should be able to be used without twisting or straining to reach a control. Using a remote control to adjust equipment settings can enhance good ergonomics and may speed up obtaining results (although the technologist or sonographer will benefit from changing positions, during and following the study).

SYSTOLIC PRESSURES

The measurement of systolic blood pressures in the limbs was one of the earliest noninvasive vascular studies performed. Since these early determinations, it was understood that relationships exist between pressure measurements recorded at various points along the arms and legs. Systolic pressures obtained correspond to the pressure in the vessels at the site of the blood pressure cuff and not to the vessels at the level of the transducer that is recording the pressure signals.

EXAMINATION TECHNIQUE

The test starts after 10 to 15 minutes of rest. This resting period allows the patient's blood pressure to normalize in cases where the patient is initially anxious upon entering the examination room. The resting period also ensures peripheral blood flow will be at a resting level and not increased due to any hyperemia, which may have occurred as a result of walking into the testing facility. During this period, the appropriate documentation, as previously mentioned, is obtained.

Blood pressure cuffs are placed around the arms and legs. An appropriate cuff size is important in order to accurately measure blood pressure. The width of the cuff should be at least 20% wider than the diameter of the underlying limb segment.[5] If the cuff is too narrow, a falsely elevated pressure will be measured. Conversely, if the cuff is too wide, a falsely lower pressure will be measured. Using 12-cm cuffs for the brachial measurements is adequate in most patients, but the cuff may need to be wider according

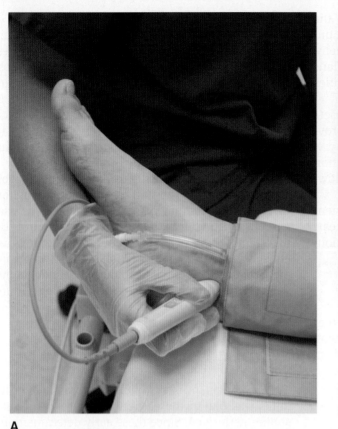
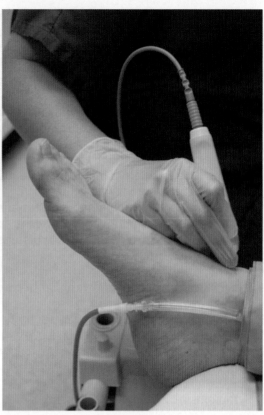

A   **B**

Figure 8-1 Correct transducer position for the insonation of pedal Doppler signals. **A:** Insonation of the posterior tibial artery. **B:** Insonation of the dorsalis pedis artery.

to body habitus. The same applies to the ankle level, where 10-cm cuffs are usually appropriate. For the measurement of an ankle–brachial index, cuffs are placed around the ankle level and around the upper arm. For a multilevel lower extremity examination, cuffs are also placed around the upper arm as well as at thigh, calf, and ankle levels. For upper extremity evaluations, cuffs can be placed around the upper arm, forearm, and wrist levels.

The measurement of a systolic pressure begins with obtaining a Doppler signal distal to the cuff. Figure 8-1 illustrates the correct positioning for insonating pedal Doppler signals. Care must be exercised not to compress the underlying artery with the Doppler transducer (Fig. 8-2), particularly at the posterior tibial, dorsalis pedis, and radial arteries because each courses just above an adjacent bone. While listening to the Doppler signal, the pressure in the cuff is inflated until the audible signal is no longer heard. If the Doppler signal output is also being displayed on a monitor or a strip-chart recorder, this will be seen as a pulsatile waveform (when a Doppler signal is audible) and thus will change to a flat line (once the Doppler signal is no longer audible). The pressure should continue to be inflated 20 mm Hg above this point. The cuff is then slowly deflated

at a rate of approximately 3 mm Hg/s. The pressure at which the audible Doppler signal (or the pulsatile Doppler waveform) returns is the systolic pressure at the level of the cuff. An incorrect pressure measurement can be recorded when a patient is arrhythmic, whereupon several measurements should be made from which to calculate an average systolic pressure.

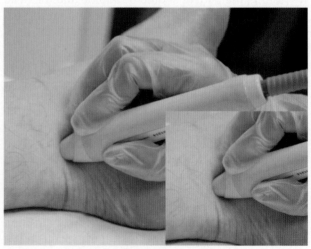

Figure 8-2 Inappropriate transducer pressure is applied to this pedal artery. Such pressure may compress the artery.

ANKLE–BRACHIAL INDICES

The association between reduced limb systolic pressures (measured using plethysmography) and PAOD affecting the lower extremities was explained in the 1950s.[6] The ratio of Doppler systolic pressures at brachial level to those at the ankle was described first in 1969[7] and was termed the ankle systolic pressure index. It is now known as the ankle–brachial index (ABI). Another less commonly used name for this ratio is the ankle–arm index (AAI). ABIs indicate the overall severity of PAOD between the heart and the ankle level.

An ABI is calculated by dividing the highest systolic pressure at ankle level measured at either the posterior tibial artery (PTA) or the dorsalis pedis artery (DPA)/distal anterior tibial artery (ATA) by the higher of the two brachial systolic pressures. An example of an ABI calculation is:

	Right	Left
Brachial	152	146
Posterior tibial artery	112	158
Dorsalis pedis artery	108	154
ABI	**0.74**	**1.04**

The right ABI was derived by dividing the highest ankle systolic pressure (posterior tibial artery pressure: 112 mm Hg) by the higher of the two brachial pressures (152 mm Hg). The left ABI was calculated by dividing 158 mm Hg by 152 mm Hg. An ABI work sheet should document systolic pressures from both brachial arteries as well as both the posterior tibial (PTA) and the dorsalis pedis (DPA)/distal anterior tibial (ATA) arteries at ankle level.

Diagnosis

Although there is variability in published interpretation criteria, those in Table 8-2 are accepted widely. Whatever criteria are used when interpreting repeat studies, an ABI must alter by at least 0.15 before such a change is considered significant.[8]

There is a normal drop of approximately 10 mm Hg in *mean* arterial pressure as blood flows from the heart to distal segments of the lower extremity[9]; however, there is a corresponding increase in the *amplitude* of distal pulses (i.e., the systolic pressure increases while diastolic pressure decreases). This results from the increased peripheral resistance and elastic recoil distally in the extremity. Thus, normal resting ankle systolic pressures tend to be higher than those in the brachial artery; however, they can be slightly lower and still be regarded as normal

TABLE 8-2

Resting Ankle–Brachial Indices Related to the Severity of Peripheral Artery Occlusive Disease (PAOD)

Ankle–Brachial Index	Severity of PAOD
>1.30	Incompressible
0.90–1.30	Normal
0.75–0.89	Mild
0.50–0.74	Moderate
<0.50	Severe
<0.35	Tissue threatening

(see Table 8-2). Initially, the lower limit of a normal resting ABI was reported as 1.0,[7] but subsequently this was modified to be 0.9,[10] especially in patients with hypertension or hypotension.

If the ABI appears to be abnormal, the higher brachial should be measured again to ensure that blood pressure has not systemically dropped enough for it to have been artifactually lowered. At ankle level, the posterior tibial artery usually has a higher systolic pressure than either the dorsalis pedis or the distal anterior tibial arteries.

A significant limitation of the measurement of systolic pressure arises in those patients with calcific vessels. Systolic pressures are invalid when the underlying artery is calcified and incompressible,[11] so interpretations must then rely solely on pulse waveforms and toe systolic pressures (to be discussed later in this chapter). Indication that the underlying artery is calcified occurs when a Doppler signal does not reappear at a clearly defined pressure and it increases in amplitude with further cuff deflation. However, even when medial calcification renders the wall of an ankle artery to be noncompressible, the influence of a *negative* hydrostatic effect (lower extremity raised above heart level) can be used to indicate a minimum systolic pressure. The systolic pressure at ankle level will be at least 50 mm Hg if Doppler signals can still be heard or plethysmographic waveforms remain even slightly pulsatile when the ipsilateral foot is raised 26 inches to 27 inches above heart level, as shown in Figure 8-3.

SEGMENTAL LIMB SYSTOLIC PRESSURES

As stated, an abnormal ABI indicates the overall severity of PAOD, but not necessarily the site(s), especially when it is at more than one level. This multisite limitation occurs when PAOD proximally causes a significant reduction in flow energy into more distal segments, which may have additional disease. In this situation, abnormal drops in systolic pressure may

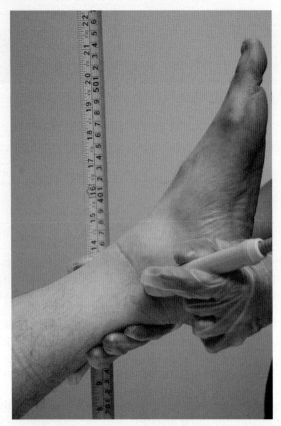

Figure 8-3 When medial calcification renders the wall of an ankle artery to be noncompressible, the influence of a negative hydrostatic effect can be used to estimate the minimum systolic pressure by raising the foot above the level of the heart.

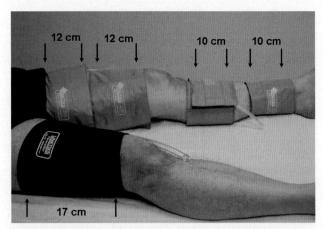

Figure 8-4 Cuff placements for lower extremity segmental pressure determinations. One leg illustrates a four-cuff technique, whereas the other leg illustrates a three-cuff technique.

not be exhibited in the distal segments, although differences in pulse waveforms may be discerned. To some degree, this can be remedied by measuring systolic pressures segmentally, at two or three levels more proximally, in addition to comparing waveforms. The same cuffs can be used for measuring segmental systolic pressures and for volume plethysmography studies, provided that the length of the connecting tubing does not invalidate the calibration of the plethysmograph instrument manufacturer.

When measuring segmental pressures, a choice must be made whether to use one wide cuff (17 or 19 cm) or two narrower cuffs (10 or 12 cm) above the knee (Fig. 8-4). This is often referred to as a three-cuff versus four-cuff method. The three-cuff method uses a single wide, contoured thigh cuff, a calf cuff, and an ankle cuff. The four-cuff method uses two narrower thigh cuffs, one placed high on the thigh around the most proximal segment and the second placed lower, just above the knee, plus a calf and an ankle cuff. Having two cuffs along the thigh allows an interpreter the ability to further define the level of disease by separating iliofemoral disease from superficial femoral artery disease. For the sonographer or vascular technologist, two cuffs present some practical problems.

Often, the thigh may not be long enough to comfortably fit two cuffs side by side along the cuff—there is simply not enough room. In this case, one cuff is usually removed or the protocol is changed to a three-cuff method. In addition, the use of the narrow 10- or 12-cm wide cuffs at the thigh level requires a higher inflation pressure to exert the same compression on the underlying tissue to obtain a systolic pressure measurement. The patient should be informed that the thigh will be squeezed tightly during this pressure measurement and should also be reassured that this should be expected in a normal or near normal limb.

Examination Technique

The technique for measuring segmental systolic pressure measurements is similar to that described earlier for measuring ABIs. Following measurement at ankle level, segmental systolic pressures are then measured at calf and then thigh levels. Although two sites are used to record the ankle pressures (the PT and DP), the technologist or sonographer typically selects the vessel with the greater pressure to insonate when recording the more proximal pressures. In the case where no signals are obtained at the ankle, one can move higher up the limb to obtain a Doppler signal. With the calf cuff in place, the ankle cuff can be removed and a mid-calf level PTA signal can be insonated. If no signal is present at the mid-calf level, a popliteal artery signal can be obtained by placing the Doppler transducer posteriorly in the popliteal fossa.

With cuffs placed around the upper arm, forearm, and wrist, segmental pressures can also be obtained for the arms. Usually both the radial and ulnar artery Doppler signals are insonated and wrist pressures are recorded from both sites. The higher of the two pressures is then used to record systolic pressure at the forearm and upper arm. As with the legs, if Doppler signals are not audible distally (at the wrist level), the Doppler transducer can be placed more proximally over the brachial artery to record the pressure in the upper arm cuff.

Diagnosis

Table 8-3 lists interpretation criteria for the lower extremity. Systolic pressures usually increase as blood flows distally along the lower extremity, although there can also be a slight drop (Table 8-3d). However, any reduction in distal pressure should be <30 mm Hg between adjacent segments (thigh level to calf, calf to ankle) (see Table 8-3i)[12] with drops greater than this being associated with the presence of proximal obstruction.

The width of the thigh cuff(s) changes the criteria when interpreting thigh pressure(s). Normal systolic pressure measured from a single large thigh cuff (17 or 19 cm width) should be equal to the higher of the two brachial pressures (see Table 8-3f). Because narrower cuffs (10 or 12 cm width) require a higher inflation pressure, the normal systolic pressure at high thigh level (using a narrow cuff) needs to be 30 mm Hg or so above the higher brachial pressure (see Table 8-3g).

PAOD is less common in the upper extremity compared with the lower but, when present, it is found most likely in the subclavian and proximal axillary arteries. Table 8-4 lists interpretation criteria for the upper extremity. A ≥75% diameter reduction in either of these arteries will cause a >20 mm Hg difference between brachial systolic pressures. Typically, segmental pressures are accompanied by abnormal

TABLE 8-3
Normal Interpretation Criteria for Lower Extremity
a. Doppler waveforms proximal to knee are triphasic/biphasic and bidirectional
b. Plethysmography waveforms exhibit a dicrotic notch
c. Pulse waveforms have a well-defined peak
d. Resting and postexercise ABIs are 0.90–1.30
e. Resting and postexercise toe-brachial indices are >0.80
f. Single (wide) above knee cuff systolic pressure equal to higher brachial
g. High thigh (narrow) cuff systolic pressure ≥30 mm Hg above higher brachial
h. All pulses have short (<135 ms, if able to be measured) systolic upstroke
i. Difference between adjacent limb segments is ≤30 mm Hg
j. Difference between brachial systolic pressures is ≤20 mm Hg

TABLE 8-4
Normal Interpretation Criteria for Upper Extremity
a. Doppler waveforms are triphasic/biphasic and bidirectional
b. Plethysmography waveforms exhibit a dicrotic notch
c. Pulse waveforms have a well-defined peak
d. Resting and postexercise digit-brachial indices are ≥0.90
e. ≤20 mm Hg systolic pressure gradient between above and below elbow levels
f. Gradient between brachial systolic pressures is ≤20 mm Hg
g. Pulse and temperature recovery time ≤10 minutes

supraclavicular pulse waveforms. Segmentally, there should not be a >20 mm Hg difference between levels above and below the elbow (Table 8-4e).

EXERCISE TESTING

Exercise testing is primarily used to investigate patients with symptoms of intermittent claudication who have normal to near normal (≥0.8) ABIs at rest. The exercise stress can be graduated on a treadmill, by walking at the patient's own pace in a corridor, or with heel raising. Bicycle ergometry and cuff-induced reactive hyperemia are rarely used as substitutes now in the vascular department.

A typical treadmill workload ranges from level to 10% grade and 1 to 2 mph, for a maximum of 5 minutes (or earlier if limited by symptoms). The degree of work is on a patient-by-patient basis. Even if an exercise component is suggested by a normal or near normal ABI, not all patients should be exercised unless they are monitored by a physician or an appropriately qualified health professional. With neither of these persons present, contraindications to treadmill exercise in the peripheral vascular department may be appropriate for patients with any of the following symptoms:

- Chest pain
- Arrhythmias
- Postmyocardial infarction/cardiac procedure and not cleared by their cardiologist
- Unsteadiness
- Hypertension >180 mm Hg

Walking at the patient's own pace and heel raising are valid alternatives to treadmill exercise, but the workload is less reproducible. The sonographer or technologist should accompany a patient being exercised at his or her own pace, walking slightly behind the patient to note the onset of any symptoms, and deciding when the patient should return to the study room. The effects of heel raising (Fig. 8-5) may be

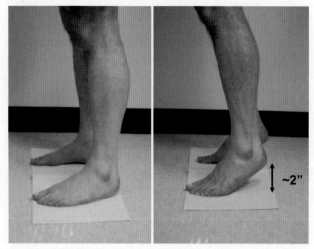

Figure 8-5 An exercise study can be conducted using heel raises as shown.

limited in the patient with arthritis and, because of the minimal effort from thigh muscles, any postexercise drop in ankle systolic pressure is likely to be more transient.

Examination Technique

Following the resting pressure measurements, cuffs can be left on (and secured with tape) or can be removed, and the patient is placed on the treadmill. Often, the initial speed is slow and the inclination is minimal at the start of the exercise study. As the patient continues to walk, the speed and inclination are increased to the protocol setting. If the patient is unable to perform the study due to the treadmill settings, a reduced setting may be used but must be recorded. The exercise study is terminated after 5 minutes, if the patient shows any signs of distress (difficulty breathing), or if the patient's symptoms become too painful to continue. The patient is immediately placed back on the examination table, ankle cuffs are quickly reapplied if they had been removed, and the immediate postexercise ankle pressures are obtained. A repeat brachial pressure is also obtained. Only the higher brachial pressure needs to be measured postexercise, which is used to calculate a postexercise ABI for designating a degree of functional severity. The pressures are typically repeated every 1 to 2 minutes until they return to baseline values or for a specific time (e.g., 10, 15, 20 minutes) according to the laboratory protocol.

Diagnosis

The lowest value of postactivity ABI categorizes functional severity (using Table 8-2) and the time to return to the preactivity level suggests whether

PAOD is single or multilevel. An ABI that returns to the preexercise level in 5 minutes or less is associated with single-level disease and an ABI that returns to the preexercise level >10 minutes is associated with it being at multiple levels.[13]

DOPPLER WAVEFORMS

Typically, nonimaging-based arterial testing modalities use a continuous wave (CW) Doppler. This is usually the same Doppler transducer used to record systolic pressure measurements.

EXAMINATION TECHNIQUE

The Doppler beam is positioned to exclude interference from an adjacent vein; however, this is largely subjective. The patient can be requested to hold his or her breath for a few cardiac cycles to reduce venous flow and thus venous interference. For the lower extremity, Doppler waveforms are recorded from the common femoral, superficial femoral, popliteal, distal posterior tibial, and dorsalis pedis arteries. For the upper extremity, Doppler waveforms are recorded from the subclavian, axillary, brachial, distal radial, and distal ulnar arteries. The Doppler transducer is placed over the general area of the underlying vessel. It is then slowly moved both medially and laterally until an arterial signal is obtained. The transducer is then adjusted so that an approximately 45° with the skin is achieved. This is varied slightly to improve the Doppler shift so that an accurate waveform with a maximum deflection is achieved.

DIAGNOSIS

Interpretation of extremity Doppler waveforms is limited to their shape (Tables 8-3 and 8-4a) because nonimaging modalities do not permit angle correction for calculating blood velocity. Waveforms from the upper extremity in Figure 8-6 show the right to be normal and the left abnormal, suggesting proximal disease. Similarly, the lower extremity waveforms in Figure 8.7 are normal on the left at the common femoral level with diastolic flow reversal and abnormal distally, suggesting femoropopliteal disease. Although it is possible to measure systolic rise time (from onset of systole to peak) and pulsatility index without imaging, this is now exclusively a duplex function (see Table 8-3h).

There have been ongoing discussions in the medical community concerning the terminology used to classify Doppler waveforms. These concerns have been raised for both duplex ultrasound-derived spectral waveforms as well as continuous-wave Doppler waveforms. Although this is still unresolved, the

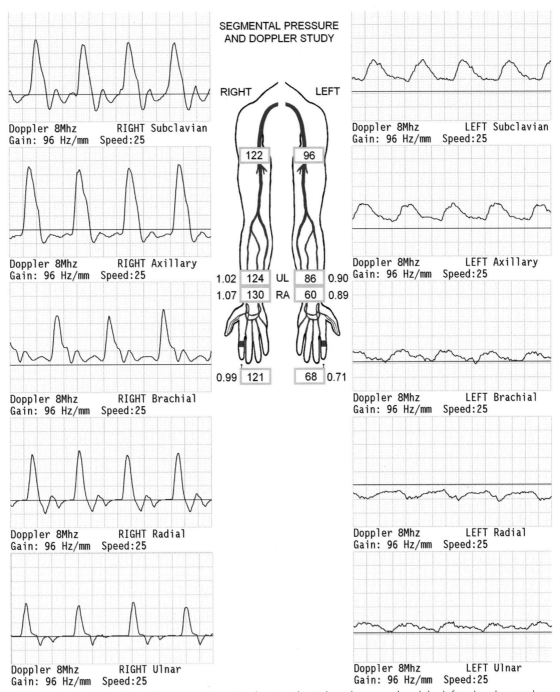

Figure 8-6 Doppler waveforms from the upper extremity showing the right to be normal and the left to be abnormal, suggesting proximal disease. (Image courtesy of Robert Scissons, RVT, FSVU, Toledo, OH.)

classic designations for waveforms that remain in use by most laboratories are as follows:

A. Triphasic
B. Biphasic: bidirectional
C. Biphasic: unidirectional
D. Monophasic: moderate/severe
E. Monophasic: severe/critical

Normal Doppler waveforms are bidirectional and exhibit a degree of flow reversal in late systole/early diastole (Fig. 8-8A,B).[14] Waveform B does not exhibit

a net return to forward flow, but this is seen frequently in older patients and those whose feet are cold and is not regarded as abnormal. Waveforms C and D are seen when PAOD progresses from mild/moderate to severe, and waveform E indicates that it is now at a critical stage; each of these three are unidirectional.

Other than from an artery feeding, a well-functioning dialysis fistula or graft, flow reversal indicates the level of peripheral resistance (PR) in the

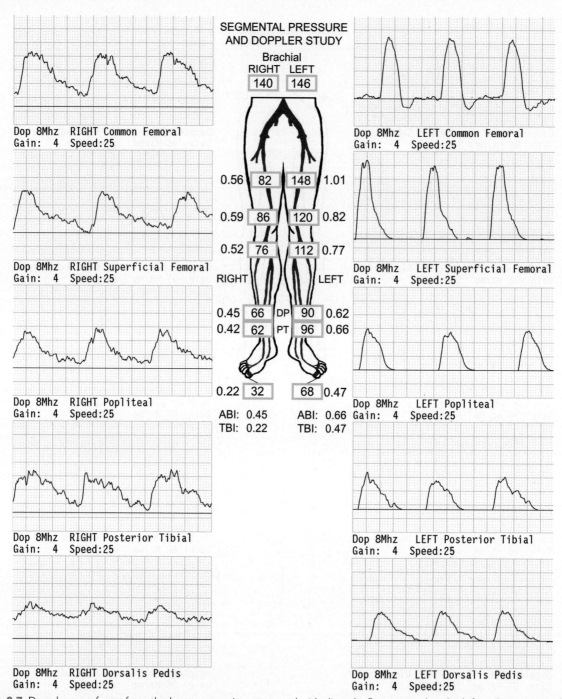

Figure 8-7 Doppler waveforms from the lower extremity are normal with diastolic flow reversal at the left at the common femoral level and abnormal distally suggesting femoropopliteal disease. The waveforms on the right are abnormal at the common femoral artery suggesting iliofemoral disease. (Image courtesy of Robert Scissons, RVT, FSVU, Toledo, OH.)

arteriolar bed, where more reversal relates to greater resistance to flow (ignoring the effects of flow reversal through an incompetent aortic valve) and less or no reversal relates to lower resistance. The normal progression of PAOD reduces flow energy distal to the lesion(s), which, without a corresponding reduction in PR, would result in lowered blood flow. However, with a PR that has reduced to the same degree as the flow energy, the volume blood flow at rest does not change. At a critical stage, the arteriolar bed

cannot dilate further and blood flow into the affected segment(s) begins to drop, whereupon the patient may start to experience forefoot pain at rest, especially when lying horizontally. Thus, a resting arterial Doppler waveform with no flow reversal (i.e., it is unidirectional) is abnormal and indicates that the PR is reduced, probably relating to the presence of PAOD. (Note: Flow reversal will be absent immediately following exercise in a normal extremity, but will reappear within 2 to 5 minutes.)

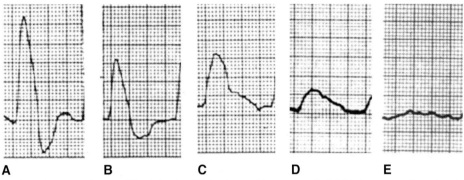

Figure 8-8 Various Doppler waveforms: **(A)** triphasic, **(B)** biphasic: bidirectional, **(C)** biphasic: unidirectional, **(D)** monophasic: moderate/severe, and **(E)** monophasic: severe/critical.

PLETHYSMOGRAPHY: PULSE VOLUME RECORDING (PVR) OR VOLUME PULSE RECORDING (VPR)

Air plethysmography (PVR or VPR) is a modality with a shorter learning curve than Doppler ultrasound and can give more consistent results in a vascular department with a low workload for this type of study (less than one per week). They reflect the total perfusion in the underlying segment of the extremity because the cuff encircles the whole limb but, unlike Doppler ultrasound, this testing modality does not identify specific arteries. Although it does not indicate the direction of blood flow, PVR has an advantage when the underlying arteries are not compressible because the waveform is relatively unchanged.

EXAMINATION TECHNIQUE

PVR techniques use either one or two cuffs above the knee (see Fig. 8-4 and Tables 8-3 and 8-4b,c) plus one each at calf and ankle levels. These are the same cuffs used for segmental pressure examinations. Some protocols also include a cuff placed across the metatarsal level of the foot. Digital studies can performed as well, which will be discussed within the section dealing with digital evaluations.

Once the cuffs are in place, each cuff is inflated to 55 to 65 mm Hg, usually with a record of the inflation volume to indicate cuff tension because inconsistent wrapping can change the waveform.[15] At this pressure, the venous outflow within the segment of the limb under the cuff is restricted. The only changes occurring under the cuff are those due to arterial inflow. With each cardiac cycle, a volume of blood enters the limb. This volume change produces a pressure change under the cuff. This pressure change is converted to a waveform, which is displayed graphically. The overall height

of the waveform is adjusted by a gain control. The gain should be set to have a waveform that is straightforward to visualize with the overall contour, which is easy to evaluate. Some protocols set the gain by first recording waveforms from the calf (these usually have the greatest amplitude as compared to the other segments) and then record the remaining segments at the same gain setting. The gain used for digital studies is usually higher due to the small volume changes occurring at this level of the vascular tree.

DIAGNOSIS

PVR waveforms relate to the moment-to-moment changes in (limb) volume, which is the difference between arterial inflow and venous outflow. Normal limb volume increases rapidly during systole, so the normal PVR waveform should exhibit a brisk upstroke with a well-defined peak (Fig. 8-9A; also see Tables 8-3 and 8-4b,c). A normal resting PVR waveform shows a "notch" on the downstroke in early diastole, which then returns to the baseline in a concave fashion (bends toward the baseline) before the onset of the next cardiac cycle. This notch is often termed the dicrotic notch and is the result of the reflected wave normally occurring in healthy vessels. As previously described, the normal high resistance peripheral arterial bed will demonstrate a brief period of reverse flow in early diastole. The reverse flow component is also known as the reflected wave. This reverse flow component adds a small volume of blood under the cuff, which produces the dicrotic notch observed on the PVR recordings. Moderate-to-severe PAOD changes the waveform, causing a delayed onset to peak, which is more rounded (Fig. 8-9B) as is also seen in an abnormal Doppler waveform. Additionally, the diastolic phase becomes convex as PAOD progresses toward the severe category.

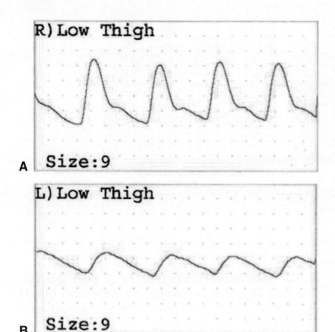

Figure 8-9 A: A normal PVR waveform from the right low thigh level exhibiting a brisk upstroke with a well-defined peak. **B:** The left lower thigh level PVR in this same patient illustrates moderate-to-severe PAOD changes in the waveform, causing a delayed onset to peak, which is more rounded.

Figure 8-10 illustrates normal PVR waveforms from the right lower extremity, exhibiting a brisk systolic upstroke and a concave (bows toward the baseline) shape in diastole. Each of those from the left extremity exhibit a delayed systolic upstroke and a convex diastolic component (bows away from the baseline), with reduced amplitude at the calf and ankle level. On the left, these findings are compatible with stenosis (or occlusion with collateralization) in the iliofemoral segment, with the suggestion of additional disease at the femoropopliteal level and certainty of severe disease below the knee. Digital waveforms are also asymmetrical, with those from the left showing slight delay in the upstroke and a more rounded appearance.

DIGITAL EVALUATIONS

Digital evaluations can include both pressures and waveforms. Waveforms can be obtained either using air PVR or photoplethysmography (PPG), although PPG is most commonly performed. There are various diseases impacting the vascular system that can be diagnosed with an examination of digital blood flow. The following section will review some of the techniques employed in digital evaluations as well as specific applications.

EXAMINATION TECHNIQUE

In terms of measuring, digit pressures can be recorded in a manner similar to other pressure measurements. Digital cuff diameters vary slightly but usually are 2.0 to 2.5 cm. Typically, PPG is the most convenient modality for measuring digital pressures, although PVR is an alternative. The use of a PVR requires Doppler to insonate the digital arteries. It is not easy to maintain the Doppler ultrasound beam within the lumen of a digital artery (which is typically only 1 to 2 mm), so using PVRs is a less convenient method for measuring digital systolic pressures.

PPGs are not true plethysmographic instruments because they cannot be calibrated in volume terms; however, they are convenient for recording arterial pulses. They operate by transmitting infrared light into tissue and detecting variations in the light reflected from underlying blood flow, from a depth of 1 to 3 mm. They are maintained in contact with the skin with double-sided tape (Fig. 8-11A), with a Velcro strap, or with a clip-style device (Fig. 8-11B). The PPG is placed on the digit and, after a brief period of 1 to 2 seconds, the sensor on the unit detects the reflected infrared light, which is then displayed as a waveform. PPG and PVR instruments provide comparably shaped waveforms and so are interpreted similarly, with normal characteristics being a brisk systolic upstroke, a well-defined peak, and a concave shape as the shape returns to the baseline during diastole (see Fig. 8-9A).

In addition to recording arterial pulses, PPGs can also be used to measure digital systolic pressures. The pulses are recorded using a slow chart or sweep speed and adjusting the gain to give an amplitude approximately one-third of the chart width (Fig. 8-12). Limb or digit movement can intrude to confuse the point at which the pulses return if the recording has greater amplitude. The cuff is inflated until pulsatility is abolished, then deflated until pulses are seen. Hands or feet can be warmed to increase pulse amplitude. This can be accomplished by heating a small towel in a microwave for 1 minute. The towel can be wrapped around each hand or foot while the history is being documented. Having the recording with an enhanced pulse amplitude enables the point of pulse return to be determined with greater confidence.

DIAGNOSIS

A toe pressure can be used to calculate a toe–brachial index (TBI), which should be ≥0.8 to be reported as normal (see Table 8-3e).[16] This is similar to measuring an ankle pressure for calculating an ABI. TBIs are particularly useful when the ankle vessels are

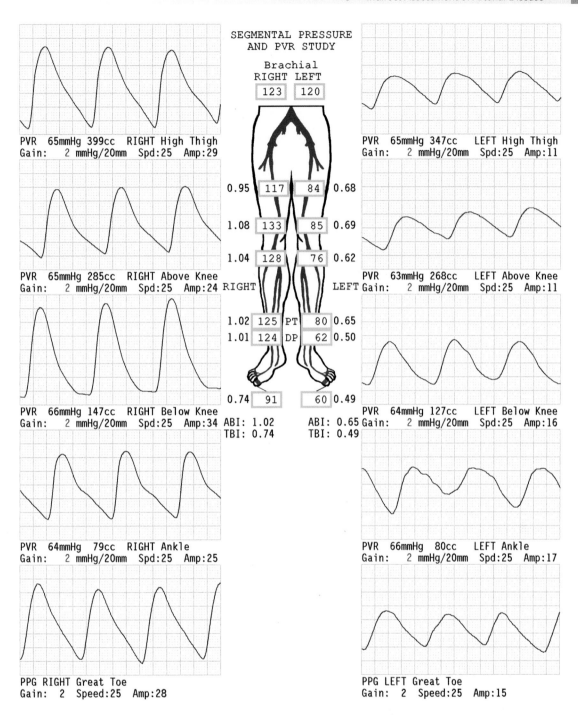

SEGMENTAL PRESSURE
AND PVR STUDY

Brachial
RIGHT   LEFT
123   120

PVR 65mmHg 399cc RIGHT High Thigh
Gain: 2 mmHg/20mm Spd:25 Amp:29

PVR 65mmHg 347cc LEFT High Thigh
Gain: 2 mmHg/20mm Spd:25 Amp:11

0.95 117   84 0.68

1.08 133   85 0.69

1.04 128   76 0.62

PVR 65mmHg 285cc RIGHT Above Knee
Gain: 2 mmHg/20mm Spd:25 Amp:24   RIGHT

LEFT   PVR 63mmHg 268cc LEFT Above Knee
Gain: 2 mmHg/20mm Spd:25 Amp:11

1.02 125 PT 80 0.65
1.01 124 DP 62 0.50

0.74   91   60 0.49

PVR 66mmHg 147cc RIGHT Below Knee
Gain: 2 mmHg/20mm Spd:25 Amp:34   ABI: 1.02
TBI: 0.74

ABI: 0.65   PVR 64mmHg 127cc LEFT Below Knee
TBI: 0.49   Gain: 2 mmHg/20mm Spd:25 Amp:16

PVR 64mmHg 79cc RIGHT Ankle
Gain: 2 mmHg/20mm Spd:25 Amp:25

PVR 66mmHg 80cc LEFT Ankle
Gain: 2 mmHg/20mm Spd:25 Amp:17

PPG RIGHT Great Toe
Gain: 2 Speed:25 Amp:28

PPG LEFT Great Toe
Gain: 2 Speed:25 Amp:15

Figure 8-10 Normal PVR waveforms from the right lower extremity, whereas the left lower extremity results indicate stenosis (or occlusion with collateralization) in the iliofemoral segment, with the suggestion of additional disease at femoropopliteal level and severe disease below the knee. (Image courtesy of John Hobby, RVT, Pueblo, CO.)

noncompressible and can be substituted for ABIs when assessing the response to exercise. Toe pressures may also be expressed directly in millimeters of mercury. To indicate the likelihood of healing following a vascular procedure in the forefoot/toe segment, 50 mm Hg is regarded as adequate even in the presence of diabetes.

Upper extremity digital pressures are important in the workup prior to the creation/revision of dialysis fistulas and grafts, and for assessing steal from the hand by the fistula/graft. The absolute pressure indicates present or potential ischemia of the hand or it can be used to calculate a digit–brachial index (DBI), similar to ABIs and TBIs. The normal value for the DBI is ≥0.9 (Table 8-4d).[17] In dialysis patients who are symptomatic for fistula steal, the digital pressures should double when the outflow side of the fistula is compressed.

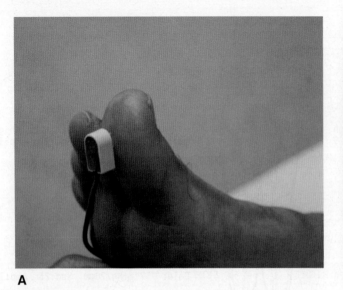
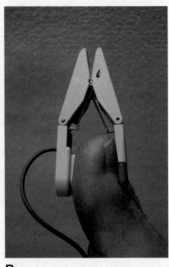

A   **B**

Figure 8-11 PPG probe placement. **A:** Using double-sided tape to maintain contact with the skin and **(B)** with a clip-style device.

THORACIC OUTLET SYNDROME

Neurovascular compression affecting the upper extremity, known as thoracic outlet syndrome, is common and, to some degree, can be found in up to 60% of persons without the patient necessarily developing symptoms.[18] Symptoms result from compression by structures in the shoulder girdle and usually they can be reproduced with the upper extremity in a specific position or when carrying out a particular activity.

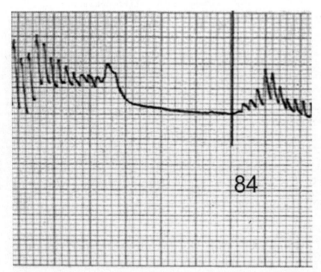

Figure 8-12 A PPG recording illustrating the use of PPG to record digital systolic pressure. The beginning of the tracing demonstrates normal pulsatile flow; pressure in an occluding cuff is increased until the pulsatile signal is obliterated; pressure is slowly released until the pulsatile signal returns; the point at which flow resumes is the systolic pressure which, in this example, is indicated at 84 mm Hg.

The most convenient method to test for TOS is to record PPG digital waveforms with the patient warm, sitting, and with arms resting comfortably in the lap (Figs. 8-13 and 8-14). Pulses are then recorded with:
- Arms resting in the lap
- Elbows to the rear and arms almost upright, palms to front (military position)
- Arms elevated above the head
- Arms abducted rearward
- Arms straight out to the sides (abducted) with head ahead, and then turned fully to the left and then to the right (Adson maneuver)
- Any other position that elicits symptoms

Finally, waveforms should be recorded with arms resting in the lap to document that pulses are present at the completion of the study. If any position causes the waveform to become flattened, maintain this position for approximately 30 seconds to establish if the patient develops symptoms (the patient may require assistance to maintain the position). Remember, up to 60% of persons can demonstrate compression without necessarily developing symptoms. For a TOS study to be reported as positive, the systolic pressures/pulse waveforms must be significantly affected by the maneuvers and the patient must develop symptoms.

COLD SENSITIVITY

As mentioned, Raynaud's disease is classified as primary or secondary and a careful history can suggest one rather than the other. Secondary Raynaud's is associated with symptoms involving one or more digits or the entire hand, with the symptoms or signs being asymmetrical. These patients often will present

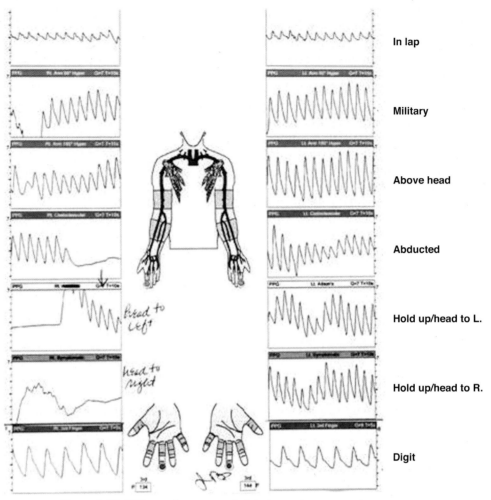

Figure 8-13 PPG waveforms recorded during various postural maneuvers.

In lap

Military

Above head

Abducted

Hold up/head to L.

Hold up/head to R.

Digit

with some tissue loss as well. The patients tend to be older, and it affects both men and women. The etiology of secondary Raynaud's is trauma from the use of vibratory tools or equipment (jackhammers, riding motorcycles, etc.), injury such as using the hand as a hammer (ulnar hammer syndrome), or severe frostbite. Other causes may include underlying medical problems such as scleroderma.

When secondary Raynaud's is suspected, the patient should not have their hands immersed in ice water in order to avoid increasing the injury. Confirmation of this, in addition to a careful history, is to record digital waveforms and digital pressures (as in recording toe pressures, PPG being the easiest method). The presence of tardus parvus waveforms (see Fig. 8-9 B) and/or abnormal pressures (DBI lower than 0.90) should alert the technologist of this possibility prior to water immersion.

The onset of primary Raynaud's is typically seen in the late preteen or early teen years, with females tending to be more affected than males. In

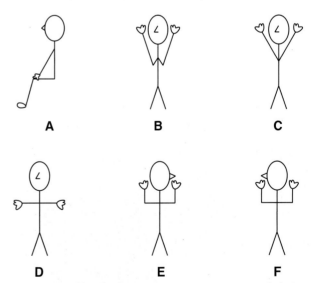

Figure 8-14 Sketch showing patient positions used during thoracic outlet testing. **A:** Neutral, resting; **(B)** arms up with elbows bent at 45°; **(C)** arms raised overhead; **(D)** arms abducted straight out, 90°; **(E)** Adson with head to the left; and **(F)** Adson with head to the right.

this instance, the hands will change color when exposed to cold. The progression of this color change is white, changing to blue, and then red when the hands are warmed. These symptoms can occur consistently when picking up a cold item, such as a glass of ice water, but are also seen when the entire body is slightly cooled, such as with seasonal changes in outside temperature. In this situation, the cool mornings in the spring or fall result in the wearing of lighter clothing, and the vasospastic response triggers the autonomic sympathetic system to constrict. This is an overreaction in those with primary Raynaud's, resulting in the color changes. This reaction can be reduced by dressing warmer than usual.

Testing for primary Raynaud's can be accomplished using waveform analysis of the digital tracings and/or a digital temperature monitoring device (Fig. 8-15). The digital pulse should be taken prior to immersion in ice water, and it may appear normal or may exhibit a "peaked pulse" on the anacrotic (systolic) portion (Fig. 8-16) that is frequently seen in primary Raynaud's.[19] There are several stress level meters or biofeedback monitors available, which are accurate to <0.1°C and are not expensive (usually less than $30). Prior to beginning the testing and challenge by immersion into ice water, the hands should be warmed to a minimum of 28°C (82°F). Immerse the hands in warm (not hot) water for several minutes, until they feel warm to the touch. In addition, the testing room should be comfortably warm at 23° to 24°C (74° to 76°F), so the patient is not cooled by the environment.

For this exam, the patient sits comfortably in a chair (one having a back will facilitate this) with a towel placed over the lap. This will avoid water

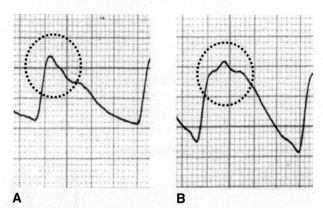

Figure 8-16 Digital PPG waveforms. **A:** A normal waveform. **B:** A "peaked pulse" waveform frequently seen in primary Raynaud's.

getting on the patient when the hands are removed from the water.

A "resting" digital pulse is then recorded from both hands and digital blood pressures are measured, if indicated, or a component of individual protocols. The PPG should be secured to the wrist to avoid "pulling" of the probe away from the digit. Securing the probe to the digit with double-stick tape (see Fig. 8-11A) will provide a clean tracing. If a thermometer is used, again the sensing probe should be secured to the digit with a Velcro strap and secured at the wrist as with the PPG probe.

It is helpful to place the hands in large disposable latex gloves (if there is no latex allergy) and secure the glove at the wrist with a strip of tape (Fig. 8-17). This will prevent the hands from getting wet and will alleviate the need to dry the hands when removed from the ice water. The hands should be immersed into the ice water, to just below the top of the gloves (Fig. 8-18).

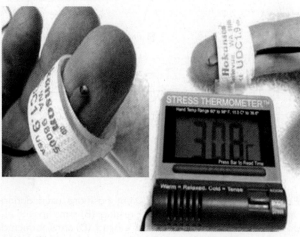

Figure 8-15 A digital temperature monitoring device used for Raynaud's testing.

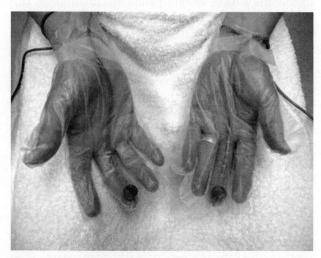

Figure 8-17 The use of disposable gloves to protect PPG sensors used during cold sensitivity testing.

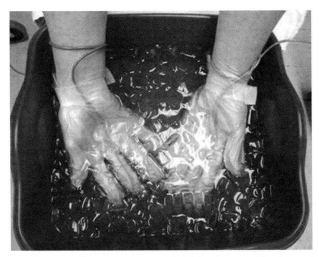

Figure 8-18 The proper patient position in an ice bath used for cold sensitivity testing.

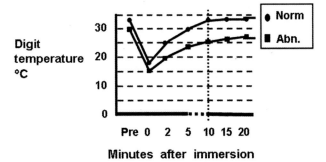

Figure 8-20 Normal and abnormal temperature measurements following cold sensitivity testing using ice water immersion. A normal response is one where temperatures return to baseline measurements within 10 minutes following removal from the cold stimulus.

A large container is needed for the hand immersion, and a "bath basin" as used routinely in hospital settings works very well. Placing the basin on a small table in front of the patient facilitates immersion and prevents accidental spills.

Cold immersion should be for 30 to 40 seconds, followed by immediate removal of the gloves. If the hands do get water on them directly, they should be "patted" dry rather than rubbed briskly. Digital waveforms (Fig. 8-19) and/or temperatures should be measured immediately at 2 minutes, 5 minutes, and 10 minutes. Normal digital tracings and/or temperatures should return to preimmersion status within 10 minutes to be categorized as normal (Fig. 8-20; also see Table 8-4f), with >10 minutes being consistent with cold sensitivity.

Time	PPG Waveform	Digital Temperature
Immediately	Reduced amplitude	≤20°C (68°F)
2 minutes	Increase in amplitude	20°–25°C (68° to 77°F)
5 minutes	Sharp peak returning	25°–30°C (77° to 86°F)
10 minutes	Return to preimmersion	30°–33°C (86° to 91°F)

If the study is abnormal, the pulse and/or temperature should be verified prior to releasing the patient.

THE ALLEN TEST

An application of the Allen test can use PPG waveforms to indicate adequacy of hand perfusion from the radial and ulnar arteries, combined and individually. It is necessary to establish the contribution to digital perfusion from each artery prior to certain surgical procedures. These procedures include the creation of a dialysis fistula or graft and radial artery harvest prior to coronary bypass procedures. The PPG transducer is affixed to the middle finger or the forefinger and pulses are recorded. The radial and the ulnar arteries are compressed sequentially to verify whether or not pulses are maintained (Fig. 8-21). The intent is to detect that pulse amplitude is not abolished when the arteries are compressed. This confirms that flow into the hand will not be interrupted if the radial artery is used to feed the fistula or graft or if harvested for bypass.

Pathology Box 8-1 summarizes some of the common arterial pathology observed in the lower and upper extremities. It also lists the indirect testing results associated with these abnormalities.

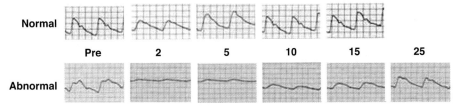

Figure 8-19 Normal and abnormal digital PPG waveforms recorded during cold sensitivity testing. *Pre* indicates initial waveforms recorded at room temperature. The numbers *2, 5, 10, 15,* and *25* indicate the minutes after removal from an ice water bath.

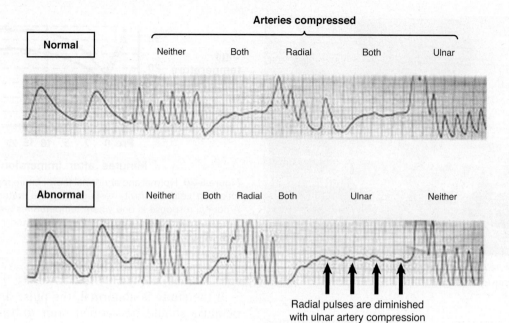

Figure 8-21 PPG waveforms recorded during an Allen test. Normal and abnormal responses are indicated with compression of the radial and ulnar arteries.

SUMMARY

Indirect arterial testing is a valuable asset when examining patients with suspected PAOD. Additionally, there are several other appropriate indications for the indirect testing of the extremities. The combination of pressures and waveforms produce both quantitative and qualitative information on extremity blood flow. The nonimaging techniques described provide an assessment of global perfusion and thus the functional status of a limb.

PATHOLOGY BOX 8-1

Lower and Upper Extremity Arterial Pathology

Pathology	Indirect Testing Results
Peripheral arterial occlusive disease (PAOD)	• ABI <0.9 • Pressure gradient >30 mm Hg between diseased segments • Loss of reflected wave (dicrotic notch) on PVRs • Loss of reverse wave component on CW waveform
Digital ischemia: Lower extremity	• TBI <0.8 • Diminished digital waveforms
Digital ischemia: Upper extremity	• DBI <0.09 • Diminished digital waveforms
Thoracic outlet syndrome	• Diminished or flat digital PPG waveforms during provocative arm/shoulder maneuvers
Raynaud's disease	• Diminished PPG waveforms at rest • DBI <0.9 • "Peaked pulse" may be present on PPG or PVR waveforms • Digital waveforms return to baseline >10 minutes following cold challenge
Incomplete palmar arch (radial/ulnar dependency)	• Positive Allen test with diminished digital waveforms during manual compression of radial or ulnar arteries

ABI, ankle–brachial index; PVR, pulse volume recording; CW, continuous wave; TBI, toe–brachial index; DBI, digit–brachial index; PPG, photoplethysmography.

Critical Thinking Questions

1. What are two important concerns about patient position for physiologic exams?

2. You perform a segmental pressure evaluation on a patient with relatively short legs. There is not enough room to place both a high thigh and low thigh cuff. You use a single contoured thigh cuff. What effect do you think this will have on your results and why?

3. You have been asked to examine the status of the common femoral artery. You can perform a PVR, CW Doppler waveform, or segmental pressure examination. Which test would you select and why?

4. Digital evaluations are commonly used to evaluate patients with thoracic outlet syndrome and Raynaud's disease. What vessels are impacted by these pathologies and why are digital studies used?

REFERENCES

1. LaPerna L. Diagnosis and medical management of patients with intermittent claudication. *J Am Osteopath Assoc.* 2001;100(10 su pt 2):S10–S14.
2. Edwards JM, Porter JM. Evaluation of upper extremity ischemia. In: Bernstein EF, ed. *Vascular Diagnosis.* 4th ed. St. Louis, MO: Mosby; 1993:630–640.
3. Sanders RJ, Hammond SL, Rao NM. Diagnosis of thoracic outlet syndrome. *J Vasc Surg.* 2007;46(3):601–604.
4. Herrick AL. Pathogenesis of Raynaud's phenomenon. *Rheumatology (Oxford).* 2005;44(5):587–596.
5. Daigle RJ. *Techniques in Noninvasive Vascular Diagnosis.* 2nd ed. Littleton, CO: Summer Publishing; 2005:142.
6. Winsor TA. Influence of arterial disease on the systolic blood pressure gradients of the extremity. *Am J Med Sci.* 1950;220:117–126.
7. Yao ST, Hobbs JT, Irvine WT. Ankle systolic pressure measurements in arterial disease affecting the lower extremities. *Br J Surg.* 1969;56:676–679.
8. Baker JD, Dix DE. Variability of Doppler ankle pressures with arterial occlusive disease: an evaluation of ankle index and brachial-ankle pressure gradient. *Surgery.* 1981;89:134–137.
9. Strandness DE Jr, Sumner DS. *Hemodynamics for Surgeons.* New York, NY: Grune & Stratton; 1975:228.
10. Stein R, Hrljac I, Halperin JL, et al. Limitation of the resting ankle-brachial index in symptomatic patients with peripheral arterial disease. *Vasc Med.* 2006;11(1):29–33.
11. AbuRahma AF. Segmental Doppler pressures and Doppler waveform analysis in peripheral vascular disease of the lower extremities. In: AbuRahma AF, Bergan JJ, eds. *Noninvasive Vascular Diagnosis.* London, England: Springer; 2000:213–229.
12. Gerhard-Herman M, Gardin JM, Jaff M, et al. Guidelines for noninvasive vascular laboratory testing: a report from the American Society of Echocardiography and the Society of Vascular Medicine and Biology. *J Am Soc Echocardiogr.* 2006;19(8):955–972.
13. vanLangen H, vanGurp J, Rubbens L. Interobserver variability of ankle-brachial index measurements at rest and post exercise in patients with intermittent claudication. *Vasc Med.* 2009;14(3):221–226.
14. Scissons R, Comerota A. Confusion of peripheral arterial Doppler waveform terminology. *J Diag Med Sonog.* 2009;25(4):185–194.
15. Daigle RJ. *Techniques in Noninvasive Vascular Diagnosis.* 2nd ed. Littleton, CO: Summer Publishing; 2005:151.
16. Carter SA, Lezack JD. Digital systolic pressures in the lower limbs in arterial disease. *Circulation.* 1971;43(6):905–914.

17. Rumwell C, McPharlin M. *Vascular Technology.* 4th ed. Pasadena, CA: Davies Publishing; 2009:110.
18. Gergoudis R. Thoracic outlet arterial compression: prevalence in normal persons. *Angiology.* 1980;31(8):538–541.
19. Mclafferty RB, Edwards JM, Porter JM. Diagnosis and management of Raynaud's syndrome. In: Perler BA, Becker GJ, eds. *Vascular Intervention: A Clinical Approach.* New York, NY: Thieme; 1998:239–247.

9 Duplex Ultrasound of Lower Extremity Arteries

Natalie Marks, Anil Hingorani, and Enrico Ascher

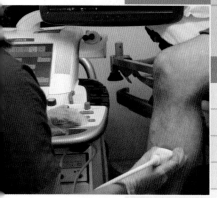

OBJECTIVES

Describe the ultrasound techniques used to image lower extremity arteries

Define normal image and Doppler characteristics of peripheral arteries

Identify peripheral arterial abnormal waveforms

Describe the use of ultrasound with arterial revascularization procedures

KEY TERMS

aneurysm | contrast arteriography | duplex arteriography | peak systolic velocity | plaque

GLOSSARY

aneurysm a localized dilation of an artery involving all three layers of the arterial wall

contrast arteriography a radiologic imaging technique performed using ionizing radiation to provide detailed arterial system configuration and pathology information

duplex arteriography ultrasound imaging of the arterial system performed to identify atherosclerotic disease and other arterial pathology proving a detailed map of the arterial system evaluated

plaque the deposit of fatty material within the vessel walls, which is characteristic of atherosclerosis

Contrast arteriography (CA) has been used for decades as the gold standard imaging tool to evaluate the peripheral arterial system particularly prior to lower extremity revascularization procedures. It is well-known that CA is associated with systemic and local complications and, nowadays, media-educated patients are demanding less invasive alternatives. Current technical advances in ultrasonographic imaging have motivated a number of authors to investigate the potential of duplex arteriography (DA) to replace standard CA in the assessment of the arterial system.[1-13] Although many authors have demonstrated a promising association between arteriography and DA,[1-9] others have been less enthusiastic and continue to promote preoperative or prebypass arteriography.[10-13] There are several factors contributing to this results discrepancy, such as: (1) lack of sonographers and vascular technologists' experience, (2) lack of commitment of time and effort to perfect the technique, (3) outdated duplex equipment with poor imaging quality, (4) surgeon's unwillingness to give up the visual effect of a complete arteriography and incorporate a perception of duplex imaging,

and (5) heavy vessel calcification and other local obstacles preventing adequate insonation in some patients.

It has been the experience of these authors to preferentially use DA since 1998. At first, the utility of DA was explored for purely diagnostic purposes in patients undergoing lower extremity revascularizations.[14-17] Over the last 6 years, DA was applied not only to diagnostic use but also for endovascular procedures such as duplex-guided angioplasties.[18-21] The use of intraoperative and postendovascular arterial ultrasound will be discussed in subsequent chapters of this text. This chapter will explore DA in the diagnosis of disease in the lower extremity arterial system.

INDICATIONS

Signs and symptoms of arterial disease, which were described in the preceding chapter on indirect arterial testing, also apply to a patient presenting for a lower extremity arterial duplex ultrasound examination. There are classic symptoms that may indicate the presence of arterial insufficiency or ischemia including intermittent claudication, rest pain, nonhealing ulcers, and gangrene. There can be some subtle changes such as hair loss, nail thickening, and skin changes. Symptoms such as pallor, pulselessness, paralysis, paresthesia, and intense pain are indicative of acute arterial ischemia. Peripheral arterial aneurysms may also be suspected if upon palpation a mass is detected in the femoral or popliteal regions. Peripheral arteries may also be examined for aneurysmal disease if the patient has a known abdominal aortic aneurysm. Atherosclerosis and aneurysmal disease are the primary pathologies suspected in most individuals. There are less frequently encountered arterial diseases, as well as traumatic and iatrogenic injuries, which may require DA for their diagnosis.

Although not an indication for testing, many of the patients will present with comorbid risk factors. These risk factors include diabetes, hyperlipidemia, hypertension, history of tobacco use, coronary artery disease, and end-stage renal disease. Additional risk factors for arterial disease are obesity, a sedentary lifestyle, heredity, gender, and age.

SONOGRAPHIC EXAMINATION TECHNIQUES

PATIENT PREPARATION

The patient should have the test procedure explained to him or her. The patient should remove all clothing from the waist down, except for undergarments, and be given a patient gown or appropriate drape.

PATIENT POSITIONING

The patient is placed in the supine position with mild knee flexion and thigh abduction for visualization of the common, superficial, and deep femoral arteries (Fig. 9-1). The same patient position can be used to examine the above-knee popliteal artery segment from a medial approach and the below-knee segment from a posterior approach. A medial approach is also used to insonate the posterior tibial artery and its plantar branches. By placing the patient in a lateral decubitus position opposite to the side of interest with slight ipsilateral knee and hip flexure, the tibioperoneal trunk and peroneal artery can be examined (Fig. 9-2). By placing the transducer just posterior to the proximal fibula, the origin of the anterior tibial artery can be assessed. The remainder of the anterior tibial artery is visualized by positioning the transducer between the tibia and the fibula. Lastly, the

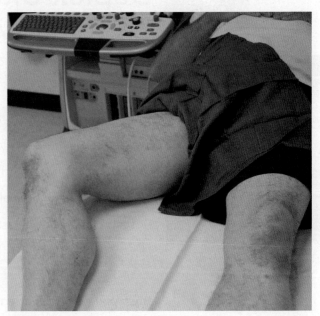

Figure 9-1 A patient positioned for a lower extremity arterial ultrasound examination with the hip externally rotated and the knee slightly flexed.

dorsalis pedis artery and its metatarsal branches are insonated with the patient in the supine position.

SCANNING TECHNIQUE

A complete evaluation for lower extremity arterial disease includes an ultrasound examination of the aortoiliac segment as well as a measurement of ankle pressures. Some laboratories include multilevel physiologic testing such as pulse volume recordings, continuous-wave Doppler waveforms, or segmental pressures as part of a routine lower extremity examination. The duplex ultrasound examination of the aortoiliac segment is discussed in Chapter 18, and the measurement of ankle pressures is described in Chapter 8.

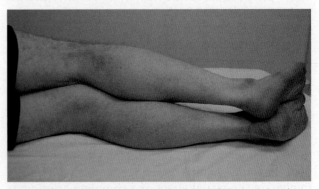

Figure 9-2 A patient positioned in the left lateral decubitus position to examine the popliteal artery, tibioperoneal trunk, and peroneal artery.

A variety of transducers are used to obtain high-quality B-mode, color, and power Doppler images as well as reliable velocity spectra. Curvilinear 5-2 MHz and phased array 3-2 MHz probes are typically used for aortoiliac scanning, but these lower frequency probes may be needed to insonate deeper lower extremity vessels in heavier limbs. Linear 7-4 MHz transducers used for visualization of the femoral, popliteal, and tibial vessels. The high resolution of a compact linear 15-7 MHz transducer allows better visualization of superficial arteries on the ankle and foot.

The duplex ultrasound examination of the infrainguinal vessels begins at the groin. At this position, the distal portion of the external iliac artery and the common femoral artery (CFA) can be identified. The transducer is moved slightly down the leg to next identify the bifurcation of the superficial femoral artery (SFA) and deep femoral or profunda femoris artery (PFA) (Fig. 9-3). Most laboratory protocols require only the first few centimeters of the PFA to be scanned. After a short distance, the PFA courses deeper in the thigh, giving rise to multiple branches. The SFA is then followed through its entire course using a medial approach. In the lower thigh, the SFA passes through the adductor canal, also known as Hunter's canal. Once through the canal, the SFA becomes the popliteal artery, which is now along the posterior aspect of the leg. This can be viewed by moving the transducer posteriorly to the knee joint and following the vessels proximally onto the lower thigh. Combining both medial and posterior approaches, the full course of the SFA and popliteal artery can be appreciated.

The popliteal artery is examined as it courses through the popliteal fossa. There are multiple small branches, including the gastrocnemius arteries, which

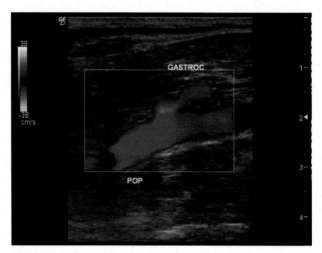

Figure 9-4 The popliteal artery, along with the gastrocnemius arteries.

can be observed (Fig. 9-4). In a complete examination, all three tibial arteries are followed throughout the calf. The anterior tibial artery can be observed with a posterior approach branching off the popliteal artery (Fig. 9-5). As this vessel courses lower in the calf, it can be followed with an anterior–lateral approach. The posterior tibial artery can be followed through the calf with a medial approach. Depending on its depth, the peroneal artery can be followed with a medial approach or with a posterior–lateral approach (Fig. 9-6). Often, the lower extremity examination includes the dorsalis pedis artery. Care should be taken when insonating the distal posterior tibial, distal anterior tibial, and dorsalis pedis arteries. These vessels are very superficial and can easily be partially compressed with the transducer if too much pressure is applied.

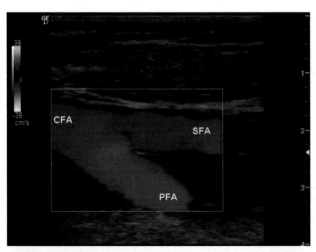

Figure 9-3 The common femoral artery (CFA) bifurcating into the superficial femoral artery (SFA) and deep femoral or profunda femoris artery (PFA).

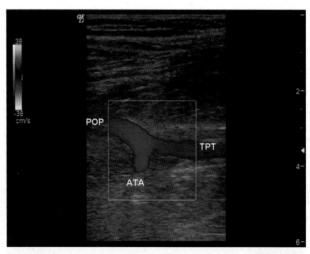

Figure 9-5 The origin of the anterior tibial artery (ATA) off the popliteal artery (POP). The tibioperoneal trunk (TPT) is also shown.

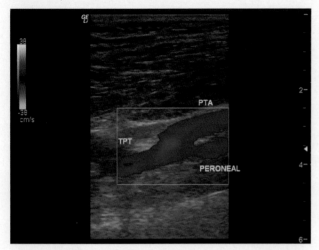

Figure 9-6 The posterior tibial (PTA) and peroneal arteries arising off the tibioperoneal trunk (TPT).

Individual laboratory protocols vary, but typically include documentation of the grayscale image, color flow image, and spectral waveforms. These images should be recorded over every major segment evaluated. Proximal, mid, and distal images of the SFA and tibial vessel are also typically recorded. The grayscale image may be documented in sagittal and transverse planes (Fig. 9-7). In the presence of pathology, it is important to document the full extent of the disease. If aneurysmal disease is suspected, diameter measurements should be recorded along the area of concern as well as just proximal to this region.

In general, color and power Doppler are used primarily to assist with localization and tracking the course of the vessels. Color can provide a rapid assessment of the flow dynamics. Color is very useful in identifying flow abnormalities associated with arterial plaque (Fig. 9-8). Color is also helpful in placing the Doppler sample volume at the area of the of the greatest velocity shift. Power Doppler should be used whenever very low flow states are encountered or when vessel occlusion is suspected.

Velocity spectra are used as the primary tool to categorize disease. The peak systolic velocity (PSV) is recorded along all the major vessels. In areas of a stenosis, the PSV should be recorded proximal to the stenosis, at the area of maximum velocity shift in the stenosis, and just distal to the stenosis (Fig. 9-9). The distal waveform should demonstrate the post-stenotic turbulence associated with hemodynamically significant stenoses. The PSV at the stenosis is divided by the PSV just proximal to the stenosis to calculate the velocity ratio (Vr). The Vr, in addition to the PSV, is used to estimate the degree of stenosis.

Because the status of the branches of the arteries can also add valuable data for the surgeon, visualization of as many tibial and pedal branches as possible including maleolar, plantars, tarsals, deep plantar arteries, and branches of the named vessels is also performed during DA. A high-frequency transducer (15-7 MHz) can be especially useful in this portion of the protocol.

A precise evaluation of arterial size, length, and degree of narrowing as well as plaque characteristics are performed for a single focal lesion or sequential lesions suitable for balloon angioplasty and/or stent placement. It is important for the sonographer or vascular technologist to possess as much information from the referring physician as possible so that all the ultrasound data required for patient management decisions can be obtained. The referring physician may be planning a specific procedure or an intervention at a specific level and require pertinent data to plan the most appropriate procedure and approach.

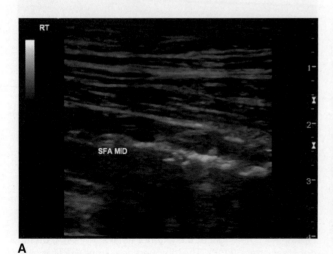

A

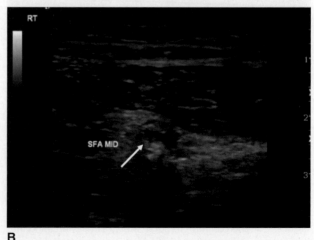

B

Figure 9-7 A: A sagittal scan of an artery with atherosclerotic plaque. **B:** A transverse view of the same plaque *(arrow)*.

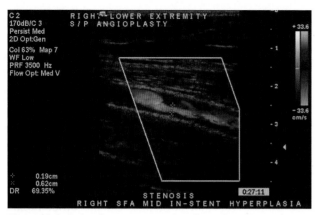

Figure 9-8 Color flow imaging identifying flow abnormalities with in-stent restenosis.

Often when an occlusion is encountered, it is helpful to note the site where the vessel is reconstituted by collateral flow.

A color-coded map of the arterial tree is drawn to facilitate reading by the surgeon in order to select optimal inflow and outflow anastomotic sites for bypasses or potential angioplasty sites (Fig. 9-10). This drawing can contain comments about the vessel walls, velocity data, and vessel size.

TECHNICAL CONSIDERATIONS

Over the years, there has been progression of preoperative DA as an integral part of revascularization procedures. In this author's institution, DA is used for procedure planning, intraoperatively and postoperatively as the first option for routine, urgent, or emergent imaging tool. This versatility stems, at large, from the duplex scanner's portability. Because DA exams can be performed at the bedside, in the operating room, or in the holding area, time and personnel used for patient transport are significantly reduced. Additionally, there is no delay associated with performance and interpretation, which can be the case with CA or magnetic resonance angiography (MRA) for a severely ischemic limb in a debilitated patient. With DA, once the patient is identified to need urgent revascularization, the machine and sonographer or vascular technologist can be brought to any part of the hospital for an abbreviated, targeted, or full examination.

Because DA is not just a luminal technology, it is essential in the assessment of the vessel wall. High-frequency duplex imaging can measure the luminal diameter and thickness of the wall with incredible precision of approximately 1/10th of a millimeter. This feature is very important because biplanar arteriography is

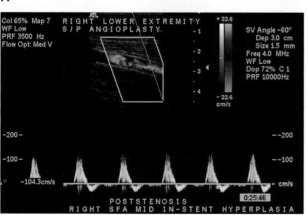

A

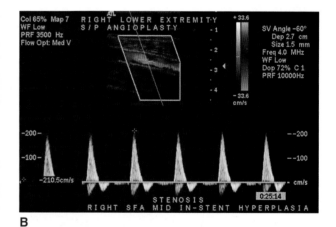

B

Figure 9-9 A: A Doppler waveform taken proximal to a stenosis. **B:** A Doppler waveform taken at the area of maximum velocity shift within a stenosis. **C:** A Doppler waveform taken distal to a stenosis, documenting poststenotic turbulence.

C

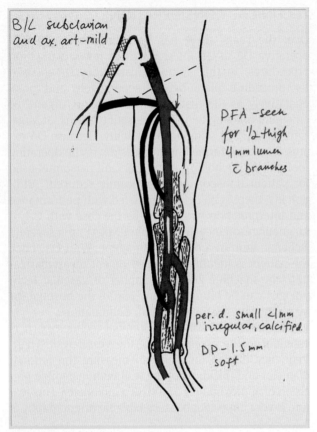

Figure 9-10 An arterial map drawing of a patient with multiple failed PTFE bypasses.

not routinely used for the entire arterial tree; therefore, eccentric arterial lesions may go undetected by CA.

Another unique advantage of DA as compared to other imaging tools is its ability to identify the softest portion of the vessel wall, which can then be marked on the skin before the intended procedure. Extensive calcification in a vessel makes for difficult suturing, so an area that is compliant with no plaque or

calcification is preferred. Skin marking of the most suitable site for outflow anastomosis, particularly for infrapopliteal segments, may limit incision size and eliminate extensive arterial dissection in search of a soft arterial segment (Fig. 9-11).

One of the strongest DA advantages is its application in the setting of acute arterial ischemia.[22] Current management of acute lower limb ischemia has evolved from simple embolectomies under local anesthesia to challenging arterial reconstructions. This dramatic change involves a more aggressive approach at limb salvage in the elderly patient by well-trained vascular surgeons. On the other hand, many of these patients presenting with acutely ischemic limbs will have underlying multisegmental occlusive arterial disease rather than a simple embolus obstructing a healthy vessel (Fig. 9-12). Although the clinical diagnosis of an ischemic leg can often be made without difficulties, the anatomical pattern of the inflow, the outflow, and the occluded arterial segment may at times be impossible to ascertain by standard preoperative imaging modalities.

Finally, during the course of a lower extremity examination, it may be necessary to evaluate other vascular segments. Routinely, venous mapping can also be performed during DA to identify usable veins for harvest. The examination of the subclavian–axillary segment may be performed as a possible inflow source for debilitated patients with severe aortoiliac disease. This is accomplished without the risk of an additional thoracic aortogram or the time needed for an additional thoracic MRA.

PITFALLS

Investigators have clearly demonstrated the feasibility and multiple advantages of DA and, as with any technology, it is important to appreciate its limitations.

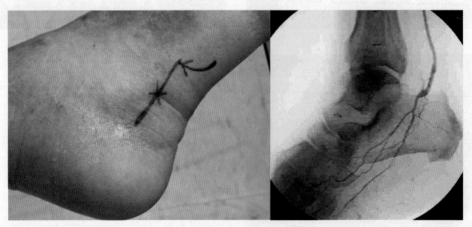

Figure 9-11 *Left:* Distal posterior tibial artery segment and a large inflow branch are marked preoperatively on the skin. *Right:* Intraoperative completion angiogram of the newly created vein bypass demonstrated a normal distal anastomosis to the distal posterior tibial artery and preserved large collateral branch on the same patient.

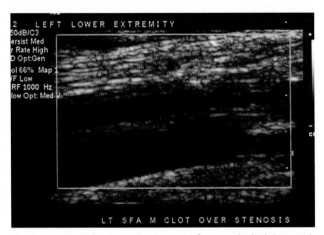

Figure 9-12 Color Doppler image of an occluded SFA with acute thrombus overlying severe chronic arterial disease.

Overall, the most common problem with DA has been with calcification. However, some techniques can be used to obtain the necessary information even within severely calcified vessel such as using multiple insonation planes, increasing color and Power Doppler gain, sensitivity and persistence, or using SonoCT imaging mode.

When an extremely low flow situation is encountered (PSV <20 cm/s, or volume flow of <20 mL/min), DA can be unreliable and alternative imaging modalities need to be employed. However, lowering the Doppler pulse repetition frequency (PRF) to 150 to 350 Hz and using the low wall filter, the highest persistence, and highest sensitivity for the color flow, imaging can be beneficial to detect flows as low as 2 cm/s, which is significantly lower than the threshold for other imaging modalities (Fig. 9-13).[23] At times, distal compression can

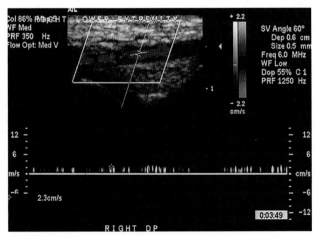

Figure 9-13 Very low flow (PSV = 2.3 cm/s) registered by duplex in the dorsalis pedis artery (appears occluded on a diagnostic contrast arteriogram).

augment arterial flow and demonstrate patency of tibial vessels.

Some obstacles encountered during DA scans may necessitate very specific approaches. When patients experience severe ischemic pain that precludes the completion of this at times, extensive exam premedication with analgesics can be helpful. Additionally, because the examination does take the cooperation of the patient, having a family member present during the examination of a confused elderly patient can comfort him or her and can allow the patient to better tolerate the examination. Visualization of the iliac arteries can be better accomplished by having the patient fast. Leg elevation for 24 to 48 hours prior to a nonemergent DA test usually decreases calf edema and provides for adequate visualization of the tibial vessels.

The depth of the tibioperoneal trunk, the origin of the proximal peroneal and posterior arteries, and the SFA at Hunter's canal may necessitate the use of a lower frequency transducer for visualization. However, this tends to sacrifice resolution details and can make significant findings in these areas difficult to interpret.

Although insonation in the area of open ulcers or excessive scarring may not be possible, this also would not be a suitable area for anastomosis. Therefore, even in those patients with poor skin condition, severe obesity, or edema (excessive vessel depth), sufficient information can sometimes still be obtained to complete the needed intervention. For example, if a claudicant is found to have a patent popliteal artery and one vessel runoff but the other tibial vessels were not fully assessed, this information will be sufficient to perform femoral–popliteal bypass regardless of the other tibial vessels condition. If a diabetic with gangrene is found to have a patent dorsalis pedis artery and an adequate conduit, but the anterior tibial artery is too calcified to visualize, one may chose to perform a bypass to the dorsalis pedis as the anterior tibial artery would not be an optimal site for the distal anastomosis.

The length of a complete DA has always been listed as one of its disadvantages and is often criticized. However, is it necessary to visualize all of the vessels from the aorta to the pedal vessels in every case? For example, the need to scan all tibial vessels for a patient with claudication, severe iliac disease, and no significant femoral disease may be questioned if the surgeon is only planning on an iliac angioplasty procedure. Thus, the DA protocol may need to be tailored for each case as a complete examination may not be absolutely necessary or additional examinations may need to be performed in certain types of patients depending on the clinical approach of the operating team.[24] With experience, DA time can be as little as 25 minutes in many simple cases.

TRAINING METHODS

To successfully achieve these results is to establish the training method for sonographers/technologists and surgeons interpreting the results and planning revascularization strategy. In an attempt to develop a training period at the author's institution, the first 25 exams completed by any new sonographer or vascular technologist are prospectively confirmed with CA or repeated DA examination by an established staff technical member. In an effort to facilitate the advancement of the DA protocol, every completion angiogram is reviewed with the staff member who performed the exam, as are the iliac angioplasties. The characteristics of the proximal and distal arteries, vein conduit, or tibial vein (in the case when an adjunctive arteriovenous fistula is performed) are discussed and any discrepancies are reviewed as a quality assurance measure. The technical staff visit the operating room to witness the intraoperative findings firsthand. In this manner, the constant feedback becomes the cornerstone for the continual improvement in the quality of the DA exams.

DIAGNOSIS

GRAYSCALE FINDINGS

Normal arterial walls appear smooth and uniform. As the atherosclerotic disease progresses, the vessel walls will thicken. Calcification may be present and will produce acoustic shadowing, limiting complete evaluation of the vessel. Vessel wall thickness and degree of calcification are reported to aid in the choice of anastomosis sites (Fig. 9-14). As stated earlier, a surgeon will want to avoid areas of heavy calcification because it is difficult to pass sutures through heavily calcified vessels. Plaque can be seen encroaching on the vessel lumen. Most plaque will appear

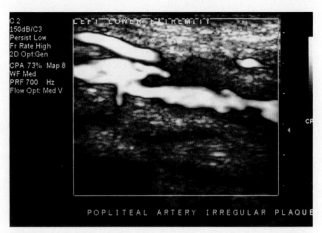

Figure 9-15 Power Doppler image of severely diseased, behind-the-knee popliteal artery with very irregular ulcerated plaque surface with high embolization potential.

heterogeneous with mixed levels of echogenicity. Occasionally, some plaque may be observed, which will appear homogeneous with similar echogenicity throughout the plaque. The surface characteristics of a plaque should be reported when possible, particularly if the plaque appeared irregular. Irregularly surfaced plaques may represent ulcerative lesions; however, many laboratories avoid reporting a plaque as "ulcerative" and simply state "irregular." High resolution DA much more clearly visualizes ulcerated and irregular plaques with potential of embolization plaques, their surface, and characteristic flow disturbance (Fig. 9-15).

DA has the ability to more accurately assess the age of the occlusion. It is possible to differentiate between an isolated chronic SFA occlusion and an acute embolism with little underlying disease or acute thrombosis with severe underlying atherosclerotic disease. The adjacent vessel walls should be closely examined to determine if atherosclerotic disease is present.

Vessel size is another component of information obtained from the grayscale image. In addition to detecting atherosclerotic disease, aneurysmal disease is another finding observed during lower extremity arterial evaluations. It is well-known that aneurysmal disease can be bilateral and multilevel. Table 9-1 illustrates diameters and velocities for lower extremity arteries.[25] A vessel is considered aneurysmal if the diameter is 1.5 times greater than the adjacent, more proximal segment. The presence or absence of thrombus within an aneurysm should also be documented as this thrombus poses an embolic risk. Aneurysmal vessels with partial thrombosis may have little-to-no luminal dilatation and may be undetectable by CA (Fig. 9-16).[26]

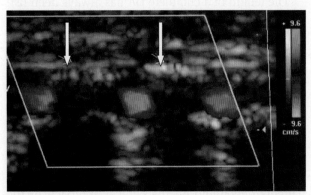

Figure 9-14 Color Doppler image of a distal posterior tibial artery with segmental heavy calcifications (*arrows*) creating shadows obscuring arterial lumen.

TABLE 9-1		
Duplex Ultrasound Mean Arterial Diameters and Peak Systolic Velocities (PSVs)		
Artery	**Diameter ± SD (cm)**	**PSV ± SD (cm/s)**
External iliac	0.79 ± 0.13	119 ± 22
Common femoral	0.82 ± 0.14	114 ± 25
Superficial femoral (proximal)	0.60 ± 0.12	91 ± 14
Superficial femoral (distal)	0.54 ± 0.11	94 ± 14
Popliteal	0.52 ± 0.11	69 ± 14

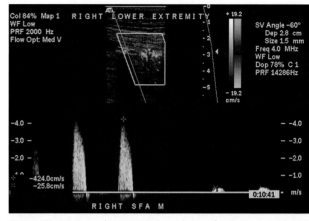

Figure 9-17 Doppler spectral analysis of a severe mid-SFA stenosis confirmed by a PSV ratio step-up of 16.4 (PSV of 424 cm/s at the stenosis over PSV of 25.8 cm/s prestenosis).

COLOR FLOW IMAGING

Normal color flow imaging will completely fill the vessels. With proper equipment settings of gain and scale, the color will appear uniform and be limited to just the lumen. In areas of disease, color aliasing will be apparent, the color flow channel within the lumen will be reduced, and a color bruit may be present within the surrounding tissue.

SPECTRAL ANALYSIS

Although the color and grayscale images are important, the PSV is the primary measurement obtained during DA that is used to determine the degree of stenosis. Table 9-1 lists values for normal velocities within the lower extremity vessels. There are some variations observed in PSV; therefore, the Vr is used for grading the stenosis. A PSV Vr ≥2 reflects

a stenosis of ≥50%, a PSV Vr ≥3 is used to confirm a severe stenosis of ≥70% (Fig. 9-17). The arterial segments are classified as normal or mildly diseased (<50%), moderately diseased (50% to 69%), severely diseased (70% to 99%), occluded, or not visualized (Table 9-2).

The hemodynamic information obtained using DA may greatly influence a patient's management. Velocity ratios can help assess whether the visualized lesion is hemodynamically significant and can determine whether repair of the lesion may be beneficial. For example, poorly visualized plaques with low PSV ratios (<2) may not be of clinical significance, whereas calcified lesions with a high PSV ratio step-up (≥2) suggest a hemodynamically significant obstruction. Other luminal imaging modalities such as CA do not provide objective hemodynamic information and the significance of lesions is often judged rather subjectively.

Waveform configuration should also be noted. Normally, the peripheral arterial bed is high resistance,

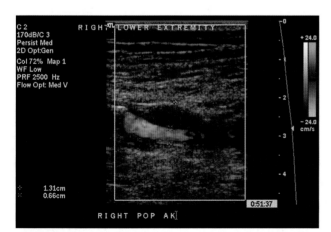

Figure 9-16 Power Doppler image of a small (13.1 mm), behind-the-knee popliteal artery aneurysm with mural thrombus by the near wall (thrombus thickness is measured 6.6 mm).

TABLE 9-2		
Arterial Disease Classification Based on Velocity Ratio		
Description	**Percent Stenosis**	**Peak Systolic Velocity Ratio (Vr)**
Normal or mildly diseased	<50%	Vr <2.0
Moderately diseased	50%–69%	Vr >2.0
Severely diseased	70%–99%	Vr >3.0
Occluded	Occluded	No flow

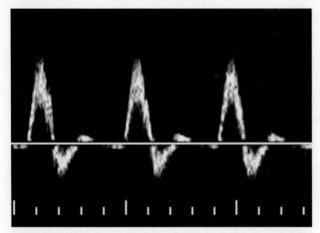

Figure 9-18 A normal multiphasic waveform taken from SFA.

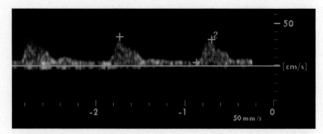

Figure 9-20 An abnormal waveform illustrating constant forward flow throughout the cardiac cycle in addition to a delayed upstroke. This is observed distal to a high-grade stenosis or occlusion.

which results in a multiphasic waveform (Fig. 9-18). There is a sharp upstroke to peak systole, a rapid deceleration, a reflected wave displayed as retrograde flow below the baseline, and often a small brief wave of antegrade flow in diastole. In situations where the peripheral resistance is lowered, constant forward flow through diastole may be observed. In the cases of a distal arteriovenous fistula, trauma, or cellulitis in the postexercise patient, antegrade flow will be observed throughout diastole (Fig. 9-19). However, in these cases, a normal sharp upstroke to peak systole will be maintained. In the event of significant arterial disease or an occlusion, the vessels distal to this disease will display a low resistance signal with antegrade flow through diastole, but there will be a delayed rise to peak systole (Fig. 9-20). Lastly, when scanning vessels proximal to an occlusion or near occlusion, the spectral waveforms can display a very high resistance pattern

with only an antegrade flow component during systole and no flow during diastole (Fig. 9-21).

Pathology Box 9-1 lists the duplex ultrasound findings with lower extremity arterial disease. Grayscale, spectral Doppler, and color imaging results are summarized.

OTHER IMAGING PROCEDURES

Standard percutaneous preoperative CA can be obtained when DA is not able to provide adequate imaging of arterial segments essential for limb revascularization or is severely disadvantaged by poor runoff. In a review of 1,023 cases at this author's institution, 112 cases (10%) were found to require CA. This was due to severe arterial calcifications present in 71 cases (63%), severe edema or morbid obesity in 23 cases (21%), extremely limited runoff with no treatment options as concluded by DA in 20 cases (18%), extensive skin wounds in 9 cases (8%), extremely low flow in 8 cases (7%), and patient's intolerance in 7 cases (6%). Eighteen of these 112 patients (16%) had undergone multiple prior revascularization attempts.

Factors associated with an increased need to obtain CA included diabetes ($P < .001$), infrapopliteal calcification ($P < .001$), older age ($P = .01$), and limb-threatening ischemia ($P < .001$). Factors not associated with the need to obtain CA included the sonographer or vascular technologist performing the examination and history of prior revascularization procedures.

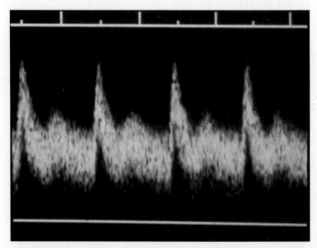

Figure 9-19 A waveform displaying a normal systolic upstroke with constant forward flow through diastole. This can be observed immediately after exercise or in the presence of a distal arteriovenous fistula, trauma, or cellulitus.

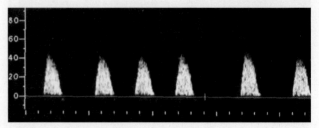

Figure 9-21 An abnormal high-resistance waveform with only antegrade flow through systole. This is observed proximal to a near occlusion or occlusion.

PATHOLOGY BOX 9-1

Lower Extremity Arterial Ultrasound Findings

	Grayscale	Spectral Doppler	Color Imaging
Normal	• Walls smooth and uniform	• No focal areas of increased PSV • Slight change in PSV across segments of arterial tree • Triphasic waveform with reverse flow component	• Uniform color filling
Stenosis	• Wall thickening • Calcification • Plaque encroaching into vessel lumen	• Focal increase in PSV • Poststenotic turbulence • Vr >2.0 • Monophasic waveform distally with no reverse flow and continuous flow in diastole	• Focal area of aliasing • Turbulence distally
Aneurysm	• Increased diameter 1.5 times larger than adjacent more proximal segment	• Turbulence within dilated area	• Turbulence in dilated area
Occlusion	• Echogenic material completely filling lumen • No patent lumen identified	• No flow identified • Increased resistance noted in waveform proximally	• No color filling

PSV, peak systolic velocity; Vr, velocity ratio.

Invasive CA has several limitations, particularly when compared to duplex ultrasound: (1) it delineates the patent arterial lumen only, (2) it misses thrombosed popliteal aneurysms, (3) it fails to visualize an outflow and inflow sources in very low-flow situations, (4) it requires potentially nephrotoxic agents, (5) it requires the use of ionizing radiation, and (6) it delays prompt treatment. Furthermore, avoidance of nephrotoxic agents and radiation, visualization of low flow arteries, and a more expeditious examination are some of the advantages of DA that are particularly important in this often sick subset of patients presenting with acute lower limb(s) ischemia.

A well-performed DA offers several practical advantages over CA in this subset of patients: (1) it is noninvasive; (2) it does not require nephrotoxic agents; (3) it is portable and can be done expeditiously; (4) color flow and waveform analysis provide a better estimation of the hemodynamic significance of occlusive disease; (5) it allows direct visualization of the entire artery and not only of the lumen thus enabling plaque characterization; (6) with color flow and power Doppler techniques, it is possible to identify patent arteries subjected to very low-flow states; and (7) it can detect occluded arterial aneurysms thereby avoiding unnecessary attempts at thromboembolectomies.

The key difference between using DA and preoperative computerized tomographic angiography (CTA) or MRA is that during DA, the sonographer or vascular technologist can identify the arterial segments where adequate visualization was not achievable and alert the surgeon that results are unreliable. In contrast, the factors that suggest when CTA or MRA are no longer supplying reliable data have yet to be identified.[27–30] Based on the present experience of the authors, about 90% of lower extremity revascularization procedures can be performed based on preoperative DA alone.

SUMMARY

Duplex ultrasound can be efficiently used for the evaluation of the lower extremity arteries and is particularly helpful in patients being evaluated for lower extremity revascularization. It is a highly operator-dependent test that demands constant optimization of the image by an operator who has mastered ultrasound technology, hemodynamics, and has a deep knowledge of pertinent anatomy. The advantages, limitations, and results of the technique are promising and may significantly improve with the use of exceptional quality imaging provided by contemporary ultrasound instruments.

Critical Thinking Questions

1. You are asked to scan the dorsalis pedis artery in a patient prior to a bypass graft. What are two technical elements of the examination that should be taken into consideration?

2. What is the most significant pitfall in imaging the lower extremity arteries, how can it be overcome, and why is it important to pay attention to this in the region of a distal anastomosis?

3. In addition to Vr calculated from the peak systolic velocity, what is another component of spectral imaging that can help identify a stenosis and what changes are expected?

REFERENCES

1. Sensier Y, Hartshorne T, Thrush A, et al. A prospective comparison of lower limb colour-coded Duplex scanning with arteriography. *Eur J Vasc Endovasc Surg.* 1996;11(2):170–175.
2. Ligush J Jr, Reavis SW, Preisser JS, et al. Duplex ultrasound scanning defines operative strategies for patients with limb-threatening ischemia. *J Vasc Surg.* 1998;28(3):482–490.
3. Sensier Y, Fishwick G, Owen R, et al. A comparison between colour duplex ultrasonography and arteriography for imaging infrapopliteal arterial lesions. *Eur J Vasc Endovasc Surg.* 1998;15(1):44–50.
4. London NJ, Sensier Y, Hartshorne T. Can lower limb ultrasonography replace arteriography? *Vasc Med.* 1996;1(2):115–119.
5. Polak JF, Karmel MI, Mannick JA, et al. Determination of the extent of lower-extremity peripheral arterial disease with color-assisted duplex sonography: comparison with angiography. *AJR Am J Roentgenol.* 1990;155(5):1085–1089.
6. Moneta GL, Yeager RA, Antonovic R, et al. Accuracy of lower extremity arterial duplex mapping. *J Vasc Surg.* 1992;15(2):275–283.
7. Wilson YG, George JK, Wilkins DC, et al. Duplex assessment of run-off before femorocrural reconstruction. *Br J Surg.* 1997;84(10):1360–1363.
8. Karacagil S, Lofberg AM, Granbo A, et al. Value of duplex scanning in evaluation of crural and foot arteries in limbs with severe lower limb ischaemia: a prospective comparison with angiography. *Eur J Vasc Endovasc Surg.* 1996;12:300–303.
9. Koelemay MJ, Legemate DA, de Vos H, et al. Can cruropedal colour duplex scanning and pulse generated run-off replace angiography in candidates for distal bypass surgery. *Eur J Vasc Endovasc Surg.* 1998;16(1):13–18.
10. Cossman DV, Ellison JE, Wagner WH, et al. Comparison of contrast arteriography to arterial mapping with color-flow duplex imaging in the lower extremities. *J Vasc Surg.* 1989;10(5):522–528.
11. Larch E, Minar E, Ahmadi R, et al. Value of color duplex sonography for evaluation of tibioperoneal arteries in patients with femoropopliteal obstruction: a prospective comparison with anterograde intraarterial digital subtraction angiography. *J Vasc Surg.* 1997;25(4):629–636.
12. Lai DT, Huber D, Glasson R, et al. Colour duplex ultrasonography versus angiography in the diagnosis of lower-extremity arterial disease. *Cardiovasc Surg.* 1996;4(3):384–388.
13. Wain RA, Berdejo GL, Delvalle WN, et al. Can duplex scan arterial mapping replace contrast arteriography as the test of choice before infrainguinal revascularization? *J Vasc Surg.* 1999;29(1):100–107.
14. Mazzariol F, Ascher E, Salles-Cunha SX, et al. Values and limitations of duplex ultrasonography as the sole imaging method of preoperative evaluation for popliteal and infrapopliteal bypasses. *Ann Vasc Surg.* 1999;13(1):1–10.
15. Ascher E, Mazzariol F, Hingorani A, et al. The use of duplex ultrasound arterial mapping as an alternative to conventional arteriography for primary and secondary infrapopliteal bypasses. *Am J Surg.* 1999;178(2):162–165.
16. Mazzariol F, Ascher E, Hingorani A, et al. Lower-extremity revascularization without preoperative contrast arteriography in 185 cases: lessons learned with duplex ultrasound arterial mapping. *Eur J Vasc Endovasc Surg.* 2000;19(5):509–515.

17. Ascher E, Hingorani A, Markevich N, et al. Lower extremity revascularization without preoperative contrast arteriography: experience with duplex ultrasound arterial mapping in 485 cases. *Ann Vasc Surg.* 2002;16(1):108–114.

18. Ascher E, Marks NA, Schutzer RW, et al. Duplex-guided balloon angioplasty and stenting for femoral-popliteal arterial occlusive disease: an alternative in patients with renal insufficiency. *J Vasc Surg.* 2005;42(6):1108–1113.

19. Ascher E, Marks NA, Hingorani AP, et al. Duplex guided balloon angioplasty and subintimal dissection of infrapopliteal arteries: early results with a new approach to avoid radiation exposure and contrast material. *J Vasc Surg.* 2005;42(6):1114–1121.

20. Ascher E, Marks NA, Hingorani AP, et al. Duplex-guided endovascular treatment for occlusive and stenotic lesions of the femoral-popliteal arterial segment: a comparative study in the first 253 cases. *J Vasc Surg.* 2006;44(6):1230–1237.

21. Ascher E, Hingorani AP, Marks NA. Duplex-guided angioplasty of lower extremity arteries. *Perspect Vasc Endovasc Ther.* 2007;19(1):23–31.

22. Ascher E, Hingorani A, Markevich N, et al. Acute lower limb ischemia: the value of duplex ultrasound arterial mapping (DUAM) as the sole preoperative imaging technique. *Ann Vasc Surg.* 2003;17(3):284–289.

23. Ascher E, Markevich N, Hingorani A, et al. Pseudo-occlusions of the internal carotid artery: a rationale for treatment on the basis of a modified carotid duplex scan protocol. *J Vasc Surg.* 2002;35(2):340–345.

24. Ascher E, Markevich N, Schutzer RW, et al. Duplex arteriography prior to femoral-popliteal reconstruction in claudicants: a proposal for a new shortened protocol. *Ann Vasc Surg.* 2004;18(5):544–541.

25. Jager KA, Risketts HJ, Strandness DE Jr. Duplex scanning for the evaluation of lower limb arterial disease. In: Bernstein EF, ed. *Noninvasive Diagnostic Techniques in Vascular Disease.* St. Louis, MO: CV Mosby; 1985:619–631.

26. Ascher E, Markevich N, Schutzer RW, et al. Small popliteal aneurysms: are they clinically significant? *J Vasc Surg.* 2003;37(4):755–760.

27. Hingorani A, Ascher E, Markevich N, et al. A comparison of magnetic resonance angiography, contrast arteriography, and duplex arteriography for patients undergoing lower extremity revascularization. *Ann Vasc Surg.* 2004;18(3):294–301.

28. Hingorani A, Ascher E, Markevich N, et al. Magnetic resonance angiography versus duplex arteriography in patients undergoing lower extremity revascularization: which is the best replacement for contrast arteriography? *J Vasc Surg.* 2004;39(4):717–722.

29. Soule B, Hingorani A, Ascher E, et al. Comparison of Magnetic Resonance Angiography (MRA) and Duplex Ultrasound Arterial Mapping (DUAM) prior to infrainguinal arterial reconstruction. *Eur J Vasc Endovasc Surg.* 2003;25(2):139–146.

30. Hingorani A, Ascher E, Markevich N, et al. A comparison of magnetic resonance angiography, contrast arteriography, and duplex arteriography for patients undergoing lower extremity revascularization. *Ann Vasc Surg.* 2004;18(3):294–301.

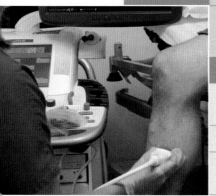

10 Upper Extremity Arterial Duplex Scanning

Aaron Partsafas and Gregory L. Moneta

OBJECTIVES

List the blood vessels imaged during an upper extremity ultrasound evaluation

Identify normal and abnormal spectral Doppler waveforms

Describe the scanning techniques used to properly insonate upper extremity vessels

Define diseases that impact upper extremity arteries

KEY TERMS

axillary | brachial | radial | Raynaud's syndrome | subclavian | Takayasu's arteritis | thoracic outlet | ulnar

GLOSSARY

Raynaud's syndrome a vasospastic disorder of the digital vessels

Takayasu's arteritis a form of large vessel vasculitis resulting in intimal fibrosis and vessel narrowing

thoracic outlet the superior opening of the thoracic cavity that is bordered by the clavicle and first rib; the subclavian artery, subclavian vein, and brachial nerve plexus pass through this opening

vasospasm a sudden constriction of a blood vessel that will reduce the lumen and blood flow rate

Upper extremity arterial examination uses components of the history and physical examination in conjunction with noninvasive and sometimes invasive studies. Duplex ultrasound examination is a key diagnostic modality when evaluating upper extremity arterial disease. Upper extremity arterial disease occurs much less frequently than lower extremity ischemia, accounting for only about 5% of extremity ischemia. Its low incidence and highly variable etiology causes considerable confusion in clinical practice. Causes of upper extremity symptoms related to arterial disease include mechanical obstruction at the thoracic outlet, embolism, trauma, digital artery vasospasm, and digital artery occlusion. In many cases, a thorough history and physical in conjunction with a duplex ultrasound examination will be sufficient to determine definitive management and minimize the use of arteriography. This chapter will review the arterial anatomy of the upper extremities, identify the important anatomic variations that may be encountered, and will discuss common clinical applications of upper extremity arterial duplex scanning. Both normal and abnormal duplex findings, some of which are unique to insonation of the upper extremities arteries, are presented. Finally, a stepwise process for examination of upper extremity arteries is presented.

ANATOMY

Arterial duplex examination of lower extremity arteries is quite common compared to the evaluation of upper extremity arteries. For some, upper extremity anatomy may be less well-known. Understanding the normal arterial anatomy of the upper extremities, along with common anatomic variants, facilitates assessment of upper extremity arteries by duplex ultrasound (Fig. 10-1). Although Chapter 1 reviewed the vascular anatomy, some additional details of upper extremity vessels are described as follows.

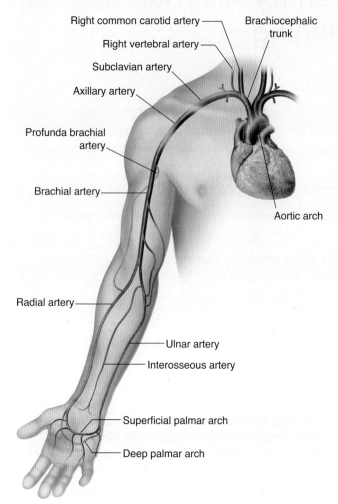

Figure 10-1 Schematic drawing of the principle upper extremity arteries.

The subclavian arteries originate in the chest, usually arising from the brachiocephalic artery on the right and directly from the aortic arch on the left. The brachiocephalic artery (also known as the innominate artery) is the first major branch of the aortic arch and divides into the right common carotid artery and the right subclavian artery. Rarely, the right subclavian artery may originate directly from the aorta distal to the left subclavian artery in what is known as a retroesophageal subclavian artery, or an aberrant subclavian artery. An aberrant right subclavian artery often arises from a dilated segment of the proximal descending aorta known as a Kommerell's diverticulum. Although most patients are asymptomatic, some may have difficulty with swallowing from compression of the esophagus (dysphagia lusoria) by the abnormally positioned subclavian artery. Palsy of the recurrent laryngeal nerve can occur with this anatomic variation and is called Ortner's syndrome.

The left subclavian artery takes its origin directly from the aortic arch as the third major branch following the left common carotid artery. The vertebral arteries are the first major branches of both the right and left subclavian arteries. The left vertebral artery may originate directly from the aortic arch in 4% to 6% of patients.[1] Also arising from the subclavian arteries are the thyrocervical and costocervical trunks. These arteries can be distinguished from the vertebral arteries by their multiple branches and lower end-diastolic flow velocities.

The subclavian arteries exit the chest through the thoracic outlet (Fig. 10-2). In the course of the subclavian artery, there are three spaces or distinct sites for potential compression. The subclavian artery passes over the first rib between the anterior and middle scalene muscles through the scalene triangle. The subclavian vein passes superficial to the anterior scalene muscle and bypasses the scalene triangle. The costoclavicular space is bound by the clavicle and first rib and is the next area of possible compression. It is traversed by all three components of the neurovascular bundle. The third (most lateral) space is the pectoralis minor space. It is infrequently involved in symptomatic compression.[2] Upper extremity arterial symptoms may be caused by impingement within the thoracic outlet. The effects on the subclavian artery may include stenosis, aneurysmal dilatation, laminar thrombus, and dynamic compression with arm abduction. The subclavian artery is renamed the axillary artery at the lateral margin of the first rib. The axillary artery lies deep to the pectoralis major and minor muscles. Within the axilla, it can be found deep to the axillary fat pad.

The axillary artery transitions to the brachial artery at the level of the inferolateral border of the teres major muscle. This muscle cannot be routinely identified by duplex ultrasound. Here, the artery takes a more superficial course in the medial arm between

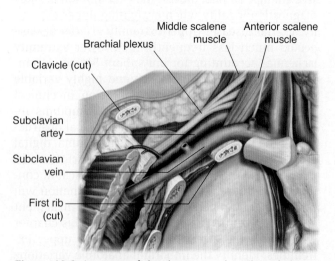

Figure 10-2 Anatomy of the thoracic outlet. The subclavian artery passes over the first rib between the anterior and middle scalene muscles.

the biceps muscle anteriorly and the triceps muscle posteriorly. The deep brachial artery is visualized in the upper arm passing posterior to the humerus. The deep brachial, radial, and ulnar recurrent arteries are important sources of collateral blood flow at the elbow. The most common anatomic variant at this level is a so-called high takeoff of the radial artery, where the radial artery originates in the mid to upper arm instead of distal to the antecubital fossa. An accessory or duplicated brachial artery is seen with a prevalence as high as 19% of some angiographic series. Less commonly, the ulnar artery may originate in the upper arm in 2% to 3% of the population.

At the elbow level, the brachial artery passes obliquely from medial to lateral, dividing into the radial, ulnar, and interosseous arteries. The radial artery continues to the wrist deep to the flexor muscles of the forearm before taking a more superficial course at the wrist between the flexor carpi radialis tendon and the radius. This is where the radial artery is readily palpated by physical exam. At the wrist, the radial artery divides into two branches. The superficial branch passes anterior to the thumb where it anastomoses with the superficial palmar arch. The main branch of the radial artery courses posterior to the thumb where it becomes the deep palmar arch.

The ulnar artery gives origin to the interosseous artery in the proximal forearm before passing deep to the forearm flexor muscles. The interosseous artery continues to the wrist as the median artery in 2% to 4% of patients.[3] The ulnar artery courses toward the wrist adjacent to the flexor carpi ulnaris tendon before crossing the wrist where it then passes deep to the hook of the hamate bone. It terminates as the superficial palmar arch. The hamate is an important landmark. Traumatic injury to the ulnar artery in this region can lead to arterial degeneration, thrombus formation, and potential occlusion. This describes the hypothenar hammer syndrome.

Branches from the superficial palmar arch, and to a lesser extent the deep palmar arch, via communicating vessels, give origin to the metacarpal arteries. These continue to the digits, forming paired digital arteries.

SONOGRAPHIC EXAMINATION TECHNIQUES

The following techniques illustrate the standard duplex ultrasound examination of the upper extremity arteries. Later in the chapter, additional methods will be discussed when describing some common disorders affecting the upper extremities. It is important to remember to keep the examination room at a comfortable temperature; too cold a room can cause peripheral vasoconstriction, which will impact Doppler spectral waveforms, particularly in the digits.

PATIENT PREPARATION

An explanation of the procedure and obtaining a pertinent history are the initial steps in upper extremity arterial duplex scanning. Clothing covering the areas to be examined should be removed and a patient gown should be provided. Any jewelry such as chains, necklaces, bracelets, and watches should be removed.

PATIENT POSITIONING

The patient is positioned supine with the head elevated to conduct the exam (Fig. 10-3). The evaluation of the axillary artery is conducted with the arm in the "pledge position," with the arm externally rotated and positioned at a 45° angle from the body.

SCANNING TECHNIQUE

Blood pressure at the brachial artery is obtained and documented for each arm. Each extremity is examined sequentially to include the subclavian, axillary, brachial, radial, and ulnar arteries. The peak systolic velocities (PSVs) are documented point to point in each major vessel using an optimal 45° to 60° transducer angle in the longitudinal plane. When irregularities are noted, Doppler signals are obtained using a "stenosis profile" consisting of a prestenosis Doppler PSV, stenosis PSV, and documentation of poststenotic turbulence. When an aneurysm is encountered, measurements are obtained in the transverse view of the proximal, mid, and distal site in both the anterior–posterior (A/P) and lateral orientations. An attempt is made to visualize intraluminal thrombosis. It is important to visualize the vessel in a true axial plane so as to not falsely overestimate the aneurysm diameter with an oblique view.

Examination of the subclavian artery can generally be accomplished with a 5-MHz transducer. The windows for insonation of the origin of the subclavian artery include the sternal notch and supraclavicular or infraclavicular approaches (Fig. 10-4A–C).

Obese patients may require a lower megahertz transducer. Using the sternal notch window, a recent study found 48 of 50 right subclavian artery origins and 25 of 50 left subclavian artery origins.[4] To use the sternal notch approach, a small footprint, 3- to 5-MHz transducer is used. The artery may be identified in the transverse view with the assistance of color Doppler. As the artery is identified, the transducer is rotated 90° to obtain a longitudinal view (Fig. 10-5).

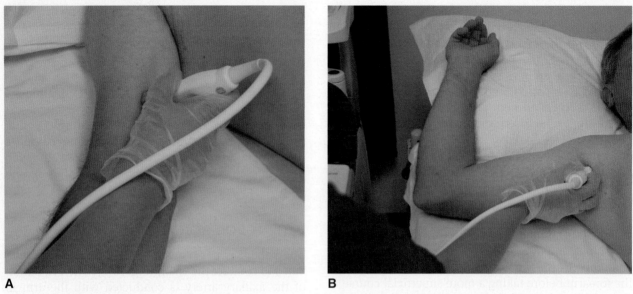

Figure 10-3 For upper extremity arterial duplex examinations, the patient is positioned supine with the head of the bed slightly elevated **(A)**; evaluation of the axillary artery can be conducted with the arm in the "pledge position" **(B).**

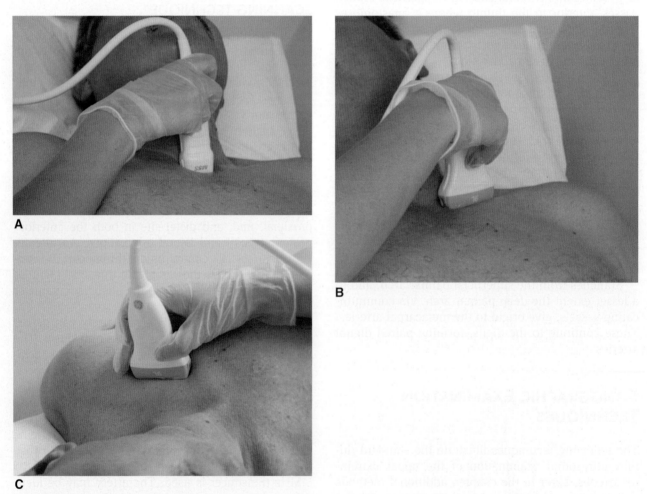

Figure 10-4 The windows for examining the proximal brachial cephalic vessels include the sternal notch **(A)** and the supraclavicular **(B)** and infraclavicular **(C)** approaches.

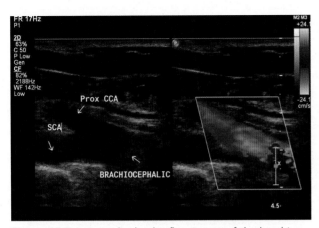

Figure 10-5 Longitudinal color flow image of the brachiocephalic artery giving rise to the right common carotid artery (CCA) and the right subclavian artery (SCA).

The subclavian artery is followed as it crosses under the clavicle and over the first rib. The axillary artery is identified in an anterior approach deep to the pectoralis major and minor muscles. In the axilla, it is seen deep to the axillary fat pad. The axillary artery becomes the brachial artery after crossing the teres major muscle. There is normally no difference noted in the artery as the subclavian artery becomes the axillary artery. The brachial artery takes a more superficial course in the medial arm between the biceps muscle anteriorly and the triceps muscles posteriorly. Views of the proximal, mid, and distal brachial, radial, and ulnar arteries are obtained. Any areas of stenosis, occlusion, or aneurysmal enlargement are documented as previously described.

TECHNICAL CONSIDERATIONS

To prevent any missed occlusions or false-negative examinations, many laboratories choose to include physiologic testing as a component of the upper extremity arterial exam. The physiologic testing performed with multilevel pressures or waveforms provide a qualitative assessment of global perfusion. The duplex ultrasound evaluation can be conducted using physiologic waveforms as a guide. When significant changes are encountered by these indirect noninvasive tests, the subclavian velocities and waveforms should be recorded with ultrasound. Chapter 8 describes these physiologic tests in more detail.

PITFALLS

Potential impediments to the examination include the presence of wounds/dressings, intravenous catheters, and orthopedic fixation devices. Multiple approaches must be used to maximize visualization around these obstacles.

DIAGNOSIS

The normal upper extremity artery waveform is triphasic with a sharp systolic peak followed by a brief period of diastolic flow reversal and then minimal continued forward flow in diastole. This is characteristic of a normal high resistance peripheral artery (Fig. 10-6).

The normal peak systolic velocities range from 80 to 120 cm/s in the subclavian arteries and 40 to 60 cm/s in the forearm arteries, with similar velocities in radial and ulnar arteries. Stenosis results in elevated peak systolic velocities (jets), poststenotic turbulence, and dampened distal waveforms with loss of end-systolic flow reversal (Figs. 10-7 and 10-8). There are no generally accepted velocity criteria to determine the degree of stenosis in upper extremity arteries.[5] Although there are no universally accepted criteria for upper extremity arterial stenosis, general guidelines are listed in Table 10-1.

Arterial duplex ultrasound was performed in 57 patients to evaluate 578 arterial segments in 66 upper extremities to determine the clinical utility of velocity criteria to detect a >50% stenosis. The criteria used for >50% stenosis was a PSV ratio of greater than 2, relating the narrowed segment to that of the artery immediately proximal to the lesion. All of the extremities underwent intra-arterial digital subtraction angiography. Duplex ultrasound correctly identified 15 of 19 hemodynamically significant stenoses giving a sensitivity of 79% and a specificity of 100%.[6] In another comparison study of duplex ultrasound and angiography, loss of diastolic flow reversal was the earliest sign of significant arterial stenosis in 21 patients with ischemic upper extremities when compared to controls.[7] The angle of insonation can be difficult to determine when

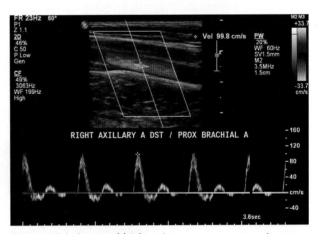

Figure 10-6 A normal high resistance upper extremity artery waveform (triphasic). There is a rapid systolic upstroke, an end-systolic reverse flow component with minimal or no flow at the end of diastole.

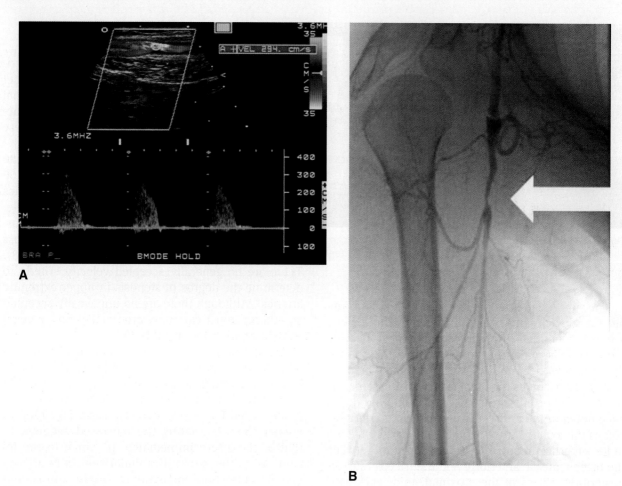

Figure 10-7 A: Duplex color flow image and velocity waveform in a patient with brachial artery stenosis and symptomatic arm ischemia secondary to a crutch injury. Note the loss of the end-systolic reverse flow component of the arterial waveform. **B:** Corresponding angiogram with brachial artery stenosis *(arrow)*.

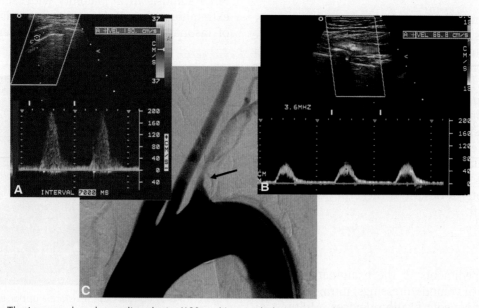

Figure 10-8 A: The increased peak systolic velocity (190 cm/s) in a subclavian artery lesion with **(B)** a dampened waveform distally in the subclavian artery suggests the patient's exercise induced arm pain is likely related to the subclavian stenosis. **C:** An angiogram illustrating proximal left subclavian artery stenosis

TABLE 10-1	
Duplex Ultrasound Criteria for the Evaluation of Upper Extremity Arterial Stenosis	
Condition	**Characteristics**
Normal	Uniform waveforms; biphasic or triphasic waveforms; clear window beneath systolic peak
<50% diameter reduction	Focal velocity increase; spectral broadening; possibly triphasic or biphasic flow
>50% diameter reduction	Focal velocity increase; loss of triphasic or biphasic velocity waveform; poststenotic flow (color bruit)
Occlusion	No flow detected

OCCLUSIONS

Occlusions are documented by demonstrating an absence of flow within the lumen of the artery by color imaging as well as the absence of spectral Doppler signals (Fig. 10-10). Power Doppler can also be used to confirm the absence of flow. Care must be taken to properly adjust equipment settings to increase sensitivity to detect low flow states.

In the forearm, there are multiple structures including tendons, nerves, and muscle fascicles that may be mistaken for occluded arteries. Fortunately, the arterial anatomy of the forearm is generally constant. The superficial location of the arteries facilitates the vascular sonographer's ability to follow these structures proximally and distally. The companion veins can also be used as a landmark to help identify the arteries. Although rarely necessary, exercise or warming the extremity can assist in the exam by increasing blood flow.

ANEURYSMS

By definition, aneurysms are a permanent localized dilation resulting in a 50% increase in the diameter of the artery compared to the diameter of the normal adjacent artery. Several regions of upper extremity arteries deserve consideration. First, aneurysms of the subclavian artery often occur in association with arterial thoracic outlet syndrome (TOS), accounting

examining the proximal brachiocephalic arteries. False elevations of peak systolic velocity may occur. The true hemodynamic significance of the stenosis may be inferred from examination of more distal waveforms. A triphasic waveform distal to a high peak systolic velocity may indicate a falsely elevated proximal peak systolic velocity. Measurement of bilateral brachial artery pressures is also useful to help sort out the hemodynamic significance of the elevated proximal peak systolic velocity (Fig. 10-9).

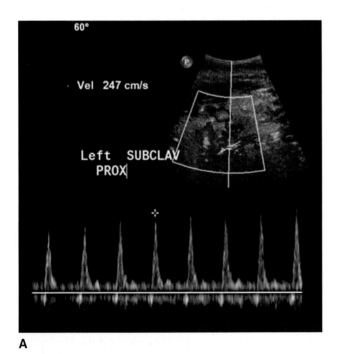

A

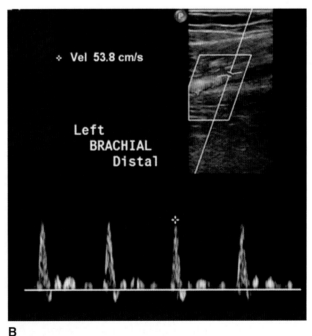

B

Figure 10-9 Angles of insonation can be difficult to determine at the origins of the brachiocephalic vessels. In this case, the elevated left proximal subclavian peak systolic velocity of 247 cm/s **(A)** may not indicate a hemodynamically significant lesion as the distal brachial artery has a normal triphasic Doppler-derived waveform **(B)**.

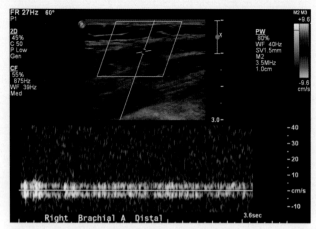

Figure 10-10 Occluded brachial artery with no flow on pulsed Doppler or color examination.

for 16 of 38 (42%) of subclavian artery aneurysms in one series.[8] Arterial thoracic outlet syndrome is not commonly associated with neurologic or venous symptoms of thoracic outlet syndrome.

The duplex evaluation of subclavian aneurysms can be challenging due to their subtle fusiform nature and location in proximity to the bony landmarks of the thoracic outlet. An examination for outer wall measurement and the documentation of a mural thrombus are important determinants of aneurysms and can be accomplished with B-mode ultrasound. Atherosclerosis and trauma are also well-known etiologies of aneurysms of the axillary, brachial, radial, and ulnar arteries. However, these lesions are infrequent. When encountered, they may present with a pulsatile mass, thrombosis, or embolization. The characterization of these aneurysms is facilitated by the ease of insonation of these arteries.

As discussed previously, the ulnar artery passes deep to the hook of the hamate bone in the hand. This is a site of arterial degeneration, which can result from repeated use of the palm of the hand as a hammer, the so-called hypothenar hammer syndrome. Patients may present with symptoms of finger ischemia from embolization to digital and palmar arteries. Vessel stenosis, thrombosis, or aneurysm may occur within this distal portion of the ulnar artery.

DISORDERS

There are multiple vascular disorders that impact the upper extremity arteries. The following sections describe various diseases and disorders, which can be evaluated with upper extremity arterial ultrasound examinations.

RAYNAUD'S SYNDROME

Many patients presenting with upper extremity ischemia demonstrate a clinical syndrome of intermittent digital ischemia from cold exposure or emotional stimuli. Primary Raynaud's syndrome is a condition of abnormal digital artery vasospasm resulting in pain and a characteristic pallor of the digits followed by cyanosis and hyperemia upon rewarming. Anatomically, the digital arteries appear normal. Primary Raynaud's syndrome generally has a benign prognosis, but Raynaud's type symptoms may be the first manifestations of an underlying systemic disease. When there is an underlying disease process responsible for the symptoms, the terms secondary Raynaud's syndrome or Raynaud's phenomenon are used.

The most common systemic condition resulting in secondary Raynaud's syndrome is the autoimmune disorder scleroderma. Other conditions associated with digital artery occlusion include mixed connective tissue disease, systemic lupus erythematosus, rheumatoid arthritis, drug-induced vasospasm, and cancer. Patients with Raynaud's secondary to a systemic disorder tend to develop occlusive lesions of upper extremity digital arteries. Even though patients with primary Raynaud's may present with a dramatic history of transient ischemic changes, they infrequently develop tissue necrosis beyond occasional mild erosions. However, in patients with Raynaud's symptoms as a result of fixed occlusive lesions of the upper extremity, digital arteries often develop tissue necrosis. The large majority of digital artery occlusive disease originating distal to the wrist is a result of a systemic disorder. Only a minority of patients have digital occlusion secondary to embolization from a proximal source. Such lesions, including subclavian artery aneurysms, stenotic lesions of the upper extremity arteries, as well as fibromuscular disease of forearm arteries, and a duplex can play a role in diagnosis.

In those with suspected pathology proximal to the digital vessel, duplex ultrasound imaging can be performed using the techniques described in the preceding section. The image should be closely examined for aneurysmal disease, thrombus, or plaque formation, which may give rise to distal embolization. Although examination of the digital vessels can be conducted with ultrasound, photoplethysmography (PPG) is often chosen to assess digital perfusion. PPG waveforms are recorded from all upper extremity digits at rest at normal room temperatures and may also be repeated following a cold sensitivity challenge. Please refer to Chapter 8 for a full description of plethysmography techniques and diagnostic criteria.

THORACIC OUTLET SYNDROME

Impingement of the neurovascular bundle as it traverses the confines of the thoracic outlet can cause symptoms related to the compression of the brachial plexus or vascular structures, but rarely both at the same time. Compression of structures in the thoracic outlet may be secondary to cervical ribs, abnormal fibrous bands, and possibly hypertrophy of the scalene muscles.

Symptoms of pure neurogenic TOS consist of pain, weakness, and muscle atrophy. A definitive diagnosis is made by appropriate history and physical combined with electromyography (EMG) or nerve conduction studies. Demonstration of positional subclavian artery occlusion with an arterial duplex is often used as "supportive evidence" of neurogenic TOS because impingement of the subclavian artery is thought to suggest impingement of the adjacent neural tissues at the thoracic outlet. However, these provocative maneuvers are not specific, and subclavian artery occlusion can be demonstrated in up to 20% of normal individuals.[9] There is no convincing evidence that arterial duplex can or should be used to confirm neurogenic TOS.

Venous TOS is another variant of thoracic outlet syndrome. Patients present with swelling of the arm due to venous obstruction and/or thrombosis. Chapter 15 discusses the venous duplex ultrasound procedures used in assessing the upper extremity venous system.

Major arterial thoracic outlet syndrome occurs primarily in younger patients. Large cervical ribs or clavicular abnormalities secondary to prior trauma can compress and damage the subclavian artery. This repeated trauma can result in a subclavian artery aneurysm, stenosis, ulceration, or occlusion of the subclavian artery. All of these abnormalities can be the source of acute or chronic distal embolization to digital and palmar arteries. In more advanced cases, even occlusion of the brachial, axillary, and/or forearm arteries can occur, all of which can be detected by arterial duplex scanning.

Arterial duplex or plethysmographic findings suggestive of asymmetric digital artery occlusion should prompt a search for a proximal embolic source. Duplex ultrasound can readily identify subclavian artery aneurysms and significant occlusive lesions. However, emboli can also result from seemingly trivial lesions. Slight areas of luminal irregularity are not definitively excluded by arterial duplex scanning. When there are unilateral digital artery occlusions and negative proximal arterial duplex studies, arteriography or intravascular ultrasound (IVUS) is indicated to definitively rule out a proximal arterial source of emboli.

Some patients with positional occlusion or stenosis of the subclavian artery may be quite symptomatic with activity, especially when working with their arms overhead. In such cases, the subclavian artery is compressed between the clavicle and first rib when the arms are abducted for overhead activity. Duplex or plethysmographic techniques can be used to demonstrate positional changes in distal arterial waveforms. It is uncommon for this so-called arterial minor form of TOS to result in damage to the arterial wall or to cause distal embolization. Treatment is only indicated in severely symptomatic patients. Treatment consists of first rib resection without arterial reconstruction.

Even though upper extremity arterial duplex is not indicated in the evaluation of neurogenic TOS, provocative maneuvers in an attempt to elicit vascular compromise as supportive evidence for possible neurogenic TOS are widely practiced. Patients are examined with a series of provocative positional changes in an attempt to provoke and therefore detect subclavian artery compromise. Other noninvasive vascular lab techniques, including segmental pressures with pulse volume recordings (PVRs) and/or digital photoplethysmography (PPG), may also be used with these maneuvers. Chapter 8 provides a complete review of these maneuvers.

TRAUMA

Currently, the standard of care for identifying a clinically significant vascular deficit in the setting of arterial trauma is arteriography or direct surgical exploration. There is a benefit in performing screening arterial duplex examinations in patients with a normal physical exam but with a history of blunt or penetrating trauma distal to the axillary crease. One study evaluated 198 patients with 319 potential vascular injuries to the neck or extremities. The mechanism of injury was gunshot wounds in 62%, stabbings in 17%, and blunt trauma in 21%. All patients were hemodynamically stable without a clinically obvious arterial injury. Arterial duplex studies correctly diagnosed 23 vascular injuries with 2 false-negative studies, neither of which required intervention, giving a sensitivity of 95% and specificity of 100%.[10]

Another study evaluated upper extremity trauma patients with diminished extremity pulses. Fifty patients underwent extremity arterial duplex ultrasound followed by confirmatory angiography and/or surgical exploration with a 100% sensitivity and specificity.[11] In a follow-up cohort of 175 patients, the same authors used duplex ultrasound as the sole imaging modality and diagnosed 18 injuries. Seventeen of these were later confirmed by angiography and/or surgery. This study gives further evidence that duplex ultrasound serves as an effective means of evaluating for occult arterial injury. If immediate operative repair is not indicated, positive findings can be followed up with arteriography. A well-performed normal arterial duplex examination essentially rules out major clinically significant injuries of upper extremity arteries distal to the axillary crease. The ultrasound techniques for examining patients with suspected arterial trauma are those used for standard upper extremity evaluation, but additional considerations should be taken. Depending on the type of trauma (particularly a gunshot wound), the arterial injury may be remote to a wound. All vessels in the region should be examined for intimal tears or dissections as these are often associated with traumatic injuries.

ARTERIAL OCCLUSIVE DISEASE

Clinically significant upper extremity atherosclerosis in the absence of renal failure or diabetes is generally confined to the proximal subclavian artery. This most often occurs in the left subclavian artery and is often an extension of atherosclerotic involvement of the aortic arch. Proximal subclavian artery stenosis rarely produces significant upper extremity symptoms. If there are symptoms, they typically manifest as exertional pain in the forearm. Progression to rest pain, ischemic ulceration, or gangrene in the absence of embolization is unusual. Atherosclerosis proximal to the origin of the vertebral artery can result in an anatomic subclavian steal syndrome. In order for there to be a true subclavian steal syndrome, there must be posterior fossa symptoms attributable to inadequate blood flow. On duplex ultrasound, this is seen as stenosis or occlusion of the subclavian artery with reversed or staccato flow in the vertebral artery (Fig. 10-11).

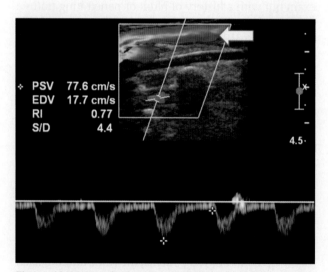

Figure 10-11 Vertebral artery with flow reversal. Flow is below the baseline in the Doppler display. Note that with color flow, vertebral artery flow is in the same direction as the flow in the internal jugular vein (*white arrow*).

Pathology Box 10-1 summarizes some of the commonly encountered upper extremity arterial pathology.

OTHER UPPER EXTREMITY DISORDERS

Takayasu's arteritis, an autoimmune disorder, affects the arteries of the aortic arch and visceral abdominal aorta, most commonly in women in their 20s and 30s. Patients have long-segment occlusions or stenosis of the affected arteries. Aortic valve insufficiency and pulmonary hypertension occur in advanced cases. In its acute phase, it is associated with fever, malaise, arthralgias, and myalgias. Laboratory studies demonstrate an elevated erythrocyte sedimentation rate and C-reactive protein. Steroids and immunosuppressive medications are the primary treatment. Arterial duplex can be used to monitor response to therapy. After the acute inflammation has subsided, patients who have not responded to medical intervention and have ongoing ischemic symptoms may benefit from vascular reconstruction.

Giant cell arteritis generally affects Caucasian women who are older than 40 years. Takayasu's arteritis and giant cell arteritis are histologically similar; however, the clinical presentation and distribution of lesions are different. Giant cell arteritis can involve the ophthalmic artery as well as the subclavian and axillary artery. In the acute phase of giant cell arteritis, duplex findings of the axillary artery, in addition to evidence of flow restriction, consist of a thickened, hypoechoic arterial wall due to edema. Anti-inflammatory and immunosuppressant medications are the mainstay treatment. Following resolution of the acute phase, B-mode images may demonstrate a hyperechoic fibrotic arterial wall.[12]

Thromboangiitis obliterans or Buerger's disease primarily involves the small vessels of the hands and feet. This condition is seen in smokers typically under the age of 50 years. Duplex ultrasound is useful to rule out proximal occlusive lesions, but a definitive diagnosis requires exclusion of other underlying causes as well as angiography. Most patients will improve with cessation of tobacco use.

It is not uncommon for patients with end-stage renal disease and dialysis grafts to present with hand ischemia and gangrene. Arterial duplex can be used to evaluate for steal phenomenon. However, in patients with end-stage renal disease and digital ischemia ipsilateral to a dialysis graft or fistula, it is most often that the distal arterial occlusive disease is not amenable to vascular reconstruction. It is frequently underlying arterial disease and not the fistula that is responsible for the occurrence of gangrene in this setting.[13]

PATHOLOGY BOX 10-1

Upper Extremity Arterial Pathology

Pathology	B-Mode Findings	Doppler Findings	Color/Power Doppler Findings
Atherosclerotic stenosis	Plaque evident along vessel walls producing narrowed vessel lumen	Focal increase in PSV; loss of multiphasic waveform	Focal color aliasing with distal turbulence
Occlusion	No visible patent lumen	Absent spectral Doppler signal; high resistance waveforms proximally	No color or power Doppler signals
Aneurysm	A localized dilation with a 50% increase as compared to the adjacent vessel	Turbulence in the dilated region	Turbulence in dilated region; dilated lumen visible on color
Raynaud's syndrome	Digital artery occlusion	Diminished digital waveforms on spectral Doppler or PPG	Poor or no color filling of digital vessels
Arterial thoracic outlet syndrome	Subclavian artery aneurysm, stenosis, ulceration, thrombus, or occlusion	Focal increase in PSV of subclavian artery or no flow seen with occlusion; spectral waveforms or PPG changes with provocative maneuvers	Reduced flow lumen at subclavian artery; no color filling seen with occlusion
Trauma	Intimal tear or dissection; vessel thrombosis or occlusion	Focal increase in PSV; turbulence in waveforms at site or distally	Poor color filling or turbulent pattern; no color filling with occlusion

PSV, peak systolic velocity; PPG, photoplethysmography.

SUMMARY

A wide range of upper extremity arterial conditions can be evaluated by duplex ultrasound reliably and effectively. Combined with the history and physical, as well as other noninvasive vascular laboratory techniques, duplex ultrasound can play a key role in the diagnosis and management of patients with upper extremity arterial disease.

Critical Thinking Questions

1. When examining the subclavian artery and its branches, what are two ways you can distinguish the vertebral artery from the other subclavian branches?

2. You are examining the left subclavian artery and obtain a PSV of 270 cm/s within the most proximal segment you can insonate. What should you do to confirm whether this is a flow-limiting stenosis?

3. You are asked to examine the upper extremities of a 28-year-old female who does not smoke. Her chief complaint is pain in the second and third digits of her right hand. What diagnostic test or tests would you perform and why?

REFERENCES

1. Rose SC, Kadir S. Arterial anatomy of the upper extremity. In: Kadir S, ed. *Atlas of Normal and Variant Angiographic Anatomy.* Philadelphia, PA: WB Saunders; 1991:55–95.
2. Sanders RJ, Cooper MA, Hammond SL, et al. Neurogenic thoracic outlet syndrome. In Rutherford R, ed. *Vascular Surgery.* 5th ed. Philadelphia, PA: WB Saunders; 2000:1184–1200.
3. Kaufman JA, Lee MJ. Upper-extremity arteries. In: Kaufman JA, ed. *The Requisites, Vascular and Interventional Radiology.* Philadelphia, PA: Mosby; 2004:144.
4. Yurdakul M, Tola M, Uslu OS. Color Doppler ultrasonography in occlusive diseases of the brachiocephalic and proximal subclavian arteries. *J Ultrasound in Med.* 2008;27:1065–1070.
5. Jager KA, Phillips DJ, Martin RL, et al. Noninvasive mapping of lower limb arterial lesions. *Ultrasound Med Biol.* 1985;11:515–521.
6. Tola M, Yurdakul M, Okten S, et al. Diagnosis of arterial occlusive disease of the upper extremities: comparison of color Duplex sonography and angiography. *J Clin US.* 2003;31: 407–411.
7. Taneja K, Jain R, Sawhney S, et al. Occlusive arterial disease of the upper extremity: colour Doppler as a screening technique and for assessment of distal circulation. *Australas Radiol.* 1996;40(3):226–229.
8. Bower TC, Pairolero PC, Hallett JW Jr, et al. Brachiocephalic aneurysm: the case for early recognition and repair. *Ann Vasc Surg.* 1991;5(2):125–132.
9. Longley DG, Yedlicka JW, Molina EJ, et al. Thoracic outlet syndrome: evaluation of the subclavian vessels by color duplex sonography. *AJR Am J Roentgenol.* 1992;158(3):623–630.
10. Bynoe RP, Miles WS, Bell RM, et al. Noninvasive diagnosis of vascular trauma by duplex ultrasonography. *J Vasc Surg.* 1991;14(3):346–352.
11. Fry WR, Smith RS, Sayers DV, et al. The success of duplex ultrasonographic scanning in diagnosis of extremity vascular proximity trauma. *Arch Surg.* 1993;128(12):1368–1372.
12. Schmidt WA, Kraft HE, Borkowski A, et al. Color duplex ultrasonography in large-vessel giant cell arteritis. *Scand J Rheumatol.* 1999;28(6):374–376.
13. Yeager RA, Moneta GL, Edwards JM, et al. Relationship of hemodialysis access to finger gangrene in patients with end stage renal disease. *J Vasc Surg.* 2002;36:245–249.

11 Ultrasound Assessment of Arterial Bypass Grafts

Peter W. Leopold and Ann Marie Kupinski

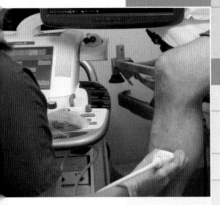

OBJECTIVES

Describe the types of common arterial bypass grafts

Define the essential components of an arterial bypass scan including B-mode, color, and spectral Doppler requirements

Describe the normal hemodynamic profiles of arterial bypass grafts

List the diagnostic criteria employed for identifying a bypass stenosis, occlusion, and other pathology

KEY TERMS

arteriovenous fistula | autogenous vein | bypass | distal anastomosis | graft | hyperemia | in situ bypass | orthograde vein bypass | prosthetic graft | proximal anastomosis | reverse vein bypass

GLOSSARY

anastomosis a connection created surgically to connect two vessels that were formerly not connected

arteriovenous fistula a connection between an artery and vein that was created as a result of surgery or by other iatrogenic means

bypass a channel that diverts blood flow from one artery to another; usually done to shunt flow around an occluded portion of a vessel

graft a conduit that can be prosthetic material or autogenous vein used to divert blood flow from one artery to another

hyperemia an increase in blood flow; this can occur following exercise; it can also occur following restoration of blood flow following periods of ischemia

in situ bypass the great saphenous vein is left in place in its normal anatomical position and used to create a diversionary channel for blood flow around an occluded artery

Duplex ultrasound evaluation of arterial bypass grafts has become a well-recognized fundamental component in postoperative follow-up and management. Careful monitoring of patients with infrainguinal bypasses has clearly shown to improve long-term patency rates.[1] There are several methods that can be used to evaluate bypass function including clinical assessment, indirect assessment with systolic pressure measurements and plethysmographic waveforms, and lastly, direct assessment with ultrasound. Clinical assessment of patient symptoms and physical examination of the limb often fails to identify problems early. Prior studies have shown that ultrasound can detect significant pathology in asymptomatic patients and before a measureable change in physiologic testing results.[2] However, there is a complementary role for ultrasound and indirect physiologic testing. Combining duplex ultrasound with physiologic testing provides both direct assessment of the bypass conduit itself as well as indirect assessment of global limb perfusion. This chapter will focus on the use of duplex ultrasound to evaluate lower extremity bypass grafts. Using these methods, disease can be detected early, prior to bypass graft thrombosis, and will thus aid the long-term maintenance of graft patency.

TYPES OF BYPASS GRAFTS

The types of bypass grafts can be categorized by the components of the graft and the surgical techniques employed. There are two main types of bypass graft materials. Prosthetic (synthetic) bypass grafts are made of various manufactured materials including polytetrafluoroethylene (PTFE) and woven composites such as Dacron. The preferred bypass graft material is autogenous vein, and this chapter will focus primarily on this type of graft. The great saphenous vein, small saphenous vein, cephalic vein, and basilic vein can all be used as bypass conduit. Vein grafts have better long-term patency than synthetic grafts by being less thrombogenic than their synthetic counterparts.[3-7] Although vein grafts are the preferred bypass of choice, they have the potential for early failure and early surveillance is recommended.[8] PTFE grafts have a low potential for early technical failure and ultrasound-detected abnormalities. However, these PTFE grafts have a distinctly worse long-term success rate due to progressive stenoses usually at the inflow or outflow arteries, which will be detectable on ultrasound usually later in the grafts' history. Another type of bypass graft is a cryopreserved human allograft. This type of material is not commonly used for lower extremity bypasses; however, ultrasound evaluation of these graft types would be similar to those outlined in this chapter.

IN SITU BYPASS GRAFTS

Because bypass grafts using an autogenous vein can be constructed using various surgical techniques, these grafts are further described based on the surgery employed. An in situ bypass graft is performed using the great saphenous vein left in place or in situ within its natural tissue bed. Branches of the vein are ligated and the valves within the vein are lyzed. This allows a downward flow of blood without the need to reverse the vein bypass and allows the larger end of the great saphenous to be anastomosed to the larger artery proximally and the smaller end of the vein to be anastomosed distally, usually to a smaller artery such as a tibial artery. This provides a conduit where one end can then be sutured to an artery proximal to the site of disease (the inflow artery), and the other end of the vein conduit is sutured to an artery distal to the distal (the outflow artery). There is often a preference for this type of orientation when the proximal and distal vein sizes match more closely the size of the arteries at the anastomotic sites.

ORTHOGRADE AND RETROGRADE BYPASS GRAFTS

The great saphenous vein and other autogenous veins can also be used as a free vein graft where the vein is completely dissected free from its natural position in the body. This conduit can be placed in an orthograde position where the proximal portion of the vein is used for the proximal anastomosis and the distal portion of the vein is used at the distal anastomosis. In this position, the valves with the vein will need to be lyzed so that blood can flow freely. A free vein graft can also be placed in a retrograde (reversed) position where the vein now has the smaller distal end of the vein anastomosed to the inflow artery and the larger proximal end of the vein is anastomosed to the outflow artery. Essentially, the vein is flipped or reversed so the valve leaflets do not need to be removed and there is no barrier to blood flow.

BYPASS GRAFT PLACEMENT

The actual position of a bypass is determined by the level of arterial disease. The proximal anastomosis is commonly performed using the common femoral or superficial femoral artery as the inflow artery source (Fig. 11-1). Less commonly, the profunda femoral, superficial femoral, or popliteal can be used as the inflow artery. The distal anastomosis is generally constructed below the level of the most distal site of arterial disease. Thus, the outflow artery can be the popliteal artery (either the above knee or below

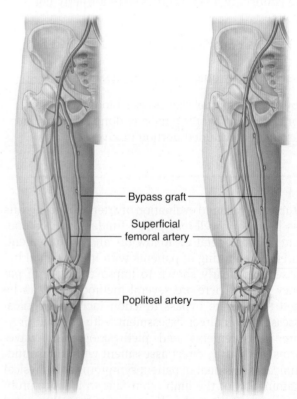

Figure 11-1 Types of vein bypass grafts. The figure on the *left* illustrates a common femoral to popliteal bypass, whereas on the *right*, the bypass is from the common femoral artery to the tibioperoneal trunk.

knee portions), the tibioperoneal trunk, or any of the tibial-level vessels (anterior tibial, posterior tibial, or peroneal arteries). Occasionally, the distal anastomosis of a bypass may be to the dorsalis pedis artery. Given the options for conduit type, orientation, and anatomical position, it can save a great deal of time if the sonographer or technologist refers to an operative note when examining a bypass graft.

MECHANISMS OF BYPASS GRAFT FAILURE

When performing ultrasound examinations on bypass grafts, it is important to have a firm understanding of normal bypass findings but equally important is knowing the types of problems that may exist. There are distinct problems that arise at specific periods during the lifetime of a bypass graft.

During the first 30 days following surgery, ultrasound scanning will identify technical problems that can lead to bypass failure. There may be a retained valve or valve leaflet, an intimal flap caused by the surgical instrumentation of the vein conduit, problems at the anastomotic sites due to suture placement, or possible graft entrapment due to improper positioning of a free vein graft. Additionally, a bypass may thrombose due to use of an inadequate venous conduit or limited run-off bed. Occasionally, early thrombosis can also occur in some patients with a hypercoagulable state. Perioperative bypass graft failure accounts for one-fourth of all failures.[9]

Between months 1 and 24, myointimal hyperplasia can develop, leading to a bypass stenosis. This is not atherosclerotic plaque and has a different ultrasound appearance. A stenosis can occur at any point within the conduit but often a stenosis develops at a valve site. A stenosis can also occur at either the proximal or distal anastomoses. Eleven percent to 33% of all bypasses will have these types of stenoses occur and often they appear within the first year, causing 75% of all revisions performed during this postoperative period.[10]

After 24 months, progression of atherosclerotic disease occurs within the inflow or outflow vessels. It is important to pay close attention to spectral waveform characteristics within the bypass itself as changes in these waveforms may help identify disease in native vessels remote to the bypass graft itself. Loss of diastolic flow is routinely seen within veins bypasses within the first few weeks of surgery particularly when carried out for critical limb-threatening ischemia. However, significant changes in diastolic flow after this early phase, in addition to possible increase in acceleration time and or decreases in peak systolic velocity, can all be signals of development of pathology elsewhere. Aneurysmal dilation of the venous conduit or at the anastomotic sites can develop during this late time, necessitating graft revision.[11] These aneurysms are rare but can result in late bypass graft thrombosis if not corrected.

SONOGRAPHIC EXAMINATION TECHNIQUES

Without any specific indications, duplex ultrasound scanning is performed at routine intervals. There are instances where duplex ultrasound can be performed, which do not follow the routine surveillance schedule. If a patient presents with acute onset of pain, diminished or absent pedal pulses, persistent nonhealing ulcers, or a recent history of loss of limb swelling (normally found in most successful vein bypass grafts) suggestive of graft failure and ischemia, a duplex ultrasound scan can be performed. Poor physiologic testing results, including an ankle–brachial index, which falls by greater than 0.15, would also be an appropriate indication for a duplex scan.

A routine surveillance protocol can consist of an ultrasound performed early in the postoperative period, usually within the first 3 months. Subsequent ultrasounds can be performed at 3-month intervals for the first year, every 6 months for the second postoperative year, and then annually thereafter. In most laboratories, the direct ultrasound scanning is performed in conjunction with indirect physiologic testing, including ankle pressures and plethysmographic waveforms. Pulse volume recordings can be safely performed over bypass grafts because the pressures are low enough not to occlude the grafts. Many laboratories choose to avoid measuring systolic pressures at levels where cuffs are placed over the grafts. In cases of grafts with distal tibial or pedal outflow vessels, toe pressures and waveforms can be recorded.

There are patients in whom surveillance should be more intense. Patients who have undergone an intraoperative revision, early postoperative thrombectomy or revision, and patients with limited venous conduits should be scanned more frequently. Many surgeons will choose to follow these patients at 2-month intervals.

The surveillance of prosthetic bypass grafts is less common. Many laboratories may follow these patients with physiologic testing and clinical evaluation. It has been shown that duplex ultrasound is more sensitive in determining failing prosthetic grafts than an ankle–brachial index or clinical examination.[12]

PATIENT PREPARATION

As with any examination, the procedures should be explained to the patient, taking into consideration the age and mental status of the patient. If relatives or caregivers are present, they can be used to assist with the explanation if necessary.

As noted earlier in this chapter, another consideration prior to the beginning of the ultrasound is review of the patient's operative notes. An operative note provides important information as to the specific course and composition of the bypass graft, which can be used as a guide to facilitate bypass graft imaging.

PATIENT POSITIONING

The patient should be positioned supine with the head of the bed slightly elevated. The limb to be examined should be externally rotated at the hip with the knee slightly bent. In those patients with various joint conditions such as arthritis, a small pillow may be placed under the knee to avoid joint pain. The patient should be resting comfortably for a few minutes prior to the recording of any velocity measurements.

EQUIPMENT

Various transducer frequencies can be used to image bypass grafts. For superficial in situ bypass grafts, a 10- or 12-MHz transducer will provide optimal near-field imaging. For deeper bypass grafts, a 5-7 MHz transducer will be needed. Technologists and sonographers must remember that many of the ultrasound transducers commonly used today have multiple imaging and Doppler frequencies. These can and should be adjusted if the course of the bypass is such that various tissue depths are encountered.

Required Documentation

Individual laboratory protocols vary slightly; however, there are several essential elements that need to be documented. The following lists the minimum suggested documentation; however, additional images are often necessary. Grayscale images should be recorded of the inflow artery, proximal anastomosis, mid-graft, distal anastomosis, and outflow artery. At each of these locations, a spectral Doppler waveform should also be recorded with the peak systolic velocity (PSV) measured. If color flow imaging is part of the protocol, color flow images should be documented at the same sites. In the case of any abnormalities, additional documentation in grayscale, spectral Doppler, and color should be recorded. For any stenotic areas, spectral Doppler needs to be noted prior

to the stenotic region, at the area of greatest velocity shift, and distal to the stenotic region.

These requirements are based on current standards established by the Intersocietal Commission for the Accreditation of Vascular Laboratories (ICAVL).

SCANNING TECHNIQUE

The examination should begin with the selection of the appropriate transducer based on body habitus and bypass depth. The ultrasound system application preset for peripheral arterial imaging should be chosen. The application preset settings for grayscale, spectral Doppler, and color will likely need to be specifically optimized for each patient.

Proper Doppler techniques should be followed during this examination. Spectral analysis should be recorded at approximately a 60° angle whenever possible. Angles greater than 60° should never be used. Angles less than 60° may need to be used depending on the course of the vessel. If this is a follow-up examination, one should try to use the same angles previously employed to avoid additional variations in data due to the angle of insonation. The sample volume placement should be in the center of the vessel or flow channel (Fig. 11-2). The sample volume should be small unless searching for a small jet or total vessel occlusion.

As mentioned in the preceding section, if disease is present within any portion of a vessel or graft, record the spectral analysis with the greatest Doppler shift as well as proximal and distal to this area, if possible. This is often referred to as "walking through" the stenosis. The PSV and end-diastolic velocities (EDVs) should be recorded. Poststenotic turbulence should be documented. All this information is helpful for the interpreting physician to properly categorize the severity of a stenosis.

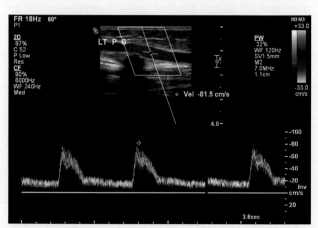

Figure 11-2 This figure demonstrates the appropriate placement of the Doppler sample volume (center stream) and alignment of the Doppler angle (parallel to the walls of the vessel).

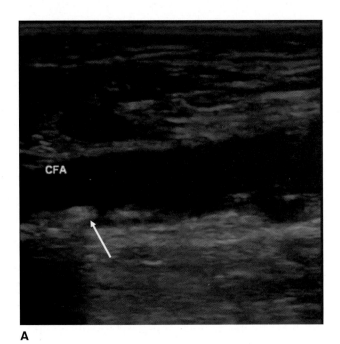

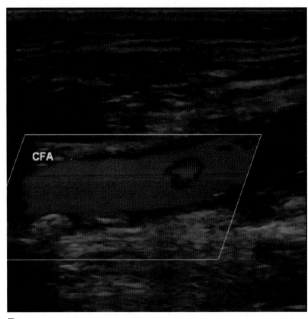

A   **B**

Figure 11-3 A: This is a grayscale image of the common femoral artery, which is the inflow source for an in situ bypass graft. A mild amount of plaque is present along the posterior wall of the vessel *(arrow)*. **B:** The same portion of the vessel with color flow imaging.

The ultrasound examination should begin within the inflow vessel. Vessels can initially be identified in transverse or sagittal views. Using a transverse view, an initial rough scan of the full length of the bypass as well as inflow and outflow vessels can help orient the vascular technologist or sonographer prior to being the formal scanning. Once the inflow artery is identified, the examination should be then performed using a sagittal orientation. A representative grayscale image should be recorded of the inflow artery (Fig. 11-3). Typically, the end of the vein conduit is anastomosed to the side of the inflow artery. This allows for flow down the bypass conduit as well as some flow to be maintained within the native distal artery. This will allow for some nutritive flow into the native arterial bed, including any collaterals that may be present. Any pathology observed should be documented in both transverse and sagittal planes. A transverse orientation is particularly helpful to identify patent tributaries of an in situ bypass graft. A spectral Doppler waveform is obtained and the PSV and EDV are recorded (Fig. 11-4).

Color flow imaging can be used to facilitate vessel identification and with following the course of a bypass graft. However, color will often mask small wall defects and other pathology. Color imaging should be documented at the various levels where grayscale and spectral Doppler images are recorded (see Fig. 11-3). Color flow imaging should also be documented in stenotic areas to illustrate the disturbed flow patterns and aliasing if present.

The scan proceeds through the proximal anastomosis. Again, at this point, grayscale, color, and spectral Doppler are recorded. It is not uncommon to observe some slight changes in velocity or minimal disturbed flow (Fig. 11-5) when there is a normal change in caliber of a vessel or graft commonly encountered at any point where blood flow changes direction, such as a branch or anastomosis between two conduits of differing size. Continuing down the leg, the entire portion of each bypass graft should be examined. Simultaneous duplex mode observing both the B-mode image and spectral Doppler analysis is the ideal method for looking and listening for any potential bypass

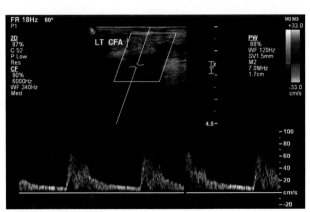

Figure 11-4 A normal Doppler spectrum obtained from the common femoral artery, which is the inflow source for an in situ bypass graft.

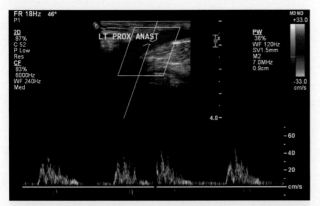

Figure 11-5 A Doppler spectrum taken at the proximal anastomosis of a bypass graft. Slight turbulence is present.

problems. When "walk through" is used, listening to the Doppler signal changes is a highly sensitive tool to localize abnormalities with an increase in velocities for more careful analysis. At a minimum, grayscale, color, and spectral Doppler should be recorded in the mid-graft region; however, a more thorough protocol would include these images documented from the proximal, mid, and distal segments (Fig. 11-6).

The examination concludes with continuing to scan through the distal anastomosis and into the outflow artery (Fig. 11-7). At both of these levels, grayscale, color, and spectral Doppler are recorded. The distal anastomosis may also exhibit mild turbulence due to the geometry of the anastomosis and the slight disruption in the laminar flow profile. One can often encounter a slight increase in PSV within the outflow artery, as this may be a small caliber as compared to the bypass itself (Fig. 11-8).

The primary goal of the examination is to document anatomic and hemodynamic characteristics of the bypass graft and adjacent vessels. It is also important to use the hemodynamic information within or near the bypass to determine if additional testing is required. Abnormal waveforms may suggest pathology remote to the region, thus justifying extending the ultrasound examination further proximally or distally. These waveforms will be discussed later in this chapter.

Even though the focus of the examination is on the bypass, the scanning protocol should include documentation of incidental findings. Other pathology such as venous thrombosis, dilated lymph nodes, hematoma, seroma, abscesses, and similar structures can be encountered. Length, width, and depth of masses, cysts, nodes, or other focal structures should be recorded. Color flow and spectral Doppler can be used to document the presence or

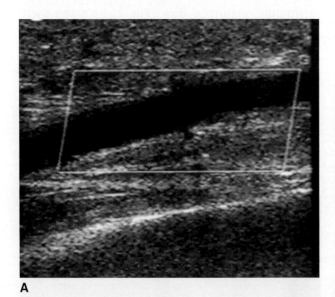

A

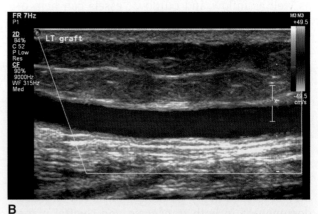

B

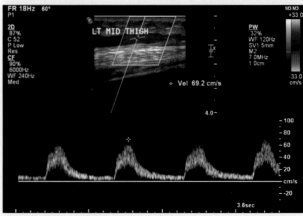

C

Figure 11-6 Normal appearance of the midportion of a bypass graft. **A:** A grayscale image, **(B)** a color flow image, and **(C)** a Doppler spectrum.

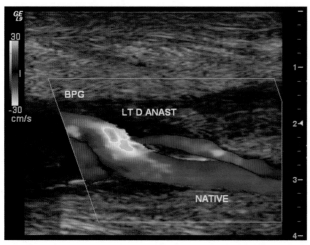

Figure 11-7 An ultrasound image of a distal anastomosis to a posterior tibial artery. (Image courtesy of Phillip J. Bendick, PhD RVT, Royal Oak, MI.)

absence of blood flow within an incidental finding. Multiple scanning planes should be used to fully document the additional pathology. Proximity to the bypass graft is also important to note, particularly in the event of an abscess.

PITFALLS

This examination can be slightly limited in a very obese patient. A bypass graft that is anatomically placed and tunneled deeply will necessitate the use of lower frequency transducers in order to penetrate deep enough to visualize the graft; however, this will result in poorer resolution. Dressings, skin staples, and sutures will also limit accessibility of portions of the bypass grafts to the ultrasound examination.

DIAGNOSIS

There are three components to analysis of the data obtained from ultrasound: the B-mode or grayscale image, the spectral Doppler waveform (which is the primary source of numerical data used to classify disease), and the color flow image.

GRAYSCALE FINDINGS

The B-mode or grayscale image should be closely examined for disease. The walls of a vein graft appear smooth and uniform. Figure 11-9 illustrates the

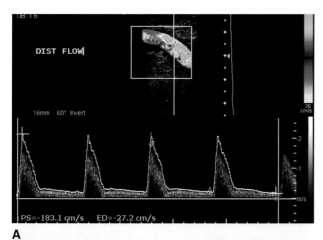

A

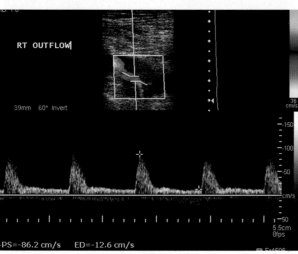

C

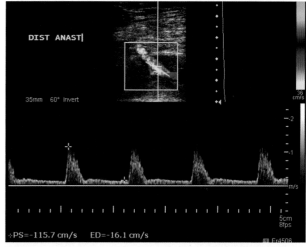

B

Figure 11-8 Spectral Doppler tracing through the distal portion of a bypass and outflow artery: **(A)** a distal bypass, **(B)** a distal anastomosis, and **(C)** an outflow artery.

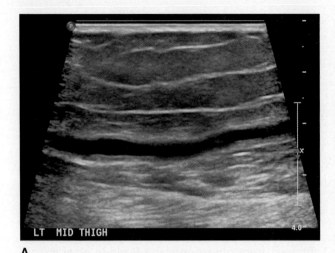

A

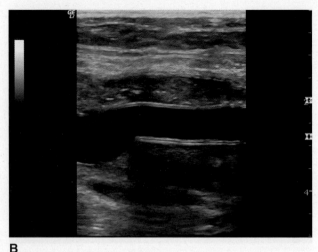

B

Figure 11-9 Normal grayscale appearance of various types of bypass grafts. **A:** An autogenous vein (Image courtesy of Debra Joly, RVT, RDMS, RDCS, Houston, TX). **B:** A PTFE (Image courtesy of William Zang, BS, RVT, RDMS, GE Healthcare, Wauwatosa, WI).

normal grayscale appearance of a vein bypass graft and a PTFE graft. The intimal-medial layer should be clearly visible if the bypass graft is perpendicular to the ultrasound beam.

Within the inflow and outflow arteries, atherosclerotic plaque may be present. Plaque should be characterized as homogeneous or heterogeneous.

Homogeneous plaques have uniform echogenicity. Heterogeneous plaques have mixed level echoes within the plaques. Calcification, which appears as bright white echoes causing acoustic shadowing, should be noted (Fig. 11-10). If possible, the surface characteristics of a plaque should be noted. This can be described as smooth surfaced or irregular surfaced.

Within the vein conduit itself, the two most common image abnormalities that can be observed are valves and myointimal hyperplasia. Valves or valve remnants may be present due to incomplete valve disruption during surgery (Fig. 11-11). Small remnants will have a minimal impact on flow through bypass. Larger remnants or completely intact leaflets will produce a flow-limiting stenosis

Figure 11-10 A grayscale image of the common femoral artery proximal to a bypass graft. The image demonstrates heterogeneous calcific plaque *(arrow)* within the common femoral artery. (Image courtesy of Debra Joly, RVT, RDMS, RDCS, Houston, TX.)

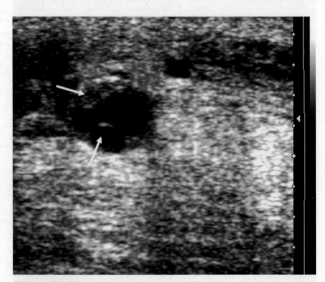

Figure 11-11 A transverse image of a retained valve *(arrows)* within an in situ bypass.

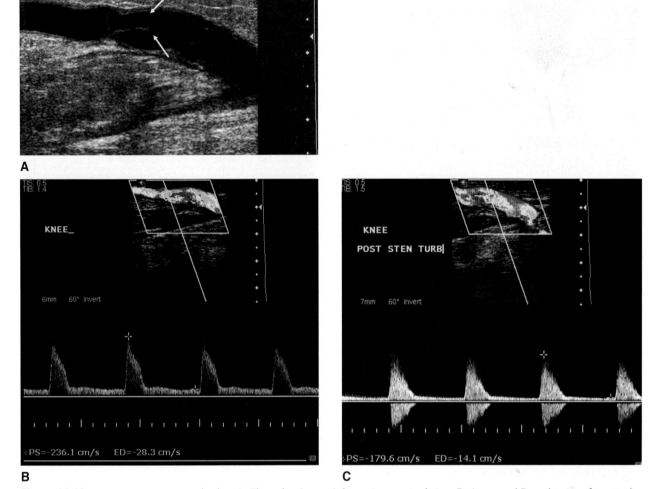

Figure 11-12 A stenosis at a retained valve. **A:** The valve *(arrows)* shown in a sagittal view. **B:** A spectral Doppler waveform at the stenosis with a PSV of 236 cm/s. **C:** A spectral Doppler waveform illustrating poststenotic turbulence.

(Fig. 11-12). Myointimal hyperplasia can occur along any point of the bypass conduit but typically takes place in areas where the vein has sustained injury or at the site of a valve sinus. Myointimal hyperplasia is a rapid proliferation of cells into the intimal layer of the cell wall, which can result in a stenosis (Fig. 11-13).

Dissections, intimal flaps, aneurysms, or pseudoaneurysms may also be present on the ultrasound image. Intimal flaps will appear as small, confined projections into the vessel lumen made up of a segment of the vessel wall that has separated from the remainder of the wall. An intimal flap may progress and extend over several centimeters, at which point it is usually referred to as a dissection (Fig. 11-14). Intimal flaps and dissections can occur early on in the life of a bypass graft due to technical problems that take place during surgery. It is not uncommon to see apparent aneurysmal dilatation at an anastomosis with the common femoral artery where the circumference of the bypass graft and common femoral artery are added

together. Occasionally in older bypass grafts, the vein wall itself can become weakened and dilate. Aneurysmal dilation can manifest as a focal dilation or diffuse dilation of the bypass graft over a long segment. As with aneurysmal native arteries,

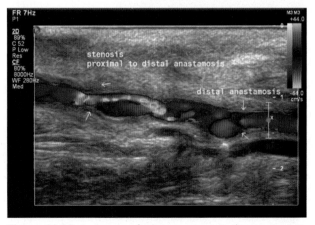

Figure 11-13 An image of a bypass stenosis due to myointimal hyperplasia.

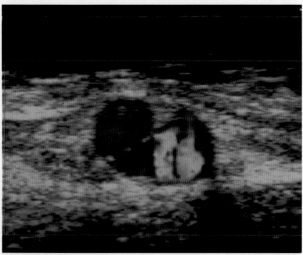

A

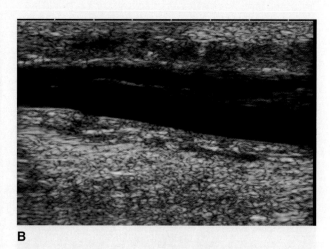

B

Figure 11-14 A: A transverse image of a vein bypass graft with a dissection. Color flow is observed in both the true lumen and the false lumen. **B:** A sagittal view of a bypass with a dissection.

a dilation equal to 1.5 times the adjacent vessel is considered aneurysmal (Fig. 11-15). Pseudoaneurysms are a rare pathology encountered and usually form at anastomotic sites. The most common site would be the common femoral artery in the groin at the outflow of a prosthetic aortofemoral or femoro-femoral crossover graft.

As previously mentioned, some findings observed on the grayscale image are not part of the bypass itself but may be contained within the tissue adjacent to the bypass. Figure 11-16A illustrates a vein bypass graft with a large perigraft fluid accumulation, which was determined to be a hematoma. Figure 11-16B

illustrates a transverse view of an accumulation of fluid surrounding a PTFE graft.

COLOR FLOW IMAGING

Color flow imaging is considered to be an adjunctive tool in the diagnosis of bypass graft pathology. Color flow imaging can indicate mild changes in flow profiles and slightly disturbed laminar flow patterns, which are consistent with mild degrees of stenosis. As a stenosis worsens, color aliasing will be evident (Fig. 11-17).

These changes in the color patterns should alert the technologist to carefully examine the grayscale image and spectral Doppler for the presence of an abnormality.

SPECTRAL ANALYSIS

Normal bypass grafts should demonstrate multiphasic waveforms with a sharp upstroke and a narrow systolic peak (Fig. 11-18A). An important component of the waveform is the reverse flow observed during early diastole. This is indicative of a normal high-resistance peripheral arterial bed. Many bypass grafts will not display a reverse flow component in diastole, particularly in the early postoperative period. These grafts will display antegrade flow throughout diastole (Fig. 11-18B). Continuous diastolic flow may be present in some bypass grafts due to hyperemia or arteriovenous fistulae. This waveform will demonstrate a normal sharp rise to peak systole with continuous forward flow in diastole indicating a decrease in resistance distally, associated with a low resistance outflow bed.

Figure 11-15 A sagittal image of a vein bypass graft with a focal aneurysmal dilation. (Image courtesy of Debra Joly, RVT, RDMS, RDCS, Houston, TX.)

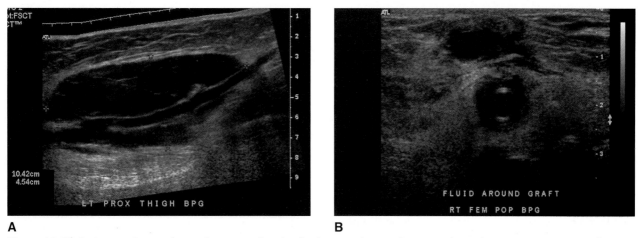

Figure 11-16 A: A sagittal view of a vein bypass graft with a fluid accumulation adjacent to the graft. **B:** A transverse view of a PTFE graft with fluid surrounding the graft. (Images courtesy of William Zang, BS, RVT, RDMS, GE Healthcare, Wauwatosa, WI.)

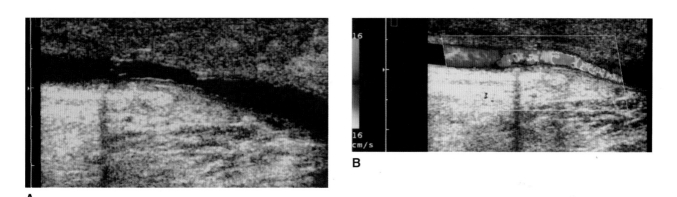

Figure 11-17 Images of a mid-bypass stenosis. **A:** The grayscale image demonstrates narrowing of the lumen with echogenic material along the bypass graft walls. **B:** The color flow image displays normal color filling within the bypass near the left of the image then color aliasing along the region of the stenosis.

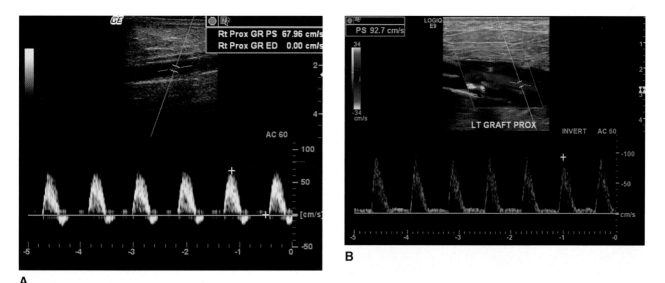

Figure 11-18 Normal multiphasic Doppler signals from vein bypass grafts. **A:** This bypass graft demonstrates reverse or retrograde flow in diastole. **B:** This bypass graft demonstrates antegrade flow through diastole.

An arteriovenous fistula is a complication unique to in situ bypass grafts. This type of fistula occurs when a branch of the great saphenous vein connects, directly or indirectly, via a perforator with the deep venous system and is left unligated after creation of the bypass. A perforating vein normally has valves that direct flow from the superficial to the deep venous system. Thus, once the great saphenous vein is arterialized as a bypass conduit, there is no impedance to blood flow through the bypass graft, into the perforating vein (now acting as a fistula), and into the deep venous system. This low resistance path can divert a great deal of blood flow into the venous system. The Doppler spectrum of the bypass graft proximal to the level of the fistula will display constant antegrade flow. Distal to the fistula, the bypass graft Doppler spectrum will exhibit little or no diastolic flow.

A blunted, monophasic pattern with zero diastolic flow is abnormal. This type of waveform indicates an abnormally high resistance to flow distally (Fig. 11-19). This is often associated with a stenosis or occlusion distally within the bypass or outflow vessels. This can sometimes progress to a staccato waveform with minimal forward flow in systole.

Another type of abnormal bypass spectrum is a waveform with continuous diastolic flow and a prolonged rise to peak systole. This dampened and delayed pattern is observed distal to a high-grade stenosis (Fig. 11-20). Energy losses across a stenosis will produce lower velocities distal to a stenosis and result in a broadened peak. The physiologic effects of an arterial stenosis are discussed in further detail in Chapter 2 of this text.

Although pattern recognition will provide clues to the overall function of a bypass graft, categorizing a stenosis depends on the measurement of PSV. Normally functioning bypass grafts have a wide range of velocities, but the PSV is typically less than

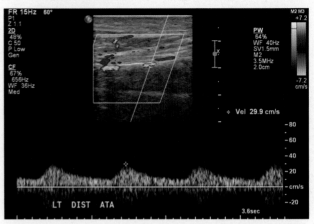

Figure 11-20 An abnormal waveform with a prolonged upstroke taken from an anterior tibial artery distal to an in situ bypass with a high-grade stenosis. (Image courtesy of Debra Joly, RVT, RDMS, RDCS, Houston, TX.)

150 cm/s. As a stenosis develops, a focal increase is noted in the PSV. A value of PSV that is greater than 180 cm/s is considered to be the cutoff for an abnormality. Another useful parameter is the velocity ratio (Vr). The Vr is measured by dividing the maximum PSV obtained at a stenosis by the PSV obtained just proximal to the stenosis. A doubling in PSV as compared to the adjacent more proximal segment (Vr = 2.0) is consistent with a ≥50% stenosis. The PSV for a stenosis in this range is 180 to 300 cm/s. A Vr of 3.5 and a PSV greater than 300 cm/s is consistent with a ≥75% stenosis[13] and associated with a high level of surgical revision.[14] A critical feature of all stenotic disease is the presence of poststenotic turbulence. Distal to a stenosis, the spectral waveforms will be disrupted with extensive turbulence and both antegrade and retrograde flow can be present. Figure 11-21 illustrates the velocity changes through a stenosis.

An additional parameter used to assess bypass graft patency is the value of mean graft flow velocity (GFV). Mean GFV is calculated by taking an average of three to four PSV values in nonstenotic segments of a bypass graft at various levels (proximal, mid, and distal). Normally, GFV is greater than 45 cm/s. A GFV of less than 40 cm/s can be present normally in large diameter grafts (>6 mm) or in grafts with limited outflow such as those to a pedal artery or isolated popliteal or tibial arteries. Trends in the GFV are also helpful diagnostic indicators. A decrease in GFV greater than 30 cm/s (compared to a previous examination) indicates that a bypass may be in jeopardy of failure.[4] This could be due to progression of disease with inflow or outflow vessels or to a stenosis within the bypass itself.

Pathology Box 11-1 summarizes the various pathologies that can be observed with bypass grafts. Grayscale, spectral Doppler, and color findings are listed.

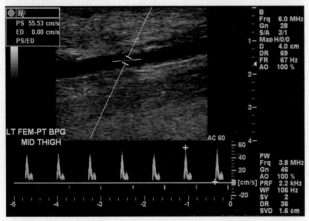

Figure 11-19 An abnormal high resistance waveform with no flow through diastole. (Image courtesy of Phillip J. Bendick, PhD, RVT, Royal Oak, MI.)

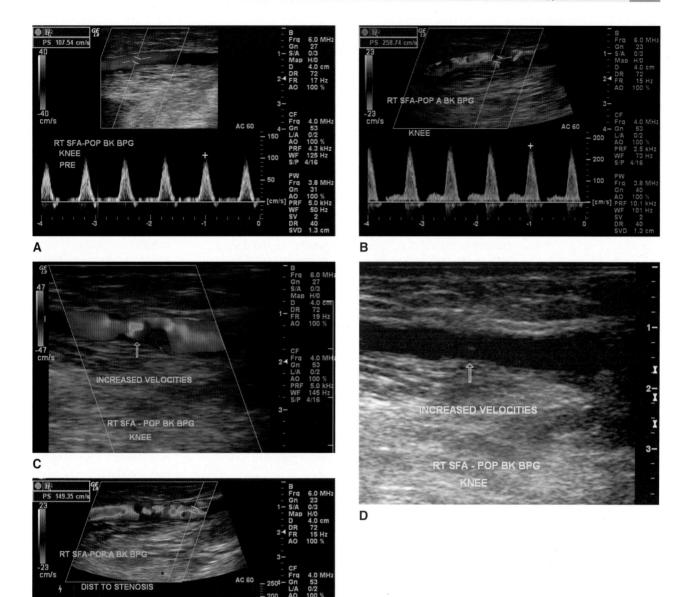

Figure 11-21 A bypass stenosis **(A)** spectral analysis proximal to a stenosis with a PSV of 108 cm/s. **B:** At the level of the stenosis, the PSV increases to 259 cm/s, Vr = 2.4. **C:** Color flow imaging at the stenosis with aliasing present. **D:** A grayscale image at the stenosis demonstrating a luminal narrowing with hypoechoic material along the walls of the graft. **E:** Distal to the stenosis, poststenotic turbulence is present.

SUMMARY

It is important to remember that there are three components to the data obtained with modern ultrasound equipment. The first data source is the B-mode or grayscale image. The second is the spectral Doppler waveform, which is the primary source of numerical data used to classify disease. The third type of data is that obtained from the color flow image. It is only by reviewing information from all three of these components that the best evaluation of the bypass will be determined. Routine surveillance of bypass grafts is a standard component of postoperative patient management. Thorough attention to ultrasound findings and the application of spectral Doppler criteria can identify failing bypass grafts prior to occlusion, thus maintaining patency.

PATHOLOGY BOX 11-1

Bypass Graft Pathology

Pathology	Sonographic Appearance		
	B-Mode	Color	Doppler
Aneurysms and pseudoaneurysms	Focal increase in diameter either along the bypass or at an anastomosis; thrombus may or may not be present	Swirling of color flow into the dilated portion; "yin-yang" appearance may be present with color changing from red to blue as flow fills the dilation	Low velocity, turbulent, disturbed flow will be present in the dilated segment; bidirectional flow in neck of pseudoaneurysm
Arteriovenous fistula	A patent branch will be present off the bypass graft; this branch may be seen to communicate into the deep venous system	Color filling will be seen within the fistula, extending to the deep venous system; aliasing is likely to be present	Flow may be slightly pulsatile to continuous within the fistula; antegrade diastolic flow will be evident in the bypass proximal to the fistula
Dissection	Linear object seen extending for several centimeters, parallel to bypass walls	Turbulent flow; red-to-blue flow may be seen in either lumen	Disturbed flow with increased resistance; flow may be bidirectional
Intimal flap	Small projection into the vessel lumen usually less than 1 cm; not associated with a valve	Disturbed flow or aliasing may be present	Disturbed flow or aliasing may be present
Myointimal hyperplasia	Occurs within the bypass or along anastomotic areas; focal increase in vessel wall thickness, which protrudes into the lumen	Disturbed flow or aliasing may be present	Increased velocities, turbulence, or aliasing may be present
Thrombus	Intraluminal echoes of varying echogenicity dependent on the age of the thrombus	No flow or reduced color filling of bypass lumen	Absent Doppler signal or, if present, increased resistance
Valve remnants	Hyperechoic structure seen protruding into bypass lumen; may be partial or complete leaflet	May demonstrate disturbed color flow patterns or aliasing in region of valve	May demonstrate elevated velocities in region of valve

Critical Thinking Questions

1. You are about to examine a patient with a bypass graft that is 4 years old. What, if anything, should you pay particular attention to and why?

2. Describe what transducer you may select to examine a femoral–popliteal PTFE graft that has been tunneled.

3. When looking for a partial retained valve or intimal tear, is color flow imaging helpful? Why or why not?

REFERENCES

1. Bandyk DR, Schmitt DD, Seabrook GR, et al. Monitoring functional patency of in situ saphenous vein bypasses: the impact of a surveillance protocol and elective revision. *J Vasc Surg.* 1989;9(2):286–296.
2. Leopold PW, Shandall AA, Kay C, et al. Duplex ultrasound: its role in the non-invasive follow up of the in situ saphenous vein bypass. *J Vasc Technol.* 1987;11:183–186.
3. Tinder CN, Chavanpun JP, Bandyk DF, et al. Efficacy of duplex ultrasound surveillance after infrainguinal vein bypass may be enhanced by identification of characteristics predictive of graft stenosis development. *J Vasc Surg.* 2008;48(3):613–618.
4. Gupta AK, Bandyk DF, Cheanvechai D, et al. Natural history of infrainguinal vein graft stenosis relative to bypass grafting technique. *J Vasc Surg.* 1997;25(2):211–225.
5. Berceli SA, Hevelone ND, Lipsitz SR, et al. Surgical and endovascular revision of infrainguinal vein bypass grafts: analysis of midterm outcomes from the PREVENT III trial. *J Vasc Surg.* 2007;46(6):1173–1179.
6. Calligaro KD, Doerr K, McAfee-Bennett S, et al. Should duplex ultrasonography be performed for surveillance of femoropopliteal and femorotibial arterial prosthetic bypasses? *Ann Vasc Surg.* 2001;15(5):520–524.
7. Brumberg RS, Back MR, Armstrong PA, et al. The relative importance of graft surveillance and warfarin therapy in infrainguinal prosthetic bypass failure. *J Vasc Surg.* 2007;46(6):1160–1166.
8. Landry GL, Liem TK, Mitchell EL, et al. Factors affecting symptomatic vs asymptomatic vein graft stenoses in lower extremity bypass grafts. *Arch Surg.* 2007;142(2):848–854.
9. Giannoukas AD, Androulakis AE, Labropoulos N, et al. The role of surveillance after infrainguinal bypass grafting. *Eur J Vasc Endovasc Surg.* 1996;11(3):279–289.
10. Mills JL, Bandyk DF, Gahtan V, et al. The origin of infrainguinal vein graft stenosis: a prospective study based on duplex surveillance. *J Vasc Surg.* 1995;21(1):16–25.
11. Reifsnyder T, Towne JB, Seabrook GR, et al. Biologic characteristics of long-term autogenous vein grafts: a dynamic evolution. *J Vasc Surg.* 1993;17(1):207–217.
12. Calligaro KD, Musser DJ, Chen AY, et al. Duplex ultrasonography to diagnose failing arterial prosthetic grafts. *Surgery.* 1996;120(3):455–459.
13. Bandyk DF, Armstrong PA. Surveillance of infrainguinal bypass grafts. In: Zierler RE, ed. *Strandness's Duplex Scanning in Vascular Disorders.* 4th ed. Philadelphia, PA: Lippincott Williams & Wilkins; 2010:341–349.
14. Mofidi R, Kelman J, Bennett S, et al. Significance of the early postoperative duplex result in infrainguinal vein bypass surveillance. *Eur J Vasc Endovasc Surg.* 2007;34(3):327–332.

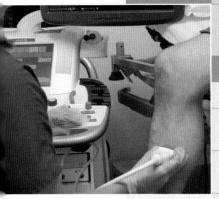

12 Ultrasound Following Interventional Procedures

Dennis F. Bandyk

OBJECTIVES

List the types of commonly performed interventions

Describe the pathology observed on ultrasound during postinterventional evaluations

Define the ultrasound criteria applied to vessels following angioplasty and stenting

Identify normal and abnormal spectral Doppler waveforms obtained from vessels following angioplasty and stenting

KEY TERMS

duplex ultrasound | peripheral angioplasty | stent angioplasty | surveillance

GLOSSARY

angioplasty a surgical repair of a blood vessel by reconstructing or replacing part of the vessel; balloon angioplasty is a specific type of angioplasty in which a balloon-tipped catheter is used to enlarge a narrowing (stenosis) in a blood vessel

atherectomy a nonsurgical procedure to remove plaque from an artery using a special catheter with a device at the tip that cuts away the plaque

dissection a tear along the inner layer of an artery, which results in the splitting or separation of the walls of a blood vessel

hyperplasia an abnormal increase in the number of cells;

myointimal hyperplasia an increase in the number of smooth muscle cells within the intima in response to vessel injury

stent a tubelike structure placed inside a blood vessel to provide patency and support

Vascular diagnostics are integral to the care of patients with peripheral arterial disease (PAD) prior to and following endovascular intervention. Care of the PAD patient includes medical treatment (atherosclerotic risk factor reduction, antiplatelet medications, exercise training, and drug therapy for claudication) and in selected patients with symptoms or signs of advanced limb ischemia, intervention by surgical reconstruction/bypass grafting or endovascular therapy.[1] The type of intervention depends primarily on disease location and extent, which can be accurately determined using duplex ultrasound, but comorbid medical conditions and the risk–benefit ratio of the proposed procedure also influence treatment decisions. Endovascular therapy has become a preferred initial intervention with a variety of techniques available to treat lower and upper limb atherosclerotic occlusive (ASO) disease (Table 12-1).[1-6] The method of lesion repair, stenosis-free patency, and failure mode varies with intervention techniques. Percutaneous transluminal angioplasty (PTA) is the most common endovascular procedure and requires passage of guide wire across a stenosis or occlusion followed by inflation of angioplasty balloon or deployment of a stent to expand the artery lumen. Other endovascular techniques such as subintimal angioplasty, mechanical atherectomy (plaque debulking or excision), or stent-graft angioplasty can treat more extensive (longer stenotic segments or occlusion, multiple lesions) atherosclerotic occlusive disease.[5-10] Often, endovascular therapy does not restore normal peripheral pulses because of multilevel disease, especially in limbs treated for critical limb ischemia (CLI). The outcome of endovascular intervention is largely dependent on the procedure indication (claudication versus CLI) and lesion severity classified using the Trans-Atlantic Inter-Society

TABLE 12-1

Endovascular Interventions for Lower Extremity Atherosclerotic Occlusive Disease

Intervention Option	Mechanism	Lesion Anatomy	Stenosis-Free Patency at 1 Year	Failure Mode
Balloon angioplasty	Lumen dilation	Focal, <5 cm stenosis or occlusion	40%–50%	Plaque dissection Myointimal hyperplasia
Stent angioplasty	Lumen dilation	Focal and longer (>10 cm) stenosis or occlusion	50%–60%	Myointimal hyperplasia Stent fracture
Atherectomy	Plaque excision	Focal and longer (>10 cm) stenosis	40%–50%	Myointimal hyperplasia Atherectomy site thrombosis
Subintimal angioplasty	Lumen dilation	>10 stenosis or occlusion	55%–60%	Myointimal hyperplasia Angioplasty site thrombosis
Stent-graft angioplasty	Lumen dilation	Long, >15 cm stenosis or occlusion	60%–70%	Myointimal hyperplasia Graft thrombosis

Consensus (TASC II) criteria based on lesion location and anatomy.[4] Endovascular intervention is the preferred therapy for focal, <5 cm in length regions of stenosis or occlusion (TASC A and B lesions) with expected 30-day technical and clinical success rates above 95%.[1,4] In claudicants, the patency of iliac angioplasty is higher (85% at 3 years) than for superficial femoral/popliteal artery angioplasty (55% at 2 years).[11,12] Treatment of CLI or TASC C and D lesions by endovascular techniques has lower stenosis-free patency rates, typically in the 25% to 40% range at 1 year.[2,8,10,13] Factors associated with angioplasty failure include lesion calcification, occlusions, poor tibial artery runoff, diabetes mellitus, and renal failure.[4–10] Approximately one-third of peripheral angioplasty sites will require reintervention to maintain stenosis-free patency during within the first year.[7]

The rationale for vascular laboratory testing following intervention is twofold: to document that the improvement in limb perfusion was sufficient to expect symptoms (claudication, rest pain) and signs (ulcer healing) to resolve and to detect angioplasty-site stenosis. Because the PAD patient is prone to disease progression, including myointimal hyperplasia producing stenosis within or adjacent to the angioplasty site, duplex ultrasound is the recommended diagnostic modality. Testing can be performed during the procedure to assess for residual stenosis, which is suited for surveillance studies and is highly accurate in the detection of angioplasty site complications versus ASO progression. Duplex testing can classify angioplasty stenosis severity and thus can provide an opportunity to retreat high-grade occlusive lesions prior to thrombosis.[7,14,15] Reliance on the patient to recognize angioplasty failure based on symptom recurrence is imperfect, especially in the sedentary patient.

SONOGRAPHIC EXAMINATION TECHNIQUES

PATIENT PREPARATION

Arterial testing after endovascular intervention mirrors the surveillance used after lower limb bypass grafting.[15–18] Patient functional status is documented, including any new or unresolved symptoms of PAD, along with limb perfusion, which is evaluated by physiologic testing and a duplex scan of the angioplasty site for abnormalities (Fig. 12-1). In the claudicant, initial indirect physiologic testing should verify improvement in the ankle–brachial index (ABI) to a normal (>0.9) or an increased (>0.2) level sufficient so that walking distance is likely to be improved. Limbs treated for CLI should have a measurement of toe pressure to verify that an increase to >30 mm Hg has been achieved. In limbs with healing foot ulcers or digit amputations, a toe pressure of >40 mm Hg predicts healing.

Duplex arterial mapping of the limb should be individualized based on whether the ABI is normal, abnormal, or if the patient has calcified tibial arteries, which preclude accurate ankle pressure measurement. If the ABI is normal and the tibial artery velocity spectra at the ankle indicate multiphasic or triphasic artery flow, angioplasty site imaging is not necessary.

PATIENT POSITIONING

Scanning is performed with the patient supine and with the lower limb positioned with the knee bent slightly. Prone or lateral decubitus positions can be used to image the popliteal artery, tibioperoneal trunk, and peroneal arteries. Imaging can be performed with a 5-7 MHz linear array transducer.

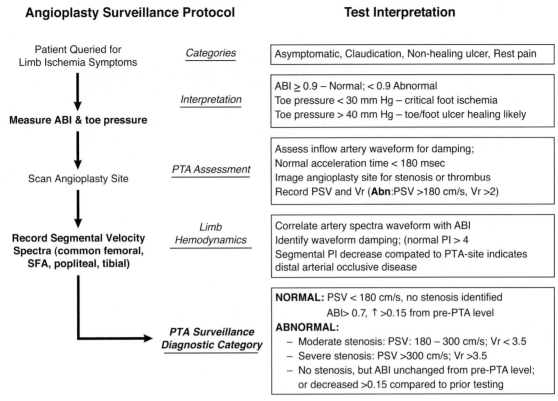

Angioplasty Surveillance Protocol

Test Interpretation

Patient Queried for Limb Ischemia Symptoms

Categories

> Asymptomatic, Claudication, Non-healing ulcer, Rest pain

Measure ABI & toe pressure

Interpretation

> ABI $\geq$ 0.9 – Normal; < 0.9 Abnormal
> Toe pressure < 30 mm Hg – critical foot ischemia
> Toe pressure > 40 mm Hg – toe/foot ulcer healing likely

Scan Angioplasty Site

PTA Assessment

> Assess inflow artery waveform for damping;
> Normal acceleration time < 180 msec
> Image angioplasty site for stenosis or thrombus
> Record PSV and Vr (**Abn**:PSV >180 cm/s, Vr >2)

Record Segmental Velocity Spectra (common femoral, SFA, popliteal, tibial)

Limb Hemodynamics

> Correlate artery spectra waveform with ABI
> Identify waveform damping; (normal PI > 4
> Segmental PI decrease compated to PTA-site indicates distal arterial occlusive disease

PTA Surveillance Diagnostic Category

> **NORMAL:** PSV < 180 cm/s, no stenosis identified
>   ABI> 0.7, ↑ >0.15 from pre-PTA level
> **ABNORMAL:**
> – Moderate stenosis: PSV: 180 – 300 cm/s; Vr < 3.5
> – Severe stenosis: PSV >300 cm/s; Vr >3.5
> – No stenosis, but ABI unchanged from pre-PTA level; or decreased >0.15 compared to prior testing

Figure 12-1 Peripheral angioplasty surveillance testing protocol and study interpretation criteria.

SCANNING TECHNIQUE

Duplex ultrasound mapping should begin at the common femoral artery (CFA) level to document the presence normal, multiphasic velocity spectra, indicating <50% proximal aortoiliac or stent stenosis (Fig. 12-2). If the CFA velocity spectra waveform is monophasic, damped compared to the contralateral CFA, or has an abnormal (>180 ms) acceleration time, duplex assessment of the iliac segment should be performed.

Duplex mapping then proceeds distal from the CFA to include the SFA and deep femoral artery origins, imaging of the SFA-popliteal arterial segment, including the angioplasty site, and recording of ankle-level, tibial artery velocity spectra. The technologist should provide sufficient duplex scan images and segmental velocity spectra recordings for study interpretation into the categories "normal" or "abnormal."

B-mode and color Doppler imaging of the angioplasty site should be performed to document vessel/stent lumen patency, artery plaque characteristics, and evidence of stent/stent-graft deformation or intimal thickening. Sites of lumen caliber reduction, flow jets, and disturbed flow identified by color or power Doppler imaging should be evaluated by pulsed Doppler spectral analysis recorded using a ≤60° angle correction relative to the vessel/stent wall. A valuable scanning tip is to "walk" the sample volume through the region of abnormality to locate and measure peak systolic velocity (PSV) changes (Fig. 12-3). The measurement of PSV proximal (PSV_{prox}) to and within the stenosis flow jet (PSV_{max}) allows for the calculation of the stenosis velocity ratio (Vr), where Vr = PSV_{max}/ PSV_{prox}. A Vr >2 indicates >50% diameter-reducing (DR) stenosis. The combination of PSV_{max}, Vr, and end-diastolic velocity (EDV) at the stenosis is used to classify stenosis severity (Fig. 12-4). Duplex findings should be recorded on a schematic of the lower or upper limb arterial tree to facilitate study interpretation and to provide a comparison baseline when evaluating for stenosis progression. In the majority of the patients, duplex testing alone provides sufficient information to inform the patient of PTA-site stenosis and to decide whether to proceed to reintervention.

TECHNICAL CONSIDERATIONS

The goal of peripheral arterial testing following intervention is to provide objective hemodynamic and anatomic information of functional angioplasty patency. The technologist should have information of the indication for intervention, the arterial site(s) treated, and the endovascular procedure performed. The measurement of limb pressures combined with

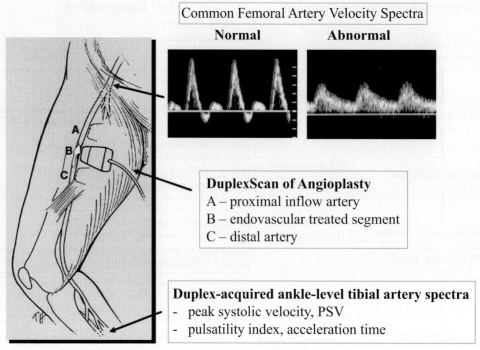

Common Femoral Artery Velocity Spectra

Normal   **Abnormal**

DuplexScan of Angioplasty
A – proximal inflow artery
B – endovascular treated segment
C – distal artery

Duplex-acquired ankle-level tibial artery spectra
- peak systolic velocity, PSV
- pulsatility index, acceleration time

Figure 12-2 Schematic-depicting sites of duplex scanning including the common femoral artery, angioplasty site, and assessment of distal tibial artery hemodynamics.

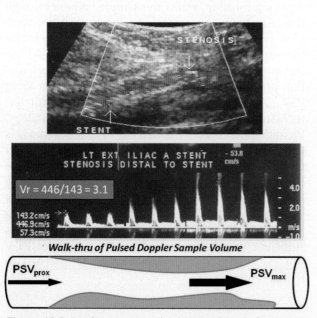

Figure 12-3 Duplex image and velocity spectra of an external iliac stent stenosis. The color duplex image *(top)* depicts an area of color aliasing at the stenosis *(arrow)*. The pulsed Doppler *(middle)* sample volume is walked through the stenosis with a measurement of peak systolic velocity proximal to (PSV_{prox}) and at the site of stenosis (PSV_{max}) for calculation of velocity ratio, $Vr = PSV_{max}/PSV_{prox}$. A schematic drawing illustrates the stenosis and PSV measurements *(bottom)*.

arterial duplex scanning enable study interpretation in categories ranging from "normal" (i.e., stenosis-free patency) to "severe stenosis," with the latter category based on threshold criteria appropriate for reintervention. Testing immediately following an endovascular intervention confirms procedural success or failure by documenting patency and whether a residual stenosis is present. Subsequent testing is based on procedure indication; it is less frequent in active individuals treated for claudication, but in patients treated for CLI, surveillance should be similar following lower limb bypass grafting.[6] Duplex surveillance after lower limb angioplasty has demonstrated >50% DR stenosis in 20% to 40% of treated limbs within 12 months of the procedure.[7,16] The most common etiology is development of myointimal hyperplasia within the angioplasty site regardless of endovascular therapy (balloon inflation, stent angioplasty, atherectomy) used. Detection of >50% residual stenosis despite a completion angiogram showing adequate lumen expansion (<30% DR) can occur, predicts angioplasty, and is the rationale for performing an intraprocedural or early (<30-day) postprocedural study.[7,16] The prevalence of duplex-detected residual stenosis following femoropopliteal angioplasty is lowest after stent-angioplasty or stent-grafting (<5%), and higher after balloon angioplasty (15% to 20%) or atherectomy (25%). Although angiogram-monitored angioplasty showing <20% to 30% residual stenosis predicts

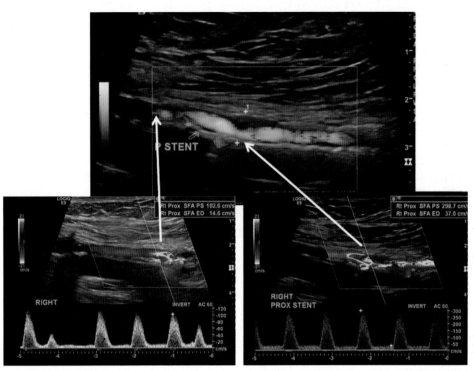

Figure 12-4 Power *(top)* and color Doppler velocity spectra images of a >50% DR stent-angioplasty site stenosis. Proximal PSV was 103 cm/s *(bottom left)* and increased to 299 cm/s at the stenosis *(bottom right)*, resulting in a calculated velocity ratio of 2.9.

30-day patency (i.e., technical success), a duplex scan of angioplasty-site hemodynamics provides a more precise assessment of functional patency. Schillinger et al.[7] documented that duplex-detected >50% stenosis developed more frequently after balloon angioplasty than after Nitinol stenting in the treatment of SFA occlusive disease at both 6 months (45% vs. 25%, $P = .06$) and 12 months (63% vs. 37%, $P < .01$). Other techniques, including cutting or cryoplasty balloon angioplasty, atherectomy, and stent-grafting, also have a high technical success rate, but similar to balloon angioplasty, angioplasty restenosis or treatment site thrombosis has been observed in 20% to 50% of limbs depending on TASC-lesion severity by 1 year.[11,15]

DIAGNOSIS

Peripheral arterial laboratory testing following PTA includes interpretation of the limb pressures and duplex ultrasound findings (see Fig. 12-1). The interpretation should comment on the severity of limb ischemia (mild, moderate, severe), changes from preintervention values, and whether adequate foot perfusion has been achieved in patients treated from CLI (i.e., toe pressure >30 mm Hg). Duplex findings at the angioplasty site are interpreted as showing no stenosis (<50% DR stenosis), moderate stenosis (>50% DR), severe stenosis (>70% DR), or occlusion (Table 12-2). A "normal study" interpretation

TABLE 12-2
Published Duplex Velocity Criteria for Classification of Angioplasty-Site Stenosis (University of South Florida)[18]

Stenosis Category	Peak Systolic Velocity (PSV, cm/s)	Velocity Ratio (Vr)	End-Diastolic Velocity (cm/s)	Distal Artery Waveform
<50% DR	<180	<2	N/A	Normal
>50% DR moderate	180–300	2–3.5	>0	Monophasic
>70% DR severe	>300	>3.5	>45	Damped, monophasic, low velocity
Occluded	No flow detected			Damped, monophasic, low velocity

DR, diameter reducing.

should indicate no stenosis was identified at the angioplasty site and the ABI is normal or unchanged if prior testing was performed. Duplex detection of a >50% DR stenosis proximal to, within, or distal to the endovascular intervention is interpreted as a "new" abnormal finding.

Velocity criteria used to interpret PTA stenosis severity relies primarily on measurements of PSV and Vr at the stenosis. Although a Vr >2 is generally accepted to indicate a >50% DR stenosis, this interpretation should also be associated with the duplex findings of lumen reduction, color Doppler imaging of disturbed flow, and a focal PSV increase to >180 cm/s. Under resting conditions, a stenosis with a Vr of 2 to 3 is associated with a minimal resting systolic pressure gradient and the ankle artery velocity spectra may demonstrate a "near-normal" multiphasic waveform. The functional significance of the stenosis can be determined by exercise testing with measurement of ABI and ankle pressure changes. Published duplex-derived criteria for the classification of an angioplasty site recommends the use of three disease categories (<50% stenosis, >70% stenosis, occlusion). This author's vascular group has used combined PSV_{max} and Vr threshold criteria of 300 cm/s and 3.5, respectively, to define the >70% DR stenosis (Fig. 12-5). The University of Pittsburgh

group reported a PPV of >95% in predicting >50% or >80% in-stent stenosis following femoropopliteal angioplasty for TASC B and C lesions (Table 12-3).[19] In patients with developed recurrent limb ischemia symptoms and a decrease of ABI >0.15, the angioplasty-site stenosis had a mean $PSV_{max} = 360$ cm/s and Vr = 3.6, with criteria of >70% DR stenosis in both classification schemes.

The presence of plaque dissection after balloon dilation, stent geometry, and the nature of myointimal hyperplasia development can affect the significance of PSV elevation and thus accuracy in predicting stenosis severity. In general, PSV values for grading an in-stent stenosis are higher than for a de novo atherosclerotic stenosis where a value >125 to 150 cm/s is an "accepted" threshold for >50% stenosis. Stent angioplasty decreases artery wall compliance, which elevates PSV within the stent and produces abnormal, nonuniform wall shear stress at stent end points, which potentiate the development of myointimal hyperplasia. This author's vascular group uses the same interpretation criteria for grading both lower limb arterial bypass graft stenosis and angioplasty-site stenosis, including the threshold criteria for reintervention (PSV >300 cm/s, Vr >3.5). This allows for uniform study interpretation between vascular laboratory staff, the diagnosis of disease

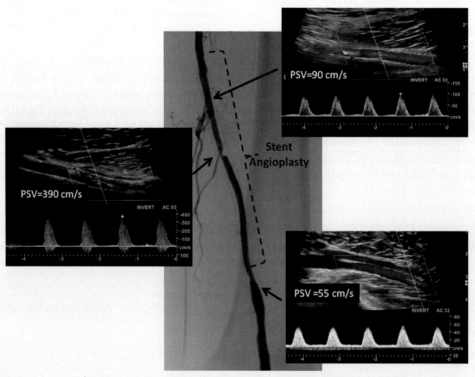

Figure 12-5 Angiogram *(center)* and duplex scan images of a focal >70% DR in-stent stenosis (PSV = 390 cm/s, Vr = 390/90 = 4.3) The image at the *top right* demonstrates the PSV proximal to the stenosis (PSV = 90 cm/s). The PSV of 390 cm/s at the stenosis is shown at the *left*. The dampened distal flow signal (PSV = 55 cm/s) is pictured at the *lower right*. ABI had decreased from 0.92 to 0.7, and the patient complained of recurrent claudication symptoms.

TABLE 12-3		
Published Duplex Velocity Criteria for Superficial Femoral Artery Stenosis (University of Pittsburgh)[14]		
Stenosis Category	Peak Systolic Velocity (PSV, cm/s)	Velocity Ratio (Vr)
<50% DR	<190	<1.5
>50% DR	190–275	1.5–3.5
>80% DR	>275	>3.5
Occluded	No flow detected	

DR, diameter reducing.

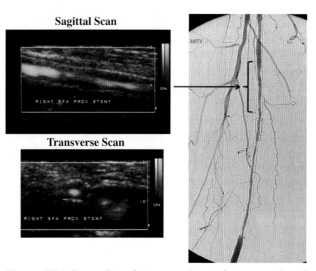

Sagittal Scan

Transverse Scan

Figure 12-6 Power Doppler images (sagittal, transverse) and an angiogram of a superficial femoral artery stent with diffuse in-stent stenosis. PSV ranged from 200 to 300 cm/s within the stent. Measured ABI was 0.56.

progression, and clinical decision making regarding a surveillance schedule or reintervention.

Angioplasty failure can manifest as an occlusion, a diffuse or multiple stenosis (Fig. 12-6), or as a focal, high-grade stenosis (see Fig. 12-5). Duplex findings of a diffuse in-stent stenosis include power Doppler lumen reduction and elevated (200 to 300 cm/s) PSV values along the entire stent length. The reduction in ABI can be similar to a high-grade focal stenosis with PSV >400 cm/s and end-diastolic velocity >100 cm/s. An important hemodynamic feature of angioplasty failure is the presence of damped, low-velocity spectra waveform in the distal arterial tree.

SURVEILLANCE PROTOCOL

The frequency of endovascular intervention failure is highest within the first 6 months, especially if a residual stenosis (PSV >180 cm/s, Vr = 1.5 to 2.5) is identified. The rationale for surveillance testing is to identify "failing" PTA sites before thrombosis occurs and, in the medically fit patient, repair of a duplex-detected >70% angioplasty stenosis should be considered. Angioplasty failure is commonly the result of myointimal hyperplasia developing within

or immediately adjacent to the treatment site. Stent fracture, a known risk factor for stenosis development and thrombosis, cannot be identified by duplex imaging, but the presence of stent deformation or kinking is abnormal and predicts stent thrombosis especially if associated with a >70% stenosis (Pathology Box 12-1).

Reporting standards of clinical improvement and procedure patency following endovascular therapy is identical to "open" surgical repair or bypass grafting. Intervention site patency documented by duplex ultrasound and an ABI increase >0.15 are minimal outcome criteria for clinical improvement.[3] Clinical success requires resolution of limb ischemia symptoms or signs and <50% DR stenosis of the arterial repair documented by duplex ultrasound or angiography. Duplex-detected >50% DR stenosis based on velocity spectra findings is an abnormal finding and if progressive to a

---

PATHOLOGY BOX 12-1

Common Postinterventional Abnormalities

Abnormality	Ultrasound Findings
In-site stenosis	Luminal caliber reduction; color flow jet with disturbed/turbulent color flow distally; focal PSV increase with turbulent Doppler spectrum distally
Stent deformation/kinking	Irregular stent walls, may protrude into vessel lumen; may be sharply angled in normally straight vessel segment; color and spectral turbulence
Myointimal hyperplasia	Homogeneous tissue growth along vessel lumen at angioplasty site or across stent walls; smooth surface contour; may appear as very thin layer along vessel or stent; may progress to in-site stenosis
Thrombosis/occlusion	No patent lumen detected; no color filling; no spectral Doppler signal

>70% DR stenosis is a criteria for a loss of "stenosis-free" patency whether repaired or selected for watchful observation in the asymptomatic patient. An open or percutaneous secondary intervention undertaken to maintain or improve functional angioplasty changes the procedural outcome to "assisted" primary patency. If the angioplasty site thrombosed and a secondary procedure is performed to restore patency, the outcome status changes to "secondary" patency. A successful surveillance program following PTA should produce an assisted-primary patency in the range of 80% to 90% at 2 years and no significant improvement in secondary patency. Failure to identify clinically significant lesions prior to thrombosis is present if the primary and assisted-primary patency rates are similar.

An abnormal or change in ABI indicates PAD, but is not diagnostic for angioplasty site failure. In many diabetic patients, the measurement of ABI is inaccurate and limb arterial testing requires pulse volume recording and duplex testing to evaluate limb perfusion and PTA functional patency. The application of objective criteria provided by duplex scanning is essential for a useful surveillance program. The use of combined threshold criteria for intervention (i.e., PSV >300, Vr >3.5) is associated with a high (>90%) positive predictive value when compared to angiogram findings for >70% DR stenosis.

The initial surveillance examination should be performed within 2 weeks, and ideally combined with an outpatient vascular clinic evaluation to assess the patient's activity level, to assess ASO risk factor modifications, and to review drug (antiplatelet, statin) therapy. If the initial PTA testing is "normal," follow-up testing in 3 months is appropriate for patients treated for CLI and in 6 months in claudicants. Subsequent testing is individualized at 6- to 12-month intervals. If initial duplex testing detects a residual 50% to 70% DR angioplasty site stenosis, a repeat evaluation in 4 to 6 weeks is safe and reliable in the detection of stenosis progression. The patient should be instructed that new limb ischemia symptoms should be evaluated in the vascular laboratory immediately. Abbreviated testing intervals (i.e., 3 months) may also be appropriate during the first year following endovascular treatment of TASC C and D lesions due to the higher likelihood of failure. The incidence of reintervention is higher following balloon (30%) than stent (20%) angioplasty.

SUMMARY

The application of duplex ultrasound surveillance following peripheral arterial interventional procedures can be useful and should be considered a part of PAD patient care. Reliance on the patient to recognize changes in limb perfusion is not reliable. Interpreting arterial testing that is performed within a surveillance protocol can be challenging, and some vascular specialists are not convinced that routine duplex surveillance is of benefit, worth the health care expense, or that the vascular laboratory is competent to execute a quality surveillance program. Duplex surveillance, when correctly performed and interpreted, should improve patency and clinical outcomes following endovascular therapy—an intervention with known limited functional patency and performed in a patient cohort subject to ASO disease progression.

Critical Thinking Questions

1. During a duplex examination of a patient with a superficial femoral artery stent, the common femoral artery ultrasound reveals an acceleration time of 210 ms. With this information, how would you augment the examination and why?

2. A patient comes in for a duplex ultrasound examination 6 months following a balloon angioplasty and stent placement. At this time interval within the follow-up protocol, where is the most likely place along the limb where a stenosis may be present?

3. When examining a patient postballoon angioplasty and stenting, do you expect the PSV within the treated site to be similar to or different from a patient who underwent an atherectomy?

REFERENCES

1. White CJ, Gray WA. Endovascular therapies for peripheral arterial disease. *Circulation*. 2007; 116:2203–2215.
2. Goodney PP, Beck AW, Nagle J, et al. National trends in lower extremity bypass surgery, endovascular interventions, and major amputations. *J Vasc Surg*. 2009;50(1):54–60.
3. Ahn SS, Rutherford RB, Becker GJ, et al. Reporting standards arterial endovascular for lower extremity. *J Vasc Surg*. 2009;49:133–139.
4. Norgren L, Hiatt WR, Dormandy JA, et al. Inter-Society Consensus for the Management of Peripheral Arterial Disease (TASC II). *J Vasc Surg*. 2007;45(suppl S):S5–S67.
5. Grimm J, Muller-Hulsbeck S, Jahnke T, et al. Randomized study to compare PTA alone versus PTA with Palmaz stent placement for femoropopliteal lesions. *J Vasc Interv Radiol*. 2001;12(8):935–942.
6. Mewissen MW. Self-expanding Nitinol stents in the femoropopliteal segment: technique and mid-term results. *Tech Vasc Interv Radiol*. 2004;7(1):2–5.
7. Schillinger M, Sabeti S, Loewe C, et al. Balloon angioplasty versus implantation of Nitinol stents in the superficial femoral artery. *N Engl J Med*. 2006;354(18):1879–1888.
8. Conrad MF, Cambria RP, Stone DH, et al. Intermediate results of percutaneous endovascular therapy of femoropopliteal occlusive disease: a contemporary series. *J Vasc Surg*. 2006; 44(4):762–769.
9. Dearing DD, Patel KR, Compoginis JM, et al. Primary stenting of the superficial femoral and popliteal artery. *J Vasc Surg*. 2009;50(3):542–548.
10. Schneider GC, Richardson AI, Scott EC, et al. Selective stenting in subintimal angioplasty: analysis of primary stent outcomes. *J Vasc Surg*. 2008;48(5):1175–1181.
11. Spijkerboer AM, Nass PC, deValois JC, et al. Iliac artery stenoses after percutaneous transluminal angioplasty: follow-up with duplex ultrasonography. *J Vasc Surg*. 1996;23(4):691–697.
12. Back MR, Novotney M, Roth SM, et al. Utility of duplex surveillance following iliac artery angioplasty and primary stenting. *J Endovasc Ther*. 2001;8(6):629–637.
13. Keeling WB, Shames ML, Stone PA, et al. Plaque excision with the Silverhawk catheter: early results in patients with claudication or critical limb ischemia. *J Vasc Surg*. 2007;45(1):25–31.
14. Mewissen MW, Kinney EV, Bandyk DF, et al. The role of duplex scanning versus angiography in predicting outcome after balloon angioplasty in the femoropopliteal artery. *J Vasc Surg*. 1992;15(5):860–866.
15. Armstrong PA, Bandyk DF. Surveillance after peripheral artery transluminal angioplasty. In: Zierler RE, Meissner MH, eds. *Strandness's Duplex Scanning in Vascular Disorders*. Philadelphia, PA: Lippincott Williams & Wilkins; 2009:302–327.
16. Abularrage CJ, Conrad MF, Hackney LA, et al. Long-term outcomes of diabetic patients undergoing endovascular infrainguinal interventions. *J Vasc Surg*. 2009;52(2):314–322.
17. Bandyk DF, Schmitt DD, Seabrook GR, et al. Monitoring functional patency of in situ saphenous vein bypasses: the impact of surveillance protocol and elective revision. *J Vasc Surg*. 1989;9(2):284–229.
18. Idu MM, Blankenstein JD, de Gier P, et al. Impact of color flow duplex surveillance program infrainguinal graft patency: a five-year experience. *J Vasc Surg*. 1993;17(1):42–53.
19. Baril DT, Rhee RY, Kim J, et al. Duplex criteria for determination of in-stent stenosis after angioplasty and stenting of the superficial femoral artery. *J Vasc Surg*. 2008;48:627–633.

13 Special Considerations in Evaluating Nonatherosclerotic Arterial Pathology

Patrick A. Washko and S. Wayne Smith

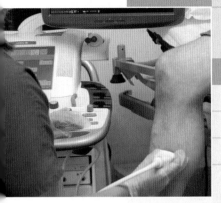

OBJECTIVES

Define the clinical presentation of nonatherosclerotic arterial disease

List the most common nonatherosclerotic arterial diseases

Identify the ultrasound presentation of nonatherosclerotic disease

Describe the most common cardiac pathologies associated with cardioembolic events

Explain the importance of clinical history before performing the arterial examination

KEY TERMS

aneurysm | arteriovenous fistula | arteritis | Buerger's disease | iatrogenic | popliteal entrapment | pseudoaneurysm | Takayasu's arteritis | traumatic

GLOSSARY

aneurysm a dilation of an artery wall involving all three layers of the vessel wall

arteriovenous fistula an abnormal communication between an artery and vein that can be the result of iatrogenic injury, trauma, or may be congenitally acquired

Buerger's disease a type of vascular arteritis also known as thromboangiitis obliterans; it affects small- and medium-sized arteries

embolism an obstruction or occlusion of a blood vessel by a transported clot of blood, mass, bacteria, or other foreign substance

giant cell arteritis a type of vascular arteritis, also known as temporal arteritis, which is associated with the superficial temporal artery and other arteries of the head and neck

pseudoaneurysm an expanding hematoma; a hole in the arterial wall that allows blood to leave the vessel and collect in the surrounding tissue

Takayasu's arteritis a type of vascular arteritis that affects the aortic arch and its large branches

vascular arteritis an inflammatory disease that affects the blood vessels

Nonatherosclerotic peripheral vascular disease is relatively uncommon. In approximately 90% of patients with peripheral arterial disease (PAD), the etiology is atherosclerosis. Nonatherosclerotic arterial pathology is often recognized by a detailed history that demonstrates the absence of any risk factors for atherosclerotic disease. Some of these typical atherosclerotic risk factors include smoking, diabetes, hypertension, and hyperlipidemia. Nonatherosclerotic arterial disease is composed of many atypical diseases that may include inflammatory diseases, congenital abnormalities, and acquired diseases or injuries. Many nonatherosclerotic arterial diseases can be assessed and properly diagnosed with vascular laboratory imaging, physiologic studies, and a detailed careful history. In this chapter, we will review imaging and physiologic tests used to assess a variety of nonatherosclerotic arterial pathology.

SONOGRAPHIC EXAMINATION TECHNIQUES

The sonographic examination of a patient with nonatherosclerotic arterial disease is similar to that employed when evaluating patients for suspected atherosclerosis (refer to Chapter 9). The portion of the vascular system interrogated is determined by the presenting symptoms and the disease suspected. In some instances, a combination of direct duplex imaging techniques along with indirect physiologic testing is employed to fully characterize the disease. Specific examination details will be included within the discussion of each disease entity. Basic ultrasound techniques are described in the following section.

DUPLEX ULTRASOUND TECHNIQUES

Generally, the grayscale image will be examined in both transverse and sagittal orientations to fully visualize any wall abnormalities or vessel defects. Images should be recorded from all major vessels examined. Additional images should be obtained from adjacent vessels when documenting wall abnormalities and should be compared to normal portions of vessels.

Spectral Doppler and color flow imaging techniques should be used to evaluate the vessels for flow disturbances and stenoses. Color can be quickly used to determine general flow patterns as well as to detect turbulent flow, increased flow, flow outside of a vessel, or the absence of flow. Spectral Doppler must be used to characterize the peak systolic velocity (PSV) from each vessel examined. End-diastolic velocity (EDV) may also need to be recorded, particularly if abnormally high or low resistance flow patterns are observed. In areas of suspected stenosis, PSV should be recorded before the area of interest, at the area of maximum PSV, and distal to this area. Poststenotic turbulence should be also documented.

VASCULAR ARTERITIS

Vascular arteritis is a phrase used to describe several inflammatory diseases that affect the blood vessels. The etiology of arteritis is unknown but often involves an immunologic condition. The inflammatory process of arteritis is associated with the media of the cell wall becoming infiltrated with a variety of white blood cells. Muscular and elastic portions of the wall are eroded and fibrosis develops. The end result is an overall weakening of the blood vessel and necrosis within the vessel wall.[1,2]

The symptoms of arteritis can often be similar to those symptoms encountered with atherosclerosis. When an arteritis involves extremity vessels symptoms such as claudication or rest, pain can be present. Several types of arteritis can impact the upper extremities. The most common upper extremity arterial pathology seen is proximal atherosclerotic subclavian artery disease. Typically these patients are referred to the vascular laboratory for asymmetrical blood pressures, dizziness, or syncope. If assessment demonstrates stenosis of the axillary or brachial artery segments, this finding is seldom due to atherosclerosis and may be more consistent with giant cell arteritis or Takayasu's arteritis.

GIANT CELL ARTERITIS

Giant cell arteritis or temporal arteritis is an inflammatory vasculitis seen in elderly patients.[3] The average age of onset is 70 years old and rarely occurs in people younger than 50 years of age. Caucasians and females are more prone to the disease than males or other races. Patients are frequently referred to the vascular laboratory because of asymmetrical upper extremity blood pressures.[3] Patients may also typically present with temporal headaches, tenderness over the superficial temporal artery (a branch of the external carotid artery), decreased pulse, or a cord-like structure over the superficial temporal artery. Other symptoms may include aching or stiffness in the neck, headaches, jaw claudication, and visual disturbances. A significant risk exists of optic nerve ischemia and blindness can occur in giant cell arteritis; hence, giant cell arteritis can be a medical emergency. The most common site for giant cell arteritis is in the superficial temporal artery but there can be involvement of multiple extracranial arteries and other arteries of the head and neck. Occasionally, arteries below the aortic arch are involved. The erythrocyte sedimentation rate is often elevated as well as another inflammatory marker, C-reactive protein. The gold standard for diagnosis is a temporal artery biopsy showing mononuclear cells and giant cells infiltrating the area around the elastic lamina within the media of the cell wall.

Scanning Technique

The sonographic examination of a patient with suspected giant cell or temporal arteritis involves imaging the region of the vascular system related to the presenting symptoms. If a patient presents with temporal pain and headaches, the temporal artery itself will be examined, usually in association with a complete carotid duplex ultrasound examination. The temporal artery is the smaller of two terminal branches of the external carotid artery. It begins behind the mandible, crosses the zygomatic process, then courses along the temporal bone. It continues for about 5 cm before it divides into the frontal and parietal branches. The temporal artery is small and superficial requiring a high-frequency transducer in order to properly insonate it.

If the patient presents with upper extremity symptoms, an upper extremity duplex ultrasound is performed, paying close attention to the subclavian, axillary, and brachial arteries. The images in Figure 13-1 were obtained from a 75-year-old Caucasian female who presented with temporal headaches. Additionally, she complained of muscle aching in shoulders and arm fatigue with physical activity. A physical examination revealed decreased pulses in both upper extremities. She underwent an upper extremity arterial duplex ultrasound. A high-grade stenosis was found within the left axillary artery with a PSV of greater than 300 cm/s (Fig. 13-1A). The grayscale image of the vessel at this level was unremarkable. Continuing distally down the arm, the brachial artery was identified. Sagittal examination revealed an irregular lumen and mural thickening. An area with echolucency surrounding the residual lumen was observed (Fig. 13-1B). The color imaging displayed several areas of poor filling and aliasing. Within the duplex ultrasound of the right upper extremity, the findings revealed a stenosis in the brachial artery (Fig. 13-1C–E). Changes in color flow were apparent at the stenosis; in addition, areas of echolucency were present within the vessel.

A stenosis due to giant cell or temporal arteritis will produce the typical ultrasound findings associated with any stenosis. The primary tool used to define a stenosis will be a focal increase in PSV. A PSV that is twice the value of the PSV in the adjacent more proximal vessel is indicative of at least a 50% stenosis. This criterion can be applied to most arteries. On B-mode image, giant cell arteritis often appears as a concentric wall thickening, which is hypoechoic. This thickening can occur over a long segment of the vessel and can lead to a tapering of the arterial lumen.[4] Additionally, an anechoic area may be present surrounding the vessel producing a "halo" around the vessel. This is thought to occur due to white blood cell infiltration. The "halo" should be present in both transverse and sagittal imaging planes.

TAKAYASU'S ARTERITIS

Takayasu's arteritis mainly impacts the aortic arch and its large branches. The subclavian arteries are involved in more than 90% of the cases, whereas the common carotid arteries are involved in approximately 60% of patients.[5] As with other forms of arteritis, the inflammatory process may be part of an immune system disorder. Takayasu's arteritis involves all three layers of the vessel wall. It can lead

to a partial obstruction of the vessel lumen or complete vessel occlusion. Vessel walls may also become weakened such that aneurysm formation may occur. The disease is most common in Southeast Asia. There is an eight to one female to male prevalence with greater than 80% of affected individuals being younger than 40 years of age. The presenting symptom of patients is often an absent peripheral pulse. There may be a brachial blood pressure gradient of greater than 30 mm Hg. Lightheadedness, vertigo, amaurosis fugax, transient ischemic attacks, hemiparesis, diplopia, and upper extremity claudication may also occur. Angiography and ultrasound can be used to diagnose the presence of this disease.

Scanning Technique

The sonographic examination of a patient with suspected Takayasu's arteritis will be similar to that employed for temporal arteritis. The portion of the vascular system interrogated is usually the carotid and subclavian vessels. The grayscale image is closely examined for evidence of wall thickening, whereas spectral Doppler and color imaging are used to detect a stenosis.

The ultrasound image typically reveals thickened walls with concentric narrowing. The thickened areas are usually homogeneous in appearance with adjacent segments of the vessels appearing normal and disease free (Fig. 13-2A–C). Often, the wall thickening will occur over long segments for several centimeters. The stenosis will produce elevated velocities within the segment with poststenotic turbulence presenting distally. In a transverse view, the circumferential thickening of the vessel wall has been termed the macaroni sign.[6] Distal to areas of stenosis, dampened arterial signals will be present (Fig. 13-2D).

THROMBOANGITIS OBLITERANS (BUERGER'S DISEASE)

Thromboangiitis obliterans or Buerger's disease is another nonatherosclerotic inflammatory disease. This disease affects the small- and medium-sized arteries involving the upper and lower extremities, including the digital, plantar, tibial, peroneal, radial, and ulnar arteries.[7] This disease typically manifests in patients younger than the age of 45 and has a three to one male to female distribution. Presenting symptoms can consist of ischemic digital ulcers. Ulcerations on the toes are slightly more common than finger ulcers. Gangrene of the digits can also occur. Superficial thrombophlebitis can be seen in one-third of patients, and half of patients have symptoms involving numbness and tingling in hands and feet. Other symptoms include claudication in the arch of the foot and also in the arms and hands.[8] This disease is always

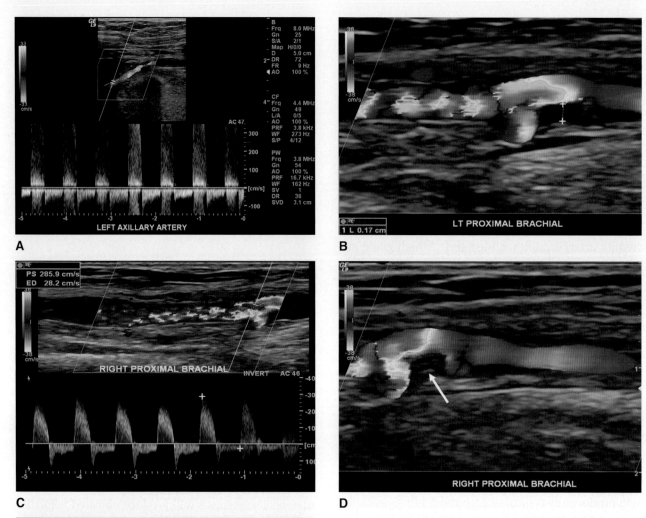

A

B

C

D

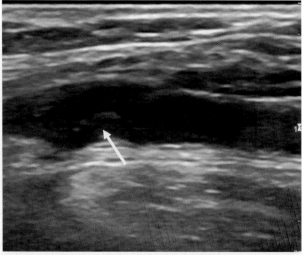

E

Figure 13-1 A: A high-grade stenosis of an axillary artery in a patient with giant cell arteritis. **B:** Irregular color filling of the brachial artery with color aliasing and echolucency observed surrounding the vessel. **C:** Doppler spectrum of the brachial artery stenosis. **D:** Color flow with irregular filling and aliasing at the stenosis (arrow). **E:** Grayscale image with diffuse wall thickening (arrow).

bilateral in nature although findings may be more pronounced in one extremity than the other. More than 80% of patients will have involvement of the disease in three of the four extremities. Because these symptoms are similar to those produced by other diseases, autoimmune diseases, hypercoagulable states, and cardioembolic disease must be excluded. Tobacco abuse is always present in the clinical history of patients with Buerger's disease and is essential to the progression of the disease. Both smoking and chewing tobacco are associated with the disease. The disease is very prevalent in India where people

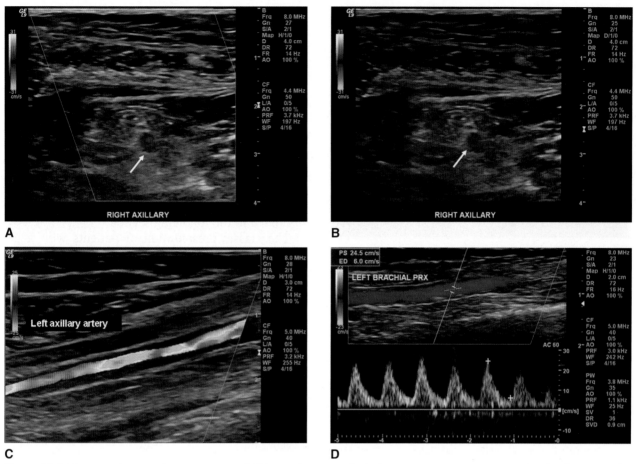

Figure 13-2 Ultrasound images from a patient with Takayasu's arteritis. **A:** Axillary artery transverse image with color illustrating the reduced flow lumen (*arrow*). **B:** Axillary artery transverse colorized grayscale image highlighting the circumferential wall thickening (*arrow*). **C:** Sagittal view of the axillary artery with color filling the reduced lumen. **D:** Dampened arterial signals from the brachial artery distal to the stenosis.

of low socioeconomic class smoke homemade cigarettes made from raw tobacco.[9] Blood tests for various inflammatory markers are often normal in these patients and thus not very helpful in the diagnosis of this disease.

Scanning Technique

Both physiologic testing and duplex ultrasound examinations are performed in order to identify Buerger's disease. Plethysmographic waveforms and pressures can be obtained from the arms (upper arm, forearm, and wrist) or legs (thigh, calf, and ankle) depending on the presenting symptoms. Digital evaluation is essential because, in some patients, waveforms recorded at the wrist or ankle levels are found to be normal. However, analysis of digital vessel waveforms will reveal the abnormality. Standard techniques for these studies have been previously described in Chapter 8.

A duplex ultrasound will be conducted on the suspected extremity to determine the level of arterial occlusion. Typically, in the upper extremity, this can include examination of the brachial, radial, and ulnar arteries. In the lower extremity, ultrasound can be performed distally along the tibial arteries. These duplex images should be carefully examined to rule out the presence of atherosclerotic plaques. Digital vessels can be evaluated with ultrasound, although this is not often the case. The digital vessels are small and superficial and, as such, require a high-frequency transducer with a small footprint in order to be adequately examined. A stenosis can sometimes be observed using digital duplex ultrasound, providing successful insonation of the digital vessels are achieved. Figure 13-3 illustrates a duplex ultrasound image from the great toe of a patient with Buerger's disease. A focal digital artery stenosis can be noted.

The preferred method to interrogate digital perfusion is with physiologic techniques. The images in Figure 13-4 were taken from a 31-year-old female that presented with pain in the first and second digits of her right hand. She was postpartum and had quit smoking during the pregnancy. She recently resumed smoking. Her medical history was also significant for

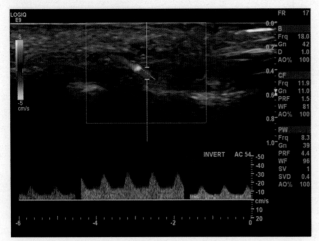

Figure 13-3 Duplex ultrasound from a digital artery of the great toe in a patient with Buerger's disease.

hypertension. Digital photoplethysmography (PPG) was performed (Fig. 13-4A). The waveforms were significantly dampened within the right second digit and slightly diminished within the right first digit as compared to the right third, fourth, and fifth digits. Clinical examination revealed an abnormal demarcation on the first and second digits, with the second digit being more severe (Fig. 13-4B). Angiography demonstrated digital artery obstruction of several vessels, which was consistent with the noninvasive vascular laboratory findings (Fig. 13-4C).

RADIATION-INDUCED ARTERITIS

Radiation-induced arteritis is a rare complication of radiation therapy for cancer. It results in perivascular fibrosis, inflammation, and acceleration of atherosclerosis. A radiation-induced arterial lesion may be difficult to distinguish from atherosclerosis. However, the localization, focal nature, and absence of atherosclerosis in other sites favors radiation as the etiology.[10,11] Typically, these patients present with claudication that may occur several months after completion of radiation treatment. Successful treatment with balloon angioplasty and stents has been performed for this condition.[12]

Scanning Technique

Duplex ultrasound evaluation includes the arterial system within the radiated region as well as adjacent vessels. Grayscale imaging is closely examined for wall irregularities and wall thickening. The appearance of these thickened areas is similar to that observed with giant cell or Takayasu's arteritis. Images from the radiated areas should be compared to those obtained from normal segments remote to the radiated area. Spectral Doppler and color waveforms are obtained from each vessel to look for evidence of stenosis. Often, physiologic tests such as an ankle–brachial index (ABI) may be performed to document global ischemia.

EMBOLIC DISEASE

An embolism is an occlusion or obstruction of an artery by a transported clot of blood or mass, bacteria, or other foreign substance. There are many sources for the clotted blood, some of which will be discussed in the following section.

The classic presentation of patients with a peripheral embolism is an abrupt onset of leg pain with no past medical history of arterial disease. Arterial embolization must be distinguished from preexisting arterial disease with thrombosis. An arterial duplex demonstrating the absence of plaque and the absence of collateral flow strongly favor acute embolization.

The site of embolization outside the cerebrovascular system includes the following locations:[13]

Upper extremity	14%
Visceral	7%
Aortoiliac	22%
Femoral	36%
Popliteal	15%
Other	6%

CARDIOEMBOLIC DISEASE

Approximately 80% to 99% of arterial emboli are from a cardiac source. This can include atrial fibrillation, postmyocardial infarction with left ventricular thrombus, mechanical heart valves, intracardiac tumors, vegetation from endocarditis, and paradoxical emboli. Cardiac embolic disease is seen across all age spectrums. The most common underlying cardiac disease seen is chronic atrial fibrillation. A thrombus forms in the left atrial appendage due to stagnation of blood then embolizes to a distal site. Although embolic stroke is the most common presentation, emboli can occur throughout the arterial tree. Figure 13-5 illustrates the spectral Doppler pattern in a patient with rapid atrial fibrillation.

Another common source is paradoxical embolization secondary to an intracardiac right-to-left shunt (patent foramen ovale or atrial septal defect). Patients who present with an acute arterial occlusion that may have deep venous thrombosis should be considered for paradoxical arterial emboli. A typical workup for these patients may include a transthoracic echocardiography or a transesophageal echocardiography with agitated saline.

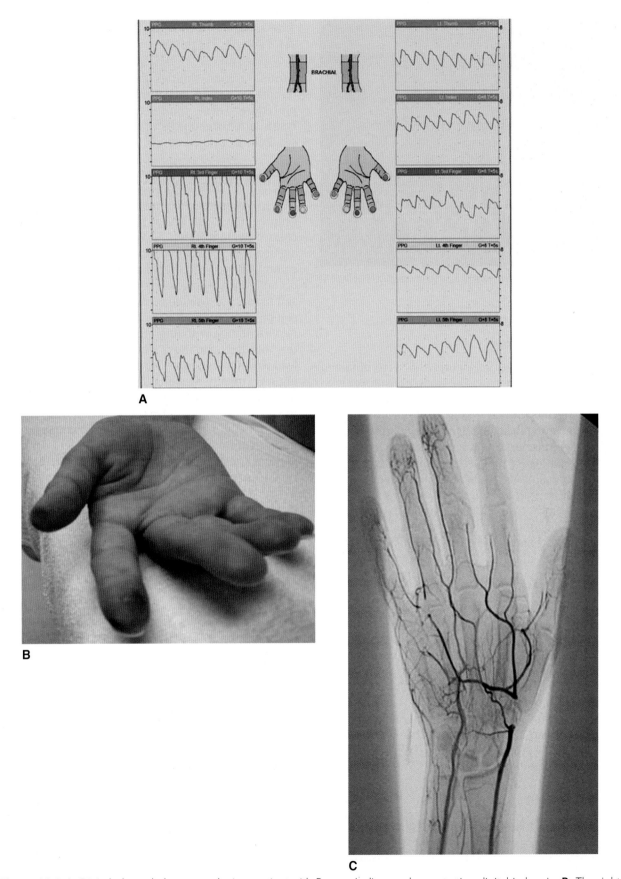

Figure 13-4 A: Digital photoplethysmography in a patient with Buerger's disease demonstrating digital ischemia. **B:** The right hand of the patient with ischemic skin changes to the first and second digits. **C:** Angiography revealing multiple areas of digital vessel occlusion.

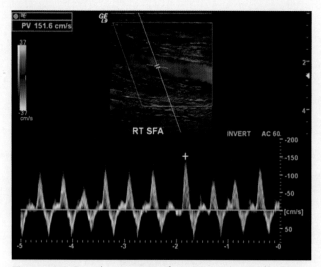

Figure 13-5 Doppler spectrum of a patient with atrial fibrillation.

Scanning Technique

The following images in Figure 13-6 were obtained from a 26-year-old female. She was a nonsmoker who was taking oral contraceptives. She had recently been treated for dehydration secondary to alcohol abuse. She presented with severe right lower extremity pain, pallor, and pulselessness. She was normotensive and in normal sinus rhythm. Figure 13-6A illustrates the presenting pallor of the patient's right foot. A duplex ultrasound examination was performed on the right lower extremity. The duplex ultrasound examination revealed an abnormal common femoral artery waveform with increased resistance demonstrated by the abrupt "spike" noted in systole (Fig. 13-6B). Continuing the ultrasound distally, echogenic material was observed within the popliteal artery (Fig. 13-6C,D). No atherosclerotic disease was present within any of the vessels imaged. Sagittal and transverse projections of the popliteal vessels revealed no flow within either the popliteal artery or vein. The patient also underwent transthoracic echocardiography, which demonstrated a right-to-left cardiac shunt. A deep vein thrombosis was present, which had embolized to the heart but passed into the systemic circulation via the cardiac shunt. This embolus occluded the right popliteal artery, resulting in the acutely ischemic right leg.

ARTERIAL EMBOLIC SOURCES

The remaining 10% to 20% of emboli arise from outside of the heart. Large upper extremity arteries such as the subclavian arteries may be a source. Disease within the aorta or iliac, femoral, or popliteal arteries may also result in emboli. This disease may be in the form of ulcerated plaques or mural thrombus aneurysms.

TRAUMATIC AND IATROGENIC ARTERIAL INJURY

Various arterial injuries can result from vascular trauma or can result iatrogenically during another procedure. These injuries can include pseudoaneurysms, arteriovenous fistulae (AVF), vessel thromboses, emboli, or dissections.

PSEUDOANEURYSMS

Due to the increased numbers of angiographic procedures, the incidence of pseudoaneurysms has increased significantly. A pseudoaneurysm or false aneurysm is a pulsating encapsulated hematoma that communicates with the adjacent artery. This process occurs from a leakage of blood after an injury into the soft tissue. The pseudoaneurysm may cause extrinsic compression of an adjacent nerve and may lead to nerve irritation with tingling or shock-like pain down the affected extremity. The pseudoaneurysm may lead to compression of the adjacent deep vein, leading to extremity swelling. The most common cause of pseudoaneurysms is the use of large-bore catheters required for endovascular procedures during cardiac or peripheral vascular interventions. The most common site for a pseudoaneurysm is the right common femoral artery. Blunt or penetrating trauma may also cause an injury and secondary pseudoaneurysm. A pseudoaneurysm can also be seen postsurgical bypass and may represent dehiscence secondary to graft infection. Pseudoaneurysms also are frequently seen in association with dialysis grafts.

Scanning Technique

Most patients with a suspected pseudoaneurysm present with a pulsatile mass. This mass may be over the site of a catheterization or traumatic injury. There may be ecchymosis and pain. A duplex ultrasound examination should be performed of both the arteries and veins in the region. Figure 13-7A illustrates a pseudoaneurysm observed in a patient who had undergone a cardiac catheterization 4 days prior. There is color outside the vessel wall with a neck or tract that connects the vessel with the pseudoaneurysm sac. The color demonstrates a red-blue swirling pattern consistent with a pseudoaneurysm. This red-blue pattern often resembles the Chinese yin-yang symbol. In this particular example, there are two pseudoaneurysm sacs that, although uncommon, does occur. Spectral Doppler patterns within the neck of the pseudoaneurysm will demonstrate a flow into the sac as well as flow out of the sac, which is referred to as a to-and-fro Doppler pattern (Fig. 13-7B).

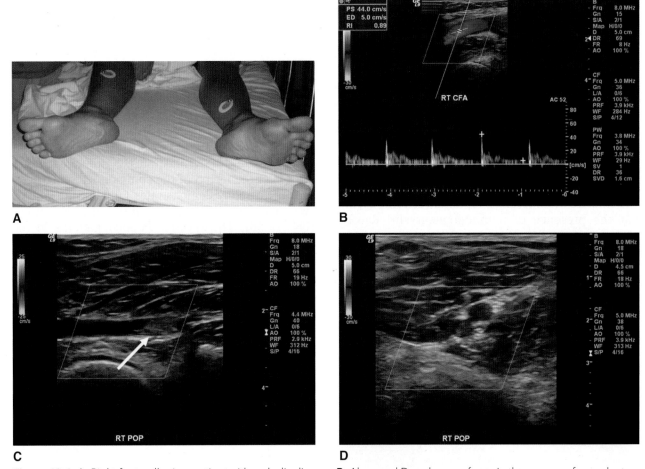

Figure 13-6 A: Right foot pallor in a patient with embolic disease. **B:** Abnormal Doppler waveforms in the common femoral artery in this patient with a popliteal artery embolus. **C:** Sagittal view of the popliteal artery embolus *(arrow)*. **D:** Transverse view of the popliteal artery and vein with no flow detected in either vessel.

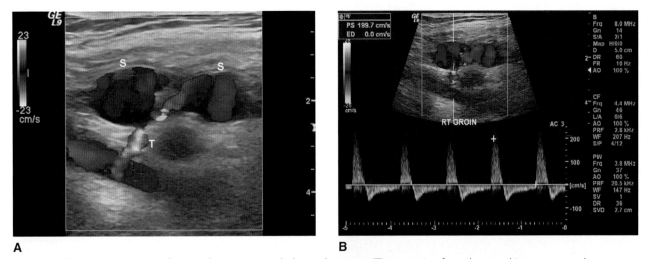

Figure 13-7 A: A color image of a pseudoaneurysm with the neck or tract *(T)* connecting from the vessel into two pseudoaneurysm sacs *(S)*. **B:** Spectral Doppler patterns within the neck of a pseudoaneurysm with a classic to-and-fro pattern.

ARTERIOVENOUS FISTULAE

Traumatic AVF can occur following arterial trauma such as a direct stab wound, gunshot wound, or blunt trauma. Most iatrogenic AVFs result as a complication of percutaneous femoral artery catheterization. Central venous catheterization occasionally leads to AVFs and rarely, AVFs are seen after total knee replacement or lumbosacral surgery. Patients with an AVF usually present with signs and symptoms at the site of intervention or injury. Typically, a new bruit is asculated, a thrill may be palpated, or a hematoma is present. The patients are often referred for an ultrasound to rule out the presence of a pseudoaneurysm. Rarely, both a pseudoaneurysm and AVF may be present at the same location.

Scanning Technique

The gold standard to detect an AVF remains digital subtraction angiography, but duplex ultrasound is a frequently used alternative for detection of an AVF. The characteristic findings on ultrasound include:

- High diastolic flow in an artery proximal to AVF
- High velocity turbulent flow (arterialized venous flow) in the vein near the fistula connection
- A color bruit may be seen at the site near the fistula connection

The following images in Figure 13-8 were taken from a 62-year-old male who presented with a palpable thrill over an arterial puncture site in the right groin. Figure 13-8A illustrates a prominent color bruit over the region of the common femoral artery. The angiography demonstrates filling of the venous system via an AVF at the common femoral artery (Fig. 13-8B). The spectral Doppler patterns in the femoral vein at the saphenofemoral junction reveal an arterialized or prominently pulsatile Doppler signal (Fig. 13-8C).

ARTERIAL OCCLUSIONS

Iatrogenic arterial occlusions can occur after various interventions or cannulations. Occasionally, an

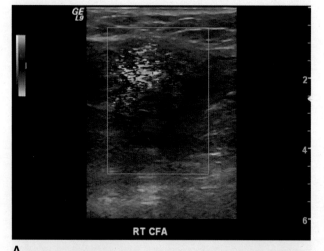

A

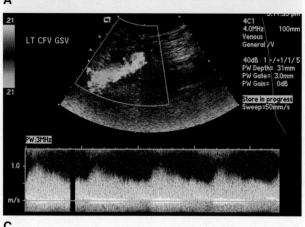

C

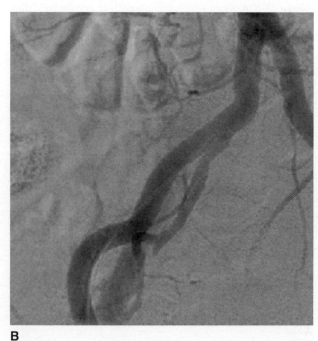

B

Figure 13-8 A: Color bruit of a common femoral artery arteriovenous fistula. **B:** An angiography demonstrating filling of the venous system via the common femoral artery arteriovenous fistula. **C:** The arterialized Doppler signal present within the common femoral vein at the saphenofemoral junction.

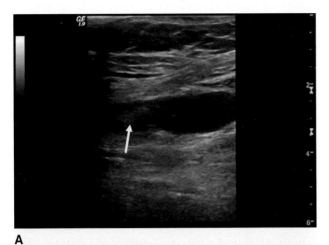

A

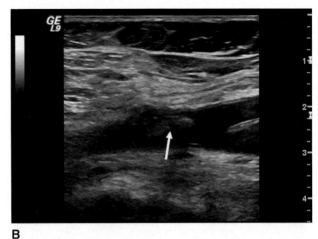

B

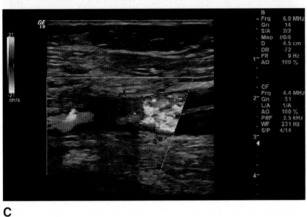

C

Figure 13-9 A: A sagittal ultrasound of a common femoral artery with echogenic material *(arrow)* present within the lumen consistent with an acute thrombus. **B:** A thrombus *(arrow)* in the common femoral artery just proximal to the superficial and deep femoral arteries. **C:** A color flow imaging demonstrating poor filling around the thrombus with filling of the vessel distal to the thrombus.

arterial occlusion may be seen following the deployment of an arterial closure device. These devices are commonly used following femoral arterial catheterization to aid with proper closure of the puncture site. The patient presentation seen with this complication is highly variable. Partial thrombosis to complete thrombosis with a cold, pulseless leg may be observed.

Scanning Technique

Duplex ultrasound can be directly performed over the puncture site. Depending on the composition of the closure device and where it was placed, it may be difficult to identify. Occasionally, only a small defect may be present in the vessel wall or a slight change in echogenicity noted at the site of the closure device. Figures 13-9A–C were taken at the common femoral artery of a patient who had a cardiac catheterization 3 days prior. A small hematoma was present in the area and weak popliteal and femoral pulses were noted on a physical examination. Echogenic material was seen in the proximal common femoral artery consistent with vessel thrombosis. Poor color filling was noted around the thrombus.

POPLITEAL ARTERY ENTRAPMENT SYNDROME

Popliteal artery entrapment is a difficult syndrome to diagnose. Popliteal entrapment occurs when the popliteal artery is compressed by the medial head of the gastrocnemius muscle or adjacent tendons.[14] This is the result of a congenital deformity of the muscle or tendon structures. The repeated extrinsic compression of the popliteal artery produces trauma to the vessel wall, which can lead to aneurysm formation, thromboembolism, or arterial thrombosis.

The presence of claudication symptoms in a young patient with no risk factors for atherosclerosis is suggestive of popliteal artery entrapment. The onset of claudication may occur after extensive exercise (such as marathon running), may be chronic with predictable claudication, or may occur with walking but not running. Rarely, symptoms may be acute if the popliteal artery has become occluded. Patients may also complain of numbness or paresthesia of the foot. There is a male to female incidence of 2:1. About two-thirds of patients may have entrapment in the contralateral limb.

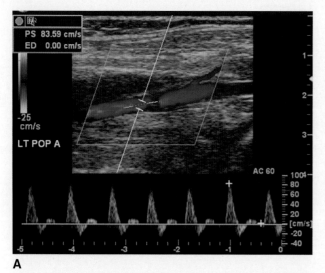
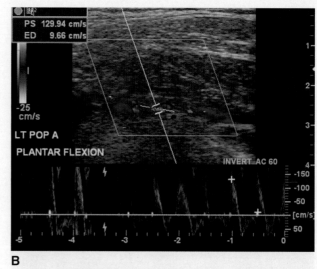

Figure 13-10 A: The left popliteal artery in a patient with popliteal entrapment. With the leg in a relaxed neutral position, the PSV is 84 cm/s. **B:** With plantar flexion, the popliteal artery velocities increase to 130 cm/s.

SCANNING TECHNIQUE

Clinical examination typically reveals that distal pulses are present at rest with the ankle in the neutral position. Pulses disappear with active plantar or dorsiflexion. Various imaging modalities can be used to aid in the diagnosis of popliteal entrapment. However, interpretation of the lower extremity vascular examination must relate to the patient's symptoms because many asymptomatic patients will partially compress the popliteal artery with provocative maneuvers.

Ultrasound can be employed to image the popliteal artery at rest and with active plantar flexion. Normal velocities at rest will become altered during the maneuver and demonstrate diminished or no flow (Fig. 13-10A,B). Digital subtraction angiography can also be performed and will demonstrate compression of the popliteal artery with active maneuvers. However, other imaging modalities such as magnetic resonance imaging or computerized tomography are often employed. These other modalities can not only provide information about the vascular system, but also can identify the skeletal/muscular features of the popliteal fossa. These anatomic details can identify those components responsible for the compression of the vessel. It can also exclude other pathology such as adventitial cystic disease of the popliteal artery.

NONATHEROSCLEROTIC ARTERIAL ANEURYSMS

Although atherosclerosis is a major cause of aneurysm formation, there are multiple other diseases that can result in aneurysm formation. Aneurysms can be associated with various inflammatory processes such as some of the arteritis diseases discussed earlier in this chapter. Takayasu's disease involves large arteries and typically causes flow-reducing stenosis of the aortic arch arteries. However, aneurysms are the most frequent fatal complication of Takayasu's arteritis. The reported incidence of aneurysms varies with one recent paper reporting a 45% occurrence of aortic aneurysms in these patients.[15] Other rare inflammatory diseases, including Behcet's syndrome, polyarteritis nodosa, and Kawasaki's disease, can also be associated with aneurysms.

Aneurysms are associated with inherited matrix defects such as Marfan's syndrome. Marfan's syndrome is a connective tissue disorder that is typically associated with aortic arch aneurysms. Ehlers-Danlos syndrome (EDS) is another well-known and often suspected cause of aneurysms. EDS patients have a congenital defect in type III collagen and this can lead to arterial rupture with or without an aneurysm.

SCANNING TECHNIQUE

Duplex ultrasound imaging has long been used to identify arterial aneurysms. Aneurysms of the aortic arch and thoracic aorta are best identified with various types of angiography. When evaluating peripheral arteries for aneurysm formation, measurements of vessel diameter should be obtained both proximal and distal to an area of suspected dilation. If a vessel diameter increases at least 50% as compared to the native, more proximal adjacent segment of artery, this vessel is considered aneurysmal. The following images in Figure 13-11 were obtained from a 51-year-old male with Marfan's syndrome. He had previously undergone an aortic arch and valve repair. He presented with left lower leg pain,

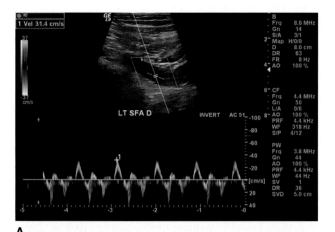

A

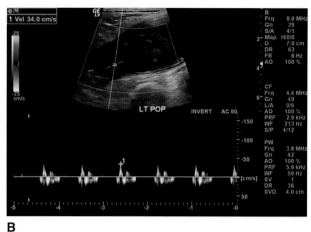

B

C

Figure 13-11 A: Abnormal distal superficial femoral artery velocities. **B:** Staccato-type flow with the proximal popliteal artery. **C:** Thrombosed popliteal artery aneurysm.

which had been worsening over the past 4 days. He had no history of smoking or peripheral vascular disease. Figure 13-11A illustrates grossly abnormal flow within the distal superficial femoral artery. Staccato-type flow was seen in the proximal popliteal artery (Fig. 13-11B). The mid-to-distal popliteal artery was

found to be aneurysmal and thrombosed (Fig. 13-11C). Popliteal artery aneurysms are rare manifestations in patients with Marfan's syndrome.[16]

Pathology Box 13-1 summarizes the nonatherosclerotic pathologies discussed in this chapter. It lists the common sites and vascular test findings.

PATHOLOGY BOX 13-1

Nonatherosclerotic Arterial Pathology

Pathology	Common Site Affected	Vascular Test Findings
Giant cell arteritis	Superficial temporal artery; extracranial arteries; occasionally, aortic arch branches	• Increased PSV at stenosis • Concentric wall thickening • Anechoic "halo" may be present
Takayasu's arteritis	Aortic arch and its branches	• Increased PSV at stenosis • Concentric wall thickening • "Macaroni" sign • Aneurysmal formation
Buerger's disease	Small- and medium-sized arteries; digital vessels	• Dampened digital PPGs • Small vessel focal stenosis with increased PSV
Radiation-induced arteritis	Any artery	• Concentric wall thickening • Increased PSV • Normal adjacent arterial segments

PATHOLOGY BOX 13-1 *(continued)*

Pathology	Common Site Affected	Vascular Test Findings
Embolic disease	Cerebrovascular vessels; any artery	• Increased resistance in Doppler signals proximal to embolus • Echogenic material within vessel • No atherosclerosis in adjacent vessel
Pseudoaneurysm	Common femoral artery; dialysis fistulae/grafts; bypass graft anastomoses	• Color flow outside normal vessel walls • Yin-yang swirling color pattern • To-and-fro signal in neck or tract
Arteriovenous fistula	Common femoral artery; any artery	• Color tissue bruit • Increased diastolic flow in artery proximal to AVF • High velocity, turbulent signals at fistula site • Prominently pulsatile venous signals
Arterial occlusion/thrombosis	Any artery	• Echogenic material in vessel at puncture site • Poor color filling • Increased PSV with partial occlusion • Increased resistance with total occlusion
Popliteal entrapment	Popliteal artery	• PSV normal in neutral, resting position • Increased PSV with active plantar or dorsiflexion
Nonatherosclerotic aneurysm	Aorta; large and medium arteries	• Diameter increase of 50% as compared to adjacent proximal vessel • No atherosclerosis • May contain thrombus • Increased resistance if completely thrombosed

PSV, peak systolic velocity; PPG, photoplethysmography; AVF, arteriovenous fistula.

SUMMARY

In summary, the majority of patients presenting for a peripheral arterial ultrasound examination will likely have atherosclerosis as the disease identified. There are numerous other pathologies that will produce peripheral arterial disease. It is important for the sonographer or vascular technologist to be familiar with these entities and their ultrasound characteristics. These uncommon causes of arterial disease should be suspected, particularly in patients without the standard risk factors for atherosclerosis.

Critical Thinking Questions

1. You are examining a patient with a 35 mm Hg brachial blood pressure difference, with the right brachial blood pressure lower than the left. Will the spectral analysis or the B-mode image be more helpful to determine the cause of a stenosis?

2. When evaluating a patient for Buerger's disease, which noninvasive vascular tests would you perform and why?

3. What are three iatrogenic arterial pathologies that can arise following catheterization of the common femoral artery for coronary artery angioplasty and stenting? Which of these problems would most impact the common femoral vein Doppler signals?

REFERENCES

1. Rigberg DA, Quinones-Baldrich W. Takayasu's disease: nonspecific aortoarteritis. In: Rutherford RB, ed. *Vascular Surgery*. 6th ed. Philadelphia, PA: W.B. Saunders; 2005:419–430.
2. Thornton J, Kupinski AM. Vascular arteritis: the atypical pathology. *Vasc US Today*. 2007;12:213–236.
3. Braunwald E. *Heart Disease*. 3rd ed. Philadelphia, PA: W.B. Saunders; 1992:1547.
4. Tatò F, Hoffman U. Giant cell arteritis: a systemic vascular disease. *Vasc Med*. 2008;13(2): 127–140.
5. Klippel JH. *The Pocket Primer on Rheumatic Diseases*. 2nd ed. London, England: Springer-Verlag; 2010:149–164.
6. Maeda H, Handa N, Matsumoto M, et al. Carotid lesion detected by B-mode ultrasonography in Takayasu's arteritis: "macaroni sign" as an indicator of the disease. *Ultrasound Med Biol*. 1991;17(7):695–701.
7. Garcia LA. Epidemiology and pathophysiology of lower extremity peripheral arterial disease. *J Endovasc Ther*. 2006;13(suppl II):II3–II9.
8. Puéchal X, Fiessinger JN. Thromoangiitis obliterans or Buerger's disease: challenges for the rheumatologist. *Rheumatology*. 2007;46(2):192–199.
9. Olin JW. Thromboangiitis obliterans (Buerger's disease). *N Engl J Med*. 2000;343(12):864–869.
10. Sacar M, Baltalarli B, Baltalarli A, et al. Occlusive arterial disease caused by radiotherapy. *Anatolian J Clin Invest*. 2006;1(1):42–44.
11. Modrall JG, Sadjadi J. Early and late presentations of radiation arteritis. *Semin Vasc Surg*. 2003;16(3):209–214.
12. Guthaner DF, Schmitz L. Percutaneous transluminal angioplasty of radiation-induced arterial stenoses. *Radiology*. 1982;144(1):77–78.
13. Kasirajan K, Ouriel K. Acute limb ischemia. In: Rutherford RB, ed. *Vascular Surgery*. 6th ed. Philadelphia, PA: W.B. Saunders; 2005:974.
14. Macedo TA, Johnson CM, Hallett JW, et al. Popliteal entrapment syndrome: role of imaging in the diagnosis. *AJR Am J Roentgenol*. 2003;181(5):1259–1265.
15. Sueyoshi E, Sakamoto I, Hayashi K. Aortic aneurysms in patients with Takayasu's arteritis: CT evaluation. *AJR Am J Roentgenol*. 2000;175(6):1727–1733.
16. Wolfgarten B, Kruger I, Gawenda M. Rare manifestation of abdominal aortic aneurysm and popliteal aneurysm in a patient with Marfan's syndrome: a case report. *Vasc Endovascular Surg*. 2001;35(1):81–84.

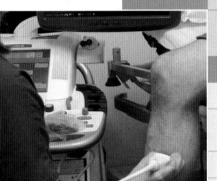

14 Duplex Imaging of the Lower Extremity Venous System

Steven R. Talbot and Mark Oliver

OBJECTIVES

Describe the components of the lower extremity venous system

Define the normal image and the Doppler characteristics of the venous system

Identify the image characteristics consistent with acute and chronic thrombus

Describe the Doppler waveform characteristics associated with various pathologies

List the risk factors associated with the formation of a deep vein thrombus

KEY TERMS

acute thrombus | chronic thrombus | deep vein | perforating vein | superficial vein | valve

GLOSSARY

acute thrombus newly formed clotted blood within a vein; generally less than 14 days old

chronic thrombus clotted blood within a vein that has generally been present for a period of several weeks or months

deep vein a vein that is the companion vessel to an artery and travels within the deep muscular compartments of the leg

perforating vein a small vein that connects the deep and superficial venous systems; a vein that

passes between the deep and superficial compartments of the leg

superficial vein a vein that is superior to the muscular compartments of the leg; travels within superficial fascia compartments; has no corresponding companion artery

valve an inward projection of the intimal layer of a vein wall producing two semilunar leaflets that present the retrograde movement of blood flow

Before the advances in ultrasound imaging that made it possible to use duplex ultrasound to look at the veins of the legs and the arms, diagnosing venous thrombosis was a complicated matter. Clinical judgment was inaccurate. The diagnostic study of choice was venography, which was painful, expensive, and carried its own set of risks.

In the 1980s, the advent of venous duplex ultrasound imaging changed all that. Since that time, duplex ultrasound imaging has become the method

of choice for imaging deep vein thrombosis (DVT).[1] Occasionally, other imaging modalities may be used for difficult or limited duplex ultrasound examinations.[2] Duplex ultrasound has the capability to diagnose, localize, and determine the age of a thrombus as well as follow the natural course of disease. Thus, it has become a mainstay in the management of DVT.[3] In addition, duplex ultrasound has the capability of discovering and diagnosing vascular and nonvascular incidental findings during the examination.[4]

However, venous duplex imaging is extremely examiner-dependent. Studies done improperly will be inaccurate. A patient who has been misdiagnosed with a venous thrombosis may be subjected to lengthy anticoagulant therapy with the risks and expenses that go with it. Conversely, a patient with an undiagnosed venous thrombosis due to an improperly performed ultrasound examination may have a life-threatening problem go undetected. This is a common tale due to the lack of standardization of qualifications for those performing venous ultrasound examinations.

The solution to this problem is to have those performing venous exams follow proper protocols and to have adequate supervised experience. The protocol in this chapter will ensure the best likelihood of performing the venous duplex ultrasound examination, using techniques that will produce accurate results.

When performing venous duplex ultrasound imaging, the examiner is trying to assess three things:

1. The presence or absence of thrombus
2. The relative risk of the thrombus dislodging and traveling to the lungs
3. The competence of the contained valves

Venous duplex ultrasound is a great tool for determining each of the items previously listed. The sonographer performing venous examinations must understand the venous anatomy.[5-8] Additionally, it is helpful to understand the pathophysiology, risk factors, and symptoms associated with DVT. This chapter will provide a comprehensive review of information pertaining to the venous duplex ultrasound examination and DVT.

ANATOMY

Chapter 1 of this text provided an anatomy review and diagrams of the vascular system. Continuing this discussion, a vascular technologist or sonographer needs to clearly understand the three main categories of veins that can be imaged:

1. The deep veins
2. The superficial veins
3. Perforators

DEEP VEINS

The deep veins are the freeways of the venous system. They are the main conduit for blood returning to the heart and are surrounded by muscle. They accompany an artery of the same name. A thrombus within the deep veins is likely to be dislodged because the muscle squeezes the deep veins with each step taken. This squeezing action is the main force that propels blood out of the leg and back to the heart, but it can also be the mechanism for dislodging a contained thrombus into the venous system, producing a pulmonary embolism (PE). A thrombus found in a deep vein is usually larger than a thrombus found in a superficial vein. This makes the thrombus from a deep vein more likely to cause a life-threatening PE because the thrombus has the potential to become lodged in a larger caliper pulmonary artery branch.

SUPERFICIAL VEINS

Unlike the deep veins, the superficial veins travel close to the skin, superficial to the muscle. These veins are usually smaller than their deeper counterparts and travel without an accompanying artery. They have an entirely different function than the deep veins. Their purpose is to get blood near the skin so as to help regulate body temperature. If the body needs to get rid of heat, the superficial veins engorge and heat from the blood-filled veins escapes into the air. If the body needs to conserve heat, the superficial veins contract and shunt blood away from the skin so the heat from the contained blood is not lost.

The traditional wisdom is that thrombi in the superficial veins do not embolize so there is often less concern about a thrombus in the superficial system. This is not true. Thrombi from the superficial venous system do embolize and travel to the lungs. However, thrombi are generally less likely to embolize from the superficial veins because they are not surrounded by muscle similar to the deep veins. Thrombi in the superficial veins are usually smaller in caliber than a thrombus in the deep veins, but their size can vary. If a thrombus is located in a superficial vein near the junction with a deep vein (the saphenofemoral or saphenopopliteal junctions), it has a greater potential to propagate into the deep veins. A thrombus in the superficial veins must be evaluated carefully to judge its potential risk to the patient.

PERFORATORS

Perforators are small bridges that connect the deep veins with the superficial veins. Their role is to keep blood from spending too much time near the skin surface by moving blood from the superficial veins to the deep veins. They have one-way valves that ensure blood is moving in the proper direction. When these valves do not function, blood can pool as the patient sits or stands too long. Over time, this can lead to chronic stasis changes and the possibility of venous ulcerations.

EPIDEMIOLOGY

Venous thromboembolism (VTE) consists of venous thrombosis (superficial or deep) and/or PE. PE is primarily a complication of DVT and a leading cause of preventable death in hospital mortality in the United States. It has been estimated that, in the United States, there are greater than 500,000 cases of DVT each year with more than 50% of those cases going unrecognized. There are also approximately 200,000 cases of fatal PE annually.[9]

In addition to acute risks from DVT, up to 30% of patients may develop symptoms of postthrombotic syndrome (e.g., pain, swelling, ulcerations).[10] This chronic condition carries a significant morbidity.

PATHOPHYSIOLOGY

The primary mechanism for the formation of venous thrombosis is Virchow's triad (circa 1856),[11] which includes venous stasis, vessel wall injury, and a hypercoagulable state. The balance between thrombogenesis (clotting factors), coagulation inhibitors, and the fibrinolytic system determines the formation of a venous thrombus. Venous stasis being one of the components of Virchow's triad allows for the increased exposure of clotting factor, which occurs in immobility. Vessel wall injury will also affect the body's normal thrombolytic system. The vessel injury could be catheter related or could include an injury such as that seen in trauma patients. Hypercoagulability is the last condition that can lead to a thrombus formation. Hypercoagulability is associated with various diseases such as cancer and patients who are on birth control pills and hormone replacement therapy. Patients with genetic factors such as factor V Leiden and prothrombic gene mutations are considered hypercoagulable.

Venous thrombi very commonly begin around small valve cusps in the calf because these are areas of slower blood flow. This slower flow may contain regions of flow stagnation—one of the features of Virchow's triad. Small thrombi can form, which can continue to develop into larger occlusive thrombi.

Risk factors for DVT can generally be associated with one or more of the elements of Virchow's triad.[12] Common risk factors are shown in Table 14-1.

SIGNS AND SYMPTOMS

Signs and symptoms of venous thromboembolism are caused by venous obstruction, vascular and perivascular inflammation, and embolization of thrombi.[13] Many patients with a venous thrombosis may be asymptomatic. Symptomatic patients may present with extremity pain, tenderness, swelling, venous distention, discoloration, or a palpable cord. Some patients may present with no symptoms within the

TABLE 14-1
Risk Factors for DVT
Age
Surgery or trauma
Immobilization
Past history of DVT
Coagulation disorders (congenital/acquired)
Malignancy
Septicemia
Birth control pills
Hormone replacement therapy
Pregnancy
Obesity
Stroke
Congestive heart failure
Long distance travel
Inflammatory bowel disease
Varicose veins

DVT, deep vein thrombosis.

extremity and only symptoms consistent with a PE such as tachypnea, chest pain, or tachycardia.

Even though the role of a sonographer or vascular technologist is to perform the venous ultrasound, it is important to be familiar with the general clinical workup of patients with suspected DVT. Many laboratories or hospitals may use clinical algorithms to assist in patient management and the scheduling of diagnostic tests such as ultrasound, particularly for after-hours studies. As mentioned at the beginning of this chapter, the clinical diagnosis of DVT is quite inaccurate with poor sensitivity and specificity. Various patient data, both demographic and clinical, are often evaluated to aid in the clinical diagnosis of DVT.[14]

Different risk factors and symptoms have been combined into the scoring algorithm known as the Well's criteria.[15] Table 14-2 lists the components of this algorithm.

Another useful clinical marker for DVT is the measurement of D-dimer. D-dimer is a breakdown product of fibrin, which will be elevated in the presence of DVT. However, false positive and false negatives do occur. Liver disease, malignancy, inflammation, trauma, or recent surgery are just a few of the conditions that may result in elevated D-dimer levels and, thus, a false-positive result for the presence of DVT. False negatives may result due to the inability of the assay to measure very low levels of the fibrin fragment. D-dimer is thought to be most useful in the setting of low probability of DVT based on clinical criteria.[15] Ultrasound in combination with D-dimer is a very useful tool for DVT determination.

TABLE 14-2
The Well's Criteria
+1 Point Each for:
Active malignancy
Paralysis, paresis, or recent plaster immobilization of lower limb
Recently bedridden for more than 3 days or major surgery/trauma in past 4 weeks
Localized tenderness along distribution of lower extremity deep veins
Entire lower limb swollen
Calf swelling more than 3 cm compared with asymptomatic leg
Pitting edema on symptomatic leg
Collateral superficial veins on symptomatic leg
−2 Points for:
Alternative diagnosis as likely or more likely than that of DVT
Probability for DVT:
High ≥3 points
Intermediate 1–2 points
Low ≤0 points

DVT, deep vein thrombosis.

SONOGRAPHIC EXAMINATION TECHNIQUES

PATIENT PREPARATION

The examination is explained to the patient. The patient's signs and symptoms along with relevant history are obtained. Lower extremity clothing should be removed. The patient can wear undergarments providing the clothing allows sufficient access to the groin area. A patient gown or drape should be provided. Some departments take this time to instruct a patient how to perform a Valsalva maneuver.

PATIENT POSITIONING

The veins of the leg in a patient lying on a flat bed are nearly closed due to low transmural pressure. This makes them extremely difficult to see. The simple solution to this problem is to tilt the bed so blood pools in the legs, thus engorging the veins. The engorged veins are large, round, and easy to see. This bed tilt maneuver is essential to doing quality venous imaging. Omitting this step is the most common reason for missing small thrombi, especially in the calf.

The entire bed should be tilted (not just elevation of the head) in a reversed Trendelenburg position. The head should be elevated in this way to an angle

of about 20°. In cases where the calf veins are still difficult to see due to their small size, the examiner can have the patient sit at the side of the bed (legs dangling) to further engorge the calf veins. This is extremely effective. It will, however, make the veins much more difficult to compress so the examiner has to be cautious not to mistake the engorged veins for thrombus-filled veins. In this position, the veins are under greater pressure, thus increased transducer pressure will be required to compress the veins.

In addition to using the proper tilt, the patient must also be positioned properly on the bed. When examining the legs, this means having the patient lie flat on his or her back with the knee slightly bent and the hip slightly externally rotated (Fig. 14-1). This allows access to the inside of the leg and creates a flat imaging surface. Omitting this subtle positioning may result in potential errors. The patient should also be moved as close to the examiner as possible for ergonomic concerns.

EQUIPMENT SELECTION

Duplex imaging equipment quality can vary dramatically. Trying to do venous duplex imaging with an ultrasound imager and transducers that are designed for other applications such as general or cardiac ultrasound can be extremely frustrating and potentially dangerous. Formatting imagers for venous work requires three specialized transducers:

- The workhorse transducer will be a midrange linear array transducer (5-10 MHz). This transducer will be used for the femoral veins, the popliteal vein, and most of the calf. In the upper extremity, the midrange transducer will be used to view the subclavian and larger arms.
- A second transducer, the high-frequency linear array transducer is indispensable. Some

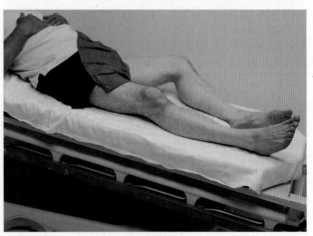

Figure 14-1 Proper patient positioning for a lower extremity venous ultrasound examination for DVT.

institutions try to do without this transducer, but this is not the best course of action. This high-frequency transducer should have a small footprint (hockey stick–type transducers are very useful). This transducer (10-18 MHz) is used for superficial veins such as the saphenous in the leg and for most of the arm veins. This transducer is a must for detailed reflux studies or upper and lower extremity mapping.

- The third transducer needed for venous imaging is the curved low-frequency transducer (2-5 MHz). This transducer is useful for the inferior vena cava (IVC) and iliac veins. It is also helpful in the heavy patient where some veins may lie deeper within the leg.

SCANNING TECHNIQUE

Recently, changes to the names of some of the veins in the leg were adopted that have unfortunately made things a bit more confusing. Some have been slow to adopt the new terms and others are not aware the changes have been made. In the following sections, both terms will be provided for those veins with new nomenclature. The protocol described here represents a summary of time-tested techniques for properly identifying the veins and evaluating them for a thrombus formation.[16-19]

Initial Examination Position

The lower extremity venous duplex examination begins at the groin crease. The common femoral vein (CFV) and common femoral artery (CFA) are located from a medial projection in a transverse plane. Moving above this area and above the level of the inguinal ligament, the CFV becomes the external iliac vein (EIV). Using the ultrasound transducer, gentle pressure is applied directly over the vein. Because the veins are under relatively low pressure, the walls of the vein will be seen to coapt or close together. The compression of the walls of the vein should be recorded. Remaining in a transverse plane, the compression and release technique is performed every 2 to 3 cm down the entire length of the leg, documenting the images at several locations along the leg. With each of the named vessels described as follows, these compression maneuvers are performed and recorded. The smaller the "cuts" (or spacing between compressions) used, the better. Spacing the cuts too far apart will allow for missing a smaller partial thrombus. After the entire vein has been imaged in the transverse plane, the examiner can then reexamine the same vein in a longitudinal plane. This will add additional information and can be used to confirm findings observed in the transverse plane.

Doppler and color imaging can be performed in the longitudinal plane.

It cannot be overemphasized, however, that one cannot omit the transverse view and do only longitudinal imaging. Doing so will result in missing nonobstructive thrombi. It is very easy to roll off a vein while in the longitudinal plane; therefore, compressions should never be performed in a longitudinal view.

In addition to compression of the veins, spectral Doppler waveforms are usually recorded from the CFV and popliteal veins. Institutions vary at which specific veins Doppler waveforms should be obtained but generally it is at least at two levels. For a DVT examination, Doppler waveforms are examined strictly for qualitative features such as spontaneity, phasicity with respiration, augmentation with distal compression, and cessation of flow with proximal compression.

Common Femoral and Great Saphenous Veins

The CFV is identified next to an accompanying artery of the same name (Fig. 14-2). Just below the level of the inguinal ligament, a large superficial vein terminates into the CFV (Fig. 14-3). This vein has been traditionally called the greater saphenous or long saphenous but has been renamed the great saphenous vein (GSV) (Fig. 14-4). The termination of the GSV into the CFV is called the saphenofemoral junction (SFJ). The GSV is the longest superficial vein in the body and travels close to the skin in the saphenous compartment. Below the SFJ, the GSV courses medially and superficially to the CFV. Below the knee, the GSV is more anterior as it courses through calf.

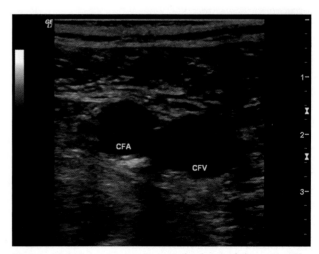

Figure 14-2 A transverse view at the level of the groin. The common femoral artery (CFA) and vein (CFV) are visualized side by side.

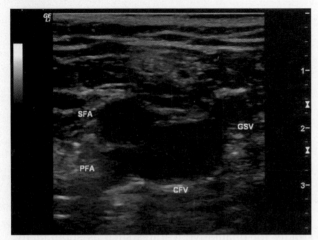

Figure 14-3 A transverse view of the bifurcation of the common femoral artery into the superficial femoral artery *(SFA)* and deep (profunda) femoral artery *(PFA)* while the great saphenous vein *(GSV)* terminates into the common femoral vein *(CFV)*.

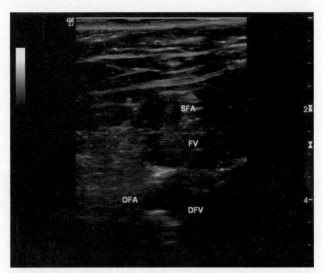

Figure 14-5 A transverse view of the femoral *(FV)* and deep femoral vein *(DFV)* in the upper thigh. Also shown is the superficial femoral artery *(SFA)* and the deep femoral artery *(DFA)*.

In the upper thigh, the CFV is formed by the junction of the femoral vein (FV) (formerly known as the superficial femoral vein) and the deep femoral vein (DFV) (also known as the profunda femoris vein) (Fig. 14-5).

Femoral Vein and Deep Femoral Vein

The FV will be more superficial than the DFV (Fig. 14-6). They will parallel each other through most of the thigh. The FV is the main venous outflow of the calf, whereas the DFV mainly drains the thigh itself. The entire length of the FV should be examined in detail (Figs. 14-7 and 14-8) with compression

images often documented in the upper thigh, midthigh, and distal thigh. The DFV should be examined as well. Most protocols include a compression of the DFV near its terminus into the CFV. The remainder of the DFV may be too deep and may have many tributaries such that complete examination of its entire length may be difficult.

The FV through the thigh may be a bifid system (Fig. 14-9). This is fairly common and simply means that the examiner must be sure to investigate each vessel. In the case of a patient with a bifid system and a venous thrombosis, it is not uncommon for one FV to be patent while the other is thrombosed.

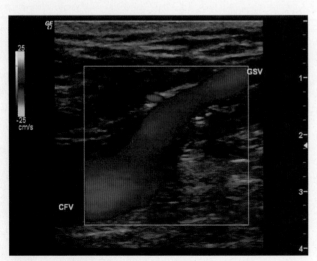

Figure 14-4 A longitudinal view of the great saphenous vein *(GSV)* terminating into the common femoral vein *(CFV)* just below the level of the inguinal ligament.

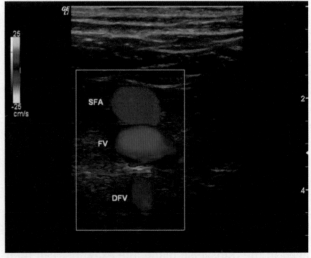

Figure 14-6 A transverse view of the femoral vein (FV) and deep femoral vein *(DFV)* in the upper thigh with color added to assist in vessel identification. The superficial femoral artery *(SFA)* is also seen.

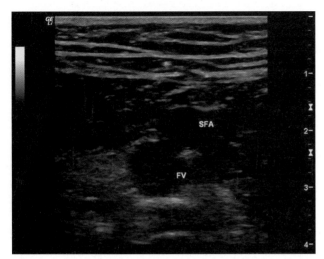

Figure 14-7 A transverse view of the superficial femoral artery *(SFA)* and femoral vein *(FV)* with the medial aspect of the thigh.

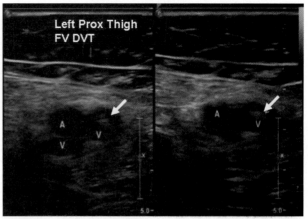

Figure 14-9 Split screen view of a bifid femoral vein *(V)* along with the superficial femoral artery *(A)*. Note how echogenic material is clearly seen in one of the two veins *(arrows)* in the noncompressed view *(left)*. The *right* image shows that the thrombus-free vein is fully collapsed when transducer pressure is exerted over it. In contrast, the thrombus-filled vein fails to fully compress in response to the same pressure. This is a reliable evidence of the presence of a thrombus in this vein.

At the adductor canal, the FV travels deep to the muscles of the thigh. Distal to the adductor canal, the vein is called the popliteal vein.

Popliteal Vein

The popliteal vein is the main drainage for blood leaving the calf (Figs. 14-10 and 14-11). In the upper portion of the popliteal fossa, the popliteal vein and artery are the only vessels visualized. As was the case with the FV, the popliteal vein can occasionally be bifid.

Anterior Tibial Vein

The anterior tibial vein (ATV) terminates into the popliteal vein in the mid to upper regions of the popliteal fossa. However, this is not commonly seen on

duplex ultrasound because of its depth and the angle of its termination into the popliteal vein. It empties into the popliteal vein as a single trunk. This single, common ATV forms at the junction of the two ATVs in the upper calf. Although the proximal calf portion of the ATVs is hard to see, the remainder of the course of the ATVs is easily imaged from an anterior–lateral projection. Because a thrombus formation in the ATVs is rare, imaging of these vessels is not a part of most protocols. Thrombi are rare in the ATVs because they do not communicate with the prime source of thrombi in the leg—the soleal sinus veins. Examination of the ATVs can be added to an existing protocol whenever there is an injury to this area or

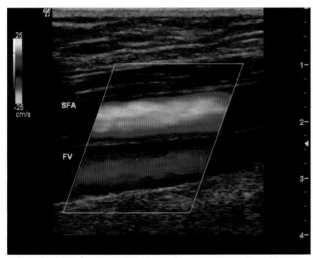

Figure 14-8 A longitudinal view in color of the superficial femoral artery *(SFA)* and femoral vein *(FV)* within the mid-thigh.

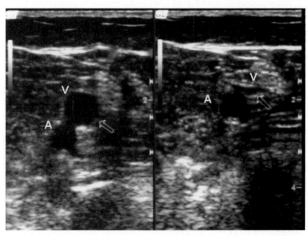

Figure 14-10 A split screen transverse view of the popliteal artery *(A)* and vein *(V)*. The *arrow* indicates the popliteal vein fully open on the *right* and completely compressed on the *left*.

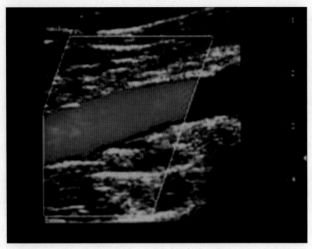

Figure 14-11 A longitudinal view in color of the popliteal vein.

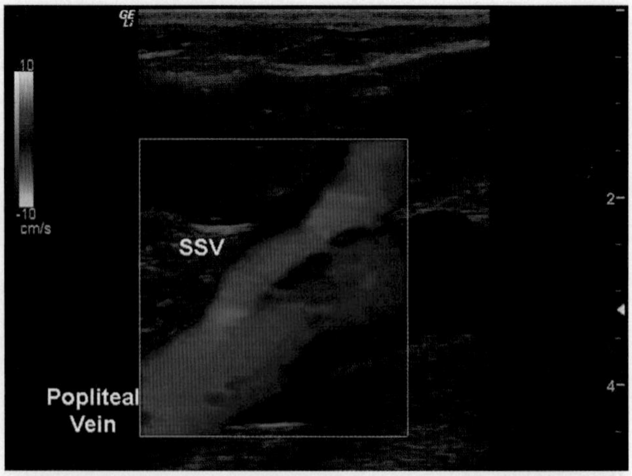

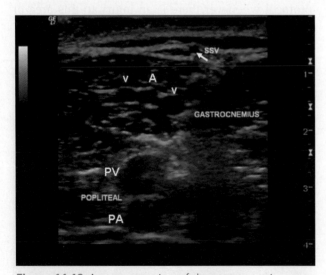

Figure 14-13 A longitudinal view of the small saphenous vein terminating into the popliteal vein.

when a patient complains of pain or other symptoms over this region.

Gastrocnemius Veins

The popliteal vein tributaries also include small muscular veins called the gastrocnemius veins (Fig. 14-12). There are lateral and medial paired gastrocnemius veins, each with an accompanying gastrocnemius artery. The paired veins often merge into a single trunk prior to emptying into the popliteal vein. These veins are deep veins but are not major deep veins of the calf. They serve to drain the gastrocnemius muscle and can be followed down the calf within the muscle.

Figure 14-12 A transverse view of the gastrocnemius artery (A) and veins (V) in the upper calf. Also in view is the popliteal artery (PA) and the popliteal vein (PV) deep to the gastrocnemius vessels. The small saphenous vein (SSV) is indicated by the *arrow* superficial to the gastrocnemius vessels.

Small Saphenous Vein

This vein was traditionally named the lesser, small, or short saphenous vein but is now only referred to as the small saphenous vein (SSV). This superficial vein terminates into the popliteal vein at about the same level as the gastrocnemius veins (Fig. 14-13). The terminus of the SSV into the popliteal vein is known as the saphenopopliteal junction. Sometimes the SSV and the gastrocnemius veins share a common trunk as they enter the popliteal. The SSV courses along the posterior calf approximately in the middle of the calf. It receives tributaries from both the medial and lateral aspects of the calf with a large tributary vein often arising from the lateral malleolus. In some patients, the SSV does not terminate into the popliteal vein. Instead, it will bypass the popliteal vein and continue up the posterior thigh, eventually joining the deep system or the GSV in the thigh. When this occurs, this extension of the SSV above the popliteal fossa is referred to as the vein of Giacomini.

Tibioperoneal Trunk

The tibioperoneal trunk receives blood from the posterior tibial and peroneal veins. These veins merge together in the upper calf to form the tibioperoneal trunk. The tibioperoneal trunk merges with the ATV to form the popliteal vein.

Common Tibial and Peroneal Trunks

The specific level at which the tibioperoneal trunk forms varies somewhat but it is usually at the distal portion of the popliteal fossa within the upper calf. The common posterior tibial and common peroneal trunks merge together to form the tibioperoneal trunk (Figs. 14-14 and 14-15). In the upper calf, the

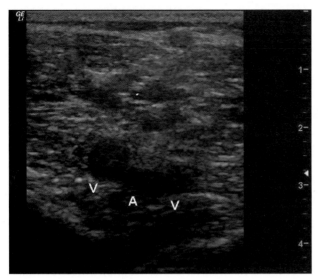

Figure 14-14 A transverse view of the common posterior tibial and common peroneal trunks.

paired posterior tibial veins unite to form the common tibial trunk, and the paired peroneal veins unite to form the common peroneal trunk. The specific length of these two common trunks is variable.

Posterior Tibial Veins

The posterior tibial veins (PTVs) will course medially in the calf near the tibia. The veins are paired following the posterior tibial artery (Fig. 14-16). They arise via tributaries between the medial malleolus and the Achilles tendon at the ankle.

Peroneal Veins

The peroneal veins are followed deeper in the calf (Fig. 14-17) as they parallel the PTVs through most

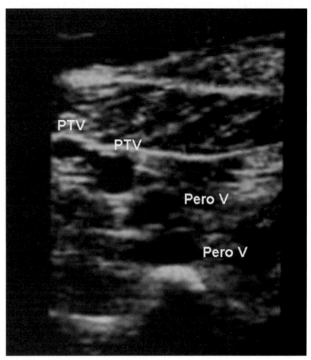

Figure 14-16 A transverse view of the medial calf with the posterior tibial veins (PTV) and peroneal veins (Pero V). The large anechoic area below the peroneal veins is the fibula.

of the calf (Fig. 14-18). They travel adjacent to the fibula along with the peroneal artery.

Soleal Sinus Veins

One of the major functions of the venous system (aside from returning blood to the heart) is to provide a storage area for blood. One of the major storage areas for blood in the calf is a network of veins called the soleal sinus veins. Because blood only moves

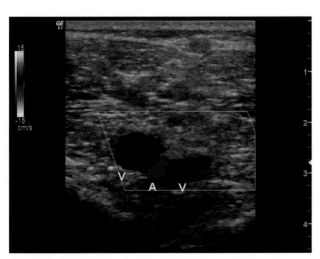

Figure 14-15 A transverse view of the common posterior tibial and common peroneal trunks with color added.

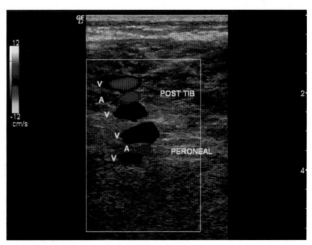

Figure 14-17 A transverse view of the medial calf showing the posterior tibial (V) and peroneal veins (V) with color added. The companion arteries are also shown (A).

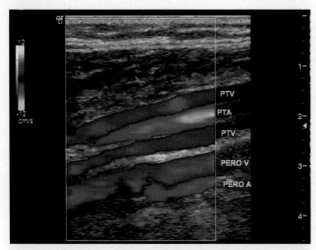

Figure 14-18 A longitudinal view in color of the posterior tibial veins *(PTV)* and posterior tibial artery *(PTA)*. This illustrates the parallel position of the peroneal artery *(PERO A)* and peroneal veins *(PERO V)* deep to the posterior tibial vessels. In this view only one of the paired peroneal veins is observed.

inside these veins when the calf muscle contracts, they are a common site for thrombi to form following surgery, a long plane trip, or anytime a person sits, stands, or is in bed for an extended period of time. The soleal veins communicate into the PTVs and peroneal veins. A thrombus that forms within the soleal veins can therefore easily extend into the major deep vein of the calf. These soleal veins are small and difficult to find but when they fill with thrombus, they enlarge and are much easier to see (Fig. 14-19).

Imaging the Iliac Veins

In most institutions, imaging above the groin is not done unless there is a clinical indication to suggest involvement of the iliac veins or the IVC. Commonly, Doppler signals obtained at the CFVs are used to provide an indirect assessment of the status of veins above the groin. If good phasic flow is detected in the CFV, it suggests the lack of an obstruction of the iliac vein or IVC. This is less sensitive in the case of a thrombus that is nonobstructive. When one suspects pathology in the iliac veins or IVC, the duplex examinations can be extended into the pelvic region and abdomen.

Imaging in the pelvic region and abdomen is difficult because of the depth of the vessels, bowel gas, and the fact that compression of the vessels is not likely to be accomplished. Because of the inability to compress the veins to determine if they are thrombus-free, the examiner may have to rely on more color and spectral Doppler techniques to determine patency—something that can lead to inaccurate results.

Detailed instruction of how to image these vessels is covered in Chapter 21. Basic guidelines for imaging in the abdomen include having the patient fast if possible to reduce bowel gas and scheduling the patient early in the morning

The examination of the iliac veins usually starts by following the CFV above the inguinal ligament into the pelvic region. The iliac veins will penetrate deep very quickly. The continuation of the CFV above the inguinal ligament is the EIV. At the level of the sacroiliac joints, the EIV will become the common iliac vein (CIV) as the internal iliac vein (IIV) merges with the EIV. The IIV may be difficult to insonate, so this transition level may be hard to determine. Eventually, the CIV (Fig. 14-20) will be joined by the CIV from the other leg to form the IVC (Fig. 14-21).

TECHNICAL CONSIDERATIONS

Compression of the vein is an essential component to this examination. However, in the presence of a venous thrombus, caution should be used when performing compressions. This is especially important if the thrombus is nonocclusive and appears as a free-flowing tail

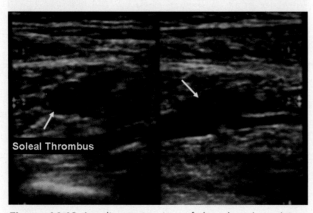

Figure 14-19 A split screen view of thrombus *(arrow)* in a soleal sinus vein. The *left* image shows the contained thrombus *(arrow)* restricting compression of the soleal vein.

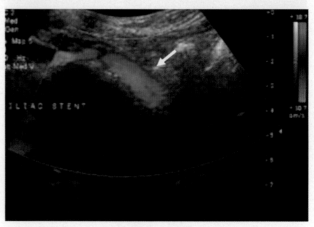

Figure 14-20 A longitudinal view of an iliac vein *(arrow)*, which is stented.

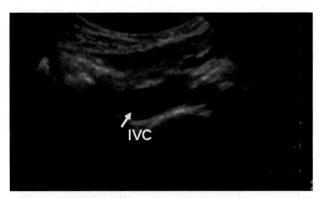

Figure 14-21 A transverse view of the inferior vena cava *(IVC)*.

of material within the vein lumen. There have been reports of dislodging loosely attached thrombi by ultrasound compressions and causing emboli.[21,22]

PITFALLS

There are several pitfalls encountered with venous imaging in the lower extremities. Most issues concern the limited visualization of the veins. Body habitus can result in veins being positioned deeply in the leg. Equipment settings should be optimized for a deeper field of view and lower frequency transducers may be used. For deep calf veins, various approaches including lateral and posterior approaches may result in a more complete visualization.

Compression of deeper veins is sometimes challenging. As it passes through the adductor canal, the femoral vein is often difficult to compress using the transducer and applying pressure from a medial approach. At this level, the examiner should take his or her free hand and press up along the posterior aspect of the thigh. Pressure applied at this point will push the vein up against the muscle and transducer (Fig. 14-22). It is more easily compressed

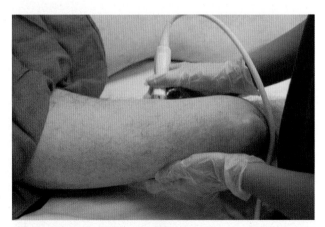

Figure 14-22 Technique used to compress distal thigh portion of the femoral vein. The examiner applies pressure with his or her free hand along the posterior aspect of the thigh.

from this approach and usually more comfortable for the patient.

There may be patients presenting for venous ultrasounds with wounds, dressings, orthopedic hardware, or surgical incisions. The veins lying under these areas may be unable to be directly assessed. Ultrasound characteristics in the veins immediately adjacent to these areas may indirectly aid in determining the patency of the veins not visualized.

DIAGNOSIS

Until the 1980s, diagnosing a venous thrombus in the extremities was done using venography. This was an accurate test but it was invasive, painful, and had some inherent risks. Attempts were being made in the early vascular laboratories to find a thrombus noninvasively, but the nonimaging techniques being employed at that time were not acceptable. When imaging quality began to improve to the point where it became possible to see the vessels well enough to consider using ultrasound imaging to find a thrombus, attempts were made to use duplex ultrasound for this purpose. Initially, those exploring this theory were convinced to abandon the idea because the wisdom of the experts at that time was that a thrombus could not be seen on ultrasound. However, those doing the initial research quickly found that veins that were thrombus-free would collapse completely when the examiner compressed over the vein being imaged.[20] This made venous imaging possible even if one could not actually see the thrombus using the ultrasound. They also found that imaging of the thrombus was possible, making this technique even more useful than its invasive counterpart because not only could one see the thrombus, but it was also possible to tell if it was old or new, stable or unstable.[23]

NORMAL, THROMBUS-FREE VEINS

After initially identifying the artery and vein, the examiner uses the transducer to compress over the vessels. The thrombus-free vein will compress, whereas the artery does not. Exerting more pressure will eventually cause the walls of the artery to close as well. The compression maneuver will aid the examiner with vessel identification. It also is the first clear indicator of the presence or absence of a thrombus in the vein. If the vein being examined closes completely in response to transducer pressure (Fig. 14-23), it can be determined that the vein is thrombus-free at that location. This complete compression of the vein (where the vein walls touch each other during compression) is the key to venous imaging. In fact, some imaging professionals refer to venous imaging as

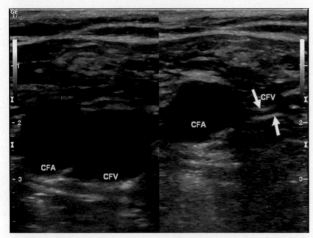

Figure 14-23 Split screen view demonstrating the full compression of the common femoral vein *(CFV)* indicating the thrombus-free status of the vein at that location. Note how the vein walls coapt together *(arrows)*. The common femoral artery *(CFA)* is also seen.

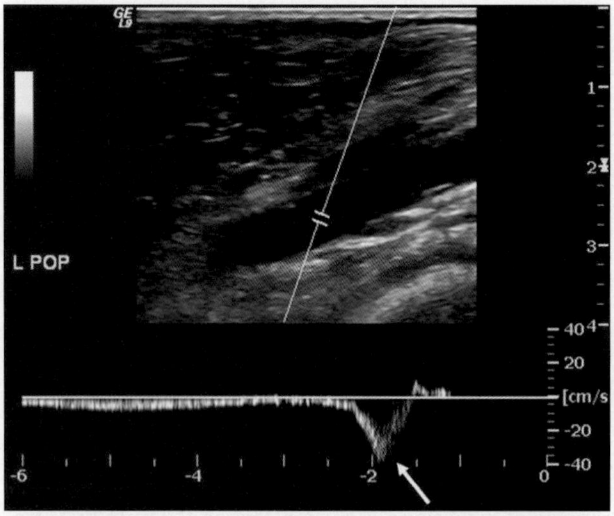

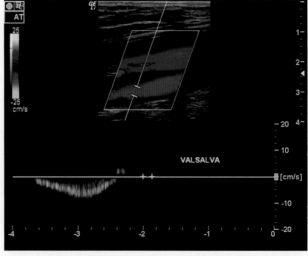

Figure 14-25 A spectral Doppler waveform obtained from the popliteal vein illustrating a normal augmentation in flow *(arrow)* with a distal compression.

"compression ultrasound." After watching the vein compress, the examiner eases up, and the vein will reopen. The walls of a normal vein appear thin and smooth. Valve sinuses may be apparent as slight dilations in the vein wall. Valve leaflets may be seen as thin white structures within the sinus freely moving in the blood stream.

NORMAL COLOR AND SPECTRAL DOPPLER

Spectral Doppler and color information can be added to the information gathered from visualizing the compressions of the veins. Laboratory accreditation protocols presently require spectral Doppler signals at key levels. Venous Doppler signals should display the following five characteristics. First, with modern ultrasound equipment, spontaneous Doppler signals should present within all major vessels. Second, spectral Doppler signals in a normal vein should be phasic with respiration (Fig. 14-24). Third, compression of the leg below the level of the transducer should augment flow (Fig. 14-25). Fourth, venous Doppler signals should cease with proximal compression or the Valsalva maneuver (Fig. 14-26). Lastly, venous Doppler signals from lower extremity veins should be unidirectional, toward the heart.

Color flow imaging should also display the same attributes as a spectral Doppler. With proper equipment setting, color should be seen completely filling the vessel lumen (Fig. 14-27).

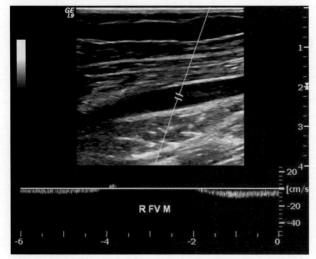

Figure 14-24 A spectral Doppler waveform obtained from the mid-thigh level of the femoral vein *(FV)* illustrating normal respiratory phasicity.

Figure 14-26 A spectral Doppler venous waveform illustrating the absence of flow during a Valsalva maneuver.

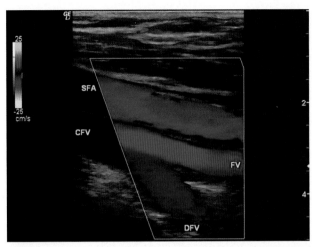

Figure 14-27 A longitudinal color image of the confluence of the femoral vein *(FV)* and the deep femoral vein *(DFV)* into the common femoral vein *(CFV)*. The superficial femoral artery *(SFA)* is also seen.

DETERMINING THE PRESENCE OF A THROMBUS

A thrombus is present when echogenic material is visualized within the lumen of a vein and the echogenic material restricts the complete compression of the vein walls (see Fig. 14-9). These two findings must occur together to definitively determine the presence of a thrombus in a vein. Too many protocols simply focus on compression ("compression ultrasound"). Failure to link compression with actual visualization of the echogenic material within the vein will result in false-positive results in cases where the vein compression is being hampered by something other than a thrombus. Examples of situations leading to false-positive results include a patient bearing down because of the discomfort of the compression, thus making the vein difficult to compress. In addition, compression of the vein may be limited by adjacent structures such as bone or dense muscle bundles. The examiner may also fail to exert sufficient pressure to coapt the vein walls and thus assume a DVT is present.

There are instances when a thrombus is present but the images are so poor that it is impossible to visually document the presence of the thrombus. In these cases, the diagnosis of a thrombus within the vein can be made by pressing harder over the vessels until the accompanying artery starts to deform, but the vein walls do not compress. When this occurs, the examiner and interpreter can be assured adequate compression has been used and that a thrombus is likely present.

Characterization of a Thrombus

One of the unique benefits of venous duplex imaging over venography is that it can be used not only to identify the presence or absence of thrombus,

but also it can be used to tell the characteristic of a thrombus that may make a difference in how it is treated. Generally, the newer the thrombus, the more likely it is to break loose and travel to the lungs. Although venous imaging does not allow one to tell the exact age of a given thrombus, there are observable clues to its age and stability that can be gleaned during venous duplex imaging.

Characteristics usually associated with *acute* thrombus include the following:
1. A lightly echogenic or hypoechoic thrombus
2. A poorly attached thrombus
3. A spongy texture of the thrombus
4. A dilated vein (when totally obstructed)

Characteristics usually associated with *chronic* thrombus include:
1. A brightly echogenic or hyperechoic thrombus
2. A well-attached thrombus
3. A rigid texture of a thrombus
4. A contracted vein (if totally obstructed)
5. Large collaterals

Acute Thrombus

A thrombus is simply the fluid and solid contents of the blood that has been captured in a thrombin net so that it becomes a solid mass. Therefore, a newly formed thrombus can be almost invisible by ultrasound (Fig. 14-28). The only clue to the presence of a DVT is the fact that the compression of the vein is being limited by the spongy thrombus and a faint reflection around its edges can be seen (Fig. 14-29). This faint reflection is created by the thrombin net that has recently formed to trap the blood (Fig. 14-30). The experienced examiner will spot this faint echo and investigate

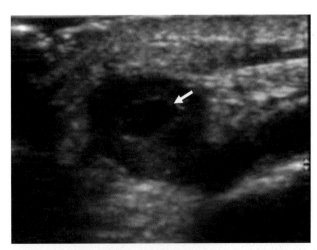

Figure 14-28 Transverse view of a vein with an extremely acute thrombus *(arrow)* forming within it. The vein was not compressing, but no thrombus was initially seen. Gains were increased so that blood flow could be seen on gray scale. Note how the thrombus is actually less echogenic than the blood flowing around it. The faint edge of the fibrin net is also visible around the thrombus.

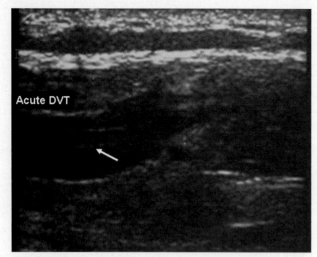

Figure 14-29 A longitudinal view of an acute thrombus. Note the faint echo of the fibrin net *(arrow)* that surrounds the newly formed thrombus.

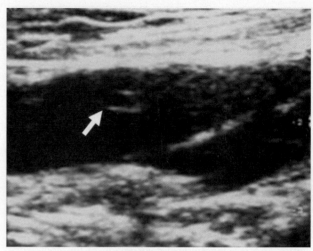

Figure 14-31 A longitudinal view of the edge of a newly formed, unstable thrombus *(arrow)*.

further. A thrombus seen at this stage will be spongy in texture, hypoechoic, and will likely be poorly attached to the vein wall (Fig. 14-31). The fact that these poorly attached acute thrombi might be more likely to embolize seems logical, although this seemingly obvious conclusion is not universally accepted.

Veins are extremely pliable and can enlarge to several times their normal size. When a thrombus forms within a vein, the movement of blood through this vein back toward the heart is reduced due to the luminal restriction produced by the thrombus. As the blood flow is reduced, pressure within the vein peripheral to the thrombus increases. As the pressure increases, the vein will enlarge. The thrombus usually will continue to expand until it has stretched the vein out to its maximum size (Fig. 14-32). At this point, the vein will be totally obstructed and will have a diameter much larger than the companion artery. This venous

dilation, which occurs during this stage of thrombus formation, aids in the confirmation of acute thrombi.

Chronic Thrombus

The human thrombolytic system is capable of dissolving a venous thrombus. In some instances, a previously completely thrombosed vein will have no residual evidence of the prior thrombus. However, the thrombus will often persist to some degree and be visible on ultrasound for several years. The thrombus that initially was relatively hypoechoic will become more echogenic as the thrombus ages (Figs. 14-33, 14-34, 14-35, and 14-36). This

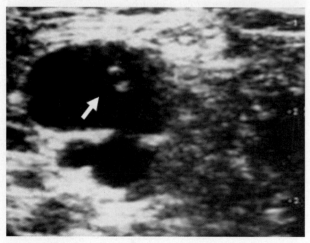

Figure 14-30 A transverse view of an unstable (poorly attached) acute thrombus *(arrow)*.

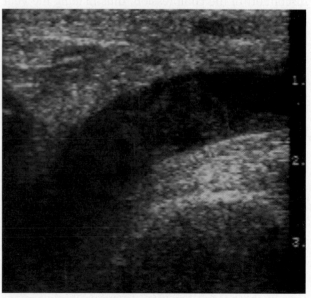

Figure 14-32 A longitudinal view of an acute thrombus that has enlarged the vein.

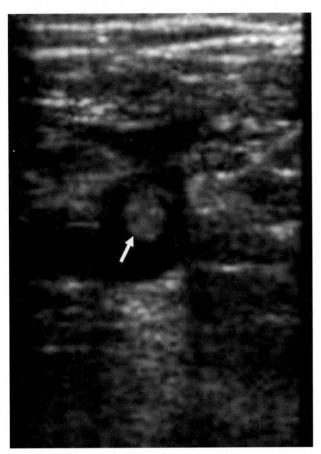

Figure 14-33 A transverse view of an acute thrombus (arrow) that has begun to gain echogenicity, making it easier to see.

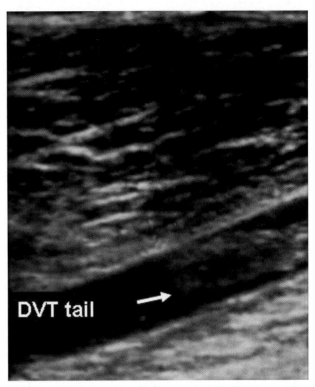

Figure 14-34 The tip or tail of an acute thrombus (arrow) that has gained some echogenicity, making it easier to see.

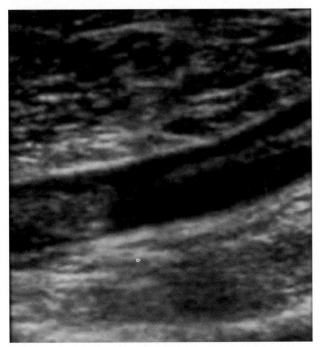

Figure 14-35 The same thrombus as was seen in Figure 14-34. Note how poorly attached the acute thrombus is.

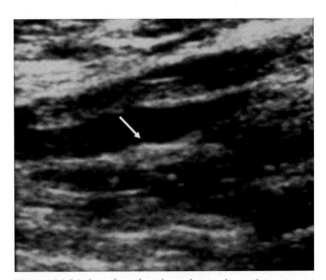

Figure 14-36 As a thrombus (arrow) ages, it continues to get brighter. This is a subacute thrombus that is not yet fully attached to the vein wall.

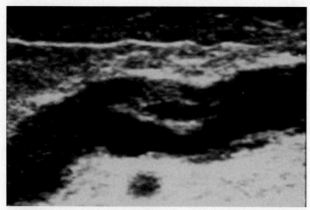

Figure 14-37 As the thrombus continues to age, it will attach to the vein wall.

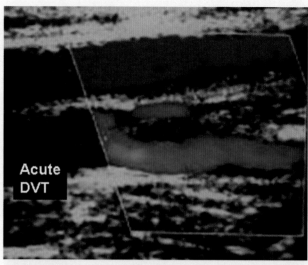

Figure 14-39 A longitudinal view of color outlining an acute thrombus. The thrombus is adhered to one wall.

increase in echogenicity aids in the identification of the vein. As the thrombus ages, the plasma or liquid component of the thrombus gets reabsorbed by the body. This results in the thrombus contracting or shrinking. The remaining material of the thrombus is more dense and composed of more solid substances such as fibrin and cellular debris (Fig. 14-37). The thrombus will now be firm, more brightly echogenic, and better attached to the vein wall (Fig. 14-38). Because of its firm attachment to the vein wall, the chronic thrombus is less likely to break loose and embolize to the lungs. Chronically thrombosed veins that have contracted may be difficult to differentiate from the surrounding tissue because the echogenicity of the vein will become similar to the tissue.

Some thrombi may not totally obstruct veins and will appear partially attached to the vein wall. This allows blood to flow through the residual lumen (Figs. 14-39 and 14-40). The contained thrombus will continue to shrink and fill less and less of the vein (recanalization). Eventually, it will appear on ultrasound like a thin scar within the vein. Its borders can be irregular and it will resemble a string inside the vein (Figs. 14-41, 14-42, and 14-43).

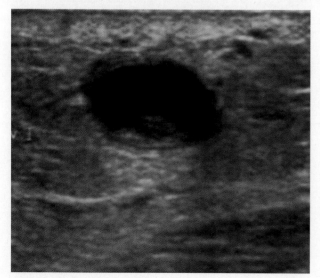

Figure 14-38 A transverse view of a thrombus attaching to the vein wall.

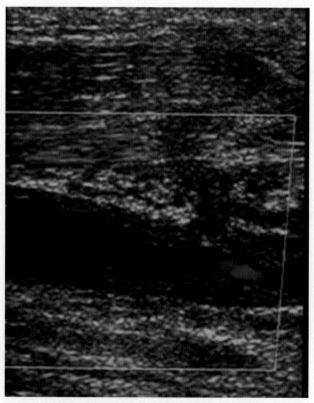

Figure 14-40 A longitudinal view of a chronic residual thrombus with blood flow moving within the center of the vein.

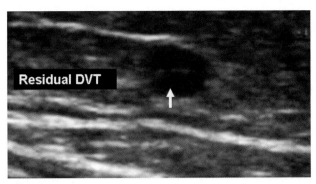

Figure 14-41 A transverse view of a residual thrombus *(arrow)* creating a septum down the middle of the vein.

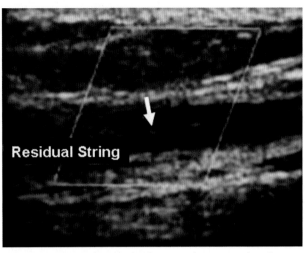

Figure 14-43 A longitudinal view showing color flowing around an old residual "string" thrombus *(arrow)*.

Whenever possible, an interpreting physician should comment on the age of a thrombus as this may alter patient treatment. Any additional information that can be described and documented by the examiner will aid the physician in rendering a final diagnosis. Pathology Box 14-1 summarizes the ultrasound findings associated with venous thrombosis.

ABNORMAL COLOR AND SPECTRAL DOPPLER

Although image characteristics are the primary ultrasound features used to make the diagnosis of DVT, a great deal of information can be obtained by evaluating the color image and spectral Doppler waveforms. In a thrombosed vein, color flow and spectral waveforms will be absent and, along with the lack of compressibility, will confirm the thrombosis. In a vein that is compressible but when performing a distal compression, no color flow is observed or no augmentation is present within the spectral Doppler waveform, an obstruction to flow between the level

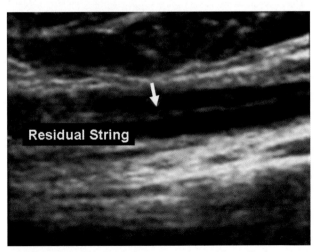

Figure 14-42 A longitudinal view of an old residual "string" thrombus *(arrow)*.

of the transducer and the site of distal compression should be suspected. This test is less sensitive with nonocclusive thrombi.

Flow that lacks respiratory phasicity and does not cease with proximal compression or the Valsalva maneuver is termed continuous (Fig. 14-44). This continuous pattern is a signal that the pressure in the vein at this level exceeds the pressure changes within the abdomen during respiration. An obstruction to flow in the venous return back to the heart will produce this pattern. If continuous flow is observed unilaterally at the CFV, this is consistent with a unilateral iliofemoral thrombus, a partial thrombus, or an extrinsic compression. If continuous flow is observed bilaterally at the CFVs, there is likely bilateral iliofemoral disease or an IVC thrombus, partial thrombus, or extrinsic compression.

Flow that is spontaneous, augments with distal compression, but appears pulsatile rather than phasic is also considered abnormal (Fig. 14-45). Unilateral pulsatile venous flow can be associated with arteriovenous fistulae (either traumatic, iatrogenic, or congenital). Bilateral pulsatile venous is diagnostic for systemic venous hypertension. Systemic venous hypertension can be the result of numerous cardiopulmonary pathologies including but not limited to right heart failure, tricuspid insufficiency, and pulmonary hypertension.

Flow in lower extremity veins that is both antegrade and retrograde is abnormal. As a thrombus becomes attached to the vein wall, it commonly will damage the vein valves. This will result in retrograde blood flow. This condition is called venous reflux or venous insufficiency. Chapter 17 will describe in detail the techniques and criteria of venous reflux testing.

PATHOLOGY BOX 14-1

Venous Thrombosis in the Lower Extremity

Abnormality	B-Mode	Ultrasound Findings	
		Spectral Doppler	Color
Acute thrombus	• Echogenic material within the veins (can be anechoic or hypoechoic) • Veins fail to fully coapt • Vein appears dilated • Thrombus is poorly attached to vein wall • Vein appears spongy	• No Doppler signals obtained with complete thrombosis	• No color flow present with complete thrombosis
Chronic thrombus	• Hyperechogenic material within the veins • Vein appears contracted • Thrombus is rigid and firmly attached • Large collaterals	• No Doppler signals obtained with complete thrombosis	• No color flow present with complete thrombosis
Partial nonocclusive thrombus	• Echogenic material within the veins • Veins will partially compress but will not be able to completely coapt walls	• Continuous signals • Slight phasicity may be noted • Will augment with distal compression • Little or no change with proximal compression or Valsalva maneuver with more central thrombus	• Color fails to fill lumen • Color will outline thrombus material

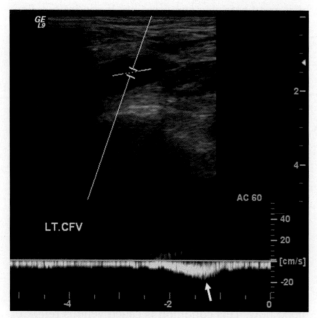

Figure 14-44 A spectral Doppler waveform from a common femoral vein illustrating an abnormal continuous pattern. Note a small augmentation in flow (*arrow*) is seen with distal compression.

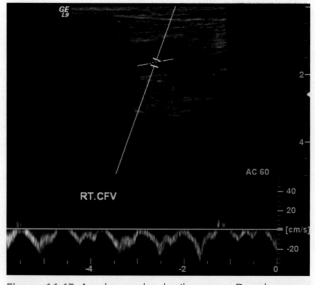

Figure 14-45 An abnormal pulsatile venous Doppler waveform from a common femoral vein.

DISORDERS

In addition to the typical venous thrombosis described previously, there are some unique disorders associated with the venous system. Within the iliac venous system, May-Thurner syndrome can develop as the left common iliac vein is compressed by the right common iliac artery. This is discussed in Chapter 21.

Two additional rare disorders arise as a result of extensive DVT, which involves the iliofemoral venous system. Phlegmasia alba dolens is a condition that is associated with marked swelling of the lower extremity, pain, pitting edema, and blanching. This has also been termed "milk leg" or "white leg" and can be associated with pregnancy. There is no ischemia associated with phlegmasia alba dolens. Phlegmasia cerulean dolens is more extensive than phlegmasia alba dolens. In addition to massive swelling, cyanosis occurs and pain is more severe. The cyanosis is produced by the extent of the venous thrombosis, which can include both deep and superficial systems. The venous outflow is completely obstructed. The extensive venous thrombosis and subsequent significant swelling may result in arterial insufficiency and venous gangrene.

INCIDENTAL FINDINGS

As with most types of ultrasound examinations, often incidental findings may be found when patients are referred to the vascular lab to rule out lower extremity DVT presenting with leg pain and/or edema. Nonvascular findings include cysts and hematomas (probably the most common), edema, abscesses, enlarged lymph nodes, and tumors. Cysts usually appear well-defined and may be oval, oblong, or crescent-shaped

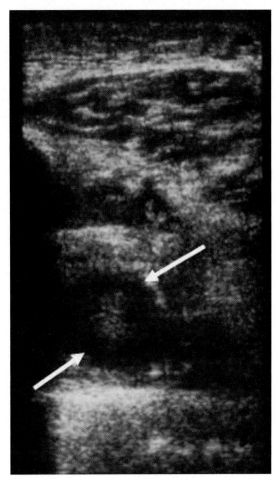

Figure 14-47 A hematoma *(arrows)* within the muscle of the mid-calf.

(Fig. 14-46). A cyst will be anechoic or hypoechoic, and septations may be present. A ruptured cyst may appear as a fluid collection that dissects along the fascia planes in the limb. The ultrasound appearance of a hematoma will vary depending on the time interval between the initial injury and the ultrasound imaging. Layering of a thrombus within the hematoma may be observed. Hematomas usually appear as a heterogeneous mass within a muscle or between muscle planes (Fig. 14-47). Vascular findings include aneurysms (venous and arterial), pseudoaneurysms, arteriovenous fistulas, or significant arterial disease (arteriosclerotic or nonatherosclerotic). Color can be used to differentiate between vascular and nonvascular structures. It is important to report these findings so that proper patient care may be implemented.

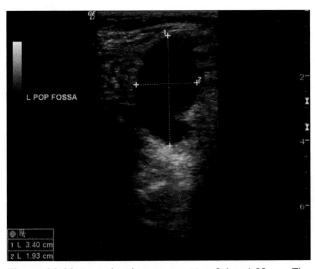

Figure 14-46 A popliteal cyst measuring 3.4 × 1.93 cm. The interior of the cyst is relatively anechoic. Posterior enhancement of the grayscale image is seen directly beneath the cyst.

OTHER IMAGING PROCEDURES

Although duplex ultrasound imaging is the preferred imaging technique to diagnose DVT, other modalities may occasionally be employed. Conventional contrast venography is uncommon but is still performed sporadically. Computed tomography venography (CTV) may be used to define the status of the iliac veins. CTV may be done in conjunction with computed tomography being performed to detect PE. Lastly, magnetic resonance venography (MRV) is also performed to detect DVT. This modality appears to be most useful when imaging veins above the inguinal ligament.

TREATMENT

At present, the primary treatment of acute lower extremity DVT is anticoagulation.[24] Heparin and warfarin are used in varying degrees to achieve initial levels of anticoagulation. After a period of 4 to 5 days, most patients remain on warfarin for several months. In some patients, depending on the level of disease and the patient's condition, the physician may also choose to treat DVT with low-molecular weight heparin. Oral anticoagulation medications will be available in the future. Other treatment methods include gradient elastic stockings, which may help to reduce lower extremity symptoms and decrease the risk of postthrombotic syndrome. Thrombolytic agents and thrombectomies (either catheter-based or surgical) may also be used to rapidly dissolve the thrombus or physically remove it. These techniques are often limited to the larger veins of the iliofemoral region.

SUMMARY

Imaging of the veins of the leg is a challenging task. However, by paying attention to sound protocols and gaining clinical experience under the supervision of an experienced mentor, one can perform accurate venous duplex examinations that will provide doctors with the information needed to safely manage their patients.

Critical Thinking Questions

1. When reviewing the relevant history of a patient, what three areas should be of the greatest concern?

2. Explain why both transverse and longitudinal imaging is used for venous DVT examinations.

3. Ultrasound is a noninvasive technique. However, venous ultrasound can have two associated negative outcomes. What are these and how can the risks be minimized?

4. What are three aspects of an acute versus a chronic thrombus that can be compared and contrasted?

REFERENCES

1. Strandness DE Jr. Diagnostic approaches for detecting deep vein thrombosis. *Am J Card Imaging.* 1994;8(1):13–17.
2. Meissner MH, Moneta G, Byrnand K, et al. The hemodynamics and diagnosis of venous disease. *J Vasc Surg.* 2007;46(suppl S):4S–24S
3. Oliver MA. Duplex scanning in the management of lower extremity DVT. *Vasc Ultrasound Today.* 2005;10:181–196.
4. Oliver MA. Incidental findings during lower extremity venous duplex examination. *Vasc Ultrasound Today.* 2008;13:77–96.
5. Hollinshead WH. *Textbook of Anatomy.* 3rd ed. New York, NY: Harper and Row; 1974:75.
6. Kadir S. *Diagnostic Angiography.* Philadelphia, PA: W.B. Saunders; 1986:541.

7. Uhl JF, Gillot C, Chahim M. Anatomical variations of the femoral vein. *J Vasc Surg.* 2010;52(3):714–719.

8. Blackburn DR. Venous anatomy. *J Vasc Technol.* 1988;12:78–82.

9. Park B, Messina L, Dargon P, et al. Recent trends in clinical outcomes and resource utilization for pulmonary embolism in the United States: findings from the nationwide inpatient sample. *Chest.* 2009;136(4):983–990.

10. Prandoni P, Lensing AW, Prins MR. Long-term outcomes after deep vein thrombosis of the lower extremities. *Vasc Med.* 1998;3(1):57–60.

11. Virchow R. *Gesammelte Abhandlungen Zur Wissenschaftli Medizia* [Collected Essays on Scientific Medicine]. Frankfurt, Germany: Medinger Sohn; 1856:719–732.

12. Meissner MH. Epidemiology of and risk factors for acute deep vein thrombosis. In: Glovicki P, ed. *Handbook of Venous Disorders.* London, England: Hodder Arnold Publishers; 2009: 94–104.

13. Ageno W, Squizzato A, Garcia D, et al. Epidemiology and risk factors of venous thromboembolism. *Semin Thromb Hemost.* 2006;32(7):651–658.

14. Dawson DL, Beals H. Acute lower extremity deep vein thrombosis. In: Zierler RE, ed. *Strandness's Duplex Scanning in Vascular Disorders.* Philadelphia, PA: Lippincott Williams & Wilkins; 2010:179–198.

15. Wells RS, Hirsh J, Anderson DR, et al. Accuracy of clinical assessment of deep vein thrombosis. *Lancet.* 1995;345(8961):1321–1330.

16. Talbot SR. B-mode evaluation of peripheral veins. *Semin Ultrasound CT MR.* 1988;9(4):295–319.

17. Sullivan ED, Peters BS, Cranley JJ. Real-time B-mode venous ultrasound. *J Vas Surg.* 1984; 1:465–471

18. Oliver MA. Duplex scanning in venous disease. *Bruit.* 1985;9:206–209.

19. Talbot SR, Oliver MA. *Techniques of Venous Imaging.* Pasadena, CA: Appleton Davies; 1992.

20. Talbot SR. Use of real-time imaging in identifying deep venous obstruction: a preliminary report. *Bruit.* 1982;6:41–42.

21. Perlin SJ. Pulmonary embolism during compression US of the lower extremities. *Radiol.* 1992;184:165–166.

22. Schroder WB, Bealer JF. Venous duplex ultrasonography causing acute pulmonary embolism: a brief report. *J Vasc Surg.* 1992;15:1082–1083.

23. Cronan JJ. History of venous ultrasound. *J Ultrasound Med.* 2003;22:1143–1146.

24. Kearon C, Kahn SR, Agnelli G, et al. Antithrombotic therapy for venous thromboembolic disease: American College of Chest Physicians Evidence-Based Clinical Practice Guidelines (8th edition). *Chest.* 2008;133(6 suppl):454S–545S.

15 Duplex Imaging of the Upper Extremity Venous System

Steven R. Talbot and Mark Oliver

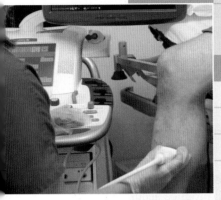

OBJECTIVES

Describe the components of the upper extremity venous system

Define the normal image and Doppler characteristics of the venous system

Identify the image characteristics consistent with acute and chronic thrombus

Describe the Doppler waveform characteristics associated with various pathologies

List the risk factors associated with venous thrombosis in the upper extremity

KEY TERMS

acute thrombus | chronic thrombus | deep vein | superficial vein | valve

GLOSSARY

acute thrombus newly formed clotted blood within a vein, generally less than 14 days old

chronic thrombus clotted blood within a vein that has generally been present for a period of several weeks or months

deep vein a vein that is the companion vessel to an artery and travels within the deep muscular compartments of the leg or arm

superficial vein a vein that is superior to the muscular compartments of the leg or arm; travels within superficial fascia compartments; has no corresponding companion artery

valve an inward projection of the intimal layer of a vein wall producing two semilunar leaflets that present the retrograde movement of blood flow

This chapter will discuss the venous duplex ultrasound examination of the upper extremity. The protocol techniques used in the upper extremity are similar to those discussed for the lower extremity in Chapter 14. However, there are three major differences to consider when moving from imaging legs to imaging the upper extremity. They are:

1. Many thrombi in the lower extremity are caused by stasis (the patient not moving). This is not true in the upper extremity. The arms do not have a counterpart to the soleal sinus veins of the legs so there is no similar place for a thrombus to spontaneously form in the arms. This is why, until modern times, thrombi in the upper extremity veins were rare. The following section on pathophysiology will discuss this further.

2. The superficial veins are affected more in the arms than in the legs. Additionally, a thrombus in a superficial vein in the arms may have greater clinical significance because superficial veins in the arms are commonly larger than their deeper counterparts. For instance, the basilic vein (a superficial vein) may be several times larger than the radial vein (a deep vein). Thus, a thrombus in the basilic vein may require treatment, whereas a thrombus in the radial vein may not. Veins like the axillary and subclavian, however, are large deep veins where a thrombus within them is more aggressively treated than a thrombus in the superficial veins.

3. Veins in the legs follow pretty reliable courses. The venous anatomy in the upper extremity can be more variable. Most of this variation occurs around the median cubital vein and how it connects with the basilic and cephalic veins.

The signs and symptoms of upper extremity venous thrombosis are similar to those described for the lower extremity venous system. These can include unilateral arm or hand swelling, a superficial palpable cord, erythema, pain, and tenderness. Some patients may present with facial swelling or dilated chest wall venous collaterals, which could be suggestive of superior vena cava thrombosis. Patients may present with indwelling catheters or a history of venous catheters.[1,2]

There may be patients presenting for an upper extremity venous ultrasound who are asymptomatic. These may be patients in whom the central veins may be required to be examined prior to catheter placement or placement of pacemaker wires or other cardiac devices.

Upper extremity veins may also be examined in those patients with suspected pulmonary embolus. These patients may present with symptoms consistent with pulmonary embolus including chest pain, tachypnea, or tachycardia.

PATHOPHYSIOLOGY

The pathogenesis of upper extremity thrombosis, as in lower extremity venous thrombosis, can be found in the components of Virchow's triad: namely, venous stasis, hypercoagulability, and vessel wall injury. Thrombosis in the upper extremity veins is now more common due to an increase in injury to the vein walls. Patients are having more frequent introduction of needles and catheters into arm veins. With few exceptions, whenever an individual has not had a venous puncture or cannulation, the incidence of upper extremity venous thrombosis will be very low. This fact makes taking a history and selecting the proper indications for study of the upper extremity veins with ultrasound much easier than with the legs. Because of the location of the subclavian and internal jugular veins, these veins are commonly used for indwelling catheters for feeding and drug administration as well as catheters used to monitor central venous pressure. Pacemaker wires are also introduced, usually through the subclavian vein, and are another common cause of upper extremity venous thrombosis.

Another type of venous catheter that can cause thrombosis is a peripherally inserted central catheter (PICC). A PICC line is not inserted into one of the large veins in the neck or shoulder region but rather via a peripheral vein, often the basilic or cephalic veins. After it is inserted via one of these arm veins, the catheter is advanced to position the tip near the right atrium.

There are patients that present with upper extremity venous thrombosis without a history of venous puncture or cannulation. These patients include a unique group that present with upper extremity venous thrombosis secondary to compression of the subclavian vein at the thoracic inlet around the area of the first rib. It is thought to be the result of years of repetitive trauma and intermittent compression of the subclavian vein. This type of thrombosis is known as effort thrombosis or as Paget-Schroetter syndrome. The patients presenting with this type of venous thrombosis are young, athletic, and muscular males but this syndrome can occur in other individuals as well.

SONOGRAPHIC EXAMINATION TECHNIQUES

The protocols described here are a summary of tried and true protocols that will produce accurate venous duplex ultrasound results.[3-7] The compression techniques employed in the examination of the lower extremity veins are also performed for the upper extremity veins. Using the ultrasound transducer, gentle compression is applied directly over the vein so that the walls of the vein coapt or close together. This compression maneuver is repeated every 2 to 3 cm along the course of each vein. Spectral Doppler waveforms are recorded from all major vessels examined.

PATIENT PREPARATION

The examination should be explained to the patient. The patient signs and symptoms, along with relevant history, should be obtained. Upper extremity clothing and jewelry should be removed and a patient gown or drape should be provided.

PATIENT POSITIONING

There is no need to tilt the bed for examination of the upper extremity. In fact, it is important to examine the jugular and subclavian veins with the patient lying flat. This will remove any impact of hydrostatic pressure, which will tend to collapse the veins with the patient upright. While imaging the subclavian and jugular veins, the arm is positioned at the side with the head turned in the opposite direction. Imaging the rest of the arm veins can be done with the bed flat or with the head elevated. To view the axillary vein, the arm may be abducted to allow access to the axilla. The arm is then repositioned to a lower angle to allow access to the remaining arm veins.

EQUIPMENT

For the examination of upper extremity veins, at least two transducers are needed. As with the examination of the legs, a midrange transducer (5-10 MHz) will be commonly used to visualize the internal jugular, brachiocephalic, subclavian, axillary, deep brachial, and brachial veins. A second transducer will be needed for proper evaluation of the superficial veins of the arm (cephalic and basilic) and it is also helpful for the small forearm vessels (radial and ulnar veins). This second transducer should be a higher frequency transducer in the 10-18 MHz range. A high-frequency transducer is extremely valuable when mapping the superficial upper extremity veins. In some instances, a midrange transducer (5-10 MHz), which is not a straight linear array, is helpful. A curved array transducer with a small footprint will be helpful in insonating vessels near the clavicle and sternum as it can be more easily maneuvered into these small spaces than a flat linear array transducer.

SCANNING TECHNIQUE

The complete examination of the upper extremity veins includes the multiple venous segments as described as follows. As previously stated, there may be indications for a limited evaluation of specific veins, such as only the internal jugular and subclavian veins prior to central line placement.

Internal and External Jugular Veins

Because a thrombus in the veins of the arms can extend into the veins of the neck, a complete upper extremity venous duplex ultrasound examination includes evaluating the jugular veins. A thrombus may also be found isolated to the jugular veins, in particular, the internal jugular vein as a result of a central line placement within this vessel. Lastly, the jugular veins are an important collateral pathway in the advent of upper extremity thrombosis, thus providing another reason for inclusion of these vessels in an upper extremity venous ultrasound examination.

The carotid artery is used as a landmark to find the internal jugular vein that runs alongside it (Figs. 15-1

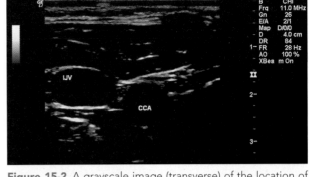

Figure 15-2 A grayscale image (transverse) of the location of the internal jugular vein *(IJV)* alongside the common carotid artery *(CCA)*.

and 15-2). The internal jugular vein will be collapsed if the patient is sitting or standing (due to hydrostatic pressure), so this part of the examination must be done with the patient lying flat. If the examiner cannot find the internal jugular vein, the head of the patient should be lowered to determine if the vein is collapsed. Documentation of patency of the internal jugular vein should include transverse grayscale images with the vein compressed and noncompressed. A spectral Doppler waveform should also be recorded from the internal jugular vein (Fig. 15-3).

The external jugular vein is found by lightening up on the transducer pressure and sliding posterior from the position used to view the internal jugular vein. The external jugular vein runs without an accompanying artery very close to the skin, and usually terminates into the subclavian vein. This vein's patency can also be documented with transverse views of the vein compressed and noncompressed as well as with a spectral Doppler waveform. Many laboratory protocols do not include routine documentation of this vein but rather, in the event of thrombosis in adjacent vessels, this vessel is then added to the examination.

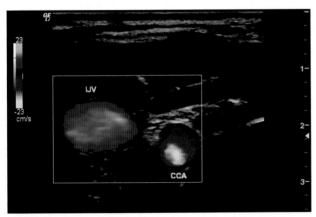

Figure 15-1 A transverse view of the internal jugular vein *(IJV)* and the common carotid artery *(CCA)* with color.

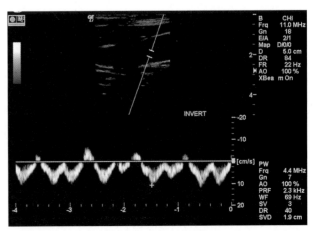

Figure 15-3 A spectral Doppler waveform from the internal jugular vein.

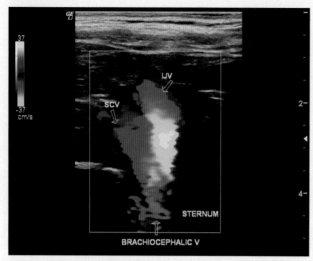

Figure 15-4 Color image of the brachiocephalic vein. The internal jugular vein (IJV) and subclavian vein (SCV) are also shown.

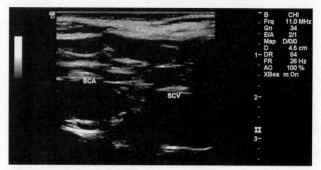

Figure 15-6 A transverse view of the subclavian artery (SCA) and subclavian vein (SCV).

Brachiocephalic Veins

Examining the brachiocephalic veins is challenging because it is difficult to position the transducer around the bony structures in the area. As mentioned earlier, a small footprint transducer may allow for partial visualization of these veins. The brachiocephalic veins come together behind the sternum to form the superior vena cava, and this portion of these veins is not usually insonated. The beginning of the brachiocephalic veins at the confluence of the subclavian and internal jugular veins is the region of this vessel that is most often examined (Fig. 15-4). Compression of the brachiocephalic veins at this level is not able to be performed. Documentation of patency of these vessels should include a grayscale image demonstrating the absence of a thrombus. A color flow image should be recorded to document full color filling of the vessel. Spectral Doppler

waveforms should also be obtained as the phasicity and pulsatility observed at this level is an important diagnostic tool (Fig. 15-5). These patterns can indirectly indicate the status of the more central veins. More about these waveforms will be discussed later.

Subclavian Vein

The subclavian vein is visualized above and below the clavicle. It is accompanied by the subclavian artery (Fig. 15-6). Just after the subclavian vein passes under the clavicle as it continues toward the arm, a vessel can be seen terminating into the subclavian vein. This is the cephalic vein (Fig. 15-7). Moving distally toward the arm beyond the terminus of the cephalic vein, the subclavian vein becomes the axillary vein. Compressing the subclavian vein to check for a thrombus can be difficult because of the clavicle. The examiner can have the patient take a quick, deep breath in through pursed lips. If done correctly, this will cause the subclavian to collapse. Spectral waveforms and color images should also be documented. As noted with the brachiocephalic veins, the spectral waveforms obtained at the subclavian vein are a helpful diagnostic tool.

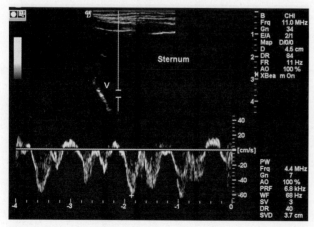

Figure 15-5 Spectral Doppler waveform from the brachiocephalic vein (V).

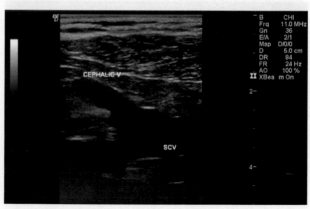

Figure 15-7 A view of the cephalic vein as it terminates into the subclavian vein (SCV).

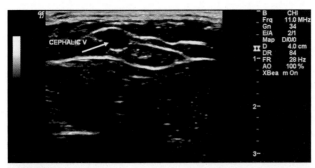

Figure 15-8 A transverse view of the cephalic vein *(arrow)* in the upper arm.

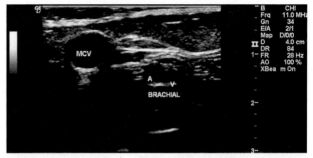

Figure 15-10 A transverse view of the median cubital vein *(MCV)* as it passes superiorly over the brachial artery *(A)* and brachial vein *(V)*.

Cephalic Vein

Before the cephalic vein terminates into the subclavian vein, it travels superficially near the skin line (Fig. 15-8) across the shoulder and along the arm at the anterior–lateral border of the biceps muscle (Fig. 15-9). At or near the antecubital fossa, it communicates with the median cubital vein. Distally onto the forearm, there are typically two veins that will unite before the antecubital fossa. One courses along the volar aspect of the forearm to the wrist, and the other travels along the dorsal aspect of the forearm. Compressed and noncompressed grayscale images are easily performed to document patency.

Median Cubital Vein

The median cubital is a vein that connects the cephalic and basilic veins. It is present in the antecubital fossa but its pattern of connection with the basilic and cephalic veins can be quite variable. It is a common site for a thrombus because it is a common site for venipuncture. The median cubital vein is a great landmark vein as it crosses directly over the brachial artery and vein (Fig. 15-10). Compressed and noncompressed images should be documented at this level, particularly if superficial thrombophlebitis is suspected.

Axillary Vein

The axillary vein terminates at the junction of the cephalic and subclavian veins. This deep vein is accompanied by the axillary artery and courses deeply as it crosses the shoulder over the axilla (Fig. 15-11). At this point, the arm is repositioned and abducted to expose the axilla. At the axilla, this vein will be seen fairly close to the skin. Usually, deep veins and their accompanying arteries are positioned side by side. In the axilla, the axillary vein and artery may not be directly adjacent to each other for a short distance (Fig. 15-12). Following the vein in the upper arm, the artery and vein will course together. Compressed and noncompressed images of the vein should be recorded along with color and spectral Doppler waveforms. In most patients, compression of the axillary vein will be possible.

Along the medial portion of the upper arm, a large superficial vein will be observed terminating into the axillary vein. This is the basilic vein. Distally in the upper arm, below the terminus of the basilic vein, the vessel is now called the brachial vein. There are usually two brachial veins at this level and each

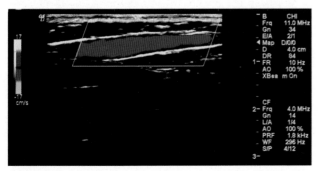

Figure 15-9 A longitudinal view of the cephalic vein with color added.

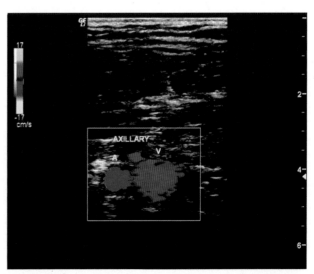

Figure 15-11 A transverse view of the axillary artery *(A)* and vein *(V)* over the shoulder.

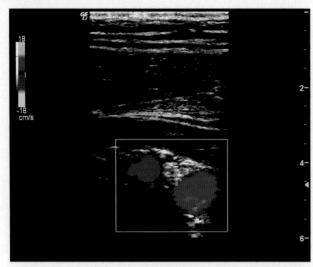

Figure 15-12 A transverse view of the axillary artery *(in red)* and vein *(in blue)* taken from the axilla. Note how there is spatial separation between the two vessels.

will be located on either side of the brachial artery. At this point, the brachial veins will be fairly small (Fig. 15-13).

Brachial Vein

The brachial vein is often a bifid system. The brachial veins will accompany the brachial artery until just below the antecubital fossa. The brachial veins are formed by the junction of two radial and two ulnar veins at the level of the antecubital fossa. The patency of the brachial veins should include clear images of both brachial veins with compressed and noncompressed views. Some laboratories also choose to document venous spectral Doppler signals at this level.

Radial Veins

The radial veins will course along the volar aspect of the forearm accompanied by the radial artery (Fig. 15-14). These vessels are very small and are

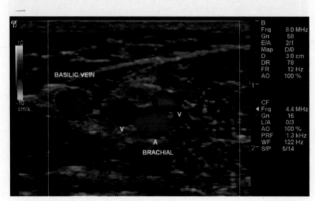

Figure 15-13 A transverse view of the brachial artery *(A)* and veins *(V)* in the upper arm. The basilic vein is also noted.

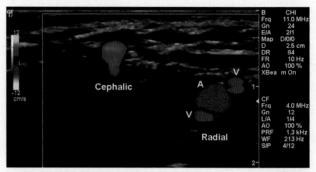

Figure 15-14 A transverse view of the radial artery *(A)* and veins *(V)*. The cephalic vein is also noted.

often not a site for venous thrombosis. They are technically deep veins but are often not included in routine upper extremity venous examinations. However, should the patient's symptoms suggest thrombosis within the forearm, the radial veins should be imaged.

Ulnar Veins

The ulnar veins are followed as they travel the volar aspect of the ulnar side of the forearm. Like the radial veins with their companion radial artery, the ulnar veins course on either side of the ulnar artery (Fig. 15-15). As with the radial veins, the ulnar veins are not examined unless indicated by the presenting symptoms of the patient.

Basilic Vein

To follow the basilic vein, the examiner can begin in the upper midportion of the upper arm and locates the level where the basilic vein terminates into the axillary vein. The basilic vein will course medially and superficially without a companion artery and will usually be the largest vein in the region (Fig. 15-16).

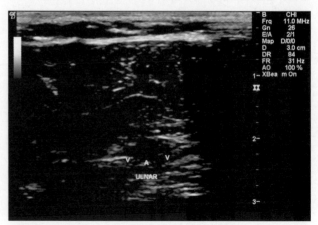

Figure 15-15 A transverse view of the ulnar artery *(A)* and veins *(V)*.

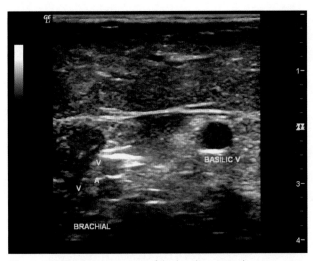

Figure 15-16 transverse view of the basilic vein in the upper arm.

At a point near the antecubital fossa, the basilic vein will communicate with the cephalic vein via the medial cubital vein. In the forearm, the basilic vein usually is comprised of two branches. One will course mostly on the volar aspect of the forearm, and the other will extend to the dorsal aspect of the forearm.

PITFALLS

There are several locations where compression of the veins is not possible. Compression of the brachiocephalic and subclavian veins is not usually performed due to the position of these vessels with respect to the sternum and clavicle. Spectral Doppler and color imaging are relied on to document venous patency in those vessels where compression of the vein is not possible. The patient may also present with dressings or intravenous catheters, which limit direct insonation of the underlying veins. Again, in these cases, spectral Doppler and color imaging of adjacent veins are important to assist in the determination of patency. If signals in adjacent vessels are normal, it is indirectly indicative of vein patency in the regions unable to be directly visualized.

DIAGNOSIS

The diagnostic criteria for the detection of the presence or absence of a thrombus, as well as distinguishing features of acute versus chronic thrombus, are the same for the upper extremity as those described in Chapter 14 for the lower extremity. Briefly, normal vein walls will be able to be completely compressed together with light transducer pressure. This compression maneuver must be performed in a transverse view and not in a longitudinal or sagittal plane of view. Normal vein walls appear thin and smooth on ultrasound. The vessel lumen should be hypoechoic. While in a transverse view, the vein diameter may be seen to change slightly with respiration, particularly with the more central veins.

If the walls fail to coapt or completely close together, a thrombus should be suspected. Echogenic material should be observed within the vein where compression fails to fully coapt the walls. There are several distinguishing characteristics associated with an acute thrombus, including visualizing a poorly attached thrombus, a thrombus that is spongy in texture, and a dilated vein (Fig. 15-17). A chronic thrombus is often brightly echogenic, well-attached, rigid, and the vein is usually contracted (Fig. 15-18).

A superficial vein thrombus will have the same appearance as deep vein thrombosis. Depending

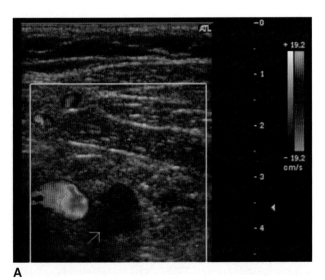

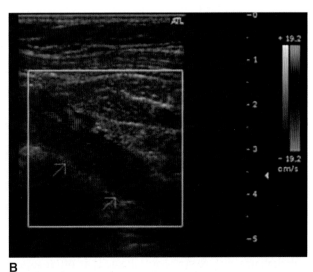

A   B

Figure 15-17 An acute thrombus in the internal jugular vein. (Image courtesy of Jean M. White, RVT, RPhS and William B. Schroedter, BS, RVT, RPhS, FSVU, Venice, FL)

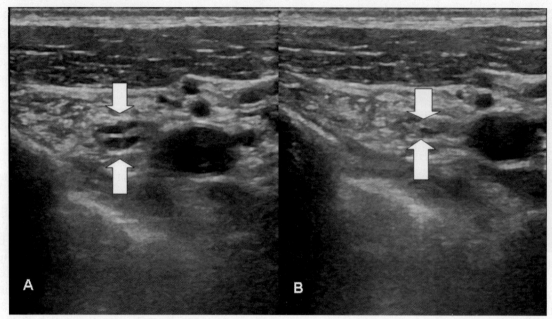

Figure 15-18 A chronic thrombus in the axillary vein. (Image courtesy of Steve Knight, BSc, RVT, RDCS, Boston, MA)

on the degree of inflammation associated with the thrombus, hypoechoic areas may be present in the tissue immediately adjacent to the veins.

COLOR AND SPECTRAL DOPPLER

In the upper extremity, in regions where the veins are not able to be compressed (near the clavicle and sternum), color and spectral Doppler characteristics are important diagnostic tools. As with normal lower extremity veins, color should be seen filling the entire vessel lumen. However, it is possible to have color overwrite grayscale information and fill in a vessel with a partial thrombus. Care should be taken to have a color-priority setting on the ultrasound equipment appropriately adjusted to avoid overwriting a partial thrombus with color. Additional color settings should be optimized in those vessels where the flow is diminished. In veins with a partial thrombus, proper color adjustments will result in color filling around the areas of a thrombus helping to outline the extent of the disease. In completely thrombosed vessels, no color filling will be seen.

Spectral Doppler criteria are similar to those used in the lower extremity as phasicity with respiration is expected. Compression distal to the position of the transducer should also augment flow. However, given the proximity of the more central veins to the right atrium of the heart, pronounced pulsatility is often observed (Fig. 15-19). It is common to observe pulsatile flow in the internal jugular, brachiocephalic, and subclavian veins. Respiratory phasicity is often superimposed on cardiac pulsatility. The lack of pulsatility in the internal jugular, brachiocephalic, or subclavian

veins is indicative of more central pathology.[8] However, depending on the patient position, volume status, cardiac function, and respiratory status, the waveform characteristics from these vessels will be affected. Thus, it is of the upmost importance to compare the symmetry of the signal between the right and left central veins to help determine patency. As one moves further away from the heart, the pulsatility dampens out so that a more phasic venous Doppler signal is obtained.

With a complete thrombus, no spectral Doppler signals will be obtained. In veins that are partially thrombosed, the spectral Doppler will be continuous but should display augmentation with distal compression. A continuous Doppler will also be observed within veins where a more central partial thrombosis is present or where there is extrinsic compression

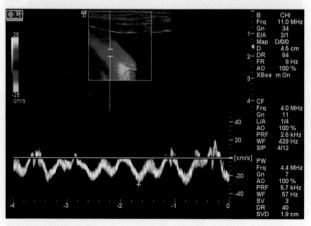

Figure 15-19 A Doppler spectral waveform taken from a subclavian vein demonstrating normal pulsatile flow.

of the more central veins. If both subclavian veins display nonpulsatile, continuous flow, disease within the superior vena cava should be suspected. It is not common to observe a reversal of venous flow in the presence of a central thrombus. Flow may be reversed in the internal or external jugular veins in association with an ipsilateral brachiocephalic vein thrombus. The venous outflow from the arm will pass through the subclavian vein but then will move cephalad up the external or internal jugular veins. Large collateral pathways exist through various routes within the neck and shoulder region.

Another type of alteration in venous Doppler signals will occur in patients with an upper extremity hemodialysis fistula or graft. This will produce pulsatile flow, which displays elevated velocities throughout the cardiac cycle. It may be difficult to assess respiratory variations; however, the signal will still augment with distal compression.

VENOUS CATHETERS

Indwelling venous catheters are commonly encountered in the arm, although they are rarely seen in the leg. Because use of these catheters is so common in the arm, this can lead to the development of a thrombus within the upper extremity venous system. Catheters will appear in the lumen of the vein as bright, straight, parallel echoes (Fig. 15-20). The exact appearance of these echoes will vary slightly depending on the number of lumens within the catheter. A thrombus can be seen as it forms

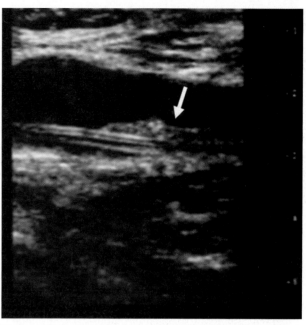

Figure 15-21 A longitudinal view of a thrombus *(arrow)* forming on a venous catheter.

on the catheter (Fig. 15-21) as echogenic material on the surface of the catheter. Left untreated, this thrombus will progress and fill the lumen of the vein. Color flow will outline the residual lumen, if any, surrounding the catheter. Spectral Doppler signals will be diminished and may be continuous depending on the degree of luminal reduction. Once a catheter with an associated thrombus has been removed, it would be expected to observe a clear anechoic vein lumen. However, commonly, there is a residual sheath of a thrombus left in the vein after catheter removal that will look as if the catheter is still present (Fig. 15-22).

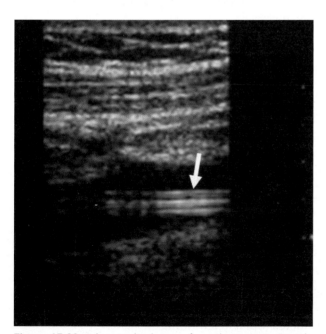

Figure 15-20 A longitudinal view of a catheter *(arrow)* inside a vein.

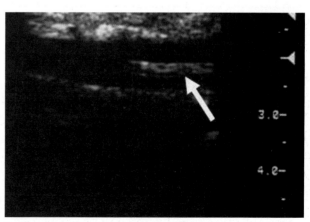

Figure 15-22 A longitudinal view of a remnant fibrous sheath *(arrow)* left in the vein after removal of a catheter. Note how this appears to resemble a catheter.

PATHOLOGY BOX 15-1

Ultrasound Findings with Upper Extremity Pathology

Abnormality	Ultrasound Findings
Acute thrombus	B-mode image: echogenic material within the veins; veins fail to fully coapt; vein appears dilated; thrombus is poorly attached to vein wall; vein appears spongy Spectral and color Doppler: no color or spectral Doppler obtained with complete thrombosis
Chronic thrombus	B-mode image: brightly echogenic material within the veins; veins fail to fully coapt; vein appears contracted; thrombus is rigid and firmly attached Spectral and color Doppler: no color or spectral Doppler obtained with complete thrombosis
Partial nonocclusive thrombus	B-mode image: echogenic material within the veins; veins will partially compress, but not able to completely coapt walls Spectral Doppler: continuous signal; slight phasicity may be noted with lesser degrees of thrombosis; will augment with distal compression; little to no cessation of flow with Valsalva maneuver Color flow: color fails to fill vessel lumen
Venous catheter–associated thrombus	B-mode image: echogenic material around brightly echogenic, straight parallel lines of catheter Spectral Doppler: diminished or continuous depending on degree of thrombosis Color Doppler: color-filling residual lumen around thrombus

Pathology Box 15-1 summarizes the ultrasound findings associated with upper extremity venous pathology.

TREATMENT

Treatment considerations for upper extremity venous thrombosis include anticoagulation, catheter removal, thrombolytic therapy, and surgical decompression of the thoracic inlet with or without venous reconstruction.[9,10] In some patients, conservative treatment may be used depending on the location of the thrombus and the patient's condition. It is important to determine the most central extent of any thrombus as this may influence the physician's treatment choices.

SUMMARY

Imaging of the upper extremity veins may seem difficult at first. However, once the examiner gets familiar with the anatomy and its variations, the upper extremity venous system becomes much easier than imaging the veins of the legs. Paying close attention to the suggestions and protocols contained in this chapter and the lower extremity chapter of this book will set the stage for accurate diagnostic imaging.

Critical Thinking Questions

1. When lower extremity veins are examined, patients can be placed in a dependent position. What position is best for an ultrasound of the subclavian and jugular veins? What is a common factor that is considered when determining the patient position for a venous ultrasound?

2. You are asked to perform an examination on a patient with a dressing in place over the subclavicular region on the shoulder. What specifically can you do to provide adequate information for determining upper extremity venous system patency?

3. You are examining a patient for an upper extremity venous thrombosis. You notice several dilated chest wall veins. The spectral Doppler signals from both subclavian and internal jugular veins are antegrade but continuous. What is the likely cause of these findings?

REFERENCES

1. Bernardi E, Pesavento R, Prandoni P. Upper extremity deep venous thrombosis. *Semin Thromb.* 2006;32(7):729–736.
2. Gaitini D, Beck-Razi N, Haim N, et al. Prevalence of upper extremity deep venous thrombosis diagnosed by color Doppler duplex sonography in cancer patients with central venous catheters. *J Ultrasound Med.* 2006;25(10):1297–1303.
3. Talbot SR. B-mode evaluation of peripheral veins. *Semin Ultrasound CT MR.* 1988;9(4):295–319.
4. Sullivan ED, Peters BS, Cranley JJ. Real-time B-mode venous ultrasound. *J Vasc Surg.* 1984;1(3):465–471.
5. Oliver MA. Duplex scanning in venous disease. *Bruit.* 1985;9:206–209.
6. Talbot SR, Oliver MA. *Techniques of Venous Imaging.* Pasadena, CA: Appleton Davies; 1992.
7. Hartshorne T, Goss D. Duplex assessment of deep vein thrombosis and upper limb disorders. In: Thrush A, Hartshore T, eds. *Vascular Ultrasound: How, Why and When.* 3rd ed. Edinburgh, Scotland: Churchill Livingston Elsevier; 2010:233–253.
8. Selis JE, Kadakia S. Venous Doppler sonography of the extremities: a window to pathology of the thorax, abdomen and pelvis. *AJR Am J Roent.* 2009;193(5):1446–1451.
9. Qaseem A, Snow V, Barry P, et al. Current diagnosis of venous thromboembolism in primary care: a clinical practice guideline from the American Academy of Family Physicians and the American College of Physicians. *Ann Fam Med.* 2007;5(1):57–62.
10. Czihal M, Hoffman U. Upper extremity deep venous thrombosis. *Vasc Med.* 2011;16(3):191–202.

16 Ultrasound Evaluation and Mapping of the Superficial Venous System

Ann Marie Kupinski

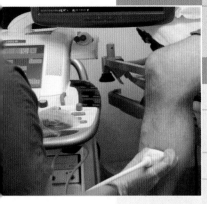

OBJECTIVES

List the indications for venous mapping

Describe the normal anatomical features of the great saphenous vein, small saphenous vein, cephalic vein, and basilic vein

Identify the pathology observed within the superficial veins

Describe the basic techniques of venous mapping

List the equipment necessary for vein mapping

Define limitations encountered during vein mapping

Describe diagnostic ultrasound criteria used in venous mapping

KEY TERMS

basilic vein | calcification | cephalic vein | great saphenous vein | mapping | perforator | planar arrangement | recanalization | small saphenous vein | varicosities

GLOSSARY

great saphenous vein a superficial vein forming at the level of the medial malleolus, which courses medially along the calf and thigh and terminates into the common femoral vein at the saphenofemoral junction

perforating vein a vein that connects from the superficial venous system to the deep venous system

recanalization a vein that was previously thrombosed

small saphenous vein a superficial vein that course along the posterior aspect of the calf, usually terminating at the popliteal fossa into the popliteal vein

varicosities dilated tortuous superficial veins

Ultrasound has been used to evaluate the venous system for more than 25 years. The use of venous ultrasound has increased greatly and its applications have also expanded. The early application of ultrasound in the venous system had centered mainly on the detection of a thrombus within the deep venous system.[1] Soon after clinicians realized the usefulness of deep venous ultrasound, they began to extend ultrasound to evaluate the superficial venous systems.[2] The superficial venous systems were of interest both to assess their competency as well as their suitability as a bypass conduit.[2,3] Superficial veins are used for a variety of types of bypass procedures, not the least of which is coronary artery bypass grafting. The autogenous vein is the preferred conduit of choice for lower extremity arterial bypass procedures. Lastly, growing interest in creating hemodialysis access fistulas in lieu of dialysis grafts presents yet another reason why the status of the superficial veins must be assessed.

When planning to use a segment of superficial vein for a procedure, surgeons gather as much information as possible to aid in the successful performance of these surgeries. Vein patency, position, depth, and size are some of the characteristics assessed preoperatively. These details provided by ultrasound imaging allow for the selection of the optimal vein. Proper knowledge of the anatomy of the superficial veins may alter the planned surgery as well as the surgical approach used. Information on the venous configuration will help to minimize the amount of surgical dissection needed.

This chapter will describe the techniques involved in ultrasonic evaluation of the superficial venous systems. Material pertaining to the great saphenous, small saphenous, basilic, and cephalic veins will be presented. Relevant anatomy, scanning techniques, tips, diagnostic criteria, and pathologic characteristics will be reviewed.

ANATOMY

THE GREAT SAPHENOUS VEIN

Prior to discussing the saphenous anatomy, it is important to briefly review the nomenclature of the venous system. A multidisciplinary panel published a consensus paper in which nomenclature was revised and standardized in an attempt to avoid some commonly confused terms.[4,5] Table 16-1 lists several of the major changes regarding saphenous vein terminology. The great saphenous vein is the standard name for the vein that had been referred to as the greater or long saphenous vein. The small saphenous vein is the correct name for the vein previously known as the lesser or short saphenous vein. Sonographers and vascular technologists should become familiar with this revised terminology.

Most anatomy textbooks display the great saphenous vein as a single trunk coursing medially along the thigh and terminating into the common femoral vein (Fig. 16-1). In the calf, the vein is often shown as traveling slightly anterior near the tibia to

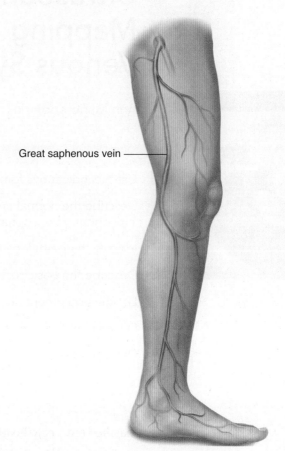

Great saphenous vein

Figure 16-1 Typical anatomic configuration of the great saphenous vein with a single medial dominant system in the thigh and an anterior dominant system in the calf.

the level of the medial malleolus. This is a common configuration for the great saphenous, but multiple variants exist. Extensive reviews of both ultrasound and venographic data have revealed complex system variability in both the thigh and calf.[6,7]

The thigh portion of the great saphenous vein has been found to have five common configurations (Fig. 16-2). In about 60% of cases, this vein is a single trunk that runs medially in the thigh. It curves slightly toward the inner thigh and typically has several large tributaries that empty into the vein before it joins the common femoral vein. These tributaries include the anterior (lateral) and posterior (medial) accessory and circumflex veins.

Less commonly, in only 8% of cases, the great saphenous is a single trunk that courses anterior–laterally in the thigh. This is likely a dominant version of the anterior accessory saphenous vein.

The remaining configurations encountered in the thigh all demonstrate some degree of duplication. The saphenous vein may have two separate systems running both medially and laterally throughout the entire length of the thigh. These double systems remain separate from each other below the knee as well. This pattern occurs in 8% of cases. Sometimes the

TABLE 16-1	
Venous Nomenclature	
Current Terminology	**Previous Terminology**
Great saphenous vein	Greater saphenous vein
	Long saphenous vein
Small saphenous vein	Lesser saphenous vein
	Short saphenous vein
Anterior accessory great saphenous vein	Accessory saphenous vein
Posterior accessory great saphenous vein	Accessory saphenous vein
	Leonardo's vein
	Posterior arch vein
Cranial extension of the small saphenous vein	Vein of Giacomini

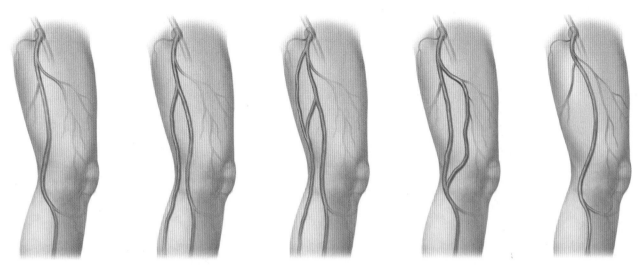

Figure 16-2 Anatomic variations in the configuration of the thigh portion of the great saphenous vein.

anterior–lateral system may be slightly larger and, in others, the posterior–medial system may be larger. It is very important to identify which vein is dominant so that the surgeon can select the most appropriate vein. Even though these systems are separate, there are often tributaries that communicate between the systems. Often, these duplicated systems may not course in the same anatomical plane (Fig. 16-3). One system may be superficial to the fascia (this is likely the superficial accessory great saphenous vein), whereas the other system may lie in the normal anatomic plane. Normally, the main trunk of the saphenous vein lies in what is termed the saphenous compartment bounded by the saphenous fascia superficially and deeply by the muscular fascia. The notation of planar arrangement on the ultrasound report will be discussed later in this chapter.

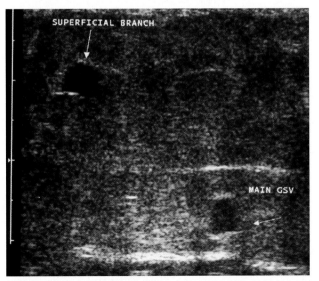

Figure 16-3 Ultrasound image illustrating the planar arrangement of a double system with deep and superficial systems.

In approximately 7% of cases, the great saphenous vein may have a loop that is contained within the thigh. This closed loop system can present the vascular surgeon with particular difficulties during an in situ bypass procedure, especially if a closed or limited vein exposure technique is used. During this form of in situ bypass, most of the thigh is kept intact (closed) and instrumentation is passed up the thigh from more distal segments to disrupt valves. In the case of a closed loop, the surgeon may inadvertently pass instruments up through the smaller vein of the loop, resulting in vein injury.

Lastly, in the remaining 17% of cases, partial double systems may be present in the thigh. Typically, there is a large posterior–medial system, which courses through the calf and terminates into the main trunk of the saphenous vein in the distal third of the thigh. This is the posterior accessory great saphenous vein that has been previously referred to as a "Leonardo's vein" or the posterior arch vein. As with the other forms of double systems, these partial double systems may share smaller communicating tributaries.

More complex variations can occur in the thigh but this is rare (usually less than 1% occurrence). Triplicate systems with multiple communicating veins have been identified. These intricate systems involve both anterior and posterior accessory veins as well as the main trunk of the great saphenous vein. Often in patients who previously had a portion or all of the great saphenous vein removed, the accessory systems in the thigh and calf dilate to accommodate venous outflow. It is important when evaluating a patient for venous conduits to always examine a leg even if a prior venous harvest or stripping has been performed. In many patients, these accessory systems are suitable for use as a conduit.

The great saphenous vein in the calf has much less variability than the thigh portion. One of three common arrangements can be found in the calf (Fig. 16-4).

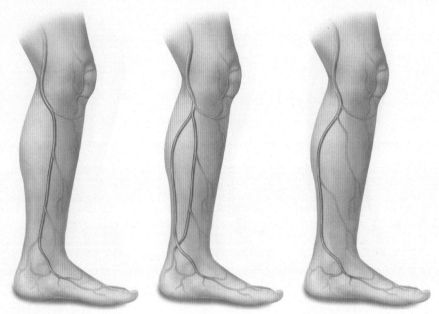

Figure 16-4 Anatomic variations in the configuration of the calf portion of the great saphenous vein.

In 65% of cases, the calf portion is a single dominant system and this is almost always positioned anteriorly near the medial border of the tibia. There is often a posterior vein, which is the posterior accessory great saphenous vein previously mentioned in the discussion of thigh anatomy. This is simply a smaller tributary that is typically not large enough to be used as a bypass conduit. In about 7% of patients, the posterior accessory great saphenous vein is dominant over the more anterior system of the calf.

Double venous systems in the calf can be seen in approximately 35% of cases. These double systems begin as a single vein at the ankle level and split into two veins in the lower calf. They remain as two separate systems and join back together into a single vein at the knee. Again, the more posterior system in these cases is likely the posterior accessory great saphenous vein, but it is just confined to the calf level. The anterior system is dominant in 85% of these cases, and the posterior system is dominant in the remaining 15%. The posterior calf system can continue up the thigh to join a duplicated thigh system or tributaries may extend further posteriorly to connect into the small saphenous vein. Table 16-2 summarizes the various anatomic distributions of the great saphenous vein.

TABLE 16-2	
Anatomic Variants of the Great Saphenous Vein	
	% Distribution
THIGH	
Single medial dominant	60%
Single lateral dominant	8%
Complete double system	8%
Closed loop double system	7%
Partial double system	17%
Triplicate/complex systems	<1%
CALF	
Single anterior dominant system	58%
Single posterior dominant system	7%
Double system, anterior dominant	30%
Double system, posterior dominant	5%

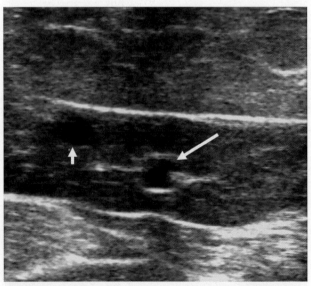

Figure 16-5 Ultrasound image illustrating the normal configuration of the great saphenous vein (*large arrow*) and a cutaneous tributary (*small arrow*).

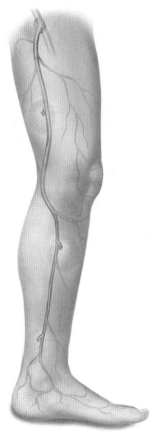

Figure 16-6 Illustration of the common levels at which deep perforating veins can be observed.

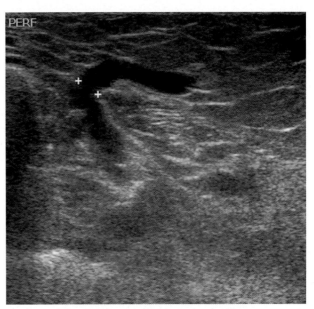

Figure 16-7 Ultrasound image illustrating the orientation of a perforating vein off the main trunk of the great saphenous vein. Note how the vein penetrates the muscular fascia (between the caliper markers).

There are multiple cutaneous tributaries of the great saphenous vein (Fig. 16-5). The exact number and level of these tributaries vary among limbs. Cutaneous tributaries are of little significance to the surgeon and are usually ligated during an open procedure. If an in situ procedure is being performed with limited vein exposure, most cutaneous tributaries can be simply left intact as they will spontaneously thrombose. Some cutaneous tributaries may be harvested if only a small segment of vein is needed as patch material. This keeps the main saphenous system intact for future use.

Of importance to surgeons is the location of deep perforating veins (Fig. 16-6). These perforating veins must always be identified and ligated. A perforating vein is a term reserved for a vein that perforates or penetrates the muscular fascia of the leg and connects the superficial system to the deep system. It initially can be seen off the saphenous vein but then dives deep into the leg (Fig. 16-7). Perforators have valves to ensure the one-way movement of blood from the superficial to the deep system. If the vein is arterialized as a bypass conduit and a perforating vein is left intact, this will create an arteriovenous fistula connecting the bypass to the deep venous system. Due to the low resistance of the venous bed, significant

blood flow can be diverted through this type of fistula. Therefore, it is important to mark the locations of these perforating veins so that a surgeon can ligate them prior to completion of the arterial bypass graft. There are several groups of perforating veins throughout the leg. Some perforating veins connect directly to the main trunk of the saphenous vein, whereas others connect to the accessory saphenous systems.

THE SMALL SAPHENOUS VEIN

The small saphenous vein is another superficial vein that can be mapped prior to surgery for use as a bypass conduit. The small saphenous vein courses in a fairly constant pattern along the posterior aspect of the calf (Fig. 16-8). Two smaller veins leave the foot and travel medially and laterally along the borders of the Achilles tendon. These two veins join together to form the small saphenous vein. The small saphenous is typically a single trunk that courses up the middle of the posterior aspect of the calf and terminates into the popliteal vein. In approximately 20% of limbs, the small saphenous vein continues above the popliteal fossa. This vein is referred to as the cranial extension of the small saphenous vein. In some cases, it terminates directly into the femoral vein or can end into the inferior gluteal vein. Sometimes, it communicates with the great saphenous vein via the posterior thigh circumflex vein and is often referred to as the vein of Giacomini. The small saphenous vein also has several cutaneous tributaries as well as deep perforating veins. It is not uncommon to

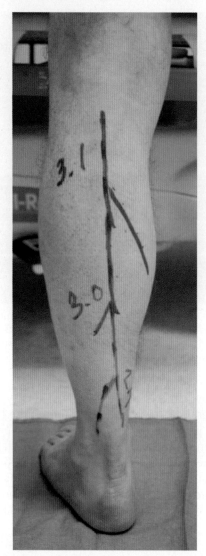

Figure 16-8 Patient leg with a completed small saphenous vein mapping.

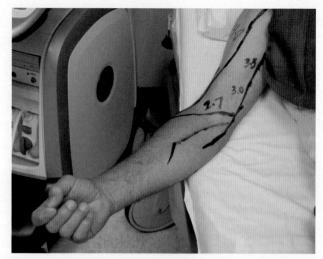

Figure 16-9 Patient arm with a completed mapping of the cephalic and basilic veins.

observe one or more intersaphenous veins connecting the small and great saphenous veins in the calf. The perforating veins may connect the small saphenous veins with the gastrocnemius or peroneal veins.

THE CEPHALIC AND BASILIC VEINS

Venous mapping techniques have extended to the superficial veins of the arm (Fig. 16-9). This has become part of the routine preoperative assessment in patients undergoing the creation of a dialysis fistula. The cephalic vein begins at the level of the wrist, coursing along the radius in the forearm and continuing through the upper arm, terminating into the subclavian vein. The basilic vein also begins at the level of the wrist, coursing along the ulnar aspect of the forearm. The basilic vein continues into the upper arm where it joins the brachial veins to form

the axillary vein. The cephalic and basilic veins communicate at the antecubital fossa via the medial cubital vein. Some variability occurs with the upper extremity superficial veins. Primarily, the branching patterns at the antecubital fossa and the position of the medial cubital vein display the most variability.

SONOGRAPHIC EXAMINATION TECHNIQUES

PATIENT PREPARATION

Vein mapping may sometimes be limited to only the ultrasound evaluation of the superficial veins with image documentation and completion of required work sheets. Often, the procedure involves the additional step of mapping the position of suitable veins directly on the patient's skin. The patient should be instructed to avoid body lotions or powders as these will impede the marking of the skin. The actual marking devices used to create the skin map vary among laboratories that perform this technique. Because the various inks used can be messy, it is recommended to cover the ultrasound transducer with a nonsterile probe cover. Ultrasound gel should be used sparingly to allow easier skin marking. It is recommended to use limited gel directly under the transducer and mark the position of the vein in front of the transducer. Limited use of gel will also reduce the amount of cooling the patient experiences as the gel evaporates from the skin surface. The marker used should be able to easily write on the skin and resist drying out with prolonged use. Some laboratories do not use a marker at all. These labs use a small plastic coffee stirrer or straw to place an indentation in the skin. These indentations remain on the skin for a short time to allow for a final map to be drawn when finished. A final map may be drawn on the skin with permanent marker, surgical markers, or permanent liquid ink commonly used by radiation therapy departments.

PATIENT POSITION

Patient position is very important when performing venous imaging, particularly when dealing with small diameter veins. Venous pressure in the superficial veins should be maximized by placing the patient's limb in a dependent position. For mapping the leg veins, the patient should be placed in a reverse Trendelenburg position with the hip externally rotated and the knee slightly flexed (Fig. 16-10). This position provides adequate access to the entire length of the great saphenous vein. For the small saphenous vein, the patient may be placed on his or her side with the posterior aspect of the calf accessible to the technologist (Fig. 16-11). In cases of small vein diameter, the patient can be asked to stand for brief periods, particularly during the measurement of vein diameter. When mapping arm veins, the patient's arm should be extended out to the side and slightly lower than the chest level (Fig. 16-12). Tourniquets are not required and often produce too much patient discomfort. They can, however, be used in select patients to help maximize vein diameter.

The examination room should be kept warm in order to limit vasoconstriction. The patient should only expose the limb being evaluated, keeping the rest of the body covered and warm. Keeping covered the foot of the leg being examined is also helpful in reducing vasoconstriction.

SCANNING TECHNIQUE

The mapping of the great saphenous vein usually begins at the groin at the saphenofemoral junction. It is important to note that very light pressure

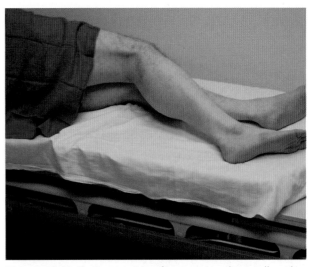

Figure 16-11 Patient position for mapping the small saphenous vein.

should be applied to the skin. Because these superficial veins are under low pressure, it is extremely easy to compress the vein with too much transducer pressure. With the transducer in a transverse orientation, the saphenofemoral junction is identified (Fig. 16-13A,B). The technologist can use either a longitudinal or transverse transducer orientation to follow the line of the vein and map its course. The technologist must be diligent in marking the correct position of the vein given the transducer orientation. With a longitudinal approach, the vein should appear to completely fill the screen from right to left. The transducer should be perpendicular to the skin surface. These techniques will ensure that the vein is not being imaged obliquely but rather, is correctly being examined. A small mark is placed in front of the ultrasound transducer along the narrow edge of the transducer (Fig. 16-14A,B). If a transverse approach is used, the vein should appear circular and

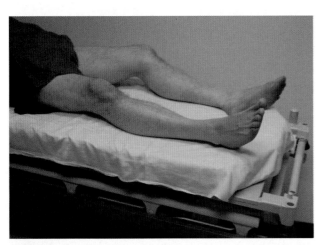

Figure 16-10 Patient position for mapping the great saphenous vein.

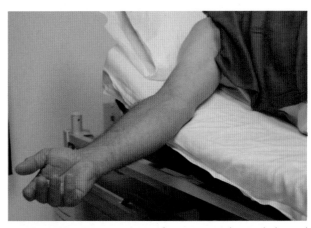

Figure 16-12 Patient position for mapping the cephalic and basilic veins.

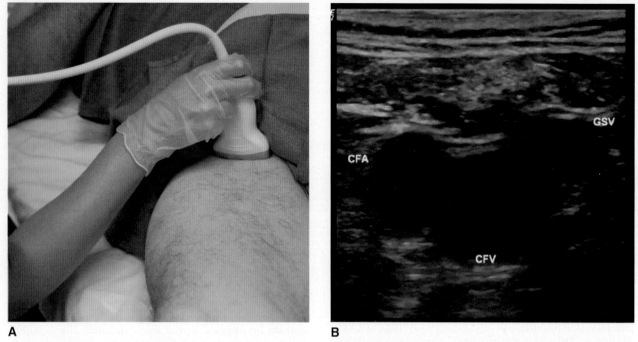

Figure 16-13 A: Transverse orientation used at the groin to identify the saphenofemoral junction. **B:** Corresponding ultrasound image at this level, CFA, common femoral artery; CFV, common femoral vein; GSV, great saphenous vein.

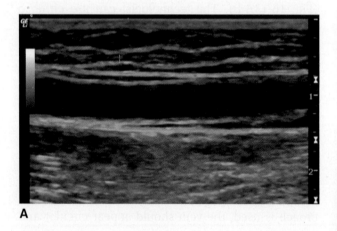

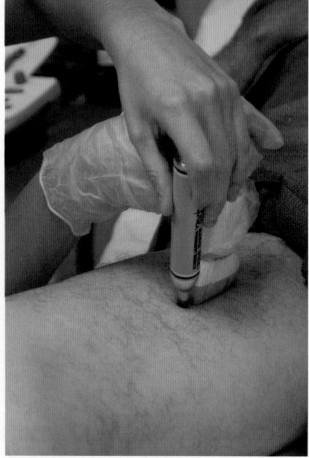

Figure 16-14 A: Longitudinal ultrasound image of the great saphenous vein. **B:** Proper position of the transducer and placement of the skin mark.

centered on the ultrasound screen. A skin mark is then placed exactly at the center of the long face of the transducer (Fig. 16-15A,B). It is this author's experience that following the vein in a longitudinal approach for the initial mapping of the course of the vein yields the most accurate results.[8,9] Once the initial skin mark is placed, the transducer is moved slightly distally toward the foot while keeping the vein in the center of view. A new mark is placed on the skin every 2 to 3 cm. This procedure is continued to the level of the ankle. The result is a line of short dashes, which mark the course of the main venous system (Fig. 16-16).

Once the main course of the great saphenous has been determined, the saphenofemoral junction is once again identified using a transverse orientation. Using the preliminary marks as a guide and remaining transverse to the vein, the main system is followed in order to identify termination points of the tributaries and measure the vein diameter. The vein should appear circular. If it appears elliptical, then too much transducer pressure is being applied to the skin. Two types of tributaries will be identified,

namely cutaneous veins and deep perforating veins. Each should be marked at the level they terminate into the main system. The orientation of these veins should also be noted. Typically, the terms anterior and posterior are used to describe the direction of branches. The examiner can simply place an "A" or "P" as a key to describe the aforementioned tributary directions. However, any type of coding system can be used as long as it results in proper placement of these veins on the final skin mapping. It is especially important to follow all significant tributaries in order to identify partial loops or double systems.

The size of the saphenous vein is measured at the proximal, mid, and distal thigh and calf. If multiple systems exist, each should be measured to determine system dominance. Additional diameter measurements may be made over any segment that appears to change in caliber. The diameter is determined by placing the calipers along the inner vein wall and blood interface (Fig. 16-17). This results in the internal diameter of the vessel being measured. Often, the boundary between the adventitial layer of the vein wall and the surrounding tissue is difficult to

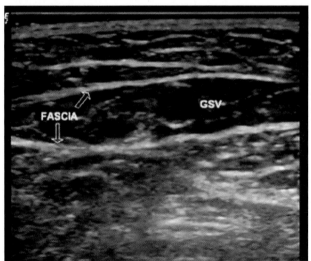

A

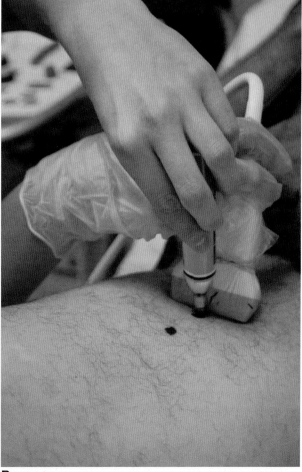

B

Figure 16-15 A: Transverse ultrasound image of the great saphenous vein (GSV). Note fascial boundaries. **B:** Proper position of the transducer and placement of the skin mark.

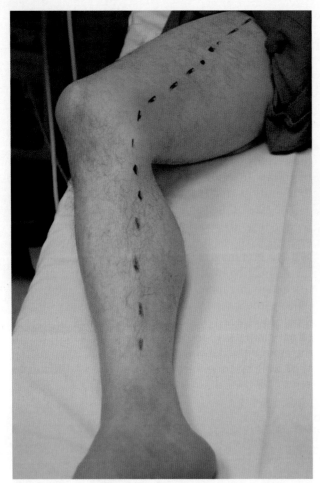

Figure 16-16 Leg with the preliminary marks of a great saphenous vein mapping.

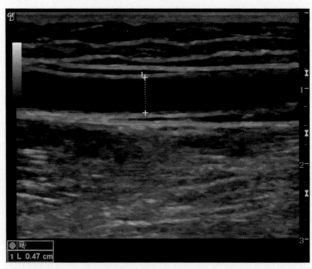

Figure 16-17 Ultrasound image illustrating a healthy vein wall with a diameter measurement.

permanent ink used. In most patients, the marks will be visible for at least 3 to 5 days.

The same scanning techniques described for the great saphenous vein can be used to map the small saphenous vein as well as the cephalic and basilic

determine; therefore, the external diameter of the vein is not measured. Surgeons may often measure the vein at time of operation, which is a measurement of the external diameter. Due to these discrepancies in techniques, the ultrasound vein diameters always underestimate the vein size as compared to the intraoperative measurements. Surgeons should always be cautioned to use the ultrasound measurements as a rough estimate.

Once the course of the vein has been marked, the tributaries have been noted and the vein diameters measured, the ultrasound gel can be wiped off the limb. Liquid marking ink (such as a carbol fuchsin stain used in radiation therapy) can be applied with a cotton-tipped applicator. The dashed marks originally placed can be connected to illustrate the course of the vein (Fig. 16-18). Termination points of the tributaries can be drawn in and diameters can be indicated at the various levels. The liquid ink requires 3 to 5 minutes to dry. During this time, a hand-drawn sketch can be made for a permanent laboratory record. This skin marking will remain on the skin for varying lengths of time depending on the type of

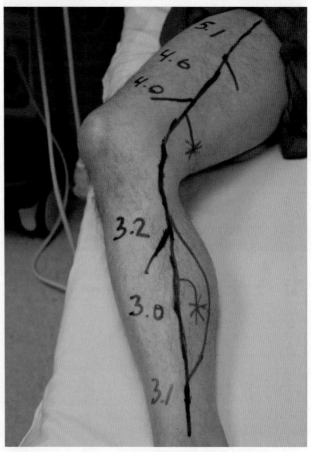

Figure 16-18 Patient with a completed great saphenous vein mapping.

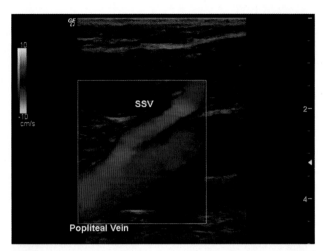

Figure 16-19 Ultrasound image of the saphenopopliteal junction.

veins. The small saphenous vein should be first identified at its confluence with the popliteal vein (Fig. 16-19). It can be then followed and mapped to the lower calf level. If there is a cranial extension of the small saphenous vein above the popliteal fossa, this can also be evaluated if the diameter meets laboratory criteria for adequacy. The small saphenous vein can often present a greater challenge to the technologist as it typically more superficial yet smaller in diameter as compared to the great saphenous vein. Vein diameters are recorded in the proximal, mid, and distal calf.

The superficial veins of the arms are usually easiest to identify in the upper arm where they are largest and have the least amount of tributaries. The basilic vein can be observed at it terminates into the axillary vein along with the brachial veins (Fig. 16-20A,B). It can be followed extending below the antecubital fossa along the ulnar aspect of the forearm and mapped from the upper arm to the wrist

level. The cephalic vein will be visualized in the upper arm over the biceps muscle (Fig. 16-21A,B). The cephalic vein can be followed centrally to its termination into the subclavian vein (Fig. 16-22). The cephalic vein can be mapped from the shoulder region then followed peripherally along the radial aspect of the forearm, mapping its position to the wrist level. Many surgeons also request the position of the medial cubital vein and its connections with the cephalic and basilic veins mapped. The arm veins present a challenge to the technologist because the veins will course over various aspects of the arm. Typically, the largest segments of vein are the ones selected for mapping. The vein diameters are measured proximally and distally in the forearm and upper arm.

Table 16-3 summarizes some of the basic strategies to follow during vein mapping. These tips will help achieve accurate vein mapping results.

TECHNICAL CONSIDERATIONS

It is imperative to optimize the ultrasound equipment for a venous mapping. Because the saphenous vein is a superficial structure, the equipment should be adjusted to provide a well-defined near-field image. The transmit power and focal zones should be adjusted to maximize the resolution of the near field. Ideally, the ultrasound transducer used should be at least 10 MHz, but a higher frequency of 12, 13, or 15 MHz can be used. A lower frequency transducer may be occasionally needed to image deeper veins in obese individuals. The pulsed Doppler frequency should be sufficient to detect the low flow states in the superficial veins, and a frequency of 4 or 4.5 MHz is adequate. Pulsed Doppler is not typically employed during venous mapping examinations unless patency is in question. Occasionally, compression of small

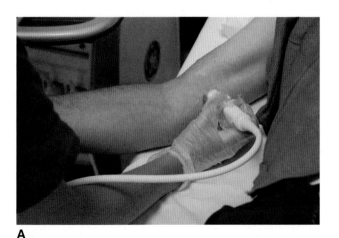

A

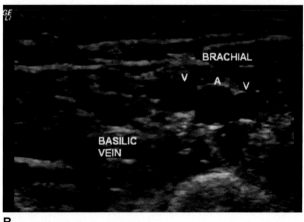

B

Figure 16-20 A: Transducer position used to identify the basilic vein in the upper arm. **B:** Ultrasound image of the basilic and brachial veins.

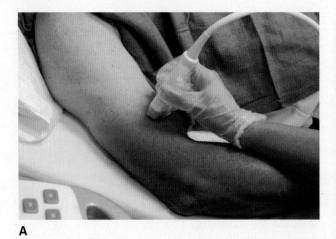

A

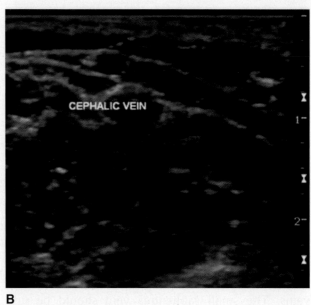

CEPHALIC VEIN

B

Figure 16-21 A: Transducer position used to identify the cephalic vein in the upper arm. **B:** Ultrasound image of the cephalic vein and adjacent tissue.

veins may be difficult to assess and, in these cases, Doppler may be helpful. The scale or pulse repetition frequency (PRF) should be adjusted to detect low flow. Color imaging can also be used to confirm vessel patency. Color flow settings should be adjusted to a low flow state with increased gain and decreased scale or PRF.

PITFALLS

Like any ultrasound examination, there are limitations to this procedure. Patient mobility, dressings, and wounds may limit scanning access to segments of the limb. It is important to make an attempt to

visualize any segments of a vein that are accessible. In some cases, only short segments of vein are required as a conduit. Even a limited examination may provide enough information to select an appropriate segment of vein.

DIAGNOSIS

Vein mapping must determine much more than the presence or absence of a vein. It must also determine the suitability of that vein for use as a bypass conduit in terms of wall status, planar arrangement, and diameter.

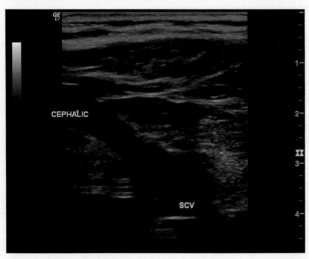

CEPHALIC

SCV

Figure 16-22 Ultrasound image of the cephalic vein terminating into the subclavian vein.

TABLE	16-3
Strategies for Successful Vein Mapping	

Action	Result
Maximize venous pressure	Increases vein diameter
Keep the patient warm	Reduces peripheral vasoconstriction
Use light transducer pressure	Minimizes extrinsic compression of vein
Use gel sparingly to facilitate marking on skin	Reduces evaporation of gel and cooling of skin, which can lead to vasoconstriction
Keep the transducer perpendicular to the skin surface	Skin mark will be most accurately placed over vein position

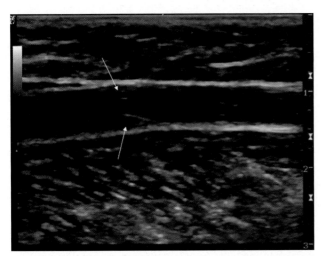

Figure 16-23 Ultrasound image of a normal healthy vein with smooth, thin walls. Valve leaflets identified at *arrows*.

A normal healthy vein should have smooth, thin walls (Fig. 16-23). The vein should be compliant and should easily compress with minimal transducer pressure. Valve sinuses may appear elliptical but in some smaller veins they may be difficult to identify. If valve leaflets are visualized, they should be freely moving without any evidence of a thrombus behind the leaflets.

As previously mentioned, the planar arrangement of the veins should be noted during the mapping procedure. This is of particular importance with mapping the great and small saphenous vein. Planar arrangement can easily be included within the written laboratory report. Figure 16-24 illustrates the normal orientation of the main trunk of the great saphenous vein within the saphenous compartment

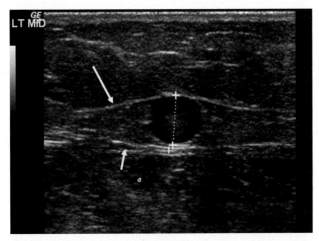

Figure 16-24 Transverse view of the great saphenous vein noting the superficial fascia *(large arrow)* above the vein and the muscular fascia *(small arrow)* below the vein. This is often referred to as an "Egyptian eye" appearance of the vein.

bounded by the saphenous fascia superficially and deeply by the muscular fascia. These layers of fascia produce the appearance of what some people refer to as the "Egyptian eye" appearance of the vein. When double systems exist, the veins often travel in different anatomic planes through the thigh as shown in Figure 16-3. The dominant vein may not be the most superficial system that exists or the larger system may not be within the normal saphenous compartment. This information is important to the surgeon so that the best vein is selected. Very superficial, subdermal veins are often encountered in limbs with extensive varicosities.

Individual laboratory criteria for suitable vein diameters vary based on surgeon preference. The adequacy of a vein diameter may also vary depending on the intended use for the vein. A cardiothoracic surgeon may prefer a certain diameter vein for a coronary bypass, whereas a general surgeon may have different diameter criteria for a dialysis fistula. Generally, most surgeons will not use a vein that is less than 2 mm in diameter. Such small diameter veins may be prone to spasm and may be difficult to suture. Many surgeons like to select a vein that is 2.5 to 3 mm, at a minimum. It is also important to instruct physicians whether internal or external vein diameters are measured during the ultrasound examination. As image resolution improves, accurate external diameter measurements may be routinely possible with ultrasound.

DISORDERS

There are several commonly observed abnormalities encountered within the superficial veins. Pathology Box 16-1 provides a quick list of superficial vein pathology.

THROMBUS

Isolated segments of a partial thrombus may be encountered during vein mapping. Often, patients cannot recall a prior occurrence of a superficial thrombophlebitis even though a residual thrombus may be present. A thrombus can be visualized adjacent to valve leaflets within the valve sinus (Fig. 16-25). A thrombus will vary in echogenicity, with acute thrombus being anechoic or hypoechoic. A chronic thrombus may be hyperechoic. Completely thrombosed veins will be noncompressible, will lack any color filling, and will not demonstrate a Doppler signal. Partially thrombosed veins will be partially compressible and will demonstrate a reduced flow lumen. Doppler signals obtained from partially thrombosed veins will display a decrease in phasicity.

PATHOLOGY BOX 16-1

Superficial Vein Pathology

Pathology	Sonographic Appearance		
	B-Mode	**Color**	**Doppler**
Thrombus	Intraluminal echoes of varying echogenicity dependent on the age of the thrombus	No flow or reduced color filling of lumen	Absent Doppler signal or, if present, diminished phasicity
Varicosities	Tortuous, dilated segments of veins	Multiple color patterns due to changes in flow direction	May demonstrate reflux
Recanalization	Hyperechoic thick walls often with an irregular surface	May demonstrate a reduced flow lumen	Continuous or diminished phasicity
Calcification	Bright white echoes within the vessel wall with acoustic shadowing	Absent color filling in area of acoustic shadow	Absent Doppler signal in area of acoustic shadow
Stenotic valves	Valve leaflet protruding into vessel lumen and frozen in place	May demonstrate disturbed color flow patterns or aliasing in region of valve	May demonstrate elevated velocities in region of valve

VARICOSITIES

Varices will appear as dilated, tortuous portions of the saphenous system. Varicosities are not an automatic contraindication to saphenous vein mapping. In many patients, the clinically evident varicose veins are subdermal tributaries of the main trunk (Fig. 16-26). The main system of the saphenous vein in these patients can often be found in the normal subfascial plane. It is often not dilated and can be used for bypass procedures. Even if the main system in the thigh is found to be varicose, sometimes the calf portion of the vein can be spared. It is always important to examine the entire length of the limb to find any suitable segments of vein.

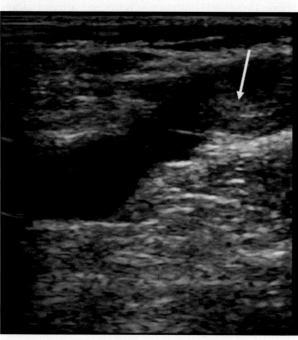

Figure 16-25 Ultrasound image of a valve leaflet with a thrombus (*arrow*) adjacent to it.

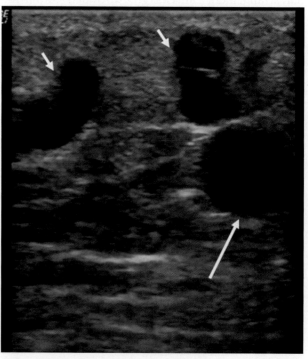

Figure 16-26 Ultrasound image of superficial varices (*small arrows*) with the main saphenous (*large arrow*) system beneath the varices.

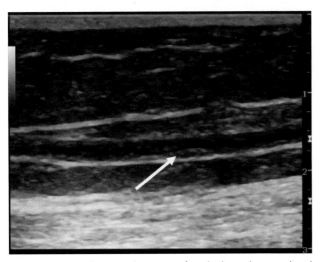

Figure 16-27 Ultrasound image of a thickened recanalized vein. The *arrow* indicates a thickened wall area.

RECANALIZATION

Veins presenting with an irregular intimal surface or wall thickening may indicate evidence of recanalization (Fig. 16-27). These veins are not usually considered to be adequate conduits for arterial bypasses. Description of the vein wall pathology is somewhat subjective but does alert the surgeon and aid in the selection of the most appropriate vein segments.

CALCIFICATION

Other wall pathology may include calcification. Although not as common as arterial wall calcification, venous calcification does occasionally present in some patients. The classic ultrasound appearance of calcification includes bright echoes within the vein wall producing acoustic shadowing. Isolated areas may not preclude the entire vein from being used as a conduit. The surgeon may simply use noncalcified segments. However, diffuse intermittent calcification renders the vein inadequate for bypass material. Venous calcification can often be observed in diabetic patients.

VALVE ABNORMALITIES

Lastly, another pathology that can be noted on the image is a stenotic or frozen valve (Fig. 16-28). This may be encountered in a vein that was previously thrombosed. All evidence of the prior thrombus can be completed resolved and the remainder of the vein wall may appear relatively normal. However, a valve sinus may be present that contains a valve leaflet that is frozen and unmoving in the blood flow stream. Again, if it is an isolated occurrence, the surgeon may simply use other healthy segments of the vein.

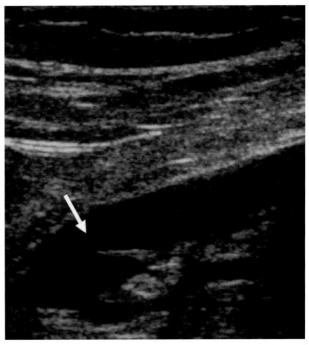

Figure 16-28 Ultrasound image of a frozen valve leaflet.

SUMMARY

Venous mapping is a valuable component in the preoperative planning of many surgical procedures. It is a highly technologist-dependent procedure. The technologist must be familiar with venous anatomy and variants and should also be familiar with the surgical procedure being performed. Proper vein mapping is highly dependent on a close working relationship between the technologist and the surgeon. Feedback from the operating room as to the accuracy of the mapping is essential for the technologist.

Preoperative mapping of the superficial venous system can provide detailed information on vein anatomy. Anatomic variants can be clearly delineated. Venous pathologies can be described so that diseased vein segments are avoided. Careful skin marking, as well as descriptive information within the vein mapping report can aid the surgeon in the placement of incisions. This can minimize the need for large skin flaps and can decrease operative time. The details provided by ultrasound vein mapping will allow the surgeon to select the optimal vein to be used as conduit material.

Critical Thinking Questions

1. A patient presents for a bilateral lower extremity mapping of the great saphenous vein. On the right leg, there is an incision that runs from the upper thigh to the mid-calf. The patient explains that he underwent a coronary artery bypass graft 4 years earlier and the surgeons used a vein from his right leg. Do you alter your planned mapping procedure? Why or why not?

2. You begin a mapping procedure of the cephalic and basilic veins. In the upper arm, both veins are found to be approximately 2 mm in diameter. What step can you take to aid in the examination of these veins?

3. You are explaining the techniques of saphenous vein mapping to a new staff member. What aspects of the ultrasound system, including specific settings and adjustments, should you review?

REFERENCES

1. Talbot SR. Use of real-time imaging in identifying deep venous obstruction: a preliminary report. *Bruit.* 1982;6:41–42.
2. Leopold PW, Shandall AA, Kupinski AM, et al. The role of B-mode venous mapping in infrainguinal arterial bypasses. *Br J Surg.* 1989;76(3):305–307.
3. Shandall AA, Leather RP, Corson JD, et al. Use of the short saphenous vein in situ for popliteal-to-distal artery bypass. *Am J Surg.* 1987;154(2):240–244.
4. Caggiati A, Bergan JJ, Gloviczki P, et al. Nomenclature of the veins of the lower limbs: an international interdisciplinary consensus statement. *J Vasc Surg.* 2002;36(2):416–422.
5. Caggiata A, Bergan JJ, Gloviczki P, et al. Nomenclature of the veins of the lower limbs: extensions, refinements, and clinical application. *J Vasc Surg.* 2005;41(4):719–724.
6. Kupinski AM, Evans SM, Khan AM, et al. Ultrasonic characterization of the saphenous vein. *Cardiovasc Surg.* 1993;1(5):513–517.
7. Shah DM, Chang BB, Leopold PW, et al. The anatomy of the greater saphenous venous system. *J Vasc Surg.* 1986;3(2):273–283.
8. Chang BB, Kupinski AM, Darling RC III, et al. Preoperative saphenous vein mapping. In: AbuRahma AF, Bergan JJ, eds. *Noninvasive Vascular Diagnosis.* London, England: Springer-Verlag; 1999:335–344.
9. Kupinski AM, Leather RP, Chang BB, et al. Preoperative mapping of the saphenous vein. In: Bernstein EF, ed. *Vascular Diagnosis.* St. Louis, MO: Mosby;1993:897–901.

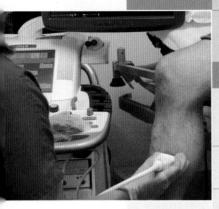

17 Venous Valvular Insufficiency Testing

Sergio X. Salles Cunha and Diana L. Neuhardt

OBJECTIVES

Define the clinical, etiological, anatomical, and pathophysiological conditions of chronic venous valvular insufficiency used as indicators for vascular laboratory venous testing

Describe both direct and indirect noninvasive vascular testing performed by vascular laboratory personnel

Describe protocol differences based on the objectives of testing for screening, definitive diagnosis, pretreatment mapping, peritreatment imaging, and procedure/patient follow-up

Define the role of duplex ultrasonography in the evaluation of patients with lower extremity venous valvular disorders

KEY TERMS

B-mode ultrasound imaging | chronic venous insufficiency | color flow ultrasound imaging | duplex Doppler | plethysmography | varicose veins | venous reflux | venous valvular insufficiency

GLOSSARY

anterior accessory saphenous vein superficial vein at the anterior thigh

CEAP clinical, etiologic, anatomical, and pathophysiological classification of chronic venous insufficiency

chronic venous insufficiency a long-lasting venous valvular or obstructive disorder

elastic compression effect of stockings used to compress the leg with the intent to compress the veins

great saphenous vein superficial vein in the medial thigh and calf

leg edema leg swelling due to the accumulation of water or fluid

lipedema swelling attributed to fat tissue

lymphedema swelling attributed to lymph channels or lymph node disorders

plethysmography graphic presentation of pulses such as changes in volume within an organ or other part of the body such as a leg

posterior accessory saphenous vein superficial vein at the posterior thigh

reflux reverse flow, usually in veins with incompetent valves

reticular veins veins with a diameter less than 3 mm

small saphenous vein superficial vein in the posterior calf

spider vein inadequate name for purple or red telangiectasias, an arteriovenous rather than a venous disorder

superficial epigastric vein tributary of the proximal great saphenous vein

telangiectasia dilation of red, blue, or purple superficial capillaries, arterioles, or venules located below the skin's surface; see *spider vein*

varicose veins veins with a diameter equal or greater than 3 mm

vein of Giacomini communicating vein between the great and small saphenous veins

Chronic venous valvular insufficiency (CVVI) is a common disorder of the modern era. The development of minimally invasive techniques has enhanced the awareness and treatment potential of superficial veins with incompetent valves and reflux. CVVI is a subset of the classical, most commonly used term "chronic venous insufficiency" (CVI). CVI includes venous obstruction and/or valvular insufficiency. This chapter focuses on valvular disorders (and not on venous obstruction), most commonly a consequence of deep venous thrombosis. Most patients with CVVI do not have a venous obstruction. The hypothesis is that patients with venous obstruction have characteristics distinct from those with venous valvular insufficiency, and the two groups deserve to be differentiated for appropriate diagnosis and treatment.

One of the philosophies behind the clinical, etiologic, anatomical, and pathophysiological (CEAP) classification of CVI recommendations is to clearly specify and differentiate types of CVI to improve the understanding of distinct disorders.[1-3] This chapter reviews CVVI with summaries of relevant anatomy, prevalence of disease, signs and symptoms, classes of disorders, quality of life questionnaires, noninvasive examinations, types of treatment, and follow-up.

ANATOMY

The sonographer must have knowledge of the deep and superficial venous anatomy as detected by ultrasound. The anatomy of the venous system has been discussed in previous chapters. Pertinent sonographic information is provided as follows.

Current knowledge about the superficial venous system has expanded, with a description of ultrasound landmarks to differentiate veins by location

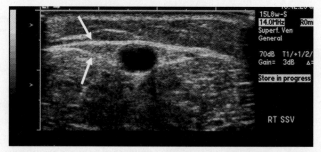

Figure 17-2 A transverse ultrasound image of the great saphenous vein within the saphenous compartment distally within the leg. *Arrows* indicate fascia both superficial and deep to the vein.

within the fascia layers of the tissue. Recently adopted nomenclature applies specifically to the superficial system: the great saphenous vein (GSV), formerly named the greater or long saphenous, and the small saphenous vein (SSV), formerly named the lesser or short saphenous.[4,5] Saphenous nomenclature follows the anatomical position and includes the anterior accessory saphenous vein (AASV), the posterior accessory saphenous vein (PASV), and the vein of Giacomini (VOG). Saphenous veins are within saphenous fascia layers, which are readily identified with ultrasound.[6,7] The saphenous "eye" differentiates the saphenous compartment from the superficial and deep compartments (Figs. 17-1 and 17-2). The GSV courses medial in the thigh and leg within the saphenous compartment. Although the AASV is within a saphenous compartment, the "alignment sign" is the anatomical landmark for its location (Fig. 17-3). The AASV is aligned with the femoral artery and vein following a vertical line perpendicular to the transducer surface in cross-sectional imaging. The AASV and PASV course anterior and posterior in the thigh, respectively. The PASV may connect to the VOG. Tributaries are veins that drain into another

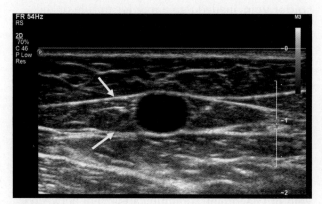

Figure 17-1 A transverse ultrasound image of the great saphenous vein illustrating the normal position of the vein within the saphenous compartment. *Arrows* indicate fascia both superficial and deep to the vein.

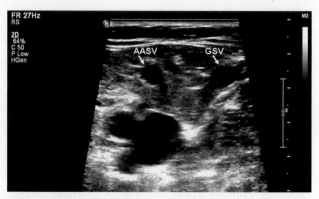

Figure 17-3 The "alignment sign" with the anterior accessory saphenous vein (*AASV*) aligned over the deep system artery and vein, whereas the great saphenous vein (*GSV*) lies more medially.

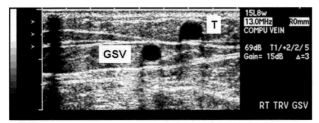

Figure 17-4 A tributary vein (T) positioned outside the saphenous compartment and superficial to the great saphenous vein (GSV).

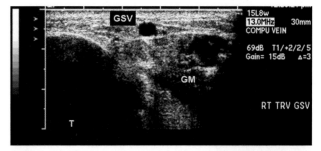

Figure 17-6 The "angle sign" of the great saphenous vein below the knee. A triangle is formed by the gastrocnemius muscle (GM), the tibial bone (T), and the great saphenous vein (GSV).

major vein. Superficial tributaries pierce the saphenous fascia, enter into the saphenous compartment, and drain into the corresponding saphenous vein (Figs. 17-4 and 17-5). Bulging varicose veins are often associated with abnormal superficial tributaries. Ultrasound identification of the GSV below the knee is aided by identification of the "angle sign" in cross-sectional imaging (Fig. 17-6). The triangular form of the gastrocnemius muscle, tibial bone, and the GSV within the fascia help to differentiate the saphenous vein from prominent tributaries. A common disagreement is about the interpretation of saphenous duplications. Most duplications are segmental; complete duplications are rare. By strict definition, duplicated saphenous veins must follow the same path and remain parallel within the fascia. The duplication demonstrates a beginning and end along the same path.

The GSV and common femoral vein (CFV) confluence is referred to as the saphenofemoral junction (SFJ). The proximal GSV has two major valves. The terminal valve is at the SFJ. The preterminal valve is distal to tributaries that join the GSV at the SFJ. The junctions of these tributaries lie in between the terminal and preterminal valves. The superficial epigastric vein (SEV), one of these tributaries, is a landmark for thermal ablation treatment. The superficial external pudendal and the superficial circumflex

iliac veins are other tributaries in the junction region. Besides the SFJ, these veins may be the most proximal source of GSV reflux, raising the suspicion of pelvic CVVI.

The SSV confluence with the deep venous system is variable and ultrasonographically challenging. The SSV may terminate into (1) the popliteal vein at the saphenopopliteal junction (SPJ), (2) the gastrocnemius vein, (3) the distal femoral vein (FV) of the thigh, (4) a small unnamed deep vein, (5) a perforating vein at the posterior thigh, or (6) the GSV via the VOG.

Venous valve leaflets are identified quite readily with B-mode imaging. Captivating to observe in motion, the bicuspid leaflets point to the direction of normal venous drainage (Fig. 17-7). Venous valves vary in number, increasing in frequency with the distance away from the heart. Venous valves open with muscular contraction (referred to as venous systole) and close with muscular relaxation (referred to as venous diastole). A series of synchronized valves regulate blood return from the skin, to tributaries, to saphenous veins, to perforating veins or junctions, and to deep veins toward the heart. Incompetent valves permit abnormal retrograde flow or reflux (Fig. 17-8).

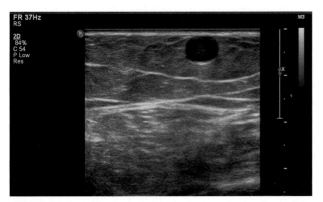

Figure 17-5 A tributary vein positioned superficially outside the saphenous compartment.

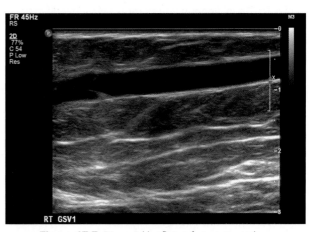

Figure 17-7 Bicuspid leaflets of a venous valve.

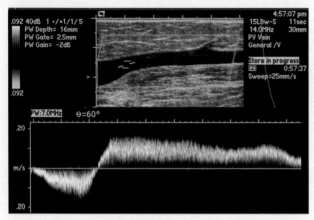

Figure 17-8 A Doppler spectrum demonstrating retrograde flow or reflux (displayed above the baseline).

PREVALENCE

CVVI is prevalent in many different populations, affecting both men and women. Prevalence of varicose veins varies between 2% and 56% in men and 1% and 60% in women.[8-11] Varicose veins were associated with valvular reflux, venous obstruction, or both. Valvular insufficiency was noted despite the absence of varicose veins. Exceptionally, varicose veins were noted more in men (40%) than in women (32%) in a general population registered in clinics of Edinburgh, United Kingdom.[12]

Screening programs funded by the American Venous Forum initially documented varicose veins in 32% and venous reflux in 40% of the subjects evaluated.[13] As the program expanded, the worst-case conditions of the subjects screened were telangiectasias (29%), varicose veins (23%), edema (10%), skin changes (9%), and ulcers (2%).[14] Telangiectasias were present in 79% of the men and 88% of the women in the Edinburgh study.[15] Varicose veins have also been linked to a higher incidence of arterial disease.[16]

Prevalence of reflux in veins of the lower extremity was 35% in a general population, 21% in superficial veins, and 20% in deep veins.[17] Prevalence of either superficial or deep vein reflux increased with severity of the CEAP classification. Prevalence of superficial reflux increased with age. The Edinburgh study described prevalence of reflux for various segments of deep and superficial veins.[18] There was no difference among prevalence on the right or left lower extremities. The great saphenous vein had the highest prevalence of reflux.

These statistics indicate that CVVI is common and demands significant efforts and resources. Education and awareness are being promoted by the American College of Phlebology and the Venous Disease Coalition; investigations are being performed among diverse population groups.

SIGNS AND SYMPTOMS

A basic concept of CVI or CVVI pathophysiology, reviewed in Chapter 3, involves the concept of venous pressure and abnormal venous hypertension. Abnormal venous pressures result in a multitude of signs and symptoms. Visual signs include spider veins, telangiectasias, reticular veins, varicose veins, edema, skin changes, and ulceration. Visual signs are the primary basis for the CEAP clinical classification.

Edema is also a palpable sign and may not be visible early on. A description of symptoms associated with temporary swelling often varies from patient to patient. Feelings of temporary leg swelling at the end of a working day, after prolonged standing, or as a consequence of certain activities or leg positioning may represent what is known as phlebedema.

A differential diagnosis of edema includes other sources besides venous obstruction or valvular insufficiency. Lymphatic obstruction results in enlarged hypoechoic channels in the lower leg and foot.[19] Edema related to cardiac disease, arterial disease, sympathetic tone, or lipid disorders (lipedema) should also be suspected in the vascular laboratory.

Skin changes can vary widely. Localized redness, either with light or dark coloration; atrophie blanche (occurs after skin injury when blood supply is poor); corona phlebectatica as a cluster of veins and skin changes; hardening of the skin as lipodermatosclerosis develops; and ulcerated wounds, healed or not, are observed with different frequencies as a function of each vascular laboratory patient population. Symptoms commonly described are heaviness, tension, aching, fatigue, restless legs, muscle cramps (primarily nocturnal), tingling discomfort, pain, burning, itching, skin irritation, tightness, or other variations of neurological sensations. Restless leg syndrome can be associated with venous disease or several other nonvascular conditions. The presence of birthmarks such as port wine stains may initiate a multifaceted study to identify the presence of vascular or nonvascular malformation.

CEAP CLASSIFICATION

An international committee organized by the American Venous Forum elaborated an initial and a subsequent advanced CEAP classification.[1-3] The initial, basic idea was to classify the patients in their worst-case condition. The advanced classification groups together with a variety of patient conditions. C, E, A, and P is an acronym for clinical, etiologic, anatomic and pathophysiologic classifications.

Clinical Classification

The clinical classification has seven classes from C_0 to C_6, pending extremity conditions:

- C_0: no venous insufficiency signs or symptoms
- C_1: telangiectasias (spider veins) and/or reticular veins (<3 mm in diameter)
- C_2: varicose veins (≥3 mm in diameter)
- C_3: edema
- C_4: skin changes, presently subdivided into:
  - C_{4A}: minor skin changes
  - C_{4B}: major skin changes such as lipodermatosclerosis
- C_5: healed skin ulcers
- C_6: open skin ulcers

The authors recommend a subdivision of C_3 into:

- C_{3A}: intermittent, functional swelling
- C_{3B}: classical, constant edema

Etiologic Classification

The etiologic classification has four classes:

- Ep: CVVI is the major cause of clinical manifestations
- Es: CVI or CVVI is secondary to deep venous thrombosis or other pathology
- Ec: CVI or CVVI has a congenital origin; for example, venous malformations or lack of valves
- En: unknown etiology, no venous etiology identified

Anatomical Classification

The anatomical classification has three abnormal classes or a combination of such classes, and the class describing no findings:

- Ad: CVI or CVVI affects the deep veins
- As: CVI or CVVI affects the superficial veins
- Ap: CVI or CVVI affects the perforating veins
- Ads, Adp, Asp, and Adsp are multiple combinations
- An: no venous anatomy identified

Pathophysiologic Classification

The pathophysiologic classification describes two primary abnormalities, combined or not, and a class without apparent findings:

- Pr: reflux or reverse venous flow
- Po: chronic venous obstruction
- Pro: a pathological combination
- Pn: no venous pathophysiology identified

One of the changes in the revised classification was to consider varicose veins as ≥3 mm rather than ≥4 mm in diameter. Most clinical articles use at least the clinical CEAP classification to describe the patients studied; the authors recommend that statistics be conducted for each class without bundling patients with different conditions in the same group. Another recommendation is a venous segmental disease score based on the veins involved.[20]

CLINICAL SEVERITY SCORE[21]

The CEAP classification is descriptive. The clinical severity score attempts to determine a numerical, quantifiable index, mostly for longitudinal research comparisons. A summary of the guidelines for venous clinical severity score lists 10 attributes:

- 1: pain
- 2: varicose veins
- 3: edema
- 4: skin pigmentation
- 5: inflammation
- 6: induration
- 7: number of active ulcers
- 8: duration of active ulcers
- 9: size of active ulcers
- 10: compressive therapy

Each attribute is then scored from 0 to 3 for a maximum of 30 points:

- 0: Absent
- 1: Mild
- 2: Moderate
- 3: Severe

Note: The clinical severity score has yet to have the acceptability and common practice of the clinical CEAP classification.

DISABILITY SCORE[21]

A summary of the guidelines for the venous disability score lists the conditions of the patient as:

- 0: asymptomatic
- 1, 2, 3: symptomatic
- 1: able to carry out usual activities without compressive therapy
- 2: able to carry out usual activities only with compressive therapy and/or leg elevation
- 3: unable to carry out usual activities even with compressive therapy and/or leg elevation

Usual activities are the activities before the onset of disability due to venous disease.

QUALITY OF LIFE QUESTIONNAIRES[22–25]

Awareness of a dual role is growing in medicine. Clinicians are concerned not only with the provision of successful physiopathological treatment, but also with improving the quality of life for patients. Patients' perceptions of successful treatment is being analyzed with quality of life questionnaires. Such questionnaires are divided according to the objectives evaluated. There are general, overall health questionnaires such as the SF-36. The Aberdeen questionnaire examines detailed peripheral venous performance. The CIVIC-2 is an example of a simplified peripheral venous performance questionnaire and has been used successfully in the evaluation of radio-frequency treatment.

SONOGRAPHIC EXAMINATION TECHNIQUES

Duplex Doppler ultrasonography (US) has become the standard technology to evaluate CVVI. Several objectives are accomplished with US of the peripheral venous system and can include:

- Screening
- Definitive diagnosis
- Pretreatment mapping
- Peritreatment mapping, guidance, and completion ultrasonography
- Posttreatment follow-up
- Patient follow-up

The US examination for CVVI has two major diagnostic goals. The first is to rule out deep venous obstruction or even acute venous thrombosis. The second is the evaluation of valvular insufficiency or reflux detection.

Screening is a concise evaluation of patients at risk or with a high probability of having CVVI. It could be the basis for prevalence studies.

A definitive diagnosis includes an evaluation of the deep veins and a segmental evaluation of reflux in the main veins. Differential diagnosis of a nonvenous disease such as types of edema (e.g., lymphedema), arterial pathology (e.g., popliteal aneurysm), masses (e.g., hematoma), among others are part of definitive diagnosis.

Pretreatment "mapping," a term typically associated with determination of superficial venous location, registers details of reflux sources and drainage, perforating vein competence, and vein diameters as a secondary variable.[26,27] Details of the report are often influenced by the technical thoroughness of perioperative US. Some reports should include detailed measurements to localize source, drainage, or perforating veins' precise location. Availability of perioperative US minimizes the need for such details. One single examination serves as screening, definitive diagnosis, and perioperative mapping in many centers.

Peritreatment US varies on the type of treatment planned. Using ultrasound guidance, some centers place skin markings with a pen or marker along the course of the vein, which creates a pretreatment "mapping." US guidance has become a standard for

thermal and chemical ablation treatment. Completion ultrasonography documents patency of the deep venous system and efficacy of superficial venous ablation or eradication.

Follow-up examinations can be subdivided into two categories: (1) direct assessment of individual veins and (2) assessment of overall pathophysiologic condition. US is used for the direct assessment of individual veins postprocedure. Air plethysmography determines overall effects caused by pathology in virtually all veins draining the lower extremity. Photoplethysmography, in its most common, simplest form, gives a compound representation of the effects of venous reflux in the region tested. These specific techniques are described later in this chapter. US has become the most popular, most used, and most mandatory examination to evaluate CVVI. Air plethysmography, however, is likely a better indicator of treatment performance, providing a global assessment of total limb venous function.

Although invasive, venography or phlebography is another diagnostic method to detect venous thrombosis, congenital venous malformations, or valvular function. The venogram (another term is phlebography) is an x-ray of the veins after dye is injected distally (ascending) or by direct puncture of the contrast into the common femoral vein or external iliac vein with the patient in a semierect position (descending). Less invasive methods are preferred by patients and ultrasonography has virtually replaced venography of the lower extremity.

TREATMENT TYPES

It is important for the sonographer to understand the various treatments for CVVI, as the use of ultrasound varies with the treatment option. Treatment options for superficial venous disease include stripping, ligation, thermal ablation, chemical ablation/sclerotherapy, and phlebectomy (microincision). Treatment for deep venous disease may include anticoagulation, valve replacement, venoplasty/stenting, and thrombolysis or chemical/physical recanalization.

Stripping and ligation of the superficial veins have been traditional treatments for decades. Ligation alone has been associated with "neovascularization." This side effect perhaps may be better described as neodilatation of small arteries and veins due to injury, fresh thrombosis, and inflammation.

Endovenous thermal ablation by radio-frequency or laser energy has become a popular choice for the treatment of saphenous and nonsaphenous trunk veins.[28-30] Thermal ablation has largely replaced

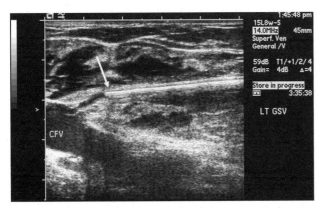

Figure 17-9 An ultrasound image of the great saphenous vein with a thermal ablation device in place just distal to the saphenofemoral junction *(arrow)*.

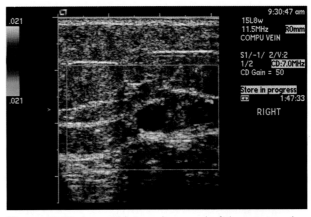

Figure 17-11 A postablation ultrasound of the great saphenous vein with no flow present.

stripping and ligation for many individuals. Thermal ablation begins with distal vein access under ultrasound guidance, step-up wires and sheaths placed, and the thermal device tip positioned in the saphenous vein at a relative distance from the confluence to the deep venous system (Fig. 17-9). Anesthesia is strategically placed in the saphenous sheath and surrounding areas (Fig. 17-10). Heating of the tip of the thermal device is activated and controlled by the physician, and the device is pulled back to the insertion site at a standard rate defined for the instrument used. Completion of the procedure is achieved once the device is successfully removed from the vein. Due to thermal injury inside the vein, the treated segment gradually shrinks and sonographically disappears over 6 to 9 months. Prior to this period, sonographic appearance of the thermally injured vein may inaccurately be termed "thrombosed" (Fig. 17-11).

Chemical ablation is the formal term for sclerotherapy, achieved with a foamed or liquid chemical (osmotic, detergent, or corrosive agent), which is injected into the vein.[31,32] A variety of superficial and saphenous veins are amenable to sclerotherapy.

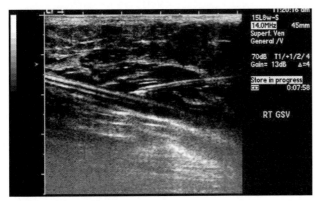

Figure 17-10 Tumescent anesthesia injected around the saphenous sheath and surrounding tissue.

Incompetent veins that are not visible from the skin are directed for injection with ultrasound guidance. Direct needle puncture into the vein and injection of the chemical is an effective treatment of small or tortuous veins, even as a complement of thermal ablation.

PATIENT PREPARATION

The patient symptoms are assessed and the basic components of the testing procedure are explained to the patient. The patient removes clothing from the waist down except for undergarments. Some laboratories instruct the patient to bring a pair of loose fitting shorts or should provide shorts for the patients. While standing, patients may wear their shoes or be provided nonslip booties. The sonographer reviews with the patient the Valsalva maneuver prior to the beginning of the examination.

PATIENT POSITIONING

The deep veins are evaluated initially in a reverse Trendelenburg position with the head and torso above the thigh, knee, and feet. The focus is to determine patency more so than unsuspected deep venous thrombosis. The classical recommendation is to evaluate lower extremity CVVI in the standing position. A platform facilitates ergonomics and patient stability (Fig. 17-12). Standing allows for optimal dilatation and venous filling. The patient shifts the weight onto the leg not being examined.

Exceptions to the standing positioning include examination of patients with advanced CVVI with obvious varicose veins and/or severe reflux of the major superficial and/or deep veins. Standing may also be contraindicated in patients susceptible to fainting, motion sickness, dizziness, nausea, discomfort during standing, and in those with a handicap. The recommended position if a standing test

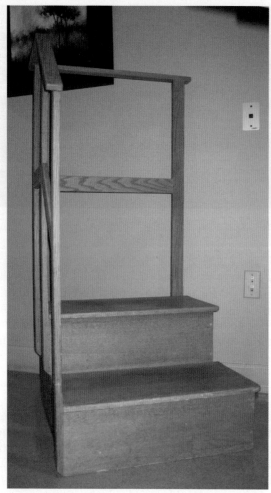

Figure 17-12 A platform device used for evaluation of patients in the standing position.

cannot be performed is a reverse Trendelenburg position.

The following order is recommended to optimize the standing examination:
1. Most symptomatic or affected thigh
2. Least symptomatic or affected thigh
3. Most symptomatic or affected calf or saphenous vein
4. Least symptomatic or affected calf or saphenous vein

Episodes of fainting or ill conditions most likely would occur after a thigh examination. Following the previous order, the thighs are examined first and the patient can then rest and recover if necessary. Veins in the calf, knee, and lower thigh can be examined in a less stressful sitting position (Fig. 17-13).

The patient rotates the knee outward during GSV examination of the great saphenous vein. The SSV can be examined with the patient facing the technologist, sideways, or with his or her back toward the technologist.

Technologist position must be addressed. Ergonometrics are paramount to a technologist's long-term professional health. The torso should be erect and not forcefully twisted because attention changes between instrument and patient. Elbows should be close to the body. One hand deals with instrument controls while the other handles the transducer. One foot controls compression/decompression maneuvers if using an automated cuff system. Positioning the patient on a platform minimizes arm extension as the veins are examined from groin to ankle. Height of the technologist's stool is accommodated to optimize body positioning differences among groin, thigh, knee, or calf examinations (Fig. 17-14).

EQUIPMENT

High-resolution duplex ultrasound with transducer frequencies ranging from 3.5 to 7.5 MHz and 7.5 to 17.0 MHz are recommended for deep and superficial venous testing, respectively. Linear transducers are ideal for extremity venous applications.

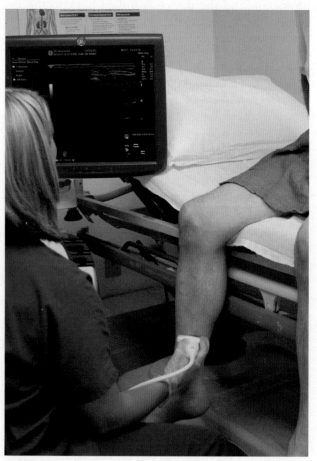

Figure 17-13 Proper patient and technologist position for a sitting CVI examination.

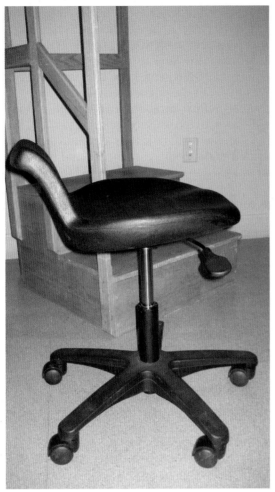

Figure 17-14 An adjustable examination stool used by technologists during venous evaluations.

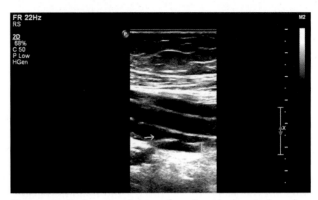

Figure 17-15 A sagittal image of a vein with chronic thrombus present *(arrow)*.

SCANNING TECHNIQUE

The essential protocol includes evaluation of patency and reflux in the deep veins, femoropopliteal veins, particularly the perforating veins, veins in the saphenous compartments, nonsaphenous superficial veins, and tributaries. Protocols also include the differential diagnoses of nonvenous pathologies such as arterial and lymphatic abnormalities and masses.

Evaluation of the deep veins precedes any CVVI testing. Detection of acute deep venous thrombosis (DVT) is rare; continuation of a CVVI examination becomes secondary and is not recommended. Interpreting and/or referring physicians should be contacted according to preestablished protocols. A preliminary report may be acceptable at certain institutions.

Detection of chronic deep venous obstruction, either total or partial, is part of a CVVI evaluation, and the examination is completed. Chronic venous obstruction is suspected in patients with a history of previous DVT (Fig. 17-15). Patients with chronic DVT deserve special hematological treatment beyond the scope of this chapter. Detection of acute superficial thrombosis or thrombophlebitis (STP) when inflammation is present does not deter continuation of CVVI examination. Protocol alternatives address the location and extension of STP. A recommendation is to treat superficial thrombosis at or near the saphenofemoral or saphenopopliteal junctions as potential DVT. Similarly, perforating or muscular vein thromboses are assessed for the potential risk of embolization before completing a CVVI examination.

The examination typically begins at the groin at or just above the level of the saphenofemoral junction. A focused evaluation of the deep veins documents the absence of a thrombus. Vein walls are imaged in a transverse plane and compressed with the transducer. Normal veins coapt completely. Chapter 14 describes techniques for a DVT examination.

Determination of Venous Flow Patterns

Once venous patency is confirmed, the examination continues with a determination of flow patterns using spectral Doppler. Various maneuvers are employed to alter venous flow in an attempt to produce retrograde flow. Color flow imaging can assist in the determination of flow directions and reflux times, but the traditional, accepted standard for reflux time measurement is via spectral Doppler. Flow recordings are localized and specific patterns of reflux can be inferred from such recordings. A complete evaluation of the GSV, for example, evaluates the terminal valve; preterminal valve; diffuse, proximal, segmental, or distal patterns of reflux; multiple sources of reflux causing multisegmental reflux; or atypical patterns involving multiple veins.[33,34] Patterns of reflux recurrence may be unusual after treatment.

Classical compression techniques using an automatic system are recommended to alter venous flow. A pneumatic cuff is wrapped around the thigh or the calf. Testing is performed in veins centrally located in relation to the cuff.

A cuff around the upper calf often provides compression sufficient to test the veins from the groin to behind the knee. Even ankle veins can be evaluated with the cuff in this position. Normal flow in a vein proximal to the cuff should increase during compression and should stop during decompression. Pathological flow or reflux occurs during decompression. Flow in a vein distal to the cuff should occur only during decompression. In this case, reflux would occur during compression.

Proper compression techniques using this cuff method require a pressure of 70 to 80 mm Hg to be applied quickly, held for a few seconds, and released quickly. Higher pressures may have to be applied to large extremities. The compressor must be filled with enough air and the hoses must be large enough, particularly if a large cuff is employed. The applied pressure may vary depending on the relative size of the cuff to the thigh or calf. The applied pressure decreases significantly with tissue depth if a small cuff is used. Tissue pressure decreases as the distance between tissue or vein and the skin increases. Large cuffs apply pressure to the deep tissues and veins more uniformly.

Reflux duration is dependent on the vein filling with blood and the vein emptying with compression. The duration of compression and the interval between compressions may affect reflux measurements. Sequential evaluations of reflux at multiple locations are also affected by compression duration and refilling time. As a standard, a minimum of 30 seconds between testing sites is recommended.

The automatic compression/decompression technique (known as rapid cuff inflation/deflation) is commonly commanded with a foot switch. This relieves the hands of the technologist to concentrate on the transducer and instrument controls. It is also considered a reproducible, standardized technique.

The "parana maneuver" presents physiological advantages. This method involves a touch provocation to force the patient to shift weight slightly forward and backward while the transducer interrogates the vein in real time. With skill and practice, the parana maneuver is reproducible and may best reflect the patient's own calf pump and valvular function.

Some examiners rely on hand compression, although this technique may introduce a large testing variability. A major justification is added variety of testing conditions. Unusual venous segments can be specifically tested. The amount and time of compression can be readily adapted to different veins, different anatomies, and different types of patients. Testing alternatives increase at the expense of consistency.

The Valsalva maneuver is commonly used to elicit reflux in the large, proximal veins of the lower extremity. Laughing, coughing, and talking are alternatives to a Valsalva maneuver.

Usually, reflux duration is measured during decompression of pressure applied distal to the site of measurement. Reflux time duration can also be measured under compression proximal to the site of observation. Reflux is then detected in a superficial vein as flow escapes to a different route in the presence, for example, of venous obstruction of the main draining channel.

Traditionally, reflux time measurement is performed using the spectral Doppler with the vein in a longitudinal image. Documentation should include this standard method as usual protocol or as validation of other methods used to detect reflux.

A greatly informative way of screening for reflux is with color flow transverse/oblique images. Multiple veins can be studied simultaneously. This technique is of great value while studying the great saphenous vein and one of its superficial tributaries at the lower thigh, for example. Another appropriate double vein evaluation is in the upper calf while observing reflux simultaneously in the GSV proper, or while differentiating the posterior and anterior arches or other tributaries. Recirculating reflux is particularly obvious while studying two veins simultaneously with color flow. Reflux time can also be screened with spectral Doppler using a transverse/oblique ultrasound image. Although this technique is adequate for detection of severe reflux, the report must validate such findings with spectral Doppler in longitudinal images.

PROTOCOL REQUIREMENTS

CVVI is concerned primarily with abnormal reverse flow, or reflux, in superficial (and deep) veins of the lower extremities. Given the scanning techniques described in the preceding section, images are obtained documenting B-mode characteristics, spectral Doppler waveforms, or color flow to demonstrate the following findings:

- Compressibility or coaptability of the femoro-popliteal veins at various levels, tested by manual compression with the transducer at the skin surface
- Patency and flow characteristics of the common femoral vein at one level, with color flow and spectral Doppler waveforms
- Patency and flow characteristics of the femoral vein at one or more levels, with color flow and spectral Doppler waveforms

- Documentation of a dual femoral vein
- Patency and flow characteristics of the popliteal vein at one level, with color flow and spectral Doppler waveforms
- Condition of calf veins in patients with localized signs and symptoms showing risk for DVT or chronic obstruction below the knee
- Flow characteristics in segmental levels of the saphenous veins including the GSV, AASV, PASV, VOG, and SSV
- Flow characteristics of nonsaphenous veins potentially associated with varicose veins or pelvic source drainage
- Possible involvement of pelvic veins or veins proximal to the groin
- Any unusual venous or nonvenous finding

Documentation may be simplified during screening protocols and may have to be more complex depending on the objectives of pretreatment mapping protocols. Peritreatment protocols are dependent on the type of treatment and the specific objectives. Follow-up protocols are also dependent on the objectives of the examination and intended treatment.

Screening for CVVI with US

The basic protocol includes image documentation of any anomaly of the femoropopliteal veins and a single documentation of the saphenous or nonsaphenous abnormality. The scans of the deep and superficial veins follow the pattern described previously but can be interrupted after the discovery of a single abnormality. The scan may also focus primarily on the region with the highest suspicion of an abnormality, for example, during the search of the source of obvious varicose veins.

DEFINITIVE DIAGNOSIS FOR CVVI WITH US

The protocol may vary depending on the objective of the test and the potential treatment. There are three common test objectives. The first is the selection of patients for thermal ablation of the GSV in the thigh. The protocol comprises a standard evaluation of the femoropopliteal veins and the GSV in the thigh. Additionally, (1) a limited evaluation of the GSV and SSV in the calf are performed, and (2) the calf deep veins may have to be studied depending on signs and symptoms.

The second is the examination of patients of a phlebology clinic with perioperative US capabilities. A complete examination included the femoropopliteal, the saphenous veins, and nonsaphenous veins related to visible varicose veins. The infrapopliteal deep veins are examined as a function of signs and symptoms. Details of the exact location of reflux

sources and drainage points are not necessary because vein mapping is performed at the time of treatment.

The third type of objective is the examination of patients for limited or extensive stripping/ligation/phlebectomy procedures. A complete examination includes a detailed drawing of refluxing and nonrefluxing veins plus segments not visualized. Perforating veins, sources, and drainage points are precisely located. Vertical and circumferential measurements are performed. Distance from the sole of the foot determines the vertical location. Distance from the tibial tuberosity, for example, determines the circumferential position of the venous finding. The physician would then perform treatment based either on a paper drawing or on a mapping on the skin of the patient. Some procedures may require measurements or skin marking very close to treatment day, often with the patient in the standing and operative position.

Saphenous sparing techniques, such as a CHIVA (French acronym for conservative and hemodynamic treatment of venous insufficiency in ambulatory care) procedure, may require additional information to determine the new flow pathways through the venous channels left open in the extremity.

Peritreatment US

The role of US in venous disease has expanded beyond a diagnostic tool and is commonly used during treatments such as thermal and chemical ablation. During thermal ablation, US is often used to map the course of the vein being treated on the patient's skin. The site of the venous incision is selected with US, and needles, introducers, guide wires, and laser or radio-frequency catheters are inserted under ultrasound guidance. The tip of the thermal ablation catheter is placed at an appropriate distance from the saphenofemoral junctions under direct US visualization. The introduction of the tumescent anesthesia is performed under ultrasound guidance. At the completion of the ablation procedure, US confirms obstruction of the treated vein and the lack of deep venous thrombosis. US can also demonstrate local recanalization of the treated vein, tributaries approaching the treated vein with potential risk for recanalization, and other superficial veins, which may need subsequent, complementary procedures.

US during Chemical Ablation or Foam Sclerotherapy

There are a few simple, primary applications of US. Imaging of the vein is performed during needle insertion. US can follow the hyperechoic foam as it flows through the treated vein and can be used to warn the physician if the foam approaches a perforating vein, the saphenofemoral junction, or saphenopopliteal junction. Transthoracic cardiac US can be used to observe the foam arrival in the right heart.[35,36] Transthoracic cardiac US may show bubbles in the left heart, indicating the presence of a right to left shunt or a patent foramen ovale (PFO). Transcranial Doppler (TCD) US may demonstrate the presence of high intensity transient signal (HITS) in the middle cerebral artery during foam sclerotherapy. Not all laboratories perform these adjunctive ultrasounds.

Follow-up US

Postablation protocols include a limited evaluation of the deep veins to ensure patency as well as a complete examination of the treated vein. US can demonstrate if segments of the treated vein are fully fibrosed or if the vein is recanalized—totally or partially in diameter as well as completely or segmentally in its longitudinal extension.[37,38] A thrombus may be detected immediately after treatment or after months or years, due to recanalization and rethrombosis.

Patients are followed primarily because venous disease is constantly reoccurring even in treated extremities. The opposite leg may develop a treatable disease with time, or the treated leg may have new veins requiring treatment. The patient follow-up study is commonly bilateral and follows the same protocols as described for definitive diagnostic US. A common problem is a lack of adequate history on previous procedures. Technologists often discover that veins are absent or that treated veins are present.

PITFALLS

Equipment settings must be properly adjusted to accurately detect venous reflux. Some technical factors affecting reflux measurement include the following:
- Gain alters the sensitivity of spectral Doppler or color flow
- High persistence may result in false-positive color flow findings
- Velocity scales (physiologic term) or PRF (engineering term) also affect the spectral Doppler or color flow sensitivity to detection of reflux
- Different instruments have different settings and different characteristics and may affect reflux detection

There are alternate explanations to retrograde flow, although initially described as "reflux." Flow from a tributary filling in a segment of the vein after a compression/decompression maneuver may produce a reverse flow pattern if this flow enters below a valve sinus. Valve leakage can occur when valves take a long time to close or if they close but do not remain closed. Valve leakage may be delayed and occur after several seconds following the testing maneuver. Sometimes the valves can close normally, but a symptomatic patient may have valve leakage with every respiration. Reverse flow may occur by surgical correction of hemodynamics to preserve drainage. Flush ligation of the saphenofemoral junction, for example, may create reverse flow through the saphenous vein until the next distal perforating vein. This perforating vein thus becomes a treatment-designed junction where flow is shunted or directed to this new drainage point. CHIVA procedures commonly create reverse flow in successfully treated veins in a similar surgical method, as described previously.

DIAGNOSIS

B-MODE ULTRASOUND FINDINGS

Normal B-mode image findings will reveal smooth, thin-walled veins with no obvious change in venous diameter. The vein is fully compressible, and the lumen is hypoechoic.

B-mode images of an acute DVT show enlarged veins, particularly when compared to a normal, contralateral, equivalent venous segment. Veins are incompressible under pressure. The lumen appears hypoechoic or even anechoic. The thrombosed vein lumen becomes more hyperechoic as the DVT progresses to a subacute thrombosis and chronic obstruction. A thrombus may be seen filling the vein either partially or completely (Fig. 17-16).

B-mode images of chronic venous obstruction show diameters smaller than normal. The vein may be partially or totally incompressible. The aged thrombus may appear hyperechoic, and fibrous strands may be observed within the lumen (see Fig. 17-15).

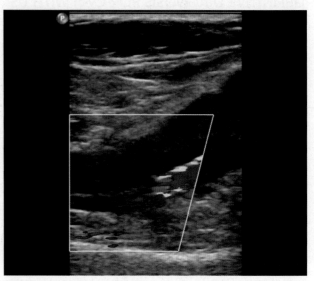

Figure 17-16 A vein with an acute thrombus present.

The veins may display possible tortuosity. Collateral veins develop and enlarge with time.

With chronic venous valvular insufficiency, the vein diameter enlarges, but the veins are completely compressible. The lumen is hypoechoic. Some of the valve sinuses may appear enlarged with flapping valve leaflets. The affected veins eventually become tortuous, varicosed, or even aneurysmal.

Immediately following thermal ablation, the vein is still anesthetized and compressed by tumescence; B-mode imaging may change rapidly or take months to reveal eventual results of treatment. In a postprocedural follow-up, typically at 6 to 9 months, the vein may be segmentally sonographically absent, fibrosed, thrombosed, or recanalized simultaneously at different sites along the course of the vein.[37,38]

SPECTRAL DOPPLER WAVEFORMS

Normal venous flow waveforms are spontaneous, phasic with respiration, and unidirectional toward the heart. Flow augments with distal compression or release of proximal compression (Fig. 17-17).

In the presence of an acute, fully occlusive DVT, the spectral Doppler waveform shows an absence of flow. Partially occlusive DVT, proximal thrombosis, or external compression can cause continuous flow. The lack of flow augmentation following distal compression or the release of proximal compression is observed in patients with acute DVT. Arterial flow waveforms can be present from within a lysing thrombus.

Flow is also absent with a complete chronic venous obstruction. A partial obstruction, a proximal obstruction, or an external compression can cause continuous flow and lack of flow augmentation, similarly to acute DVT. Spectral analysis may also reveal flow through small, tortuous channels within the diseased vein. Arterial, venous, or fistula-like flow may be observed in small vessels near the obstructed vein, and these may be a possible sign of

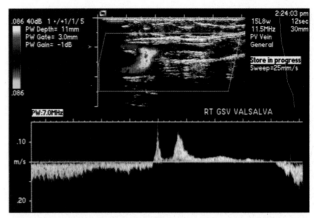

Figure 17-18 A venous Doppler signal demonstrating reflux during a Valsalva maneuver.

recanalization, neovascularization, or inflammation. Flow via dilated, collateral veins is common.

In patients with CVVI, chronic venous valvular insufficiency reverse flow or reflux are noted following proximal compression (includes Valsalva maneuver) or release of distal compression (Fig. 17-18). Turbulent flow may also be present within enlarged valve sinuses.

COLOR FLOW

Color flow shows the respiratory phasicity and flow augmentation of normal veins, findings better perceived with Doppler spectral analysis. Colors usually become lighter with increased flow and may alias.

Color detects no flow if DVT completely occludes the vessel. If a partial thrombus exists, color flow demonstrates flow around the thrombus. Perception of color flow augmentation depends on instrument settings and visual acuity.

Color flow has several advantages during the evaluation of chronic venous obstruction. Color flow through small, tortuous channels inside a chronically obstructed vein may be present. Arterial, venous, or fistula-like flow in small vessels near the obstructed vein may be present and may represent a possible sign of recanalization, neovascularization, or inflammation. Perception of collateral flow is dependent on venous dilatation or neoformation, flow patterns, and instrument settings.

Chronic venous valvular insufficiency will demonstrate retrograde color flow away from the heart. This may occur spontaneously, under proximal compression, or following the release of distal compression. Turbulent or multiple color flow patterns may be displayed within enlarged valve sinuses. An advantage of using color flow in transverse and longitudinal planes prior to spectral Doppler is to optimize the location of the sample volume in the region of the most perceived flow or reflux.

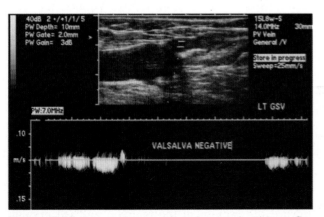

Figure 17-17 A normal venous Doppler signal with no reflux present.

PATHOLOGY BOX 17-1

Ultrasound Finding of CVVI

B-Mode (Grayscale)	Spectral Doppler	Color Flow Imaging
• Vein diameter enlarged • Valve sinuses enlarged • Tortuosity, varicosities, or venous aneurysms may be present	• Saphenous veins and tributaries retrograde flow >500 ms • Deep veins retrograde flow >1.0 s • Perforating veins retrograde flow >0.350 ms	• Retrograde flow color • Turbulent or multiple color patterns seen within valve sinuses

QUANTIFICATION OF REFLUX

Measurement of reflux duration is commonly preferred to measurement of peak reverse velocity or reflux volume flow rate. A classical, commonly referenced study was originally designed to describe normal values.[39] In the vast majority of normal subjects, saphenous vein valves close in less than 500 ms. The valves of the deep femoropopliteal veins close in less than 1 second. Perforating vein valves close in less than 350 ms. Longer durations are commonly considered as an abnormal reflux. A severely abnormal GSV typically has reflux durations longer than 2 seconds. The actual duration of reflux may depend on the diameter, the amount of venous blood volume stored distally, the strength and duration of distal compression, and characteristics of the distal venous network. Pathology Box 17-1 summarizes the duplex ultrasound findings of CVVI.

OTHER NONINVASIVE DIAGNOSTIC PROCEDURES

Two classical technologies, photoplethysmography (PPG) and air plethysmography (APG), have been used as a screening tool and as a quantifier of venous abnormality, respectively. Recently, another indirect test has been employed in this patient population. This newer test employs a "red" light detector to aid in superficial vein mapping.

VENOUS PHOTOPLETHYSMOGRAPHY

PPG testing should be considered a screening procedure for the detection of reflux.[40] Source of reflux is mostly undetermined. A PPG transducer emits infrared light and detects the signal reflected back from the blood within the cutaneous vessels.

Compression/decompression maneuvers alter the quantity of blood under detection by the PPG. The amount of blood detected by the PPG is reduced when blood is pumped back toward the heart. Upon completion of the maneuvers, blood volume returns and the sensor displays the return.

Patient Position

The patient is examined in a sitting position with legs dependent. The PPG is placed against the skin in the medial aspect of the calf. A common placement is about 10 to 15 cm above the medial malleolus. Other positions may be used for additional testing. The PPG positioned on the posterior aspect of the lower calf would provide information about small saphenous vein reflux.

Technique and Required Documentation

Once the patient and the PPG transducer are appropriately positioned, the examination begins with recording a baseline tracing while the limb is relaxed and no muscular contractions are occurring. The next step is to produce emptying of the calf venous blood volume. This is done using muscular contractions with flexion/relaxation of the foot. About 5 to 10 ft flexion maneuvers are common practice. The PPG tracing is recorded during these maneuvers. A resting horizontal line is usually placed near the top of a 5-cm wide strip paper. The tracing falls to the bottom of the strip paper during the flexion/relaxation of the foot. The tracing returns to the baseline position during the recovery period with the foot at rest and leg relaxed. The timing of blood return to the region indicates the presence or absence of reflux. Tracings may be observed on a monitor, but paper graphic registration is recommended. A common recording speed is 25 mm/s or about 0.5 to 1 cm/min.

The test can be repeated with the use of a tourniquet in an attempt to differentiate a superficial reflux from a deep system reflux. A tourniquet can be placed around the thigh or other location over the great saphenous vein. The tourniquet can also be used to occlude the small saphenous vein by placing the tourniquet around the upper third of the calf. Changes in the recording both with and without the tourniquets in place may indicate different portions of the venous system are incompetent.

Paper registry should be filled with information about (1) the instrument used; (2) the time scale; (3) the anatomical location of the PPG; (4) the resting trace showing arterial pulses and stable baseline; (5) the clear tracing during foot flexion, usually toward the bottom of the registry; and (6) enough paper length documenting recovery time.

Diagnostic Criteria

Venous recovery time or refilling time (VRT) is the parameter measured during PPG. VRT is usually measured from the end of flexion/relation period to about 90% to 95% of the distance between the bottom of the curve and the baseline tracing. Recovery time is usually greater than 20 seconds.

Venous reflux is suspected if the PPG tracing takes less than 20 seconds to return to baseline. Severe reflux may be suggested if the recovery time is less than 10 seconds.

If results are abnormal, the use of a tourniquet proximal to the PPG location may indicate a superficial or deep vein source for reflux. With a tourniquet in place over the GSV in the thigh, if the VRT returns to normal, then GSV incompetence is suspected. If the recovery time remains abnormal with the use of the tourniquet, then a deep vein reflux is suspected. Similar principles are applied to the detection of a small saphenous vein reflux. With a tourniquet placed in the upper third of the calf, if VRT normalizes, then SSV reflux is likely.

AIR PLETHYSMOGRAPHY

APG is a recommended technique for quantification of chronic venous insufficiency.[41] Clinically, APG can be used to detect physiologic abnormalities to clearly differentiate a pathophysiologic condition from an apparent aesthetic problem. A comparison between serial APG testing can demonstrate and quantify disease evolution. A comparison between pretreatment and posttreatment APG testing can demonstrate immediate quantifiable improvement, particularly in patients in the C4B, C5, and C6 clinical CEAP categories showing skin changes that are not readily modifiable. Immediate and long-term posttreatment APG testing can be used to demonstrate either improvement due to treatment or disease evolution.

Patient Position

Patient training and performance is paramount to obtaining reliable results. The patient is asked to perform a series of maneuvers requiring the movement from supine to standing positions. The specific positions are described in the following section that discusses these particular techniques.

Technique and Required Documentation

An APG examination is conducted as follows with particular care in the use of specific patient position sequencing:
- The subject rests supine to relax while receiving instructions and providing information pertinent to the test
- The sensing cuff is wrapped around the calf and is inflated to 10 mm Hg
- The leg is elevated to optimize emptying of venous volume
- The leg is brought back to a horizontal position; pressure in sensing cuff is readjusted to 10 mm Hg; in and out 100 mL calibration is performed with syringe
- The patient stands over the nontested leg holding onto a support structure and relaxing the leg being tested (a difficult task in this standing position)
- The patient rests the foot of the leg being tested on the floor and performs one toe raise, then relaxes; this movement is optional in a short protocol
- The patient performs 10 toe raises and relaxes
- The patient returns gently to the horizontal position

The following simplified APG measurements are recommended:
- Blood venous volume (VV; in milliliters) accumulated in the veins once the patient moves from a supine to a standing position
- Filling time (FT) demonstrating how long it takes to accumulate blood in the calf to 90% of VV once the patient stands
- Volumetric filling rate indicating blood accumulated per unit time (90% VV/FT in mL/s) as complement to filling time
- Residual volume (RV) measured as a percentage of venous volume (100 × RV/VV in %) indicating how much volume is pumped from the calf after 10 toe raises.

An extensive APG testing would also include:
- Measurement of the ejection fraction as a complement to a "residual volume" testing following one toe raise
- Total blood volume accumulated in the calf of a supine patient once a pneumatic cuff placed around the thigh is inflated to 80 mm Hg
- Volumetric emptying rate measured after the pneumatic cuff is deflated
- Differentiation of data from superficial and deep veins by repeating tests with a tourniquet applied around the knee, for example, to minimize the influence of the superficial veins.

Required documentation for the APG testing includes the tracings obtained during the various maneuvers. The tracing should illustrate the stable baseline at the bottom of the chart; the 100 mL calibration pulse; the exponential filling curve with the estimate of the venous volume VV, FT, and filling rate (90% VV/FT); the one toe raise curve for calculation of the ejection fraction (optional in the limited protocol); the 10 toe raise curve with the estimate of the RV; and the return to the baseline showing a posttest baseline curve deviating from the pretest baseline curve by no more than 5% to 10% of the VV.

Diagnostic Criteria

Normal values for VV are variable and will be dependent on gender, age, and other characteristics. Normal FT should be longer than 25 seconds. The venous filling rate (FR) should be less than 2 mL/s. The RV is normally less than 20% to 35%.

Abnormal findings include a very low VV, which may indicate a calf venous thrombosis or chronic obstruction. A high venous volume greater than for example, 100 mL should indicate abnormally high venous pooling due to large veins or numerous veins. An FT shorter than 10 seconds indicates severe reflux, whereas an FT shorter than 25 seconds suggests mild-to-moderate reflux. An FR greater than 2 mL/s indicates venous insufficiency, and ranges of this variable have been coarsely related to severity of venous diseases. An RV greater than 20% to 35% has been associated with increased ambulatory venous pressures, suggesting severity of disease according to the inability to empty the calf veins. Pathology Box 17-2 summarizes CVVI findings with PPG and APG.

Extensive APG evaluation may give parameters suggesting (1) proximal venous obstruction in the pelvic and abdominal regions, (2) differentiation between superficial and deep venous pathologies, (3) a nonfunctional calf muscle pump, (4) the

---

PATHOLOGY BOX 17-2

APG and PPG Results with CVVI

PPG	VRT >20 seconds
APG	FT >25 seconds FR <2 mL/s RV <20%–35%

VRT, venous refilling time (recovery time); FT, filling time; FR, filling rate; RV, residual volume.

---

effectiveness of elastic compression, and (5) venous versus nonvenous edematous changes.[41,42]

NEAR-INFRARED IMAGING[43,44]

Several imaging technologies are being developed to show superficial veins on the skin. These are not commonly employed, but some centers are using this technology to aid in venous imaging in this patient population. Imaging in the near-infrared range (880 to 930 nm) demonstrates subcutaneous veins with a diameter of 0.5 to 2 mm at a depth of 1 to 3 mm. This technology may help with guidance of venous access, phlebotomy, injection sclerotherapy, and control of laser interstitial therapy.

A highly processed method detects veins as deep as 8 mm from the skin. The vein is detected with near-infrared technology and is projected on the skin with green light.[44] The green light does not affect the infrared signal. Appropriate projection is the key to localizing veins that are going to be treated.

SUMMARY

Chronic venous valvular insufficiency is one of the most prevalent diseases. Proper clinical, etiological, anatomical, and pathophysiological descriptions of the patient being studied and/or treated are recommended. Color flow duplex ultrasonography has become the most useful technology for definitive diagnosis, pretreatment and peritreatment imaging, and procedure/patient follow-up.

Critical Thinking Questions

1. What is an anatomic feature that differentiates an anterior accessory saphenous vein (AASV) from the great saphenous vein (GSV)?

2. A patient is old and reports episodes of dizziness in the past. Your examination table cannot be put into a reverse Trendelenburg position. What can you do to accurately complete your CVVI examination?

3. You are having difficulty demonstrating retrograde flow in a patient with extensive varicose veins. What equipment settings should you check and why?

REFERENCES

1. Eklöf B, Rutherford RB, Bergan JJ, et al. Revision of the CEAP classification for chronic venous disorders: consensus statement. *J Vasc Surg.* 2004;40(6):1248–1252.

2. Beebe HG, Bergan JJ, Berggvist D, et al. Classification and grading of chronic venous disease in the lower limbs—a consensus statement. Organized by Straub Foundation with the co-operation of the American Venous Forum at the 6th annual meeting, February 22-25, 1994, Maui, Hawaii. *Vasa.* 1995;24(4):313–318.

3. Porter JM, Moneta GL. International consensus committee on chronic venous disease. Reporting standards in venous disease: an update. *J Vasc Surg.* 1995;21(4):625–645.

4. Caggiati A, Bergan JJ, Gloviczki P, et al. Nomenclature of the veins of the lower limbs: an international interdisciplinary consensus statement. *J Vasc Surg.* 2002;36(2):416–422.

5. Kachlik D, Pechacek V, Baca V, et al. The superficial venous system of the lower extremity: new nomenclature. *Phlebology.* 2010;25(3):113–123.

6. Coleridege-Smith P, Labropoulos N, Partsch H, et al. Duplex ultrasound investigation of the veins in chronic venous disease of the lower limbs—UIP consensus document. Part I. Basic principles. *Eur J Vasc Endovasc Surg.* 2006;31(3):83–92.

7. Cavezzi A, Labropoulos H, Partsch S, et al. Duplex ultrasound investigation of the veins in chronic venous disease of the lower limbs—UIP consensus document. Part II. Anatomy. *Eur J Vasc Endovasc Surg.* 2006;31(3):288–299.

8. Robertson L, Evans C, Fowkes FG. Epidemiology of chronic venous disease. *Phlebology.* 2008;23(3):103–111.

9. Cesarone MR, Belcaro G, Nicolaides AN, et al. "Real" epidemiology of varicose veins and chronic venous diseases: the San Valentino Vascular Screening Project. *Angiology.* 2002;53(2):119–130.

10. Carpentier PH, Maricq HR, Biro C, et al. Prevalence, risk factors, and clinical patterns of chronic venous disorders of lower limbs: a population-based study in France. *J Vasc Surg.* 2004;40(4):650–659.

11. Maffei FH, Magaldi C, Pinho SZ, et al. Varicose veins and chronic venous insufficiency in Brazil: prevalence among 1755 inhabitants of a country town. *Int J Epidemiol.* 1986;15(2):210–217.

12. Evans CJ, Fowkes FG, Ruckley CV, et al. Prevalence of varicose veins and chronic venous insufficiency in men and women in the general population: Edinburgh Vein Study. *J Epidemiol Community Health.* 1999;53(3):149–153.

13. McLafferty RB, Lohr JM, Caprini JA, et al. Results of the national pilot screening program for venous disease by the American Venous Forum. *J Vasc Surg.* 2007;45(1):142–148.

14. McLafferty RB, Passman MA, Caprini JA, et al. Increasing awareness about venous disease: the American Venous Forum expands the National Venous Screening Program. *J Vasc Surg.* 2008;48(2):394–399.

15. Ruckley CV, Evans CJ, Allan PL, et al. Telangiectasia in the Edinburgh Vein Study: epidemiology and association with trunk varices and symptoms. *Eur J Vasc Endovasc Surg.* 2008;36(6):719–724.

16. Mäkivaara LA, Ahti TM, Luukkaala T, et al. Persons with varicose veins have a high subsequent incidence of arterial disease: a population-based study in Tampere, Finland. *Angiology.* 2007;58(6):704–709.

17. Maurins U, Hoffmann BH, Lösch C, et al. Distribution and prevalence of reflux in the superficial and deep venous system in the general population—results from the Bonn Vein Study, Germany. *J Vasc Surg.* 2008;48(3):680–687.

18. Evans CJ, Allan PL, Lee AJ, et al. Prevalence of venous reflux in the general population on duplex scanning: the Edinburgh vein study. *J Vasc Surg.* 1998;28(5):767–776.

19. Drinan KJ, Wolfson PM, Steinitz D, et al. Duplex imaging in lymphedema. *J Vasc Technol.* 1993;17:23–26.

20. Rutherford RB, Padberg FT, Comerota AJ, et al. Venous severity scoring: an adjunct to venous outcome assessment. *J Vasc Surg.* 2000;31(6):1307–312.

21. Moura RM, Gonçalves GS, Navarro TP, et al. Relationship between quality of life and the CEAP clinical classification in chronic venous disease. *Rev Bras Fisioter.* 2010;14(2):99–105.

22. Darvall KA, Sam RC, Bate GR, et al. Changes in health-related quality of life after ultrasound-guided foam sclerotherapy for great and small saphenous varicose veins. *J Vasc Surg.* 2010;51(4):913–920.

23. Shepherd AC, Gohel MS, Brown LC, et al. Randomized clinical trial of VNUS ClosureFAST radiofrequency ablation versus laser for varicose veins. *Br J Surg.* 2010;97(6):810–818.

24. Garratt AM, Macdonald LM, Ruta DA, et al. Towards measurement of outcome for patients with varicose veins. *Qual Health Care.* 1993;2(1):5–10.
25. Launois R, Reboul-Marty J, Henry B. Construction and validation of a quality of life questionnaire in chronic lower limb venous insufficiency (CIVIQ). *Qual Life Res.* 1996;5(6):539–554.
26. Engelhorn C, Engelhorn A, Salles-Cunha S, et al. Relationship between reflux and greater saphenous vein diameter. *J Vasc Technol.* 1997;21:167–172.
27. Morrison N, Salles-Cunha SX, Neuhardt DL, et al. Prevalence of reflux in the great saphenous vein as a function of diameter. Paper presented at: 21st Annual Congress, American College of Phlebology; November 8–11, 2007; Tucson, AZ. Congress Syllabus 111.
28. Morrison N. Saphenous ablation: what are the choices, laser or RF energy. *Semin Vasc Surg.* 2005;18(1):15–18.
29. Lurie F, Creton D, Eklof B, et al. Prospective randomized study of endovenous radiofrequency obliteration (closure) versus ligation and vein stripping (EVOLVeS): two-year follow-up. *Eur J Vasc Endovasc Surg.* 2005;29(1):67–73.
30. Tzilinis A, Salles-Cunha SX, Dosick SM, et al. Chronic venous insufficiency due to great saphenous vein incompetence treated with radiofrequency ablation: an effective and safe procedure in the elderly. *Vasc Endovasc Surg.* 2005;39(4):341–345.
31. Morrison N, Neuhardt DL, Rogers CR, et al. Comparisons of side effects using air and carbon dioxide foam for endovenous chemical ablation. *J Vasc Surg.* 2008;47(4):830–836.
32. Morrison N, Neuhardt DL, Rogers CR, et al. Incidence of side effects using carbon dioxide-oxygen foam for chemical ablation of superficial veins of the lower extremity. *Eur J Vasc Endovasc Surg.* 2010;40(3):407–413.
33. Engelhorn CA, Engelhorn AL, Cassou MF, et al. Patterns of saphenous reflux in women with primary varicose veins. *J Vasc Surg.* 2005;41(4):645–645.
34. Engelhorn CA, Engelhorn AL, Cassou MF, et al. Patterns of saphenous venous reflux in women presenting with lower extremity telangiectasias. *Dermatol Surg.* 2007; 33(3): 282–288.
35. Hansen K, Morrison N, Neuhardt DL, et al. Transthoracic echocardiogram and transcranial Doppler detection of emboli after foam sclerotherapy of leg veins. *J Vasc Ultrasound.* 2007;31(4):213–216.
36. Morrison N, Neuhardt DL. Foam sclerotherapy: cardiac and cerebral monitoring. *Phlebology.* 2009;24(6):252–259.
37. Salles-Cunha SX, Rajasinghe H, Dosick SM, et al. Fate of the great saphenous vein after radio frequency ablation: detailed ultrasound imaging of the treated segment. *Vasc Endovasc Surg.* 2004;38(4):339–344.
38. Salles-Cunha SX, Comerota AJ, Tzilinis A, et al. Ultrasound findings after radiofrequency ablation of the great saphenous vein: descriptive analysis. *J Vasc Surg.* 2004; 40(6): 1166–1173.
39. Labropoulos N, Tiongson J, Pryor L, et al. Definition of venous reflux in lower-extremity veins. *J Vasc Surg.* 2003;38(4):793–798.
40. Beraldo S, Satpathy A, Dodds SR. A study of the routine use of venous photoplethysmography in a one-stop vascular surgery clinic. *Ann R Coll Surg Engl.* 2007;89(4): 379–383.
41. Christopoulos DG, Nicolaides AN, Szendro G, et al. Air-plethysmography and the effect of elastic compression on venous hemodynamics of the leg. *J Vasc Surg.* 1987;5(1):148–159.
42. Pizano RN. Guias Colombianas para el Diagnostico y el Manejo de los Desordenes Cronicos de las Venas (Columbian Guidelines for the Diagnosis and Management of Chronic Disorders of the Veins). Editor Guadalupe S.A, Bogota, D.C., 2009, 247.
43. Zharov VP, Ferguson S, Eidt JF, et al. Infrared imaging of subcutaneous veins. *Lasers Surg Med.* 2004;34(1):56–61.
44. Miyake RK, Zeman HD, Duarte FH, et al. Vein imaging: a new method of near infrared imaging, where a processed image is projected onto the skin for the enhancement of vein treatment. *Dermatol Surg.* 2006;32(8):1031–1038.

18 | Aorta and Iliac Arteries

Kathleen A. Carter and Jenifer F. Kidd

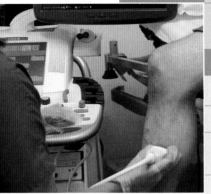

OBJECTIVES

Identify the characteristics of a complete aortoiliac duplex imaging exam

Define aortic and iliac aneurysms

Describe the importance of orthogonal orientation in the measurement of aneurysms

Identify three key characteristics that should be evaluated when assessing iliac stents

List three frequent complications associated with aortic endograft repair (EVAR)

List four types of endoleaks and their frequency

KEY TERMS

aneurysm | aortoiliac | aortoiliac disease | atherosclerosis | endoleak | endovascular aneurysm repair (EVAR) | fusiform | iliac stent | long-term surveillance | saccular

GLOSSARY

aneurysm a localized dilatation of the wall of an artery

endoleak the continued blood flow into an excluded aneurysm after endovascular placement of a stent graft

endovascular aneurysm repair a form of minimally invasive surgery in which a stent graft

is placed inside an aneurysm providing a new channel for blood flow and excluding flow from the dilated walls of an artery

fusiform elongated, spindle-shaped

saccular a saclike or pouch-like bulging

stent a tubelike structure placed inside a blood vessel to provide patency and support

Color duplex ultrasonography (CDU) can be an important modality for the diagnosis and postintervention follow-up of pathology in the aorta and iliac arteries. Ultrasound has been used for many years to detect and follow the presence of abdominal aortic aneurysm (AAA).[1] The first use of ultrasound to demonstrate the size of an AAA was reported in 1961 by Donald and Brown.[2] Studies have also shown excellent correlation of ultrasound with arteriography in the detection of aortoiliac atherosclerotic disease.[3,4] CDU provides both anatomic as well as physiologic information, is noninvasive,

nontoxic, and well tolerated by patients. It allows the examiner to make both qualitative as well as quantitative assessment of blood flow using a combination of pulsed wave and color Doppler.

Ultrasound can rapidly differentiate aortic aneurysmal disease from tortuosity, adjacent visceral aneurysms, or retroperitoneal lymphadenopathy.[5] The incidence of AAA in the US population is 60/1,000.[6] It is the 12th leading cause of death, with approximately 15,000 deaths from ruptured aortic aneurysms in the US annually.[7] AAA occurs with more frequency in older men and is found most often inferior to the renal arteries. Aortic aneurysms are commonly associated with iliac, femoral, and popliteal aneurysms with some reports of almost a 20% incidence of associated popliteal aneurysms.[8] The most common abnormality of the iliac arteries noted on ultrasound is aneurysmal dilatation with an incidence one-tenth as common as aneurysms of the aorta.[9,10]

SONOGRAPHIC EXAMINATION TECHNIQUES

A complete aortoiliac duplex ultrasound or a limited aortoiliac duplex ultrasound is performed based on the indication for the study and whether the exam is preintervention or postintervention. Indications for aortoiliac duplex ultrasound include pulsatile abdominal mass, suspected or known aortic or iliac aneurysm disease, claudication (usually of the hip or buttock areas) that interferes with the patient's occupation or lifestyle, ischemic rest pain, decreased femoral pulses, abdominal bruit, and emboli in ischemic digits (also known as blue toe syndrome). Additionally, a duplex may be performed following lower extremity physiologic studies indicating inflow disease, after intervention (postoperative angioplasty or poststent evaluation), or as a follow-up to iliac revascularization.

PATIENT PREPARATION

Patients should fast overnight (8 to 12 hours) to minimize the amount of scatter and attenuation from bowel gas. Medication or bowel prep is usually not necessary. Patients can take morning medications with water. Gum chewing or smoking the morning of the exam is discouraged because this may increase the swallowing of air that could further obscure the field of view. The procedure and its length should be explained to the patient.

PATIENT POSITIONING

The patient should be supine in a comfortable position with the head elevated. The examiner should be seated comfortably, slightly higher than the patient with the scanning arm supported. In patients with large abdominal girth, it may sometimes be necessary for the sonographer to push on the abdomen to bring the aorta and iliac arteries into better view. Considerable transducer pressure on the abdomen can help displace abdominal contents and bowel gas without too much discomfort to the patient. When using this technique, inform the patient and request that he or she report if there is any discomfort. In addition, it is ergonomically important that the examiner shoulder

be positioned over the transducer so as to allow the examiner's body weight to help push rather than to put strain on the arm or elbow. It is often helpful to place the patient in a lateral decubitus view when an anterior–posterior approach is obscured by abdominal contents, bowel gas, or scar tissue.

EQUIPMENT

High-resolution ultrasound equipment using robust color flow and spectral Doppler capability is necessary for good assessment of the aortoiliac segments deep in the abdomen. The system must have the penetration ability to clearly image deep vessels and structures with good tissue differentiation as well as adequate color Doppler sensitivity. Low frequency transducers with imaging and Doppler carrier frequencies ranging from 2-5 MHz are used most often. Curved linear transducers are best for optimum resolution. However, based on patient girth and condition, the sector transducers with frequencies of 2-4 MHz can be used. Additionally, gel, wipes, and hardcopy documentation apparatuses and supplies are needed.

SCANNING TECHNIQUE

AAA Protocol

When an ultrasound study is performed for the assessment of AAA, evaluation is performed of the subdiaphragmatic aorta and the common iliac arteries. Beginning at the level of the celiac axis and extending to the femoral bifurcation, examine the aorta and iliac arteries with B-mode in both transverse and sagittal planes. The iliac arteries are usually easier to follow in a longitudinal plane. The normal aorta lies immediately adjacent to the spine, has smooth margins, no focal dilatation, and tapers toward the terminal aorta at about the level of the umbilicus (Fig. 18-1). Transverse images with diameter measurements are

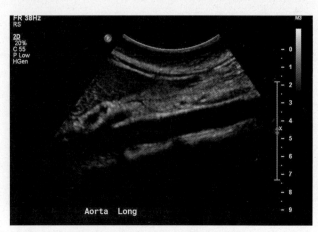

Figure 18-1 Normal tapering aorta in longitudinal view.

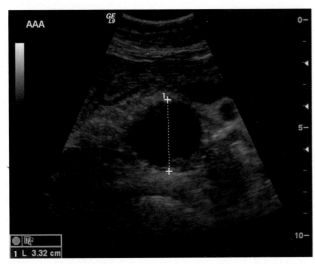

Figure 18-2 Transverse view of the aorta with an AP diameter measurement.

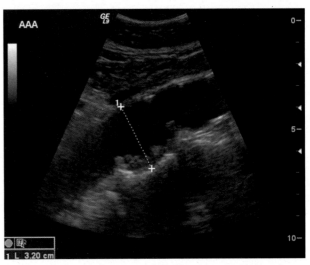

Figure 18-3 Longitudinal view of the aorta with calipers placed perpendicular to the long axis or the aorta.

documented from the proximal aorta (near the diaphragm), mid-aorta (near the renal arteries), and distal aorta above the bifurcation of the iliac arteries. The diameter measurements may include both anterior-to-posterior (AP) wall measurements as well as left-to-right lateral wall measurements; however, it is the AP measurement that is most reliable. The lateral wall edges are subject to acoustic dropout and thus are less accurate (Fig. 18-2). Measurements of the proximal common iliac arteries are also documented. Longitudinal images with AP diameter measurements are taken from the outer wall to outer wall of the aorta, taking care that the measurements are perpendicular to the long axis of the aorta (Fig. 18-3).[11] This is particularly important in those patients with angulation of the aortic neck. Angulation can occur as the aorta enlarges in diameter, when it often elongates. This elongation results in angulation of the proximal neck, with larger diameter aneurysms having more angulated necks.[12] Studies comparing three-dimensional (3D) computed tomography (CT) reconstruction with ultrasound have shown that both allow for the assessment of the aorta in the orthogonal plane and both avoid oblique cuts due to aortic neck angulation that would overestimate the diameter.[13] Because the decisions for management of abdominal aortic aneurysms depend on the precise determination of aneurysm size, it is critically important that the sonographer makes sure that the transducer is orthogonal or perpendicular to the aorta itself, and not necessarily transverse or parallel to the long axis of the body. Typically, a transverse approach to the aorta, as shown in Figure 18-2, will provide the most accurate orthogonal assessment of the aorta. In addition to aortic measurements, in the presence of a focal aneurysm, it is important to note its length, its proximity to the renal arteries, and the

presence and extent of any intraluminal thrombi. The presence of a thrombus, residual lumen, dissection, flaps, pseudoaneurysms, wall defects, stenoses, and/or occlusion should be documented. When plaque is encountered, characterize the plaque as to its echogenicity and presence of calcification.

An additional segmental Doppler sampling of velocities along the course of the aorta and iliac arteries will reveal any concurrent atherosclerotic disease of hemodynamic significance. All spectral Doppler waveforms are collected, maintaining an angle of 60° or less, parallel to the wall, and with the sample volume placed in the center stream of the vessel. This often requires manipulation of the transducer to avoid angles greater than 60°. The peak systolic velocity (PSV) should be recorded from the proximal, mid, and distal aorta as well as from each common iliac artery.

Preintervention Aortoiliac Protocol

The increasing use of endovascular therapy has changed the role of the vascular laboratory in many centers. In addition to having a diagnostic role, the vascular laboratory is often used today to assist in determining what type of treatment the patient may undergo. The scope of the stenoses and the disease identified should be noted. This careful duplex assessment can determine whether the disease is focal or diffuse; can determine the location, length, and severity of lesions; and with good visualization, can assist in determining residual diameters. Whether disease is present proximal or distal to the inguinal ligament is an important differentiation in the management of patients with lower extremity ischemia. In addition, duplex ultrasound can also determine the important distinction between severely stenotic iliac lesions from occlusion. These data will aid the physician in planning potential angioplasty/stent procedures and will help determine what type of intervention will be appropriate for the patient.

When the duplex is performed preintervention for atherosclerotic disease, symptoms of claudication, follow-up to known stenosis, or based on a positive physiologic exam, a comprehensive study is done. The general techniques described for an AAA evaluation are used for the preintervention evaluation. A combination of transverse and longitudinal views should be employed. The study should include the entire aorta (proximal, mid, and distal); the visceral vessel origins (celiac, superior mesenteric artery, inferior mesenteric artery [IMA], and renal artery origins); proximal, mid, and distal common iliac arteries (CIAs); proximal, mid, and distal external iliac arteries (EIAs); the internal iliac (hypogastric) arteries; the common femoral arteries (CFAs); and the superficial femoral and profunda femoral artery (SFA, PFA) origins. The internal iliac artery origin is important to identify as a landmark ending the CIA segment and beginning the EIA. The internal iliac artery is not always seen in the same plane as the external iliac artery. Diameter measurements and velocities are recorded from each of these segments.

Postintervention Aortoiliac Protocol

The rationale of following patients after intervention is based on several indications. First, identification and treatment of restenosis prior to complete occlusion may improve patency rates. Second, it is thought that stenoses are technically easier to manage than occlusion. Finally, percutaneous transluminal angioplasty (PTA) and stent procedures are associated with a significant restenosis rate. The follow-up of aortic and iliac arteries postendovascular intervention requires knowledge of the location and extent of the angioplasty treatment area and/or stent placement. The stent structure within the arteries is not always easily visible by B-mode evaluation. Therefore, it is important to know where the stents have been placed to ensure the Doppler cursor is carefully walked throughout the entire length of the stent. The stent should be evaluated for alignment, full deployment, and relationship to the vessel wall (Fig. 18-4). Images of the stent and adjacent vessels should be recorded. As mentioned in preceding sections, the Doppler angles ideally should be 45° to 60° and always should be parallel to the vessel wall in the longitudinal plane when collecting peak systolic and end-diastolic waveforms. A limited duplex exam for postintervention patients typically may include assessment of the terminal aorta, common iliac arteries, external iliac arteries, and internal iliac arteries. The assessment can also include the

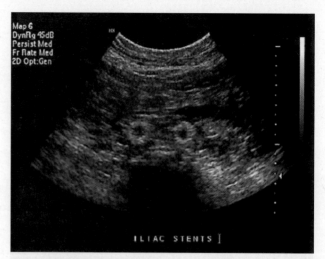

Figure 18-4 Transverse view of common iliac stents with normal stent deployment.

CFA, SFA, and PFA origins, depending on what type of intervention has been done. A general rule of thumb is to image several centimeters above and below any area treated by PTA and/or stenting as well as a thorough assessment of the treated segment(s). The PSV should be documented in the terminal aorta; the proximal, mid, and distal common iliac artery; the proximal internal iliac artery; and the proximal, mid, and distal external iliac artery.

TECHNICAL CONSIDERATIONS

Color flow imaging is a useful component to aortoiliac ultrasounds because it assists with vessel localization and aids in following these vessels. Color flow imaging is especially helpful in assessing the iliac arteries. The iliac arteries are often deep and tortuous as they travel within the pelvis. It may be helpful to place patients in a lateral decubitus position in order to evaluate the length of the iliac arteries. Using color flow imaging in a sagittal view can help obtain properly aligned spectral Doppler waveforms. Care should be taken to adjust the color scale or pulse repetition frequency (PRF) appropriate to the segment being assessed in order to identify areas of increased velocity.

PITFALLS

Although all abdominal duplex ultrasound examinations have challenges (e.g., bowel gas, obesity, and tortuosity of vessels), in most instances the aortoiliac segments can be adequately assessed using thorough use of protocols, proper technique, and adequate time allowance. There are certain limitations that may prevent complete evaluation of the aortoiliac segments such as recent abdominal surgery, open wounds, indwelling abdominal catheters, or pregnancy in the second or third trimester.

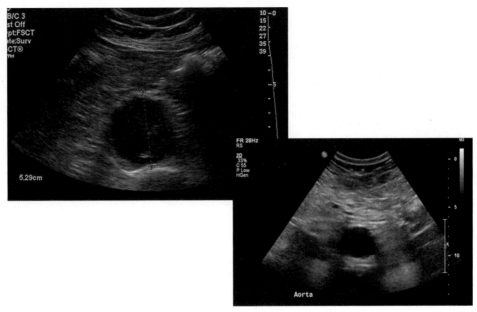

Figure 18-5 Transverse image of fusiform aneurysm.

DIAGNOSIS

The normal aortic diameter is usually less than 2 cm and tapers as it courses distally. Abnormalities are usually defined as a focal dilation of the aorta involving all three layers of the aortic wall that exceeds the normal diameter by more than 50%, usually 3 cm or larger. The larger the dilation, the more risk there is for potential rupture. Focal diameter measurements greater than 3 cm are considered to be consistent with AAA. Ectasia is present when there are areas of dilation less than 3 cm or when there are irregular margins and a nontapering profile. Most aortic aneurysms are fusiform (Fig. 18-5), which involve the entire circumference of the affected portions of the aorta, whereas fewer aneurysms are saccular (Fig. 18-6). Saccular aneurysms are asymmetric outpouching dilations and are often caused by trauma or penetrating aortic ulcers.

The iliac artery is also considered to be aneurysmal when the diameter increases by 50% as compared to the adjacent segment. Generally, when the iliac arteries exceed a diameter of 1.5 cm, they are considered aneurysmal. Iliac aneurysms are usually associated with atherosclerotic disease and are often bilateral. Complications of iliac aneurysms can include rupture, hydronephrosis secondary to compression of the ureter, or even bladder compression in the presence of large bilateral iliac aneurysms.[14]

Thrombus, plaque, and calcification can also be identified within the aortoiliac system and will have the same ultrasound appearance as observed elsewhere within the vascular system. Plaque may appear heterogeneous or homogeneous with either smooth or irregular borders. Calcification will appear as bright hyperechoic areas that produce an acoustic shadowing. A thrombus is often homogeneous with smooth borders and is found within the sac of the aneurysm.

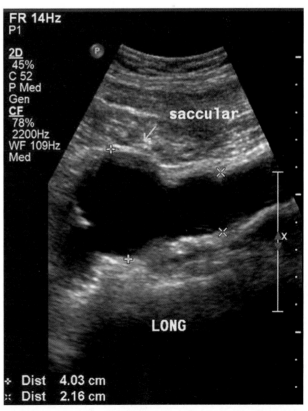

Figure 18-6 Longitudinal view of a saccular aneurysm.

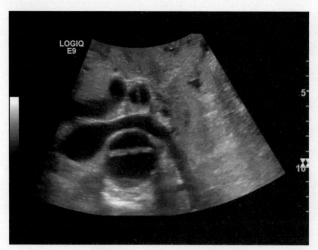

Figure 18-7 Transverse view of an aortic dissection.

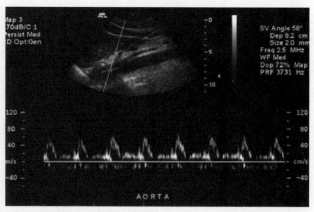

Figure 18-8 Lower resistance aortic spectral waveform superior to visceral vessel origins.

Wall defects can be encountered within the aorta and iliac arteries. Intimal tears may appear as small isolated defects on the vessel wall where a short piece of the vessel wall is separated from the remaining wall. This small piece of the wall will protrude into the vessel lumen. Dissections occur when a tear forms between the layers of the wall, usually at the intimal medial interface and then extends for several centimeters (Fig. 18-7). The initial tear weakens the wall of the aorta, which may enlarge. Existing aneurysms can also dissect. Acute dissections are readily identified by two channels of flow. Chronic dissection may be more challenging to identify when the false lumen has thrombosed and can be confused with stenosis or atherosclerotic disease.

In postinterventional patients, stents should be observed completely expanded to fill the vessel lumen. The walls of the stent should be opposed to the walls of the vessel. The stents should be closely examined to document any irregularities or changes in the shape. The stents should appear circular in transverse view. Elliptical-shaped stents may indicate partial stent compression. A kink within a stent may appear as a sharp angulation of the stent walls in an otherwise straight vessel segment.

Hemodynamics in the proximal aorta will have different waveform characteristics than the distal aorta. This is because the proximal aorta supplies the visceral arteries, which supply lower resistant vascular beds like the liver and kidneys. This is reflected in the waveform as shown in Figure 18-8. The distal aorta should be reflective of the higher resistant peripheral vascular bed, which normally has a reverse flow component in early diastole (Fig. 18-9). The hemodynamics in normal iliac segments should also be multiphasic with reversal of flow below the baseline in early diastole, reflective of the normally high resistant peripheral vascular system.

If a stenosis is identified, it is important to carefully assess the lesion throughout with spectral Doppler and document poststenotic turbulence. When a stent is in place, the spectral Doppler is "walked" through the proximal, mid, and distal ends of the stent. The sonographer should be aware of the location of all stents to ensure a complete assessment. The examination is completed with an evaluation of the CFA, the SFA, and the PFA origins. Their accompanying hemodynamics should validate the more proximal findings. For example, severe proximal disease will often result in turbulent or multiphasic-to-monophasic distal signals (Fig. 18-10A). Be sure to clearly denote any areas not well visualized. This is important because iliac arteries can have focal severe stenoses or occlusions with multiphasic flow distally, including the reverse flow component below the baseline if good collateralization is present. If a stenosis is encountered, the PSV of the prestenotic signal prior to the stenosis, the maximum PSV within the stenosis (Fig. 18-10B), and the poststenotic signal should be documented. When a ratio of 2:1 (or a 100% increase in velocity) with poststenotic turbulence is documented, there is at

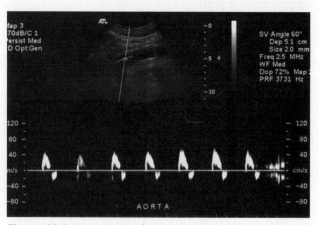

Figure 18-9 Spectral waveform of a normally high resistance distal aortic signal.

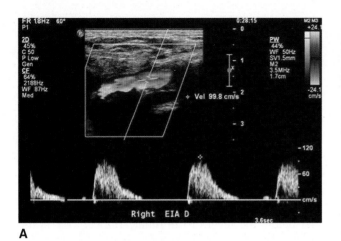

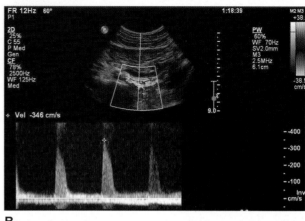

Figure 18-10 A: Abnormal spectral waveform associated with hemodynamically significant proximal disease. **B:** A LEIA spectral waveform within stenosis with a PSV of 346 cm/s.

least a 50% stenosis present. Care should be taken to remain in the artery of interest because elevated velocities in collateral vessels could be mistaken for stenosis. Tortuosity can also cause elevated velocities. In the absence of a stenosis, however, there is usually no poststenotic turbulence associated with the elevated velocity. Chronic iliac occlusions can be difficult to identify. The artery can become contracted and echogenic, and differentiation with the surrounding tissue may be challenging. It is helpful to identify and follow the companion vein when chronic occlusion is suspected (Fig. 18-11A,B).

AORTOILIAC DUPLEX ULTRASOUND FOLLOWING ENDOVASCULAR AORTIC STENT GRAFT REPAIR (EVAR)

The endovascular stent graft repair method of treating AAA has proven to be a much less invasive alternative procedure with lower incidences of perioperative mortality and improved survival rate compared

with conventional open surgical repair.[15] Recovery from this procedure is considerably shorter than with the traditional method, and there is no abdominal incision.

The endovascular aneurysm method of repair (i.e., EVAR) involves the placement of a stent graft device within the aortic aneurysm sac via a catheter-based delivery system through small groin incisions into the common femoral artery, and deployment is under angiographic guidance. The goal of this minimally invasive treatment is to achieve exclusion of the aneurysm sac from the general circulation, thereby reducing its risk of rupture.[16,17] Failure to isolate the aneurysm from the circulation where persistent blood flow is demonstrated outside the graft lumen but within the aneurysm sac has been defined as *endoleak* and is a common complication associated with many of the commercially available aortic stent graft devices.[18–20] Close surveillance, therefore, is mandatory after EVAR, as rupture is still possible if an endoleak is present because the aneurysm continues to be perfused at near-systemic arterial pressure. This has been

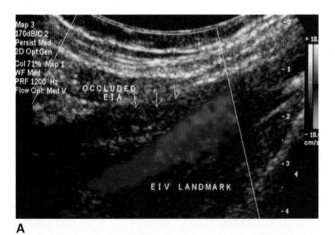

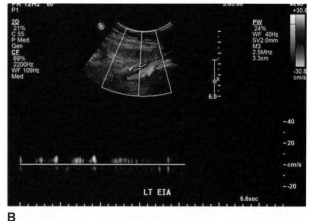

Figure 18-11 A: Identification of an iliac vein in the presence of an iliac artery occlusion. **B:** A spectral analysis documents an iliac artery occlusion.

shown to be true even with very small endoleaks. It is long-term surveillance and patient compliance that have become the key issues following the repair of AAAs by the endovascular method. Both CT angiography and CDU imaging have been the imaging modalities of choice postoperatively to evaluate and monitor stent grafts.

CDU has emerged as a low-cost and low-risk alternative imaging modality that is widely available without the exposure to ionizing radiation or the risk of nephrotoxicity in patients with marginal renal function. In many institutions, CDU is now used as a first choice method of surveillance post-EVAR, thus allowing CT scanning and aortography to be used more selectively to plan a secondary intervention. CDU can accurately monitor the residual aneurysm sac size, demonstrate graft and limb patency, has the ability to identify endoleaks and to determine the leak source, detect graft limb dysfunction and kinking, and in some cases, detect the migration of the stent graft device. It can provide the examiner with hemodynamic information that is not available with other imaging modalities.[21-25] Other complications associated with the procedural graft deployment that can cause iatrogenic injury due to the use of large bore catheters in the groin include arteriovenous fistulas, hematomas, intimal flaps, dissection, or pseudoaneurysms.

EVAR DEVICES

Prior to commencing the examination, it is important for the examiner to have a good working knowledge and understanding of the endovascular technique, as well as the aortic stent graft designs, and configurations that are currently available. The examiner should have the relevant patient information about what type of endograft device has been deployed and details of the operative procedure performed.

There are three basic types of aortic stent grafts currently used: bifurcated, straight tube, and uni-iliac grafts. These may be used in conjunction with side-branch occluding devices, coil embolization of branch vessels, extension grafts, and femoro-femoral crossover grafting. It is, however, the bifurcated modular stent graft that is most frequently deployed. The examiner should also be aware of the recent development and implantation of fenestrated grafts where there is transrenal aortic endograft fixation with renal artery stenting. The examiner will observe the graft material and metal struts extending above the usual position (below the renal arteries), and it is essential to identify renal artery patency after graft deployment to evaluate the technical success of the proximal fixation, which could adversely affect renal perfusion.

SCANNING TECHNIQUE

The examination is performed with the patient lying in the supine position. The examiner commences the study using B-mode imaging in the transverse plane, identifying the aorta at the level of the celiac axis and superior mesenteric arteries. The reflective metal struts of the aortic stent graft should be identified; as previously discussed, in some grafts these struts can be visualized above the level of the renal arteries. The proximal extent of the graft fabric is seen as a hyperechoic signal along the anterior and posterior walls of the aortic lumen (Fig. 18-12); it can be visualized just below the level of the renal arteries. This is the proximal attachment or fixation site. If the stent graft is bifurcated or uni-iliac, then the distal attachment or fixation site(s) would be the native common or external iliac artery. Often, the reflective struts or dilatation of the distal end of the graft limb to the native vessel can be readily observed (Fig. 18-13A,B).

The examiner then uses the caliper measurement on the ultrasound machine to measure the aorta at the level of the renal arteries in the both the anterio-posterior and transverse diameters as a baseline for comparison on follow-up studies to assess for possible dilatation of the aneurysm neck. The distance should be measured from landmarks such as the superior mesenteric or renal arteries in the longitudinal plane to the proximal attachment site for the detection of possible graft device migration. The assessment should be repeated along the entire length of the aorta, taking maximum orthogonal diameter measurements of the residual aneurysm sac. The vessel axis should be followed with measurements made perpendicular to the aorta, accommodating for vessel tortuosity so as to accurately obtain baseline transverse measurements that will be used for ongoing serial follow-ups of the residual sac (Fig. 18-14). The B-mode characteristics of the excluded sac should be noted, paying particular attention to any areas of hypoechogenecity or heterogeneity, as these

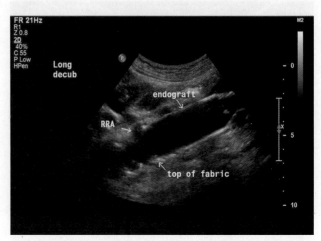

Figure 18-12 A hyperechoic signal of the endograft fabric along the anterior and posterior walls of the aortic lumen.

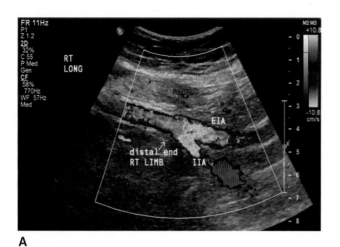

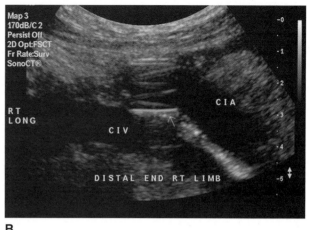

A **B**

Figure 18-13 A: A CDI demonstrates distal end of right limb aortic endograft; the graft limb ends just proximal to the internal iliac and external iliac bifurcation. **B:** A B-mode image illustrating the reflective struts at the distal end of the right graft limb to the common iliac artery.

may be associated with an endoleak. Transverse and sagittal views of the distal attachment/fixation site(s) are obtained to identify any evidence of graft kinking or graft limbs that appear crossed due to device rotation during deployment. The additional use of harmonic imaging by the examiner will assist in facilitating the accurate identification of the attachment sites and will characterize the thrombus within the sac by improving overall quality and contrast resolution of the image.

With spectral Doppler, record a PSV measurement in the suprarenal aorta and confirm patency of the renal arteries. For all velocity measurements, the Doppler angle is maintained at 60° or less, and the angle cursor is aligned parallel to the vessel wall in the longitudinal approach. Using color and spectral Doppler, the stent graft is assessed from the proximal attachment site throughout the body of the graft and the graft limbs to the distal attachment site(s) looking for any perigraft flow, graft stenosis, thrombosis, or kinking, recording waveforms and velocities throughout. It is important to have a small color box so as to incorporate the entire

residual aneurysm sac and to fill the lumen of the graft and graft limbs, thus avoiding excessive artifact (Fig. 18-15). If flow is identified within the sac, it is easier to differentiate between a true endoleak and a color artifact from bowel gas or excessive color gain. Any suspected color endoleak should be confirmed with spectral Doppler.

The examination continues distally beyond the distal attachment/fixation site(s) with color and spectral Doppler to assess the patency of the native iliac and femoral arteries. Any complications following endograft placement (i.e., stenosis, occlusion, hematoma, or pseudoaneurysm at access site) should be thoroughly documented.

DIAGNOSIS

Over time, there should be a decrease in the size of the aneurysm sac. Therefore, any increase in the sac size, pulsatility of the sac, or any areas of echolucency within the sac on B-mode should alert the examiner

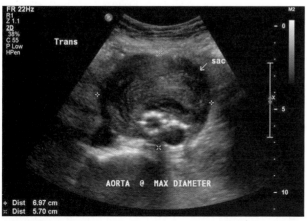

Figure 18-14 Transverse and AP measurements of the residual AAA sac.

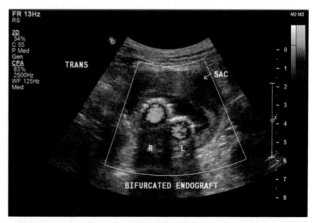

Figure 18-15 Color duplex imaging of normal bifurcated endograft with a color box appropriately placed to include the excluded AAA sac.

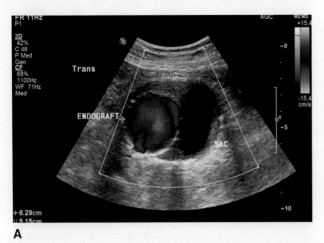

A

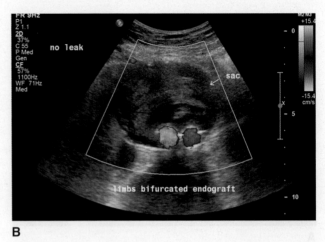

B

Figure 18-16 A: A residual AAA sac that appears very heterogeneous ("spongy") in texture with hypoechoic areas. **B:** An unstable sac; hypoechoic areas above bifurcated limbs.

to probable sac instability (Fig. 18-16A,B). A residual sac that appears very heterogeneous ("spongy") in texture with hypoechoic areas combined with an increase in size or a sac size that has not decreased since the last assessment would suggest an impending endograft complication and a possible endoleak.[26]

Flow patterns will normally be multiphasic in the aortic stent graft and outflow vessels of the iliofemoral segment arteries. This is due to the normally high-resistance lower extremity arterial bed.

It is essential for the examiner to recognize flow patterns associated with perigraft leaks and their potential sites (Fig. 18-17). A real leak will have reproducible arterial waveforms with *different* spectral Doppler characteristics compared to flow within the aortic endograft. The examiner should try to determine the source(s) of the leak and should identify the flow direction (e.g., a leak arising from a lumbar artery and exiting via the inferior mesenteric artery). Endoleaks may result from an inadequate or ineffective seal at the proximal or distal attachment site (type I) or an endoleak originating from a branch vessel (Fig. 18-18A–F) resulting in retrograde flow may include the inferior mesenteric, lumbar, accessory renal, or internal iliac arteries (type II). Both type I and II endoleaks are the most common endoleaks observed with implanted EVAR devices now in current use. Less common causes of endoleaks are flow from modular disconnection, an inadequate seal at the modular junction or through a defect in the graft fabric (type III), or flow in the sac due to graft porosity or microleak (type IV). Another form of unstable AAA sac where the aneurysm continues to expand due to persistent or recurrent pressurization in the absence of an endoleak has been termed endotension.[27]

The ability for the examiner to recognize B-mode characteristics of an unstable AAA sac and then identify any endoleak may depend on using other diagnostic maneuvers to determine if there is perigraft flow. In some instances, an endoleak may be very subtle or intermittent, and these maneuvers can include changing the position of the patient from supine to left and right decubitus positions, optimizing the color settings by decreasing the color PRF and increasing persistence and gain to ensure there is no flow in the residual sac.[28] The additional use of power Doppler can facilitate the detection of low-flow amplitude endoleaks that may course off axis to the sound beam. This may be seen as an atypical signal on the stent graft wall in the presence of a type IV endoleak. Pathology Box 18-1 summarizes the various findings with endoleaks.

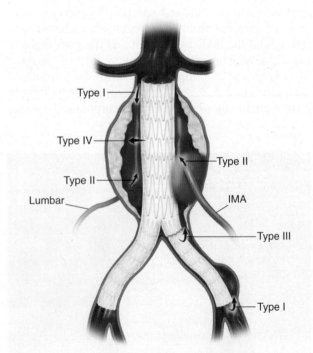

Figure 18-17 A diagram of potential sites of perigraft leaks (types I–IV).

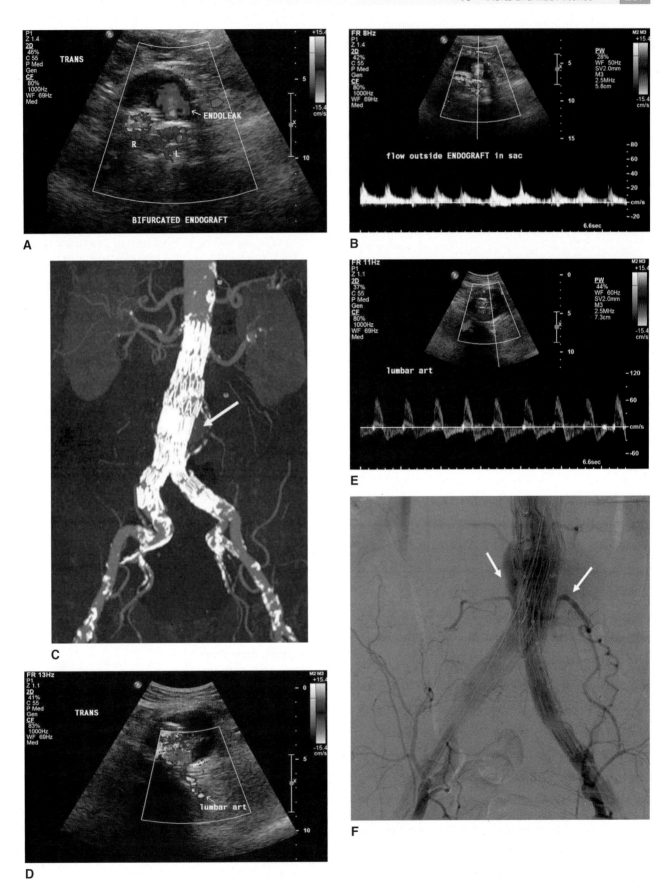

Figure 18-18 **A:** A B-mode and color appearance of a type II endoleak. **B:** Spectral waveforms from a type II endoleak. **C:** A type II endoleak (*arrow*) demonstrated on CT. **D:** A type II endoleak from a posterior lumbar artery. **E:** A spectral waveform of a type II endoleak from a posterior lumbar artery. **F:** A type II endoleak (*arrows*) from a posterior lumbar artery demonstrated on CT.

PATHOLOGY BOX 18-1

Classification of Endoleaks

Type	Cause of Perigraft Flow	Usual Hemodynamics
I	Inadequate seal at endograft attachment or fixation site(s)	Because the endoleak originates from the graft, the Doppler waveform morphology should be the same as that within the graft. Usually high flow rates.
II	Branch vessel flow without communication with attachment site (lumbar, IMA, occasionally accessory renal artery, hypogastric [internal iliac]) artery	Can be monophasic or multiphasic but most often is **bidirectional**. Can be very slow flow or higher flow rates. Doppler waveform morphology reflects the end source (e.g., a single branch vessel entering the sac will be bidirectional or "to-and-fro"). If there is entering IMA and exiting lumbar, the waveform morphology would likely be multiphasic, reflective of the peripheral vascular bed.
III	Flow from modular disconnect* between segments of the endograft** Flow from fabric disruption	Similar waveform morphology as to the graft flow because that is the source. Usually high flow.
IV	Flow from fabric porosity (more than 30 days after placement)	Similar waveform morphology as to the graft flow because that is the source. Can be very subtle and difficult to define.
Undefined source	Flow identified but source undetermined	Varies.

*Would only be seen in devices with modular configuration.

**These can occur in isolation or in combination with type II branch vessels.

SUMMARY

The long-term outcome of the endovascular method of AAA repair and the durability of the prosthesis is unknown. Structural device failure and complications have been reported in the literature. Duplex ultrasound imaging with color and power Doppler is an accurate modality to detect early and late endoleaks and device complications following endoluminal aortic surgery. The test has emerged as a reliable tool for follow-up surveillance and is the diagnostic test of first choice that is cost-effective, non-invasive, and can be repeated without exposure to ionizing radiation. It is, however, a very operator-dependent and operator-driven modality that requires experience and a sound knowledge of the endovascular technique with standard laboratory imaging protocols and good quality equipment to achieve a thorough and optimal examination.

Critical Thinking Questions

1. You are examining a patient in follow-up to an infrarenal abdominal aortic aneurysm (AAA). As you are scanning in transverse, the AAA appears to be fusiform but is not round but rather ovoid. What can you do to ensure that you are measuring this AAA transverse measurement most accurately?

2. When an increase in velocity is encountered when performing an aortoiliac duplex ultrasound, what are the three most important pieces of information to collect in order to determine whether this is a hemodynamically significant stenosis versus some other reason for increased velocity?

3. "Endoleak" is the term used to describe what complication following endograft implantation in the treatment of abdominal aortic aneurysm (AAA)?

4. Draw a diagram of an aortic endograft and discuss the potential sites of an endoleak the examiner should be aware of.

5. What are the ultrasound features that are suggestive of graft or sac instability?

REFERENCES

1. Kohler TR, Nance DR, Cramer MM, et al. Duplex scanning for diagnosis of aortoiliac and femoropopliteal disease: a prospective study. *Circulation*. 1987;5:1074–1080.
2. Donald I, Brown TG. Demonstration of tissue interfaces within the body by ultrasonic echo-sounding. *Br J Radiol*. 1961;34:539–546.
3. Yehuda GW, Otis SM, Bernstein EF. Screening for abdominal aortic aneurysm in the vascular laboratory. In: Bernstein EF, ed. *Vascular Diagnosis*. 4th ed. St. Louis, MO: Mosby; 1993: 645–651.
4. Currie JC, Jones AJ, Wakeley CJ, et al. Non-invasive aortoiliac assessment. *Eur J Vasc Endovasc Surg*. 1995;9:24–28.
5. Rizzo RJ, Vogelzang RL, Bergan JJ, et al. Use of imaging techniques for aortic evaluation. In: Bergan JJ, Yao JS, ed. *Aortic Surgery*. Philadelphia, PA: W.B. Saunders; 1989;48.
6. Melton LJ III, Bickerstaff LK, Hollier LH, et al. Changing incidence of abdominal aortic aneurysms: a population based study. *Am J Epidemiol*. 1984;120(3):379–386.
7. DuBost C, Allary M, Oeconomos N. Resection of an aneurysm of the abdominal aorta: re-establishment of the continuity by a preserved human arterial graft with results after five months. *AMA Arch Surg*. 1952;64(3):405–408.
8. Grimm JJ, Wise MM, Meissner MH, et al. The incidence of popliteal artery aneurysms in patients with abdominal aortic aneurysms. *J Vasc Ultrasound*. 2007;31(2):71–73.
9. Gooding GAW. Aneurysms of the abdominal aorta, iliac and femoral arteries. *Semin Ultrasound*. 1982;3(2):170–179.
10. Marcus R, Edell SL. Sonographic evaluation of iliac artery aneurysms. *AM J Surg*. 1980;140: 666–670.
11. American College of Radiology, American Institute of Ultrasound in Medicine, Society of Radiologists in Ultrasound. Practice guideline for the performance of diagnostic and screening ultrasound of the abdominal aorta. http://www.acr.org/SecondaryMainMenuCategories/quality_safety/guidelines/us/us_abdominal_aorta.aspx. Published 2005. Amended 2006. Accessed June 11, 2011.
12. Veith FJ, Hobson RW, Williams RA, et al., eds. *Vascular Surgery: Principles and Practice*. New York, NY: McGraw Hill; 1994:372.
13. Sprouse LR II, Meier GH III, Parent FN, et al. Is ultrasound more accurate than axial computed tomography for maximal abdominal aortic aneurysm? *Eur J Vasc Endovasc Surg*. 2004;28(1):28–35.
14. Gooding GAW. B-mode and duplex examination of the aorta, iliac arteries and portal vein. In: Zweibel WJ, ed. *Introduction to Vascular Ultrasonography*. 2nd ed. Grune and Stratton, Orlando; 1986;433.
15. May J, White GH, Yu W, et al. Concurrent comparison of endoluminal versus open repair in the treatment of abdominal aortic aneurysms: analysis of 303 patients by life table method. *J Vasc Surg*. 1998;27:231–222.
16. Parodi J, Palmaz JC, Barone HD. Transfemoral intraluminal graft implantation for abdominal aortic aneurysms. *Ann Vasc Surg*. 1991;5:491–499.
17. May J, White GH, Harris JP. Endoluminal repair of abdominal aortic aneurysms- state of the art. *Eur J Radiol*. 2001;39:16–21.
18. White GH, Yu W, May J, et al. Endoleak as a complication of endoluminal grafting of AAA: classification, incidence, diagnosis and management. *J Endovasc Surg*. 1997;4:152–168.
19. White GH, May J, Petrasek P, et al. Type III and type IV endoleak: toward a complete definition of blood flow in the sac after endoluminal repair of AAA. *J Endovasc Surg*. 1998;5: 305–309.
20. Buth J, Laheij RFJ. Early complications and endoleaks after endovascular abdominal aortic aneurysm repair: report of a multi-centre study. *J Vasc Surg*. 2001;34:98–105.

21. Wolf YG, Johnson BL, Hill BB, et al. Duplex ultrasound scanning versus computed tomographic angiography for postoperative evaluation of endovascular abdominal aortic aneurysm repair. *J Vasc Surg.* 2000;32:1142–1148.

22. Zannetti S, De Rango P, Parente B, et al. Role of Duplex scan in endoleak detection after endoluminal abdominal aortic aneurysm repair. *Eur J Vasc Endovasc Surg.* 2000;19:531–535.

23. Carter KA, Gayle RG, DeMasi RJ, et al. The incidence and natural history of type I and II endoleak: a 5 year follow-up assessment with color duplex ultrasound scan. *J Vasc Surg.* 2003;35:595–597.

24. May J, Harris JP, Kidd JF, et al. Imaging modalities for the diagnosis of endoleak. In: Mansour M, Labropoulos N, eds. *Vascular Diagnosis.* Philadelphia: Elsevier Saunders; 2005: 407–419.

25. Berdejo GL, Lipsitz E. Ultrasound imaging assessment following endovascular aortic aneurysm repair. In: Zweibel W, Pellerito J, eds. *Introduction to Vascular Ultrasonography.* 5th ed. Philadelphia: Elsevier Saunders; 2005;553–570.

26. Nelms C, Carter K, DeMasi R, et al. Color duplex ultrasound characteristics: can we predict aortic aneurysm expansion following endovascular repair? *J Vasc Ultrasound.* 2005;29(3): 143–146.

27. White GH, May J, Petrasek P, et al. Endotension: an explanation for continued AAA growth after successful endoluminal repair. *J Endovasc Surg.* 1999;6:308–315.

28. Busch K, Kidd JF, White GH, et al. What are the duplex ultrasound signs that characterize an "unstable abdominal aortic aneurysm sac" after endograft implantation? *J Vasc Ultrasound.* 2007;31(3):143–146.

19 The Mesenteric Arteries

Anne M. Musson, Jack I. Siegel, and Robert M. Zwolak

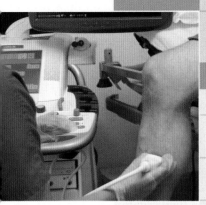

KEY TERMS

celiac artery | inferior mesenteric artery | mesenteric ischemia | postprandial | splanchnic | superior mesenteric artery | visceral

GLOSSARY

collateral flow relating to additional blood vessels that aid or add to circulation

postprandial occurring after a meal

splanchnic relating to or affecting the viscera

visceral relating to internal organs or blood vessels in the abdominal cavity

The mesenteric duplex examination is a widely accepted and accurate test to identify stenosis or occlusion in the mesenteric arteries. Less common indications for this study include the identification of aneurysms and dissections of the visceral arteries and the evaluation of patients with suspected median arcuate ligament compression syndrome. Patients with abnormal findings may require open surgical or percutaneous endovascular repair, and another excellent application of this noninvasive test is to monitor patients following these procedures for patency and restenosis.

The most common application in the noninvasive vascular laboratory is evaluation of the celiac and superior mesenteric arteries (SMAs) for chronic mesenteric ischemia. Attempts should be made to visualize the inferior mesenteric artery (IMA) as well. The diagnosis of chronic mesenteric ischemia is difficult because the disorder is rare and the symptoms are nonspecific, so it is often overlooked for prolonged periods of time as the patient is worked up

for malignancy, ulcer, gallbladder, and psychological etiologies. Duplex ultrasound remains a reliable noninvasive test to identify pathologic blood flow patterns in patients with chronic mesenteric ischemia. Although symptomatic mesenteric ischemia is rare, atherosclerotic stenosis or occlusion of the visceral arteries is not uncommon. In one study, 27% of patients undergoing aortic angiography for the evaluation of aortic aneurysm or lower extremity arterial occlusive disease were found to have ≥50% stenosis of either the celiac or the superior mesenteric arteries.[1] The duplex examination holds an advantage over computed tomography (CT) or computed tomography angiography (CTA) in that the duplex examination provides physiological information about a stenosis. Only a small fraction of these patients develop chronic intestinal ischemia because these arteries are interconnected by a rich collateral network. It is in patients with extensive disease involving two or all three of these vessels that symptoms generally develop and can become life threatening.

The importance of evaluating the IMA increases if disease is identified in the celiac or mesenteric artery. An exception to this multivessel standard is the patient in whom previous abdominal surgery has interrupted the collateral network. The indications for duplex screening for chronic mesenteric ischemia include abdominal pain and cramping associated with eating, the presence of an abdominal bruit, and weight loss. In effect, eating is the "stress test" for the mesenteric circulation. Similar to the cramping pain in the leg that occurs with exercise, there is insufficient visceral blood flow following a meal to support the increased oxygen demand required to support intestinal functions of motility, secretion, and absorption. Typically, epigastric or periumbilical pain starts approximately 30 minutes after eating and lasts for 1 to 2 hours. Because of this postprandial pain or mesenteric angina, patients often develop sitophobia or "food fear," and limit the size of meals. It is primarily the decreased nutritional intake, rather than malabsorption, which leads to weight loss. The latter can occur, but is not a consistent feature. Patients with chronic mesenteric ischemia are predominantly female (ratio of females to males is 3:1) between the ages of 40 and 70 years. Although diarrhea is frequently mentioned, constipation and normal bowel habits have also been described in patients with well-documented chronic intestinal ischemia.

The first case report describing the use of ultrasound in the diagnosis of mesenteric artery disease was published by Jager and associates from the University of Washington in 1984.[2] Subsequently, many researchers reported the use of ultrasound to describe normal splanchnic blood flow and the physiologic response to eating.[3-5] In 1991, two large retrospective studies identified duplex flow velocities that allowed for the accurate identification of mesenteric artery stenosis.[6,7] Since then, the mesenteric duplex examination has been adopted by many laboratories, and prospective studies have established the accuracy of the velocity thresholds.[8,9]

ANATOMY

As with any duplex exam, it is important to know the expected anatomy of these arteries (Fig. 19-1) as well as the common variants. The celiac artery is the first abdominal branch arising from the abdominal aorta, and its origin from the anterior aspect of the aorta usually lies 1 to 2 cm below the diaphragm. The celiac

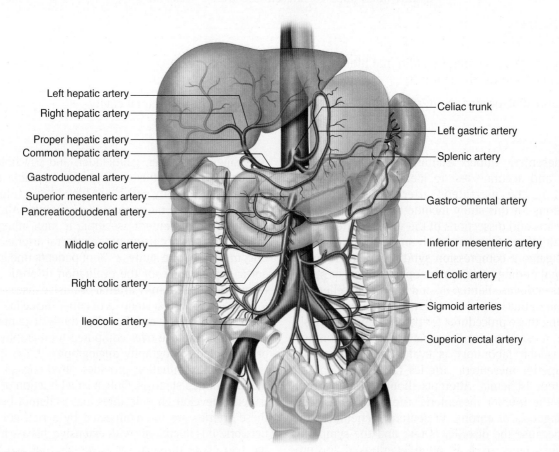

Figure 19-1 The abdominal aorta and mesenteric branches. (Original drawing by F. Elizabeth LaBombard, RVT, Dartmouth-Hitchcock Medical Center Vascular Lab; reproduced with permission.)

is usually only 2 to 4 cm long, branching into the common hepatic and splenic arteries. The SMA typically originates from the anterior surface of the aorta 1 to 2 cm below the celiac artery. The IMA arises from the distal aorta just above the aortic bifurcation.

The extensive collaterals that enable patients to tolerate significant occlusive disease in these mesenteric vessels, with the vast majority remaining asymptomatic, are primarily the superior and inferior pancreaticoduodenal arteries (pancreaticoduodenal arcade) bridging the celiac and SMA, and the arc of Riolan, or meandering mesenteric artery, between the inferior and superior mesenteric arteries. There are also collaterals between the internal iliac arteries and the inferior mesenteric artery.

ANATOMICAL VARIANTS

Anomalous mesenteric artery anatomy has been reported in approximately 20% of the general population, and this can increase the complexity of a mesenteric duplex examination substantially. Awareness of the possible anomalies facilitates recognition of unusual ultrasound findings (Table 19-1). A right hepatic artery originating from an artery other than the celiac artery is described as a replaced right hepatic artery. This is the most common anomaly, with a prevalence of approximately 17%. Most often a replaced right hepatic originates from the SMA (approximately 10% to 12%), with the remainder originating from a variety of alternative sites.[10] This finding should be suspected when a low-resistance flow pattern (flow throughout diastole) is found in an otherwise normal-appearing proximal SMA. Occasionally, a replaced right hepatic artery may be seen arising from the SMA and arching back toward the liver. The SMA distal to the takeoff of the hepatic artery will revert to the normal high resistive pattern. Other important mesenteric artery anomalies include the common hepatic artery originating from the SMA, the common hepatic artery originating from the aorta, and a common origin of the celiac artery and SMA (celiacomesenteric artery) originating from the aorta.

SONOGRAPHIC EXAMINATION TECHNIQUES

PATIENT PREPARATION

An important difference in this scan from all others performed in the vascular laboratory is that it is essential that the patient has fasted for at least 6 hours because the SMA velocity waveform changes dramatically from a low-flow, high-resistance pattern to a high-flow, low-resistance pattern after eating. Velocity thresholds for identifying stenosis of the celiac artery and SMA have been established for patients in the fasting state, so application of these standard criteria requires that the examination be performed in fasting patients. Typically, the patient is asked not to eat or drink anything starting at midnight and is then scheduled for a duplex scan in the early morning to minimize abdominal gas and disruption of the patient's meal and medication cycles. Regular medications can be taken with sips of water. Diabetic patients are instructed to consult with their primary care provider to alter insulin or other medications appropriately, and all patients are asked to refrain from smoking or chewing gum on the morning of the examination.

If scanning a nonfasted patient, it is important to state in the report that the standard criteria for determining stenosis do not apply and report only on the patency of the vessels. The results should include an explanation that criteria for stenosis identification in the celiac and SMA are based on data obtained from patients in a fasting state.

PATIENT POSITION

The examination is performed with the patient supine. A slight reverse Trendelenburg position or head elevation may be helpful. As with the renal duplex scan, low-frequency transducers (2-5 MHz) are required, with the frequency range determined by the body habitus of the patient.

REQUIRED DOCUMENTATION

Current minimum requirements for image and Doppler waveforms include samples from the following vessels:
- Adjacent aorta
- Celiac artery origin
- Splenic and hepatic arteries when appropriate
- SMA origin
- Proximal SMA
- IMA

TABLE 19-1	
Anatomic Variants of the Mesenteric Arteries	
FOUR MOST COMMON CELIAC AND MESENTERIC VARIANTS	
Variant	**% Incidence**
Replaced right hepatic originating from the SMA	10%–12%
Replaced common hepatic originating from the SMA	2.5%
Common hepatic originating from the aorta	2%
Common origin of the celiac and SMA—celiacomesenteric	<1%

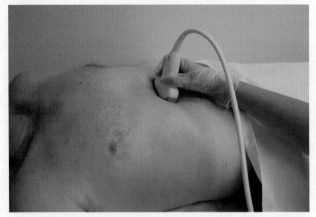

Figure 19-2 Photo showing patient and technologist position and probe position.

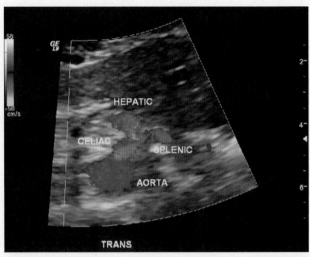

Figure 19-3 Color flow image in transverse view of the origin of the celiac artery from the aorta. The "seagull sign" is formed by the celiac artery bifurcation into the common hepatic and splenic arteries.

These requirements are based on current standards established by the Intersocietal Commission for the Accreditation of Vascular Laboratories (ICAVL).

SCANNING TECHNIQUE

The transducer is initially placed just below the xiphoid process for identification of the proximal abdominal aorta (Fig. 19-2). The aorta, celiac artery, proximal common hepatic and splenic arteries, the SMA, and the IMA should be interrogated thoroughly by pulsed Doppler, and spectral waveforms should be recorded from these vessels. This will require a combination of sagittal and transverse scanning. The Doppler sample volume should be "walked" from the aorta through the origin and proximal celiac, the SMA, and the IMA to identify the highest peak systolic velocity (PSV) and end-diastolic velocity (EDV). In the case of a suspected stenosis, care should be taken to document the present of poststenotic turbulence to aid in the confirmation of a flow-limiting stenosis.

Celiac, Hepatic, and Splenic Arteries

From its origin off the aorta to the bifurcation into the common hepatic artery and the splenic artery, the celiac artery is usually best viewed in a transverse plane. This image of the celiac bifurcation is often referred to as the "seagull sign" and provides adequate angles for Doppler interrogation (Fig. 19-3). The "seagull" has its "wings" formed from the common hepatic artery (coursing toward the liver and the patient's right) and splenic artery (coursing toward the spleen and the patient's left). The normal Doppler waveform from the celiac artery has a low-resistance pattern with antegrade flow continuing throughout systole and diastole. This Doppler waveform morphology occurs because the celiac artery supplies two low-resistance solid organs—the liver and the spleen (Fig. 19-4). Careful attention to Doppler angle

correction for velocity determination is necessary, as these vessels may be very tortuous. It is not unusual for the celiac to have a sharp anterior and superior angulation as it exits from under the crus of the diaphragm. The splenic and common hepatic arteries should also display low resistance signals with flow through the entire cardiac cycle.

Superior Mesenteric Artery

The SMA is best visualized in a sagittal plane as it courses parallel to the aorta. The normal fasting SMA Doppler waveform is triphasic (high resistance), with a brief phase of reversed flow and little or no flow in the second half of the cardiac cycle, similar to the pattern found in the major upper and lower extremity arteries (Fig. 19-5). The SMA should be scanned as far distally as possible, obtaining Doppler waveforms from the proximal, middle, and distal segments.

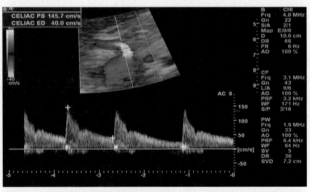

Figure 19-4 Color flow image and Doppler spectral waveform from a normal celiac artery. The flow pattern is typical of a low-resistance vascular bed, with forward flow throughout the cardiac cycle.

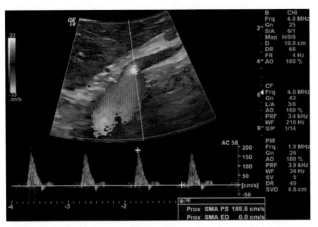

Figure 19-5 Normal high-resistance, triphasic superior mesenteric artery (SMA) spectral waveform flow pattern in a fasting patient. The color flow image shows the origin of the SMA in sagittal view. Note placement of the angle cursor for Doppler angle correction along the curve near the vessel origin.

Inferior Mesenteric Artery

The IMA is most easily identified in a transverse view by locating the aortic bifurcation and then scanning proximally up the distal abdominal aorta for 1 to 3 cm. The IMA usually originates from the anterior aorta slightly to the left of the midline (Fig. 19-6). Normal Doppler waveforms from the IMA resemble those from the fasting SMA, with a high-resistance waveform pattern.

TEST MEAL

Researchers have studied the dynamic effects of the mesenteric blood flow in normal subjects following a test meal, demonstrating substantial changes in normal SMA flow, with the PSV nearly doubling and the EDV nearly tripling compared to the baseline velocities.[11] In the diseased, stenotic SMA, there is a failure of the postprandial SMA PSV to increase substantially beyond the already elevated levels. The question of whether adding postprandial scanning to the mesenteric study provides important additional information was addressed by Gentile et al. who studied 25 healthy controls and 80 patients with vascular disease undergoing aortography. The minimum normal hyperemic response to test feeding was an increase in PSV of ≥20%. They concluded that adding postprandial duplex scanning offered no definite improvement over fasting scans in the identification of >70% stenosis.[12] A test meal may be included on a selective basis, but generally is not justified in routine clinical practice, as the combination of fasting and postprandial duplex results increased specificity and positive predictive value slightly but did not improve overall accuracy.

TECHNICAL CONSIDERATIONS

Positive Vessel Identification/Accurate Angle Determination

Attempts should be made to visualize the origins of both the celiac artery and SMA in the same duplex image to confirm correct identification of these vessels (Fig. 19-7), particularly when both arteries have elevated velocities and abnormal Doppler waveforms. This may require rotating the transducer slightly or moving laterally and angling the transducer back toward the midline. As with the renal duplex examinations, there is movement of these arteries with respiration. Asking the patient to suspend

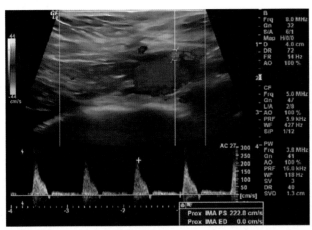

Figure 19-6 Color flow image showing a normal inferior mesenteric artery (IMA) originating from the distal aorta slightly to the left of the anterior midline (usually seen at 1 to 2 o'clock off the aorta on a transverse image). The spectral waveform shows a high-resistance flow pattern. The angle correction is aligned to the vessel origin.

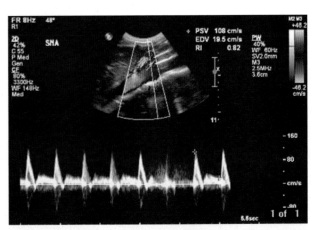

Figure 19-7 Duplex image showing the origins of both the celiac artery and superior mesenteric artery (SMA) from the aorta in a sagittal view. The pulsed Doppler sample volume is positioned in the SMA, just distal to the origin of the celiac artery. The corresponding SMA spectral waveform shows a normal high-resistance flow pattern.

breathing momentarily to record the Doppler waveform and determine the correct angle can increase accuracy. The angulation of the proximal SMA is acute, and Doppler angles change quickly in a short distance. If breathing is not suspended, it is possible for the angle of the Doppler sample volume to change significantly from where it was first placed or even to inadvertently slip between the celiac and the SMA. To avoid potential errors due to incorrect Doppler angles, particularly in tortuous segments, ask the patient to suspend respiration in order to keep these vessels as still as possible during acquisition of the Doppler spectrum. As with other types of arterial spectral Doppler evaluation, angles of 60° or less should always be used.

Use of Color Features for Aliasing, Turbulence, and Flow Direction

A color bruit frequently offers an instant clue to the presence of a significant stenosis. Once observed, inspect thoroughly with Doppler to find the maximum velocity (Fig. 19-8).

Close attention should also be given to the Doppler pulse repetition frequency (PRF) and the orientation of the color-scale bar. The PRF scale should be adjusted (usually increasing the frequency range to limit aliasing of the color scale) to more reliably determine flow direction. The color on the top half of the color bar scale is assigned to flow coming toward the transducer, whereas the colors on the bottom half represent flow away from the transducer. This feature allows the technologist to identify and track antegrade flow in tortuous vessels and more readily identify retrograde flow. Flow direction becomes particularly important when the celiac artery is occluded or severely stenotic. In this situation, low pressure in the celiac artery induces SMA collaterals to divert blood toward the liver and spleen through

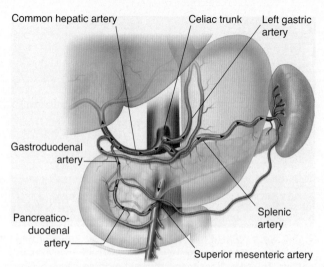

Figure 19-9 When the celiac artery is occluded or severely stenotic, collaterals from the SMA divert blood through the gastroduodenal artery toward the liver and spleen. Retrograde flow in the common hepatic artery fills the splenic artery. (Original drawing by F. Elizabeth LaBombard, RVT, Dartmouth-Hitchcock Medical Center Vascular Lab; reproduced with permission.)

the gastroduodenal artery (GDA). The GDA backfills the common hepatic artery such that retrograde flow in the common hepatic crosses the celiac artery origin to perfuse the splenic artery (Figs. 19-9 and 19-10). The finding of retrograde flow direction in the common hepatic artery is always (100% predictive) associated with severe celiac artery stenosis or occlusion.[13] Thus, even when the celiac artery cannot be well visualized, the finding of retrograde flow in the hepatic artery is a significant finding, as long as the examiner is confident that flow direction has been determined accurately.

Turn Color Off: Inspect with B-Mode

Color can mask important features. Although there are distinct color cues in arterial dissections, the thin echogenic line seen in the grayscale image is an

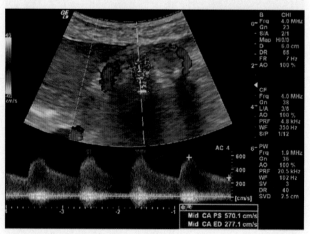

Figure 19-8 Color bruit in celiac artery. Doppler velocities indicate significant stenosis, with PSV 5 570 cm/s and EDV 5 277 cm/s.

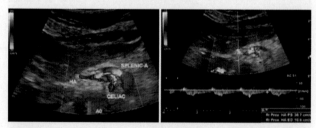

Figure 19-10 Color flow image *(left)* and Doppler spectral waveform *(right)* illustrating the importance of color-scale and pulse repetition frequency (PRF). The pulsed Doppler sample volume is positioned in the common hepatic artery, and both the spectral waveform and color flow *(blue)* image indicate flow away from the transducer. This represents retrograde collateral flow in the common hepatic artery and antegrade flow *(red)* into the splenic artery.

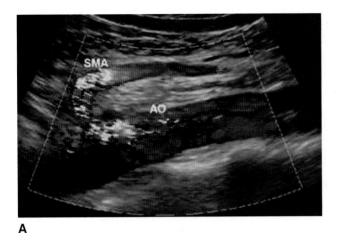

A

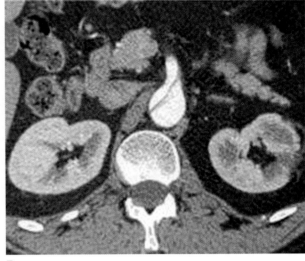

B

Figure 19-11 Color flow abnormalities with definite separation of red and blue channels is classic for dissection. Dissections of the visceral arteries frequently start in the aorta. **A:** Illustrates a color picture of an aortic dissection extending into the SMA with associated turbulence. **B:** The CT image shows the echogenic line produced by the dissection that can also be seen by B-mode duplex of the aorta.

important piece of the puzzle (Fig. 19-11). As stents are echogenic and tend to "light up" with B-mode ultrasound (Fig. 19-12), turning color off can help locate the stent.

Prepare for Scan by Reading Operative Report

Revascularization with bypass grafts is a common procedure for the treatment of mesenteric ischemia. It is important to know the locations of the proximal and distal anastomoses, as these are quite variable in their configurations. The inflow artery may be the supraceliac aorta, in which case the flow will be antegrade. Flow will be retrograde if the proximal anastomosis is from the infrarenal aorta or iliac artery. Prepare for the duplex scan by reading the operative report, which will include information about the location of the proximal and distal anastomoses, whether the bypass is to a single artery or bifurcated to supply two arteries, and to know the graft material (prosthetic or vein). The inflow artery supplying the bypass graft should be evaluated, and the Doppler sample volume "walked" through the proximal anastomosis, the body of the graft, the distal anastomosis, and into the outflow artery (Figs. 19-13 and 19-14). It is difficult, if not impossible, depending on the length of the bypass to show the entire graft in one image (e.g., ilio-SMA bypass graft) and is often necessary to concentrate on one segment at a time, with particular attention to the proximal and distal anastomoses.

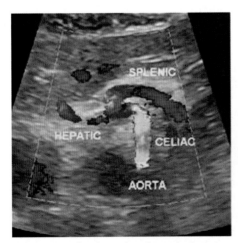

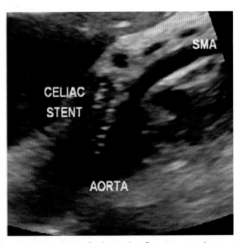

Figure 19-12 Turning color off aids in identifying the location of a stent. On the *left*, the color flow image demonstrates adequate filling of the celiac artery but masks the stent, which is more clearly visualized in the grayscale image on the *right*.

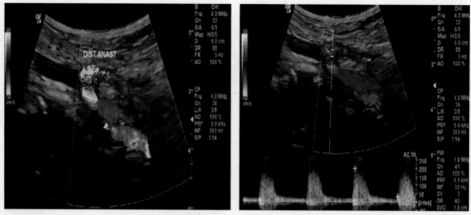

Figure 19-13 Duplex images of an external iliac artery to the superior mesenteric artery (SMA) bypass graft. The distal anastomosis to the SMA is shown on the *left*. The image on the *right* shows a high-resistance spectral waveform. This bypass was too long to visualize in one image.

Liem et al. reviewed 167 duplex scans from 38 patients to characterize duplex findings in mesenteric bypass grafts with respect to type of revascularization, graft caliber, and changes over time.[14] They found that mid-graft mean PSV, typically 140 to 200 cm/s, may be affected by graft diameter, but is not significantly affected by the choice of inflow artery, whether antegrade or retrograde. If the PSV ≥300 cm/s or <50 cm/s in the bypass, the recommendation is to decrease the time between surveillance scans to less than 6 months or to use secondary imaging (CTA or angiography).

Compensatory Flow

Elevated velocities may be noted in a normal mesenteric artery when compensatory flow through collaterals occurs due to critical stenosis or occlusion of one of the other visceral vessels. This is common in the mesenteric circulation due to the extensive collateral pathways that often develop when there is arterial occlusive disease in the SMA, IMA, or celiac artery. For example, flow through the SMA might be increased, resulting in increased Doppler velocities when the celiac artery has a critical stenosis or occlusion. In certain patients, it may be difficult to distinguish increased velocities associated with a pathological stenosis from compensatory flow in a widely patent artery. Doppler waveform analysis may be helpful in this situation. A stenosis usually elicits a flow disturbance with high velocities and poststenotic spectral broadening, whereas with compensatory flow, there is little spectral broadening; an absence of a prestenotic, stenotic, poststenotic velocity profile; and velocities may be elevated throughout the main portion of the artery. A prominent IMA may suggest occlusion or stenosis of the SMA with collateralization through a meandering mesenteric artery, although only the very experienced technologist is likely to have a good baseline perception of the normal IMA appearance.

PITFALLS

Poor visualization is sometimes present with all types of ultrasound but can be particularly challenging with abdominal examinations. If there is air in the epigastrium, a light massage with the transducer will sometimes move it out of the way. If midline scars from an abdominal surgery cause shadowing, sliding the transducer to the right or left and angling

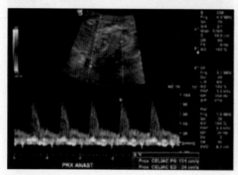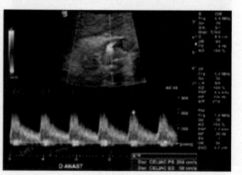

Figure 19-14. Duplex images of an aorto-celiac bypass graft with Doppler spectrum of the proximal (*left image*) and distal (*right image*) anastomoses. This bypass graft was able to be visualized in one image.

TABLE 19-2

Summary of Velocity Thresholds for Diagnosis of Celiac Artery and Superior Mesenteric Artery (SMA) Stenosis by Duplex Scanning

Author	Artery	% Stenosis	PSV	EDV	Sensitivity	Specificity
Moneta[6,8]	Celiac	≥70%	≥200 cm/s		87%	80%
	SMA	≥70%	≥275 cm/s		92%	6%
Zwolak[7,9]	Celiac	≥50%		≥55 cm/s	93%	100%
	SMA	≥50%		≥45 cm/s	90%	91%

PSV, peak-systolic velocity; EDV, end-diastolic velocity.

it toward the midline may help with visualization. Having the patient turn into a slight right lateral decubitus position occasionally provides an adequate acoustic window through the liver, although positive identification of these vessels may require reorientation. When in doubt, one should always go back to an image of the aorta, identify known standard landmarks, and work from there again.

DIAGNOSIS

The normal SMA Doppler spectral waveform has a sharp systolic upstroke with a narrow band of frequencies or velocities (clear systolic window). As noted previously, the normal SMA flow pattern reflects a high-resistance outflow bed in the fasting state. This typically includes a brief reverse flow phase at the end of systole and little or no forward flow at the end of each cardiac cycle. The PSV in the normal SMA is usually <125 cm/s. Diagnostic velocity data focusing on PSV criteria were determined retrospectively and then tested prospectively, as reported by Moneta et al.[6,8] In their prospective study, these authors found excellent accuracy for the diagnosis of a ≥70% angiographic stenosis in the SMA by using a threshold PSV of ≥275 cm/s, with 92% sensitivity and 96% specificity. In parallel studies, the Dartmouth group focused on EDV for diagnosis of a ≥50% angiographic SMA stenosis.[7,9] These values were also established by retrospective analysis then tested prospectively. An EDV >45 cm/s in the SMA resulted in 90% sensitivity and 91% specificity in the prospective study.

Doppler waveforms recorded from the normal celiac artery also demonstrate a sharp systolic upstroke and PSV <125 cm/s, but with a low-resistance flow pattern characterized by forward flow throughout the cardiac cycle. The PSV criterion reported by Moneta et al. for ≥70% angiographic celiac artery stenosis is ≥200 cm/s, a lower threshold than that determined for the SMA. When tested prospectively, this threshold demonstrated a sensitivity of 87% and

a specificity of 80%. The Dartmouth criterion for celiac artery stenosis is an EDV ≥55 cm/s, with 93% sensitivity and 100% specificity in a prospective study. These criteria are summarized in Table 19-2.

There are no commonly accepted velocity criteria applied to the IMA. Flow velocities through this vessel will vary widely depending on the patency of the celiac artery and the SMA. However, the pattern of elevated velocity and poststenotic turbulence can be used to identify stenosis.

STENTED VISCERAL ARTERIES

As has been reported for stented internal carotid arteries and renal arteries, one study provides evidence that the duplex velocity criteria for native SMAs may overestimate the severity of stenosis after the vessel has undergone stent placement.[15] Mitchell and coworkers from the Oregon Health and Science University followed 35 patients who underwent SMA stent placement. Despite confirmation of improvement by anatomic (poststent angiographic residual stenosis <30% in all patients) and physiologic measures (significant reduction in pressure gradient), mean early poststent duplex scanning in 13 patients revealed SMA velocities ranging from 279 to 416 cm/s, with a mean posttreatment SMA PSV of 336 cm/s. Based on these early data, the authors concluded that SMA duplex velocity criteria developed for native vessels will likely overestimate the prevalence of recurrent or residual disease after stenting. This is important to keep in mind when the results are interpreted, as standard velocity thresholds may need to be adjusted. More investigation will be required to confirm this observation, but this issue will be of increasing importance as percutaneous intervention for mesenteric occlusive disease gains wider acceptance.

Duplex scanning is an ideal monitoring method for these stents. As with other tests, it is important to compare findings with the previous study to report whether there has been an improvement in peak systolic velocity and whether the velocity increases in sequential follow-up studies.

DISORDERS

There are several vascular disorders that can be identified with mesenteric duplex ultrasound scanning. In addition to atherosclerotic disease, median arcuate ligament compression syndrome, aneurysm, and dissection can be identified on duplex ultrasound. Rarely, an ultrasound is performed to detect thromboembolic disease.

MEDIAN ARCUATE LIGAMENT COMPRESSION SYNDROME

Individuals with median arcuate ligament compression syndrome have transient compression of the celiac artery origin by the median arcuate ligament of the diaphragm during exhalation, which is relieved by descent of the diaphragm with inhalation. Thus, the PSV of the celiac artery is increased during exhalation and decreased during inhalation. This is a controversial diagnosis with patients often having poorly defined symptoms and inconsistent results

following surgery. Autopsy studies have indicated that one-third of people demonstrate significant compression of the celiac axis. Duplex interrogation can identify changes in celiac artery velocity with inhalation versus exhalation. When scanning patients with possible median arcuate ligament compression syndrome, representative Doppler waveforms should be obtained from the celiac artery during deep inhalation and compared with waveforms obtained during complete exhalation (Fig. 19-15A,B).

ANEURYSM

Visceral artery aneurysms are rare, occurring in 0.1% to 0.2% of routine autopsies.[16] Most are identified incidentally during CT and magnetic resonance imaging (MRI) studies, although there are several case studies reporting identification by duplex ultrasound. Among visceral artery aneurysms, the greatest incidence occurs in the splenic artery at 60%, with female patients affected four times more often than male patients.

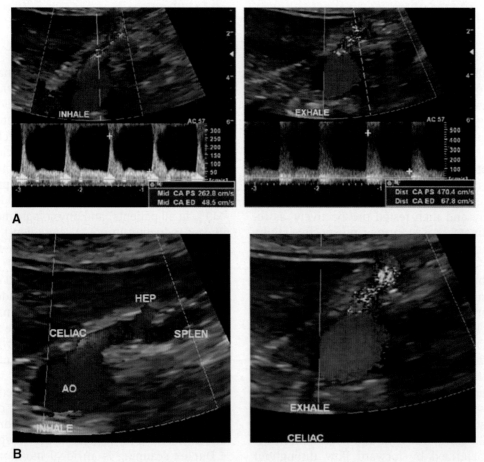

Figure 19-15 A: Doppler spectral waveforms from a celiac artery during inhalation *(left)* and exhalation *(right)* illustrate the findings in median arcuate ligament compression syndrome. Note the change in peak systolic velocity (PSV) from 263 (inhalation) to 470 cm/s (exhalation) and end-diastolic velocity (EDV) from 49 (inhalation) to 68 cm/s (exhalation). These changes are due to transient compression of the celiac artery by the median arcuate ligament during exhalation. **B:** The visual color changes were apparent before interrogation with Doppler. These images demonstrate the color increase in velocity and turbulence associated with compression of the celiac artery with exhalation *(on the right)*.

TABLE 19-3	
Relative Incidence of Visceral Artery Aneurysm	
Visceral Artery	**% Incidence**
Splenic	60%
Hepatic	20%
Superior mesenteric	5%
Celiac	4%
Gastric and gastroepiploic	4%
Jejunal ileal colic	3%
Pancreaticoduodenal	2%
Gastroduodenal	1.5%
Inferior mesenteric	Rare

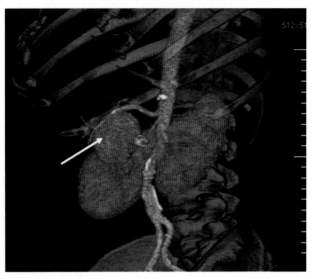

Figure 19-16 A CT scan of 5.5 cm superior mesenteric artery aneurysm *(arrow)*.

Medial degeneration of the splenic artery most often occurs due to arterial fibrodysplasia, portal hypertension with splenomegaly, and repeated pregnancies. Although the incidence of splenic artery aneurysm is rare, rupture can be catastrophic. A 95% rupture rate has been reported in the splenic aneurysm recognized during pregnancy, with an associated 70% maternal mortality rate and 95% fetal mortality rate.[17] Other locations of visceral artery aneurysms most commonly include the hepatic (with men affected twice as often as women), superior mesenteric, or celiac arteries (with men and women affected equally) (Table 19-3, Figs. 19-16 and 19-17). Treatment options for visceral artery aneurysms include open surgery and endovascular repair, with the goal of preventing aneurysm expansion and/or rupture. Duplex imaging can be used for follow-up scans after treatment.

DISSECTION

Causes of celiac, superior, and inferior mesenteric artery dissections include atherosclerosis, fibromuscular dysplasia, mycotic infection, trauma, connective tissue disorders, vasculitis, and iatrogenic-induced dissections. Some dissections occur without any identifiable etiology. Superior mesenteric artery dissections are the most frequent type of visceral artery dissection, and many are associated with aortic dissection. Treatment of superior mesenteric artery dissection may include conservative management with anticoagulation, or more aggressively with endovascular stent placement and surgical procedures. The choice among these depends on the degree of intestinal ischemia.

Dissections provide a unique pattern of color separation with antegrade flow along one wall of the artery and retrograde flow along the other wall (Figs. 19-11A,B and 19-18). Duplex ultrasound can be used to monitor dissections and for treatment follow-up. Pathology Box 19-1 summarizes the common pathology observed during a mesenteric duplex ultrasound examination.

ACUTE MESENTERIC ISCHEMIA

Acute mesenteric ischemia can result from an embolus to the mesenteric arteries or a thrombosis of an artery with existing chronic disease. Approximately two-thirds of these patients are women, with a median age of 70 years. The nature of the pain varies, but generally is described as "pain out

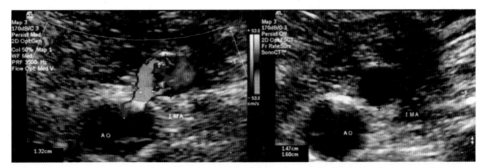

Figure 19-17 An inferior mesenteric artery aneurysm as seen on duplex exam. The typical color pattern of an aneurysm is demonstrated on the *left*. Measurements, obtained in grayscale on the *right*, were 1.5 × 1.6 cm.

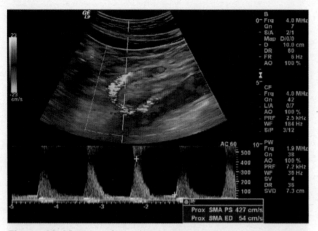

Figure 19-18 Taken from the same patient as in Figure 19-11, high velocities consistent with stenosis were documented in the proximal SMA. The stenosis was likely the result of thrombosis of the false lumen of this portion of the dissection extending into the SMA from the aorta.

of proportion to physical findings." Time spent in the vascular laboratory is generally not useful and should be discouraged. If the diagnosis is not made quickly, bowel necrosis rapidly ensues, with a high mortality rate. In an analysis of 103 cases of acute occlusion of the SMA at Massachusetts General Hospital, the mortality rate was 85%.[18] In addition to the critical time factor, there is a possibility that a distal embolus in the SMA may go undetected by ultrasound. It is important for the requesting provider to understand that although patency of the proximal SMA may be verified, an embolus to the more distal branches cannot be excluded and the provider should consider alternative imaging, such as CTA. The majority of visceral emboli lodge in the SMA, often 3 to 8 cm beyond the SMA origin and first several branches at the origin of the middle colic artery.

PATHOLOGY BOX 19-1

Celiac and Mesenteric Artery Pathology

Pathology	Sonographic Appearance Color	Doppler
Stenosis >50%	High velocity flow with aliasing, color bruit	High velocity flow with poststenotic turbulence
Celiac artery occlusion	No color filling at the origin, retrograde hepatic artery flow	No Doppler flow signal at the origin, retrograde Doppler flow velocity in the hepatic artery
Celiac artery compression syndrome	Increase color velocity with exhalation	Increase in velocity with exhalation and decrease with inhalation
Superior mesenteric artery occlusion	No color filling at the origin, reconstitutes distally	Absent Doppler signal in proximal artery
Aneurysm	Focal dilation with mixed color filling observed in dilated region	Disturbed flow usually present in dilated regions
Dissection	Color separation with both antegrade and retrograde flow	Disturbed or stenotic signals may be present with both antegrade and retrograde flow

SUMMARY

The mesenteric arteries can be successfully interrogated by duplex ultrasound. In an era where CT and CTA are used frequently, many appropriate clinical situations remain wherein duplex scanning is a valuable and appropriate test. Screening patients for suspected chronic mesenteric ischemia and median arcuate ligament syndrome are two such clinical situations. This test also provides a reasonable noninvasive method for monitoring revascularization procedures, although criteria for diagnosis of in-stent restenosis are yet to be accurately determined. Duplex ultrasound remains a cost-effective alternative to CTA and avoids the small but real incidence of complications related to CT contrast injection.

Critical Thinking Questions

1. A patient arrives for a mesenteric duplex exam and was not instructed to remain NPO, having just eaten a large breakfast. The patient lives 2 hours away, is unhappy she was not told to be NPO, and wants to get the test done. Do you proceed with the duplex exam?

2. During your mesenteric duplex scan, you can identify only one artery coming off the aorta that appears to be the SMA, as it parallels the more distal aorta. Scanning more proximally, you identify the splenic and hepatic artery "seagull" sign, but are unable to demonstrate flow in the celiac artery by color or Doppler. Flow in the hepatic artery is toward the splenic artery. How do you interpret these findings?

3. You are scanning a patient and find a celiac artery stenosis with PSV = 435 cm/s, EDV = 70 cm/s, and poststenotic turbulence beyond this high velocity. The SMA PSV = 325 cm/s and EDV = 50 cm/s. The SMA waveform demonstrates a "window," and no poststenotic turbulence is identified. Do you conclude that the patient has significant celiac and SMA stenoses? Why or why not?

4. A patient in whom you found a significant stenosis of the celiac artery returns to the lab for follow-up scan s/p stenting of the celiac artery stenosis. On your exam, you find the celiac PSV = 220 cm/s and EDV = 55 cm/s, which are above your lab's standard criteria for stenosis. The prestent velocities were PSV = 450 cm/s and EDV = 75 cm/s. Do you conclude that there is a residual stenosis? How might you write an interpretation of this?

5. A young woman is referred to your lab for a mesenteric duplex study with a question of median arcuate ligament syndrome. Do you alter your standard protocol for identifying significant mesenteric artery stenosis? Why or why not?

REFERENCES

1. Valentine RJ, Martin JD, Myers SI, et al. Asymptomatic celiac and superior mesenteric artery stenoses are more prevalent among patients with unsuspected renal artery stenoses. *J Vasc Surg.* 1991;14:195–199.
2. Jager KA, Fortner GS, Thiele BL, et al. Noninvasive diagnosis of intestinal angina. *J Clin Ultrasound.* 1984;12:588–591.
3. Jager K, Bollinger A, Valli C, et al. Measurement of mesenteric blood flow by duplex scanning. *J Vasc Surg.* 1986;3:462–469.
4. Moneta GL, Taylor DC, Helton WS, et al. Duplex ultrasound measurement of postprandial intestinal blood flow: effect of meal composition. *Gastroenterology.* 1988;95:1294–1301.
5. Flinn WR, Rizzo RJ, Park JS, et al. Duplex scanning for assessment of mesenteric ischemia. *Surg Clin North Am.* 1990;70:99–107.
6. Moneta GL, Yeager RA, Dalman R, et al. Duplex ultrasound criteria for diagnosis of splanchnic artery stenosis or occlusion. *J Vasc Surg.* 1991;14:511–518; discussion 8–20.
7. Bowersox JC, Zwolak RM, Walsh DB, et al. Duplex ultrasonography in the diagnosis of celiac and mesenteric artery occlusive disease. *J Vasc Surg.* 1991;14:780–786; discussion 6–8.
8. Moneta GL, Lee RW, Yeager RA, et al. Mesenteric duplex scanning: a blinded prospective study. *J Vasc Surg.* 1993;17:79–84; discussion 5–6.
9. Zwolak RM, Fillinger MF, Walsh DB, et al. Mesenteric and celiac duplex scanning: a validation study. *J Vasc Surg .*1998;27:1078–1087; discussion 88.
10. Kadir S. *Atlas of Normal and Variant Angiographic Anatomy.* Philadelphia, PA: W.B. Saunders; 1991.

11. Jager K, Kehl O, Ammann R, et al. [Postprandial hyperemia of the superior mesenteric artery]. *Schweiz Med Wochenschr.* 1985;115:1826–1829.
12. Gentile AT, Moneta GL, Lee RW, et al. Usefulness of fasting and postprandial duplex ultrasound examinations for predicting high-grade superior mesenteric artery stenosis. *Am J Surg.* 1995;169:476–479.
13. LaBombard FE, Musson A, Bowersox JC, et al. Hepatic artery duplex as an adjunct in the evaluation of chronic mesenteric ischemia. *J Vasc Technol.* 1992;16:7–11.
14. Liem TK, Segall JA, Wei W, et al. Duplex scan characteristics of bypass grafts to mesenteric arteries. *J Vasc Surg.* 2007;45:922–927; discussion 7–8.
15. Mitchell EL, Chang EY, Landry GJ, et al. Duplex criteria for native superior mesenteric artery stenosis overestimate stenosis in stented superior mesenteric arteries. *J Vasc Surg.* 2009;50:335–340.
16. Grotemeyer D, Duran M, Park EJ, et al. Visceral artery aneurysms—follow-up of 23 patients with 31 aneurysms after surgical or interventional therapy. *Langenbecks Arch Surg.* 2009; 394(6):1093-1100.
17. Stanley JC, Wakefield TW, Graham LM, et al. Clinical importance and management of splanchnic artery aneurysms. *J Vasc Surg.* 1986;3:836–840.
18. Ottinger LW. The surgical management of acute occlusion of the superior mesenteric artery. *Ann Surg.* 1978;188:721–731.

20 The Renal Vasculature

Marsha M. Neumyer

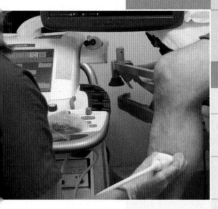

OBJECTIVES

Describe the anatomy of the renal vasculature

Relate the most common pathologies found during a sonographic examination of the renal circulatory system

Describe patient preparation and positioning used for sonographic evaluation of the renal arteries, renal veins, and kidneys

Define the technical applications of the B-mode, spectral, color, and power Doppler evaluations of the renal vasculature

List the validated diagnostic criteria used for defining renal artery stenosis, occlusion, and renal parenchymal dysfunction

KEY TERMS

renal–aortic velocity ratio | renal artery stenosis | renal artery stent | renal cortex | renal hilum | renal medulla | renal ostium | renal parenchymal disease | renal sinus

GLOSSARY

poststenotic signal a Doppler spectral waveform recorded immediately distal to a flow reducing stenosis; the waveform exhibits decreased peak systolic velocity and disordered flow during systolic deceleration and diastole as a result of the pressure-flow gradient associated with the lesion

renal–aortic velocity ratio the peak systolic renal artery velocity divided by the peak systolic aortic velocity recorded at the level of the celiac and/or superior mesenteric arteries; the ratio is used to identify flow-limiting renal artery stenosis

renal artery stenosis narrowing of the renal artery most commonly as a result of atherosclerotic disease or medial fibromuscular dysplasia

renal artery stent a tiny tube inserted into a stenotic renal artery at the time of arterial dilation (angioplasty); the stent, usually a metallic mesh structure, helps to hold the artery open

renal cortex the outermost area of the kidney tissue lying just beneath the renal capsule, the fibrous covering of the kidney

renal hilum the area through which the renal artery, vein, and ureter enter/leave the kidney

renal medulla the middle area of the kidney lying between the sinus and the cortex; the medullary tissue contains the renal pyramids

renal ostium the opening of the renal artery from the aortic wall

renal parenchymal disease a medical disorder affecting the tissue function of the kidneys

renal sinus the central echogenic cavity of the kidney; it contains the renal artery, renal vein, and collecting and lymphatic systems

suprasternal notch the visible indentation at the base of the neck where the neck joins the sternum

symphysis pubis/pubic bones the prominence of the pelvic bones noted in the lower abdomen

The true prevalence of renovascular hypertension is unknown but is estimated to affect approximately 50 million people in the United States alone.[1,2] As many as 6% of hypertensive patients have underlying renal disease as the cause of their elevated blood pressure.[2,3] In patients with severe diastolic hypertension, the prevalence of renal artery stenosis approaches 40%. Progression of stenosis occurs in 31% to 49% of patients depending on the initial severity renal artery narrowing.[3-5] Renal artery stenosis should be suspected in adults with sudden onset or worsening of chronic hypertension; azotemia, which is induced by angiotensin-converting enzyme inhibitor; unexplained renal insufficiency or pulmonary edema; and in hypertensive children.[6] In the majority of patients, renal artery disease is correctable with treatment providing control or cure for renovascular hypertension, retention of renal mass, and stabilization of renal function in patients with chronic renal failure.[7]

For identification of renovascular disease, contrast arteriography has historically been the procedure of choice. Although it provides anatomic information, this diagnostic test does not identify the functional significance of renal artery disease in hypertensive patients, nor does it provide hemodynamic information. Because of its associated, albeit low, morbidity, this invasive test is most often reserved for defining therapeutic intervention. Magnetic resonance angiography (MRA) and computed tomography angiography (CTA) offer less invasive diagnostic testing and excellent sensitivity and specificity, but are relatively expensive and require the injection of intravenous contrast.[8] It should be noted that in the case of CTA, the contrast agent may be nephrotoxic and is, therefore, unsuitable for use in patients with renal insufficiency. Given these deficiencies, many clinicians reserve MRA and CTA for use as secondary confirmatory studies and have focused their attention on duplex sonography as a primary diagnostic tool. Sonographic imaging can be performed on an outpatient basis at low cost without the risk of ionizing radiation or the use of nephrotoxic contrast agents. This modality has the additional advantages of being noninvasive and painless and has demonstrated an overall accuracy of 80% to 90% for identification of renal artery stenosis and definition of its hemodynamic significance.[9]

ANATOMY

The kidneys are located retroperitoneally in the dorsal abdominal cavity between the 12th thoracic and the 3rd lumbar vertebrae with the right kidney usually lying more inferior to the left (Fig. 20-1). The normal organ length is 8 to 13 cm with a width of 5 to 7 cm. The kidneys decrease in size with increasing age. An uncommon finding is a horseshoe kidney, which occurs in less than 1% of the population. In an excess of 90% of cases of horseshoe kidney, the organs are joined at their lower poles by an isthmus of tissue, which lies anterior to the aorta at the level of the fourth or fifth lumbar vertebrae.

For the purpose of sonographic interrogation, the kidneys are segmented into four main areas

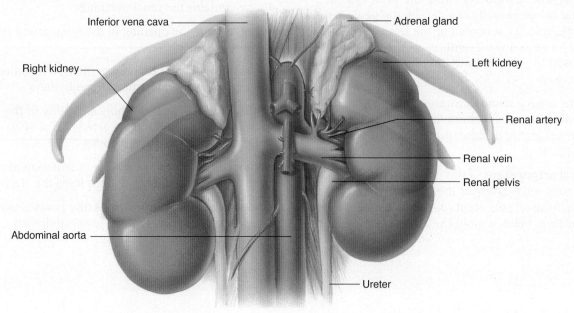

Figure 20-1 Diagram illustrating the anatomic location of the kidneys.

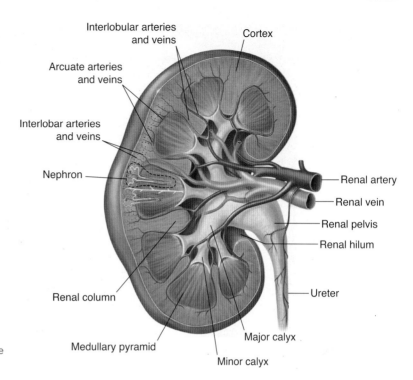

Figure 20-2 Diagram illustrating the vasculature of the kidneys.

(Fig. 20-2). The *renal hilum* is the area through which the renal artery, vein, and ureter enter and leave the kidney. The hilum forms a cavity called the *renal sinus*, which contains the renal artery and vein, and the collecting and lymphatic systems. The sinus is in large part made up of fat and fibrous tissue. For this reason, it is normally brightly echogenic on sonographic imaging (Fig. 20-3). The tissue of the kidney is referred to as the renal parenchyma. The parenchyma is divided into two parts: *the medulla* and *the cortex*. The renal pyramids, which appear triangular-shaped when the kidney is imaged longitudinally, carry urine from the cortex to the renal pelvis. The cortex is the outermost area of the kidney and lies just beneath the renal

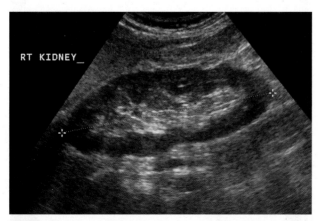

Figure 20-3 B-mode longitudinal image of a kidney, which illustrates the echogenic sinus, the medulla, the cortex, and the renal pyramids.

capsule. This is the area in which urine is produced. Cortical tissue, called columns of Bertin, lies between the medullary pyramids. The 12 to 18 pyramids generally have lower echogenicity than the cortex and are usually seen well in the normal adult patient.

The transpyloric plane serves as an important surface anatomic landmark for sonographic localization of the renal arteries (Fig. 20-4). This transverse plane is located halfway between the suprasternal notch and the symphysis pubis cutting through the lower border of the first lumbar vertebrae, the ninth costal cartilages and the pylorus. The renal arteries can be identified approximately 2 cm below the transpyloric plane arising from the anterior, lateral, or postero-lateral wall of the abdominal aorta. The left renal artery usually originates slightly more cephalad than the right. The right renal artery initially courses anterolaterally and then moves posterior to the inferior vena cava (IVC) and the right renal vein. In a small number of cases, the right renal artery will originate from the aortic wall anteriorly and course superior to the IVC (Fig. 20-5) The left renal artery courses on a slightly inferior path from the aortic wall, passes posterior to the left renal vein, and is crossed by the inferior mesenteric vein. Between 12% and 22% of patients have duplicate main renal arteries, which enter the kidney through the renal hilum or accessory polar arteries, a feature found more often on the left than on the right[10] (Fig. 20-6). Most often the accessory renal arteries arise from the aortic wall below the main renal artery and course to the polar surfaces of the kidney instead of entering

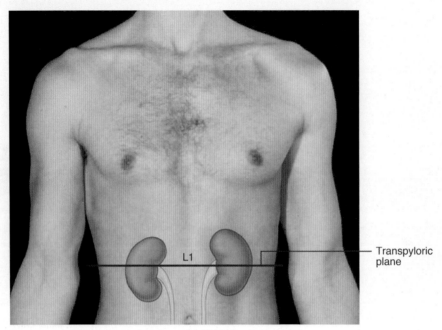

Figure 20-4 Diagram illustrating the anatomic location of the renal arteries and the transpyloric plane.

the renal hilum. Occasionally, accessory renal arteries originate from the common or internal iliac arteries.

Along its course, the renal artery normally gives rise to two to five branches, which supply blood to segments of the kidney. At the level of the renal hilum, the renal artery divides into a large anterior and a smaller posterior branch, which give rise to interlobar, arcuate, and interlobular arteries within the renal parenchyma (refer to Fig. 20-2).

On each side, the renal vein courses anteriorly from the renal hilum with the ureter arising posteriorly. The renal artery normally lies between the vein and the ureter. The right renal vein has a short

course from the hilum of the kidney to the IVC, whereas the left renal vein courses anterior to the aorta just below the origin of the superior mesenteric artery (refer to Fig. 20-1). In 2% to 5% of patients, the left renal vein takes a retroaortic path. Approximately 9% of patients will demonstrate a bifid left renal vein with both a retroaortic branch and another branch coursing anterior to the aorta. It is important to be aware of these anatomic anomalies because the left renal vein is used as a major anatomic landmark for locating the renal arteries during the sonographic examination.

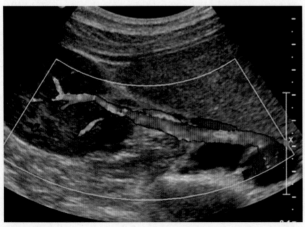

Figure 20-5 Color flow image demonstrating the right renal artery lying anterior to the inferior vena cava.

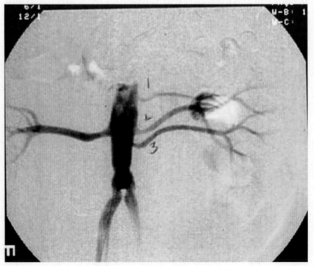

Figure 20-6 Arteriogram demonstrating multiple renal arteries on the left side.

ETIOLOGY OF RENAL ARTERY DISEASE

In a majority of cases, renovascular disease is caused by atherosclerotic renal artery stenosis.[7,11] As noted in Pathology Box 20-1, these lesions primarily affect the ostium and the proximal third of the renal artery, but may be found in any segment of the vessel including the interlobar and smaller branches within the renal medulla and cortex.[12] For reasons that are not well understood, renal artery stenosis is found more often in men than in women with lesions occurring bilaterally in more than 30% of patients.[13] Those most at risk for atherosclerotic renal artery stenosis include the elderly, hypertensive patients, smokers, and patients with coronary and/or peripheral arterial disease, hyperlipidemia, or diabetes.

Medial fibromuscular dysplasia is the second most common curable cause of renovascular disease. This nonatherosclerotic disease entity commonly affects the mid-to-distal segment of the renal artery in females aged 25 to 50 years. Although the disease is most often found bilaterally, it may involve one side only with the right side being affected more frequently than the left.[14] As noted sonographically and angiographically, the lesions produce segmental concentric narrowing and dilation, resulting in a "string of beads" appearance (Fig. 20-7A,B).[15,16] An intimal form of this disease, found more commonly in males, produces focal narrowing of the mid- or distal segment of the renal artery.

Although atherosclerotic stenosis and fibromuscular dysplasia are the most commonly observed renal artery pathology, other complications must be considered during the sonographic examination. These include aortic dissection extending into the renal arteries, aneurysms of the main or segmental renal arteries, aortic coarctation proximal to the renal artery origins, arteriovenous fistulae, arteritis, and extrinsic compression of the renal artery and/or vein by tumors or other masses.[12,17]

SONOGRAPHIC EXAMINATION TECHNIQUES

PATIENT PREPARATION AND POSITIONING

To reduce excessive abdominal gas that may obviate adequate visualization of the renal arteries and veins, patients are asked to fast for 8 to 10 hours prior to their examination. Elective studies are scheduled in the morning, and diabetic patients are prioritized according to their insulin schedules. To prevent the development of hypoglycemia while awaiting their renal duplex examination, diabetic patients are permitted to have dry toast and clear liquids. Patients are permitted to take morning medications with sips of water and are asked to refrain from smoking or chewing gum to reduce the amount of swallowed air.

PATIENT POSITIONING

Prior to initiating the examination, patients are asked to lie supine on the examination table with their head slightly elevated. The examination table is placed

---

PATHOLOGY BOX 20-1

Characterization of the Most Common Types of Renal Artery Pathology Encountered during Sonographic Evaluation of the Renal Arteries

Pathology	Location	Sonographic Appearance	Spectral Doppler
Atherosclerosis	Usually ostial or proximal Any segment of main renal Parenchymal arteries	Acoustically homogeneous or heterogeneous Smooth or irregularly surfaced	High velocity with poststenotic turbulence if >60% diameter-reducing stenosis Low velocity if stenosis is preocclusive
Medial fibromuscular dysplasia	Mid-to-distal renal artery Parenchymal arteries	Segmental narrowing and dilation of the renal artery Alternating regions of forward and reversed flow	High velocity compared to proximal arterial segment
Occlusion	Focal or entire length	Intraluminal echoes of varying echogenicity dependent on chronicity Kidney length <8–9 cm	Absent Doppler signal in imaged artery Low velocity, low amplitude signals in the renal parenchyma

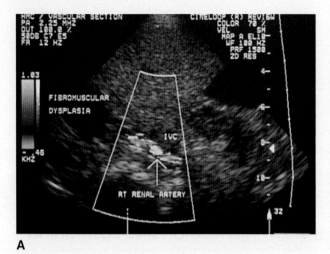

A

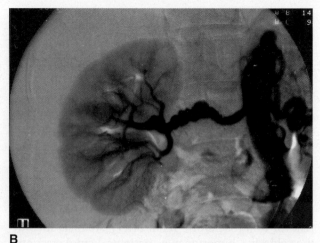

B

Figure 20-7 A: Color flow image of a renal artery with fibromuscular dysplasia (FMD). Note the regions of forward and reversed flow associated with the segmental concentric narrowing and dilation **(B)**. Arteriogram illustrating FMD in the mid-to-distal renal artery segment on the right.

in the reverse Trendelenburg position with the patient's feet 15° to 20° lower than his or her heart. This allows the visceral contents to descend into the lower abdomen and pelvis, enhancing the acoustic windows used for access to the renal arteries and kidneys. From the supine position, the sonographer is able to examine the aorta, celiac trunk, proximal superior mesenteric artery, the renal ostia, and the proximal-to-mid segment of the renal arteries. To facilitate visualization of the mid-to-distal segment of the renal arteries and the kidneys, the patient may be moved to the right or left lateral decubitus position with his or her arm placed over the head and the legs extended to elongate the body. In some cases, the patient may be asked to lie prone with his or her midsection flexed over a pillow or foam wedge. This position allows access to the kidneys and distal renal arteries through an intercostal image plane.

The sonographer should be positioned on either side of the examination table, which is elevated to a height that allows scanning without overextension of his or her arm. It is also important to ensure that the patient is lying close to the sonographer's side of the table. This facilitates ease of movement of the transducer from the midline of the patient's abdomen to the flank while allowing the sonographer to maintain correct ergonomic positioning. If at all possible, sonographers should learn to scan with both hands, moving the ultrasound system to the opposite side of the bed as appropriate to the study.

EQUIPMENT

Examination of the abdominal vasculature is performed using a high-resolution ultrasound system with phased or curved array transducers ranging in frequency from 2.0 to 5.0 MHz. The grayscale image

is used to localize vessels and organs, and to identify atherosclerotic plaque, aneurysmal dilation, and dissections. Color and power Doppler imaging facilitate visualizing arteries and veins, identifying anatomic landmarks, detecting regions of disordered flow, and confirming vessel occlusion. Differentiation of normal and abnormal flow patterns is based on Doppler velocity spectral waveform parameters. A diagnosis of renal artery stenosis or occlusion requires an accurate interpretation of Doppler spectral waveform data and the integration of all accompanying sonographic information. Throughout the study, careful attention must be given to optimizing spectral and color Doppler pulse repetition frequency (PRF, velocity scale), gain, wall filters, and most importantly, angle of insonation.

SCANNING TECHNIQUE[18]

Interrogation of the Aorta, and the Mesenteric and Renal Arteries

With the patient lying supine, a sagittal image of the aorta is obtained from the left paramedian scan plane beginning at the level of the xiphoid process and continuing through the aortic bifurcation to include the common iliac arteries. Care is taken to identify atherosclerotic plaque, duplicate main and accessory renal arteries, aneurysmal dilation, dissection, and regions of flow disturbance using B-Mode, color, and power Doppler imaging. Using a small Doppler sample volume size and an appropriate angle of insonation less than 60°, spectral waveforms are recorded from the abdominal aorta at the level of the celiac and superior mesenteric arteries. The peak systolic velocity (PSV) from the aorta is retained to calculate the renal–aortic velocity ratio.

Because branches of the celiac and superior mesenteric arteries may course in proximity to the main or accessory renal arteries, it is important to recognize the mesenteric arterial flow patterns. To achieve this goal, representative Doppler spectral waveforms should be obtained from the proximal celiac and superior mesenteric arteries. A secondary benefit may be identification of flow-limiting mesenteric artery stenosis. This is most likely to occur in patients where atherosclerotic plaque is noted along the aortic walls in the region of the mesenteric artery origins.

A cross-sectional image of the aorta is obtained at the level of the superior mesenteric artery (SMA). Just inferior to the SMA, the left renal vein is identified as it crosses either anterior to the aorta or in a retroaortic position (refer to Fig. 20-1). Optimized B-mode and color flow imaging should be used to determine the presence of renal vein thrombosis or entrapment of the renal vein by small bowel or the SMA. Extrinsic compression of the vein may result in "nutcracker" or mesenteric compression syndrome.

The renal arteries normally lie immediately inferior to the left renal vein. Visualization of the proximal segments of these vessels may be facilitated by moving the transducer upright so that it is perpendicular to the patient's abdominal wall (Fig. 20-8). This position allows compression of the left renal vein. While remaining upright, the transducer is then angled slightly to the right or left to create a sagittal image of the renal artery (Fig. 20-9). Color flow imaging may facilitate the identification of the vessels and optimal visualization of the renal artery origins and accessory renal arteries. From this scan plane, the renal arteries can most often be visualized from the ostium to the mid-segment. To rule out orificial renal artery stenosis, the Doppler sample volume is swept slowly from the aortic lumen through the renal ostium. Demonstration of the change in spectral

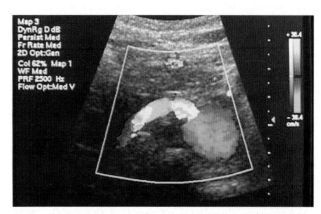

Figure 20-9 Sagittal color flow image of the right renal artery.

waveform pattern from high-resistance, low-diastolic aortic flow to low-resistance, high-diastolic renal artery flow allows for the recognition of abnormal flow patterns and ostial lesions (Fig. 20-10). Thereafter, Doppler spectral waveforms are obtained continuously throughout all visualized segments, and representative signals are then recorded taking care to ensure that all waveforms are obtained at appropriate angles of insonation.

To interrogate the mid-to-distal segment of the renal arteries and parenchymal flow, the patient is moved to the lateral decubitus or prone position. With the patient lying in the decubitus position, a transverse image of the kidney can be obtained through an intercostal window using a coronal plane from the patient's flank. The right renal artery is relatively easy to follow from the renal hilum to its origin at the aortic wall. The left renal artery may be more difficult to

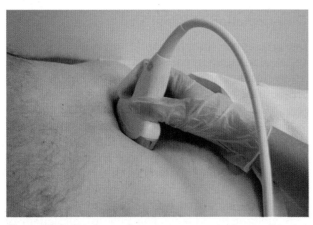

Figure 20-8 This figure demonstrates appropriate positioning of the ultrasound transducer for the acquisition of images and Doppler spectral waveforms from the ostium and proximal renal artery.

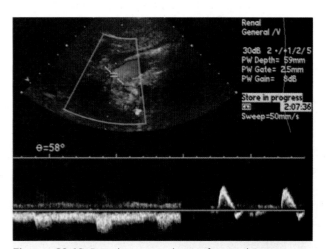

Figure 20-10 Doppler spectral waveforms demonstrating the transition from the high-resistance (low-diastolic flow) aortic signal to the low-resistance (high-diastolic flow) signal obtained as the sample volume is slowly swept from the aortic lumen into the renal artery ostium. Because the renal arteries often originate from the aortic wall at angles between 70° and 90°, it may be difficult to have a correct angle when collecting the transition signals.

visualize. It is helpful to image from a posterolateral plane, using the left kidney as an acoustic window. Assuming the positions of the hands on a clock, an image of the left kidney is obtained so that the renal pelvis is positioned at either 5, 6, or 7 o'clock. From the 5 o'clock position, the left renal artery will be noted to course slightly to the right before entering the kidney (Fig. 20-11). At the 6 o'clock position, the renal artery will enter the hilum on a straight course. When imaged from the 7 o'clock position, the artery will course slightly to the left just before entering the pelvis of the kidney.

Access to the distal segment of the renal artery can also be obtained by having the patient lie prone and flexed in the midsection over a pillow or foam wedge. Using an intercostal window, excellent images of the kidney and distal-to-mid segments of the renal artery are readily obtained. With both approaches, attention must be given to appropriate angle correction, taking care to use a range of angles similar to those used for Doppler spectral interrogation of the proximal-to-mid segments of the artery.

Identification of Accessory Renal Arteries

Several imaging approaches may be used to facilitate the identification of accessory or multiple renal arteries. Duplicate renal arteries may be detected on a longitudinal, oblique image of the aorta or from a transverse view of the kidney where the arteries can be noted coursing to the polar surfaces rather than to the renal hilum (Fig. 20-12). Although color flow imaging is helpful in highlighting these small vessels, power Doppler imaging has shown value because of the lower angle dependence of this modality compared to color flow imaging. Clues to the presence of additional renal arteries can also be obtained by increasing the sample volume size and scanning in the para-aortic region from the level of the SMA through the aortic bifurcation. As the renal arteries are the only low resistance vessels distal to the SMA,

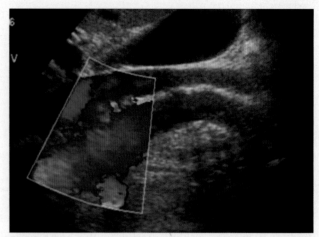

Figure 20-12 Longitudinal color flow image of the abdominal aorta demonstrating duplicate right renal arteries.

detection of multiple low-resistance Doppler signals should encourage the examiner to pursue one or more of the previously mentioned acoustic planes.

Evaluation of Blood Flow within the Kidney

Blood flow patterns are recorded at a 0° angle of insonation throughout the upper, mid, and lower poles of the renal sinus, medulla, and cortex. Color and/or power Doppler imaging may facilitate the detection of regions of absent or disturbed flow or increased signal amplitude. The Doppler spectral waveforms with the highest PSV and end-diastolic velocity (EDV) from each segment of the organ should be retained. In addition to evaluating the renal vasculature, the parenchyma of the kidney should be examined for cortical thinning, renal calculi, masses, cysts, or hydronephrosis. The presence of perinephric fluid collections should also be noted.

Determination of Renal Size

Because renal atrophy could preclude successful revascularization in patients with flow-limiting renal artery lesions, it is important to document kidney size during every examination. The normal renal length is between 9 and 13 cm. Comparing the sides, a difference in renal length greater than 3 cm suggests compromised flow on the side with the smaller kidney. With the patient lying in the lateral decubitus position and the transducer angled antero-laterally just below the costal border, a coronal or lateral flank approach can be used to obtain a long axis view of the kidney. The pole-to-pole length of the kidney is measured during deep inspiration. Accuracy is enhanced by averaging three separate measurements.

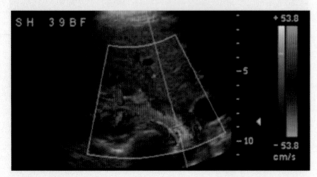

Figure 20-11 Transverse color flow image of the left kidney obtained from a coronal image plane demonstrating the renal artery entering the renal hilum at the 5 o'clock position.

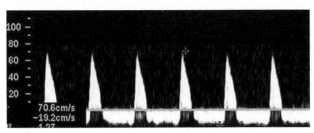

Figure 20-13 Doppler spectral waveforms recorded within the renal parenchyma in a patient with renal vein thrombosis. Note the reversed, blunted diastolic flow component.

Evaluation of Renal Vein Thrombosis

Patients may be referred to the vascular laboratory to rule out renal vein thrombosis. Patients with acute renal failure may present with pain and hematuria. Other patients may be suspected of renal cell carcinoma with extension of the tumor into the renal veins or IVC. The renal veins and IVC should always be examined in patients with an IVC filter or thrombosed IVC because retrograde thrombosis may extend into the renal veins.

Confirmation of renal vein thrombosis can be technically challenging. It is important to optimize the grayscale image because acute thrombus may have acoustic properties similar to flowing blood. Although venous dilation suggests acute thrombosis, the renal vein may be contracted when the condition is chronic. The absence of an optimized spectral, color, or power Doppler signal suggests thrombosis of the renal vein. In this setting, Doppler spectral waveforms with retrograde, blunted diastolic flow

components are usually recorded throughout the arteries of the renal parenchyma (Fig. 20-13).

Use of Contrast-Enhanced Imaging

There are many factors that may influence the ability to visualize the entire length of the renal artery including excessive bowel gas, patient body habitus, and an inability to adequately position the patient to gain optimal acoustic windows.[9] Quite often, imaging can be improved and diagnostic accuracy increased by employing intravenous ultrasound contrast agents to enhance visualization of the renal arteries. Although not yet approved by the U.S. Food and Drug Administration for clinical vascular evaluations, investigators have shown improved diagnostic accuracy when these agents are used in the liver and in the mesenteric and peripheral vessels.[17,19]

A recent study has shown improved ability to identify the renal ostium, the length of the renal artery, accessory renal arteries, and flow-limiting renal artery stenoses in select cases following intravenous injection of contrast (Fig. 20-14A,B).[20] A further discussion of ultrasound contrast agents will be found in Chapter 27 of this text.

DIAGNOSIS

THE ABDOMINAL AORTA AND THE COMMON ILIAC ARTERIES

B-mode images of the normal abdominal aorta and common iliac arteries should demonstrate anechoic lumens with smooth arterial walls. Care should be

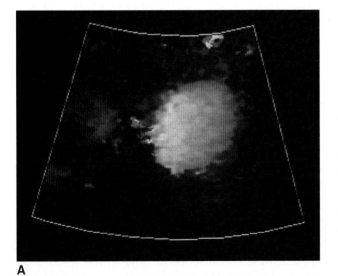
A

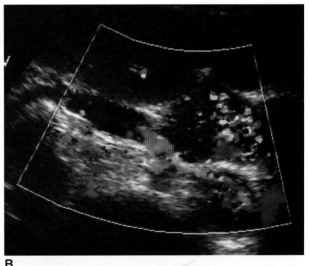
B

Figure 20-14 Color flow images of a renal artery prior to **(A)** and following **(B)** intravenous injection of an ultrasound contrast agent. The image obtained prior to injection of the contrast agent was created from a cross-sectional aortic approach at the renal ostium. Following contrast enhancement, the length of the renal artery could be visualized from an intercostal approach using the liver as an acoustic window. (Courtesy of John Pellerito, MD, North Shore University Medical Center, Long Island, NY.)

taken to identify aneurysmal dilation, dissection, and/or atherosclerotic plaque with particular attention to the regions surrounding the aortic branch vessels. Recognition of narrowed or tortuous arterial segments may be facilitated by using color flow or power Doppler imaging.

The proximal abdominal aorta carries blood to the low resistance vascular beds of the liver, spleen, and kidneys. This flow demand is reflected in the Doppler spectral waveform morphology. At this level, the Doppler spectral waveform is characterized by rapid systolic upstroke, sharp systolic peak, and forward diastolic flow. The PSV ranges from 60 to 100 cm/s. Distal to the renal arteries, the aortic waveform exhibits slightly lower velocity and a triphasic flow pattern. This waveform pattern reflects the elevated vascular resistance of the lumbar arteries and lower extremity circulation.

Flow should be laminar throughout the normal proximal abdominal aorta with the exception of slight flow disturbance, which may be evident at the ostia of the renal and mesenteric arteries. Increased velocity may be noted in tortuous vessels in the absence of disease, but high velocity, turbulent signals suggest significant arterial narrowing.

THE NORMAL RENAL ARTERY

The lumen of the normal renal artery should be anechoic, and the vessel should have smooth walls throughout its length. Color flow and/or power Doppler imaging may demonstrate regions of narrowing caused by tortuosity, kinking, or extrinsic compression.

The Doppler spectral waveform from the normal renal artery is characterized by rapid systolic upstroke, a slightly blunted peak, and forward diastolic flow. An early systolic peak (ESP) or compliance peak may be seen on the upstroke to systole (Fig. 20-15). It is thought that the ESP or compliance peak is a reflection of the elasticity of the arterial wall and, therefore, its presence is usually variable throughout the renal artery and smaller vessels within the

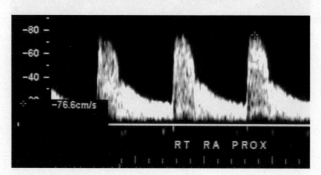

Figure 20-15 Doppler spectral waveforms illustrating normal renal arterial waveform morphology.

kidney. The PSV of the renal artery ranges from 90 to 120 cm/s with EDV exceeding one-third of the systolic value. Normally, PSV and EDV decrease proportionately from the main renal artery to the level of the renal cortex. The PSV in the distal renal artery ranges from 70 to 90 cm/s, decreasing to 30 to 50 cm/s in the renal sinus, and 10 to 20 cm/s at the level of the renal cortex.

RENAL ARTERY STENOSIS OF LESS THAN HEMODYNAMIC SIGNIFICANCE (<60%)

B-Mode imaging may demonstrate atherosclerotic plaque extending from the aortic wall into the orifice or proximal segment of the renal artery. Color flow imaging is helpful in identifying regions of disordered flow and narrowing of the arterial lumen.

As the diameter of the renal artery decreases, the flow demands of the kidney increase. Narrowing of the renal artery diameter by 30% to 60% results in an increase in renal artery PSV in excess of 180 cm/s. The degree of narrowing is not yet severe enough to cause a decrease in pressure or flow distal to the lesion. Therefore, poststenotic turbulence is not present with this degree of luminal compromise.

FLOW-REDUCING RENAL ARTERY STENOSIS (>60%)

When the diameter of the renal artery is reduced by more than 60%, the PSV increases significantly above 180 cm/s and poststenotic turbulence develops immediately downstream (Fig. 20-16A–D). Beyond this region, in the absence of tandem or critical lesions, flow will gradually return to a normal laminar profile. It is important to confirm the poststenotic signal, which differentiates a flow-reducing stenosis from one that is of less than hemodynamic significance (<60%). When the degree of arterial narrowing exceeds 80%, systolic upstroke will be delayed, the compliance peak will be lost, and the PSV will decrease distally (parvus tardus signal). In the absence of elevated renovascular resistance, diastolic forward flow will be maintained.

RENAL ARTERY OCCLUSION

Occlusion of the renal artery is confirmed by using optimized spectral, color, and power Doppler to demonstrate the absence of flow in the main renal artery. Multiple image planes may be required to ensure complete visualization of the full length of the vessel. Because the kidney is supplied by adrenal and ureteral collaterals, low-amplitude and low-velocity

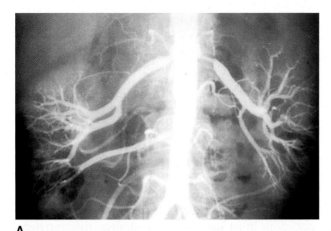

A

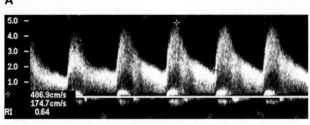

```
5.0 –
4.0 –
3.0 –
2.0 –
1.0 –
    486.9cm/s
    174.7cm/s
RI    0.64
```

B

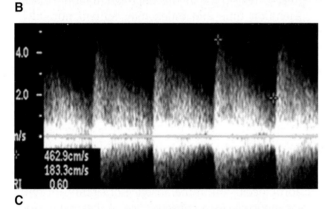

```
4.0 –

2.0 –

n/s –
    462.9cm/s
    183.3cm/s
RI    0.60
```

C

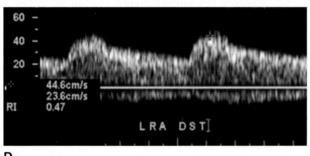

```
60 –
40 –
20 –
    44.6cm/s
    23.6cm/s
RI  0.47
```

LRA DST

D

Figure 20-16 Arteriogram demonstrating a proximal left renal artery stenosis **(A)** and the associated Doppler spectral waveforms demonstrating high velocity at the site of stenosis **(B)**, poststenotic turbulence **(C)**, and dampening parvus tardus signal] **(D)** distally.

Doppler signals are usually noted throughout the renal medulla and cortex. With chronic renal artery occlusion, the PSV in the cortex will be less than 10 cm/s, and pole-to-pole length of the kidney will be less than 9 cm.

INTRINSIC PARENCHYMAL DYSFUNCTION

Using a 0° angle of insonation, Doppler spectral waveforms should be recorded throughout the parenchymal vessels in the medulla and cortex of the kidney. The spectral pattern differentiates normal renovascular resistance from intrinsic parenchymal dysfunction (medical renal disease). In the normal kidney, the Doppler spectral pattern demonstrates continuous high diastolic flow throughout all segments of the kidney. In the absence of parenchymal disease, diastolic flow normally approximates 40% to 50% of the systolic velocity. Surprisingly, elevated diastolic flow is sustained even in normal kidneys with flow-limiting renal artery stenosis. It is most likely that the reduction in flow triggers compensatory vasodilation and renovascular resistance remains low.

Parenchymal disease most often results in the accumulation of interstitial cellular infiltrates and edema, resulting in impedance to arterial inflow to the kidney and increased renovascular resistance. This finding is associated with a broad spectrum of renal disorders including glomerulonephritis, polycystic disease, acute tubular necrosis, obstructive hydronephrosis, and diabetic nephropathy. In 1979, Arima et al.[21] and Norris and his colleagues[22] demonstrated that increased renovascular resistance is associated with decreased diastolic flow in native and transplanted kidneys. A diastolic-to-systolic velocity ratio less than 0.3 (resistive index greater than 0.8) is predictive of medical renal disease; further decline in diastolic flow is associated with elevated blood urea nitrogen and serum creatinine levels.[23] Most modern ultrasound systems include the calculation of end-diastolic to peak systolic ratio (EDR) or resistive index (RI). The equation for EDR is EDV/PSV, whereas the equation for RI is (PSV − EDV)/PSV.

INDIRECT RENAL HILAR EVALUATIONS

Based on the knowledge that in peripheral arteries pulsatility decreases and systolic upstroke is delayed as a consequence of more proximal significant disease, several investigators have advocated use of a limited, indirect assessment of the arteries within the renal hilum. This approach is attractive because it overcomes the technical challenges associated with interrogation of the entire length of the renal artery and decreases the time required to perform the study. Handa et al. demonstrated an accuracy of 95%, a sensitivity of 100%, and a specificity of 93% for identification of proximal flow-reducing renal artery stenosis using an *acceleration index (AI)* of less than 3.78.[24] The AI is defined as the slope of the systolic upstroke (kilohertz per second) divided by the transmitted frequency. When translated into velocity units, an AI equal to or greater than 291 cm/s^2 is suggestive of proximal flow-reducing renal artery stenosis. Martin and his colleagues found an *acceleration time* (AT)—defined as the time interval between the onset of systole and the initial compliance peak—greater than 100 ms to be more predictive of significant proximal renal artery disease in their patient population than an AI.[25] The AT can be calculated automatically on most high-end ultrasound systems by indicating with calipers the onset of systole and the early systolic (compliance) peak. The value can also be determined by manual calculation by using handheld calipers to measure the distance between these two points. Because the smallest time interval measured on most state-of-the art ultrasound systems is 40 ms, 2.5 time intervals demonstrated on the spectral display is equal to 100 ms. Stavros et al. combined the AI and AT with loss of the compliance peak to identify proximal flow-limiting renal artery lesions and to differentiate 60% to 79% stenosis from more critical lesions as detailed in Figure 20-17.[26] Other investigators have found low diagnostic sensitivity using hilar waveform evaluation for the detection of significant renal artery disease.[27,28]

As noted previously, the main renal artery divides into several segmental branches proximal to the renal hilum. Because each of these branches originates from the main renal artery, in theory it should not matter which branch is used for Doppler signal analysis. Inaccurate information could be obtained if Doppler waveforms were recorded in accessory, polar renal arteries as each of these could give rise to segmental branches with varying Doppler spectral waveform contours.

The indirect renal hilar examination is performed with the patient lying in the lateral decubitus or prone position. Using an intercostal approach, a transverse image of the kidney is obtained at a depth

between 4 and 8 cm in most patients. From this plane of view, the renal hilum and distal segmental branches of the main renal artery can be interrogated using a 0° angle of insonation. It is important to record a strong Doppler signal in order to optimize waveform clarity. This is accomplished by using the highest possible transducer frequency to improve Doppler sensitivity,[26] a large (3 to 5 mm) Doppler sample volume, and a sweep speed of 100 ms.

It has been estimated that hypertension affects 10% of the U.S. population and that less than 6% of this group has renal artery disease. In order to detect disease that has such a low prevalence, a diagnostic test procedure must have high sensitivity. Unfortunately, although indirect hilar assessment is an attractive option, investigators report varying results ranging from high sensitivity to lack of correlation between the duplex sonographic findings and angiography.[10,26,29-35] There are multiple reasons for this variation in accuracy. Doppler waveform contour is affected by arterial compliance, obstruction to arterial inflow, and the degree of resistance in the microcirculation.[36,37] The acceleration time and index may remain normal in patients with elevated renovascular resistance (e.g., parenchymal dysfunction, medical renal disease) or systemic arterial stiffness. Although delayed systolic upstroke and loss of a compliance peak are common findings in cases of renal artery stenosis exceeding 80% diameter reduction, the Doppler spectral waveform may remain normal when there is stenosis in the range of 60% to 79%. To complicate matters further, we have also noted low velocity, dampened intrarenal spectral waveforms in patients with aortic coarctation, or aortic occlusion in the absence of significant renal artery stenosis. As a consequence of these and other issues, indirect renal hilar assessment is not recommended as the sole diagnostic tool for the detection of renal artery disease. As long as the deficiencies of this approach are recognized, it does serve as a valuable tool to complement direct renal artery interrogation, particularly in cases where the direct examination is technically limited. It is important to keep in mind that hilar studies do not define the anatomic location of proximal renal artery lesions nor can they differentiate a well-collateralized renal artery occlusion from a high-grade stenosis.[25] Care must be taken to ensure that spectral waveforms are recorded in the distal main renal artery and its hilar branches and not in segmental branches of accessory renal arteries.

RENAL–AORTIC RATIO AND CURRENT CRITERIA

Current diagnostic criteria for identification of renal artery stenosis are based on the renal–aortic ratio (RAR), which is the ratio of the renal artery PSV to

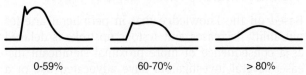

0-59%   60-70%   > 80%

Figure 20-17 Diagram illustrating a comparison of Doppler waveform morphology recorded in the distal main renal artery and segmental renal artery branches in normal and stenotic renal arteries. Note that rapid systolic upstroke and the compliance peak or ESP are commonly found in arteries with a less than hemodynamically significant stenosis (0% to 59%). Some investigators have noted the loss of the compliance peak or ESP with renal artery stenosis in the range of 60% to 79%. The most validated observation is the dampened waveform found with renal artery stenosis exceeding 80%. (Modified from Stavros TA, Parker SH, Yakes YF, et al. Segmental stenosis of the renal artery: pattern recognition of the tardus and parvus abnormalities with duplex sonography. *Radiology.* 1992;184:487–492.)

the aortic PSV recorded at the level of the mesenteric arteries. Narrowing of the renal artery diameter by more than 60% to 70% results in a significant increase in PSV, whereas the velocity in the aorta remains relatively unchanged. Kohler and his colleagues demonstrated excellent sensitivity for confirming the absence of flow-limiting renal artery stenosis (>60% diameter reduction) using an RAR <3.5.[38] Similarly, an RAR >3.5 has shown excellent value to identify significant renal artery stenosis. As such, the RAR may be used as a primary diagnostic criterion as long as caveats are recognized. In patients with increased cardiac output or significant abdominal aortic stenosis, the aortic PSV may exceed 100 cm/s. In such cases, the calculated renal–aortic velocity ratio will be too low and the severity of renal artery stenosis will be underestimated. For example, if the aortic velocity is 140 cm/s and the renal artery velocity is 320 cm/s, the renal–aortic velocity ratio is 2.3, mistakenly suggesting the absence of significant renal artery stenosis. Similarly, in cases with low cardiac output, aortic occlusion, coarctation, or aortic aneurysm, the aortic PSV will be lower than normal (<40 cm/s). Use of the calculated RAR could result in overestimation of the severity of renal artery stenosis.

Elevated renal artery velocity accompanied by poststenotic turbulence has been shown to be a sensitive predictor of flow-limiting renal artery stenosis.[39–41] Hoffman et al. used a renal artery PSV greater than 180 cm/s as an indicator of stenotic renal artery disease.[42] A pressure-flow gradient results when the diameter of the artery is reduced by more than 60% and poststenotic turbulence is apparent immediately distal to the site of narrowing. Renal artery stenosis of less than hemodynamic significance is identified by an elevated PSV (>180 cm/s), an RAR <3.5, and most notably, the absence of a poststenotic signal. Inclusion of these criteria should be used in addition to or in place of the RAR to increase diagnostic accuracy. Table 20-1 summarizes the commonly used diagnostic criteria for renal artery stenosis.

EVALUATION OF THE RENAL VEINS

The duplex examination should demonstrate an anechoic lumen and respirophasicity throughout all visualized segments of the normal renal vein. Intraluminal echoes will be apparent when the vein is obstructed. Care must be taken to optimize B-mode, spectral, and color Doppler parameters to ensure identification of acute thrombus, partial venous obstruction, recanalization, collateralization, and/or extrinsic compression. Continuous, nonphasic low velocity flow will be noted proximal to thrombosed venous segments. Minimally phasic flow is often recorded distally if the thrombosed segment has recanalized or if venous collaterals have developed. If the kidney has been severely damaged by the thrombotic process, renal atrophy may be apparent and the kidney may demonstrate increased echogenicity compared to the acoustic pattern of the contralateral organ. If the left renal vein is compressed by the mesentery or superior mesenteric artery, a high velocity signal associated with a color bruit may be noted in the vein as it crosses anterior to the aorta.

SONOGRAPHIC EXAMINATION OF RENAL STENTS

Several technical and interpretive considerations must be applied to an evaluation of renal arteries with stents.[43] Although a majority of stents will be placed in the ostium or proximal renal artery, the number and location of stents may be variable. Proximal renal artery stents are most readily visualized from a cross-sectional image of the aorta at the level of the renal artery origins (Fig. 20-18). Harmonic and/or real-time compound imaging is used to improve the resolution and conspicuity of lesions and to decrease artifacts. A slight velocity increase is to be expected in stented arterial segments due to the reduction in arterial compliance. Increased velocity may also be

TABLE 20-1				
Classification of Renal Artery Stenosis Based on the Renal–Aortic Velocity Ratio, Peak Systolic Renal Artery Velocity, and Kidney Length				
CLASSIFICATION OF RENAL ARTERY STENOSIS				
% Stenosis	RAR	PSV	PST	Kidney Length
Normal	<3.5	<180 cm/s	Absent	9–13 cm
<60%	<3.5	>180 cm/s	Absent	9–13 cm
>60%	>3.5	>180 cm/s	Present	Variable
Occluded	N/A	N/A	N/A	<8 cm

RAR, renal–aortic ratio; PSV, peak systolic velocity; PST, poststenotic turbulence.

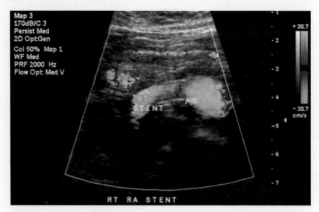

Figure 20-18 Transverse aortic color flow image illustrating a proximal renal artery stent

noted at the distal end of the stent when the diameter of the stented segment exceeds the diameter of the native renal artery. This most often occurs when the stent is placed in the smaller diameter distal renal artery.

It is important to note whether elevated velocity is focal or associated with downstream propagation of flow disturbance. Diameter mismatches are more likely to produce focal elevation in velocity without associated turbulence, whereas the flow profile of a flow-reducing stenosis exhibits high velocity, poststenotic turbulence, and dampening of the distal waveform. Additionally, temporal changes in velocity will likely be noted when stenotic disease is present but velocity elevations should remain stable if related to a diameter mismatch.

At present, diagnostic criteria have not been well validated for the classification of renal artery stent stenosis, and native renal artery criteria are being applied with special consideration to the issues of compliance, diameter mismatch, and stent location.[44-47] Recently, Mohabbat et al. reported a sensitivity of 93% and a specificity of 99% when using a PSV >280 cm/s and an RAR >4.5 to determine a significant in-stent stenosis.[46]

PREDICTION OF SUCCESSFUL RENAL REVASCULARIZATION

Although duplex sonography has been accepted as a valued noninvasive tool for the identification of renal artery stenosis and renal parenchymal dysfunction, it has been difficult to define parameters that can be used to successfully select patients whose blood pressure or renal function will improve following renal revascularization. In 2001, Radermacher and his colleagues investigated the use of a resistive index (1-end-diastolic velocity divided by the highest peak systolic velocity) in 138 patients with unilateral or bilateral significant renal artery stenosis to predict successful revascularization.[48] They also documented creatinine clearance and ambulatory blood pressure prior to the procedure and at three-month intervals throughout the first year and yearly thereafter with a mean follow-up of 32 months. They found that a resistive index of 80 or greater could be used to predict which patients would be unlikely to benefit from either renal artery angioplasty or surgical bypass.

Numerous studies have shown that severe renal artery stenosis is associated with renal atrophy.[49-54] Caps et al. demonstrated a high risk for progression to renal atrophy in patients with a renal artery PSV greater than 400 cm/s and a cortical EDV equal to or less than 5 cm/s.[55] If renal artery stenosis is recognized before it critically affects blood flow to the kidney, it is likely that intervention may salvage or improve renal function.[54,56] Conversely, revascularization is most often unsuccessful in kidneys with a pole-to-pole length less than 8 cm.[57] As such, the measurement of kidney length should be a component of the scanning protocol whenever renal artery stenosis is suspected.

SUMMARY

Duplex sonography of the renal vasculature and kidneys has become the initial primary diagnostic procedure for evaluation of renovascular hypertension and suspected renal artery pathology. Although technically challenging, renal vascular sonography provides noninvasive, cost-effective, and accurate diagnostic information. Duplex technology allows for the definition of vessel and tissue pathology, detection of altered blood flow patterns, and quantitation of hemodynamic disturbances. The length of the abdominal aorta, the renal arteries, and the kidneys can be evaluated with B-mode imaging to localize atherosclerotic disease, fibromuscular dysplasia, aneurysms, dissections, cysts, and masses, and to demonstrate extrinsic compression of the renal vessels due to masses or entrapment. This modality has also shown value as a tool for confirming progression of renal artery stenosis and defining therapeutic options based on kidney size. Color flow and power Doppler imaging facilitate recognition of regions of flow disturbance, stenosis, occlusion, and anatomic anomalies. Visualization of the blood flow vectors eases placement of the Doppler sample volume for waveform analysis and measurement of velocities. The determination of disease severity is based on the PSV and the presence or absence of a poststenotic signal in the main renal artery. The assessment of velocity waveform parameters recorded within the renal parenchyma yields clues to the presence of intrinsic renal disease and the likelihood of successful revascularization. The role of indirect renal hilar duplex for the identification of flow-limiting renal artery disease remains controversial. At present, studies have shown that it is best used to complement direct and complete examination of the renal arteries and kidneys. Given the broad scope of diagnostic information that can be obtained using ultrasound to interrogate the renal vasculature, it is not surprising that duplex sonography is recognized as the ideal technology for the identification of renal vascular disease and for follow-up after endovascular or surgical intervention. The technical success of each study is influenced by the experience of the examiner and the physician interpreter. Complete and accurate examinations of the renal vasculature are possible in more than 90% of patients when the study is performed in high volume laboratories by experienced, credentialed sonographers and interpreted by qualified physicians, both of whom have a knowledge of renal vascular disease, the validated techniques used for assessment of the renal vasculature, and the current diagnostic criteria used for the classification of renal artery stenosis.

Critical Thinking Questions

1. A patient presents for a renal duplex scan. Prior to initiating the examination, you can determine the approximate location of this patient's renal arteries by noting several body surface landmarks. What are the most important landmarks to use to accomplish this goal?

2. During the renal sonographic examination, there are other important anatomic landmarks to use for locating the renal arteries. Which of the landmarks are most commonly used?

3. It is always important to consider the patient's clinical presentation. If a 40-year-old hypertensive female presents for renal duplex examination, what would be the most likely pathology responsible for her renovascular hypertension?

4. A patient of large body habitus presents for a renal duplex examination. With the patient lying supine, you are able to image the abdominal aorta in both sagittal and cross-sectional planes but you cannot visualize the right renal artery. What steps can you take to determine if the renal artery is patent or occluded?

5. A PSV of 220 cm/s is recorded in the proximal segment of a tortuous right renal artery. How would you determine whether the elevated velocity was the result of flow-limiting stenosis or vessel angulation?

REFERENCES

1. Berglund G, Anderson O, Wilhelmensen L. Prevalence of primary and secondary hypertension: studies in a random population sample. *Br Med J.* 1976;2(6035):554–556.
2. Dunnick NR, Sfakianakis GN. Screening for renovascular hypertension. *Radiol Clin North Am.* 1991;29:497–510.

3. Holley KE, Hunt JC, Brown AL, et al. Renal artery stenosis: a clinical-pathologic study in normotensive and hypertensive patients. *Am J Med.* 1964;37:14–18.

4. Eyler WR, Clark MD, Garman JE, et al. Angiography of the renal arteries including a comparative study of renal arterial stenoses in patients with and without hypertension. *Radiology.* 1962;78:879–882.

5. Caps MT, Perissinotto C, Zierler RE, et al. A prospective study of atherosclerotic disease progression in the renal artery. *Circulation.* 1998;98:2866–2872.

6. Chobanian AV, Bakris GL, Black HR, et al. The seventh report of the Joint National Committee on Prevention, Detection, Evaluation, and Treatment of High Blood Pressure. *JAMA.* 2003;289:2560–2572.

7. Safian RD, Textor SC. Renal artery stenosis. *N Engl J Med.* 2001;344(6):431–442.

8. Johnson PT, Halpern EJ, Kuszyk BS, et al. Renal artery stenosis: CT angiography—comparison of real-time volume rendering and maximum intensity projection algorithms. *Radiology.* 1999;211(2):337–343.

9. Hansen KJ, Tribble RW, Reavis SW, et al. Renal duplex sonography: evaluation of clinical utility. *J Vasc Surg.* 1990;12:227–236.

10. Kliewer MA, Tupler RH, Hertzberg BS, et al. Doppler evaluation of renal artery stenosis: interobserver agreement in the interpretation of waveform morphology. *Am J Roentgenol.* 1994;162:1371–1376.

11. Stanley JC. Natural history of renal artery stenosis and aneurysms. In: Calligaro KD, Dougherty MJ, Dean RH, eds. *Modern Management of Renovascular Hypertension and Renal Salvage.* Baltimore, MD: Williams & Wilkins; 1996:14–45.

12. Detection, evaluation, and treatment of renovascular hypertension. Final report. Working Group on Renovascular Hypertension. *Arch Intern Med.* 1987;147:820–829.

13. Bookstein JJ, Maxwell MH, Abrams HL, et al. Cooperative study of radiologic aspects of renovascular hypertension. *JAMA.* 1977;237:1706–1709.

14. Stanley JC, Gewertz BL, Bove BL, et al. Arterial fibrodysplasia: histopathologic character and current etiologic concepts. *Arch Surg.* 1975;110:561–566.

15. Treadway KK, Slater EE. Renovascular hypertension. *Am Rev Med.* 1984;35:665–692.

16. Harrison EG, McCormack U. Pathological classification of renal artery disease in renovascular hypertension. *Mayo Clin Proc.* 1971;46:161–167.

17. Cotter B, Mahmud E, Kwan OL, et al. New Ultrasound agents: expanding upon existing clinical applications. In: Goldberg BB, ed. *Ultrasound Contrast Agents.* St. Louis, MO: Mosby; 1997:31–42.

18. Neumyer MM, Thiele BL, Strandness DE Jr. *Techniques of Abdominal Vascular Sonography* [videotape]. Pasadena, CA: Davies Publishing, Inc.; 1996.

19. Goldberg BB, Liu JB, Forsberg F. Ultrasound contrast agents: a review. *Ultrasound Med Biol.* 1994;20(4):319–333.

20. Blebea J, Zickler R, Volteas N, et al. Duplex imaging of the renal arteries with contrast enhancement. *Vasc Endovasc Surg.* 2003;37:429–436.

21. Arima M, Ishibashi M, Usami M, et al. Analysis of the arterial blood flow patterns of normal and allografted kidneys by the directional ultrasonic Doppler technique. *J Urol.* 1979;122:587–591.

22. Norris CS, Pfeiffer JS, Rittgers SE, et al. Noninvasive evaluation of renal artery stenosis and renovascular resistance. *J Vasc Surg.* 1984;1:192–201.

23. Neumyer MM, Wengrovitz M, Ward T, et al. Differentiation of renal artery stenosis from renal parenchymal disease using duplex ultrasonography. *J Vasc Technol.* 1989;13:205–216.

24. Handa N, Fukunaga R, Etani H, et al. Efficacy of echo-Doppler examination for the evaluation of renovascular disease. *Ultrasound Med Biol.* 1988;14:1–5.

25. Martin RL, Nanra RS, Wlodarczyk J. Renal hilar Doppler analysis in the detection of renal artery stenosis. *J Vasc Technol.* 1991;15(4):173–180.

26. Stavros TA, Parker SH, Yakes YF, et al. Segmental stenosis of the renal artery: pattern recognition of the tardus and parvus abnormalities with duplex sonography. *Radiology.* 1992;184:487–492.

27. Isaacson JA, Neumyer MM. Direct and indirect renal arterial duplex and Doppler color flow evaluations. *J Vasc Technol.* 1995;19:309–316.

28. Isaacson JA, Zierler RE, Spittell PC, et al. Noninvasive screening for renal artery stenosis: comparison of renal artery and renal hilar duplex scanning. *J Vasc Technol.* 1995;19:105–110.

29. Baxter GM, Aitchison F, Sheppard D, et al. Colour Doppler ultrasound in renal artery stenosis: intrarenal waveform analysis. *Br J Radiol.* 1996;69:810–815.

30. Kliewer MA, Hertzberg BS, Keogan MT, et al. Early systole in the healthy kidney: variability of Doppler US waveform parameters. *Radiology.* 1997;205:109–113.

31. Helenon O, Rody FE, Correas JM, et al. Color Doppler US of renovascular disease in native kidneys. *Radiographics.* 1995;15:833–854.

32. Postma CT, Bijlstra PJ, Rosenbusch G, et al. Pattern recognition of loss of early systolic peak by Doppler ultrasound has a low sensitivity for the detection of renal artery stenosis. *J Hum Hypertens.* 1996;10:181–184.

33. Nazal MM, Hoballah JJ, Miller EV, et al. Renal hilar Doppler analysis is of value in the management of patients with renovascular disease. *Am J Surg.* 1997;174:164–168.

34. Kliewer MA, Tupler RH, Carroll BA, et al. Renal artery stenosis: analysis of Doppler waveform parameters and tardus-parvus pattern. *Radiology.* 1993;189:779–787.

35. Patriquin HB, LaFortune M, Jequier JC, et al. Stenosis of the renal artery: assessment of slowed systole in the downstream circulation with Doppler sonography. *Radiology.* 1992;184:470–485.

36. van der Hulst VPM, van Baalen J, Kool LS, et al. Renal artery stenosis: endovascular flow wire study for validation of Doppler US. *Radiology.* 1996;100:165–168.

37. Bude RO, Rubin JM, Platt JF, et al. Pulsus tardus: its cause and potential limitations in detection of arterial stenosis. *Radiology.* 1994;190:779–784.

38. Kohler TR, Zierler RE, Martin RL, et al. Noninvasive diagnosis of renal artery stenosis by ultrasonic duplex scanning. *J Vasc Surg.* 1986;4:450–456.

39. Taylor DC, Kettler MD, Moneta GL, et al. Duplex ultrasound scanning in the diagnosis of renal artery stenosis: a prospective evaluation. *J Vasc Surg.* 1988;7:363–369.

40. Taylor DC, Moneta GL, Strandness DE Jr. Follow-up renal artery stenosis by duplex ultrasound. *J Vasc Surg.* 1989;9:410–415.

41. Neumyer MM, Wengrovitz M, Ward T, et al. The differentiation of renal artery stenosis from renal parenchymal disease by duplex ultrasonography. *J Vasc Technol.* 1989;13:205–216.

42. Hoffman U, Edwards JM, Carter S, et al. Role of duplex scanning for the detection of atherosclerotic renal artery disease. *Kidney Int.* 1991;39:1232–1239.

43. Neumyer MM. Duplex scanning after renal artery stenting. *J Vasc Technol.* 2003;27(3):177–183.

44. Rocha-Singh K, Jaff MR, Kelley Lynne. Renal artery stenting with noninvasive duplex ultrasound follow-up: 3-year results from the RENAISSANCE renal stent trial. *Catheter Cardiovasc Interv.* 2008;72(6):853–862.

45. Chi YW, White CJ, Thomton S, et al. Ultrasound velocity criteria for renal in-stent restenosis. *J Vasc Surg.* 2009;50(1):119–123.

46. Mohabbat W, Greenberg RK, Mastracci TM, et al. Revised duplex criteria and outcomes for renal stents and stent grafts following endovascular repair of juxtarenal and thoracoabdominal aneurysms. *J Vasc Surg.* 2009;49(4):827–837.

47. Girndt M, Kaul H, Maute C, et al. Enhanced flow velocity after stenting of renal arteries is associated with decreased renal function. *Nephron Clin Pract.* 2007;105(2):c84–c89.

48. Radermacher J, Chavan A, Bleck J, et al. Use of Doppler ultrasonography to predict the outcome of therapy for renal artery stenosis. *N Engl J Med.* 2001;344(6):410–417.

49. Moran K, Muihall J, Kelly D, et al. Morphological changes and alterations in regional intrarenal blood flow induced by graded renal ischemia. *J Urol.* 1992;148:1463–1466.

50. Truong LD, Farhood A, Tasby J, et al. Experimental chronic renal ischemia: morphologic and immunologic studies. *Kidney Int.* 1992;41:1676–1689.

51. Gob'e GC, Axelsen RA, Searle JW. Cellular events in experimental unilateral ischemic renal atrophy and regeneration after contralateral nephrectomy. *Lab Invest.* 1990;63:770–779.

52. Sabbatini M, Sansone G, Uccello F, et al. Functional versus structural changes in the pathophysiology of acute ischemic renal failure in aging rats. *Kidney Int.* 1994;45:1355–1361.

53. Shanley PF. The pathology of chronic renal ischemia. *Semin Nephrol.* 1996;16:21–32.

54. Guzman RP, Zierler RE, Isaacson JA, et al. Renal atrophy and renal artery stenosis: a prospective study with duplex ultrasound. *Hypertension.* 1994;23:346–350.

55. Caps MT, Zierler RE, Polissar NL, et al. The risk of atrophy in kidneys with atherosclerotic renal artery stenosis. *Kidney Int.* 1998;53:735–742.

56. Cambria RP, Brewster DC, L'Italien GJ, et al. Renal artery reconstruction for the preservation of renal function. *J Vasc Surg.* 1996;24:371–380.

57. Hallett JW Jr, Fowl R, O'Brien PC, et al. Renovascular operations in patients with chronic renal insufficiency: do the benefits justify the risks? *J Vasc Surg.* 1987;5:622–627.

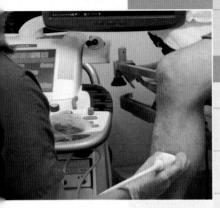

21 | The Inferior Vena Cava and Iliac Veins

Michael Costanza

OBJECTIVES

Describe the anatomy and physiology of the inferior vena cava and iliac veins

Identify the most useful positions for the patient and sonographer for conducting an ultrasound exam of the inferior vena cava and iliac veins

Recognize useful maneuvers to improve the ergonomics and imaging quality of an ultrasound exam of the inferior vena cava and iliac veins

List the required images for an ultrasound exam of the inferior vena cava and iliac veins

Understand the most common pathologic conditions and anatomic variants of the inferior vena cava and iliac veins

Describe how color, spectral, and power Doppler evaluations are complementary to each other and grayscale images

List the grayscale, color, and spectral Doppler characteristics of the most common pathologic conditions and anatomic variants of the inferior vena cava and iliac veins

KEY TERMS

confluence | inferior vena cava | pulmonary embolus | retroperitoneum | thrombosis

GLOSSARY

confluence the union of two or more veins to form a larger vein; the equivalent of a bifurcation in the arterial system

inferior vena cava filter a typically cone-shaped medical device designed to prevent pulmonary embolism; an inferior vena cava filter is placed into the inferior vena cava so that it can trap venous thromboemboli from the lower extremities before they travel to the heart and lungs

pulmonary embolus the obstruction of the pulmonary arteries usually from detached fragments of a blood clot that travels from the lower extremity veins

retroperitoneum the space between the abdominal cavity and the muscles and bones of the posterior abdominal wall; vascular structures in the retroperitoneum include the inferior vena cava, the iliac veins, and the abdominal aorta

thrombosis partial or complete occlusion of a blood vessel due to clot

The retroperitoneal location of the inferior vena cava (IVC) and iliac veins make them challenging to examine sonographically. Successful imaging of the IVC and iliac veins requires knowledge of their anatomy and physiology as well as appropriate preparation and patient positioning. Because these vessels can be the source of a pulmonary embolus, careful evaluation is essential. In addition to detecting a thrombus, ultrasound has proven to be a useful tool to aid in the placement of IVC filters and their follow-up.

ANATOMY

The external iliac veins drain the lower extremities as a continuation of the common femoral veins. They begin at the inguinal ligament and course cephalad as they dive deep into the pelvis. The internal iliac veins drain the pelvic viscera and musculature and join the external iliac veins at the level of the sacroiliac joints to form the common iliac veins. The IVC begins at the junction of the right and left common iliac veins at the level of the fifth lumbar vertebra. It ascends in the retroperitoneum to the right of the abdominal aorta and courses through the deep fossa on the posterior surface of the liver between the caudate lobe and bare area. After passing through the diaphragm at the level of the eighth thoracic vertebra, the IVC terminates in the right atrium. The venous tributaries of the IVC are listed in Table 21-1.

The IVC receives blood from all organs and tissues inferior to the diaphragm. It returns the deoxygenated blood to the heart for oxygenation and recirculation. The diameter of the IVC depends on the hydration status of the patient. In well-hydrated patients, the IVC appears distended and the mean diameter at the level of the renal veins is 17 to 20 mm.[1] Megacava (excessively large IVC diameter) is a rare condition that tends to occur only in patients of very large stature or in patients with congestive heart failure. Most large series reported that less than 3% of examined patients had an IVC larger than 28 mm in diameter.[2] Dehydration causes collapse of the IVC, making it narrow and difficult to detect and evaluate with ultrasound. In these situations, having an assistant elevate the patient's legs often increases the caliber of the vein, making it easier to visualize.[3]

ANATOMIC VARIANTS

Because several precursor veins contribute to its formation during embryogenesis, the IVC can display a wide spectrum of anatomic variation. Persistence of the left precursor of the IVC can result in paired venae

cavae or a left-sided IVC. In the case of paired venae cavae, the duplication typically terminates at the level of the renal veins when the left IVC drains into the left renal vein. A completely left-sided IVC can either terminate in the left renal vein or can extend cranially to drain into the azygos vein in the chest.[4]

Anomalies of the IVC may also involve its intrahepatic portion. When the intrahepatic portion of the IVC is congenitally absent, blood is returned to the heart via the azygos or hemiazygos veins. Although ultrasound may not detect this anomalous collateral venous pathway, the diagnosis can be made by demonstrating direct drainage of the hepatic veins into the right atrium as well as absence of the intrahepatic IVC. In membranous obstruction of the intrahepatic IVC, ultrasound demonstrates a fibrous septum in the IVC just cephalad to the insertion of the right hepatic vein. Flow may be reversed in the IVC, and flow in the distal hepatic veins is sluggish and continuous.

SONOGRAPHIC EXAMINATION TECHNIQUES

PATIENT PREPARATION

Extensive bowel gas represents the most common impediment to a successful sonographic examination of the IVC and iliac veins. The bowel gas prevents transmission of the ultrasound signal and precludes accurate identification of any deep abdominal structures. Having the patient fast for 8 hours prior to the exam can decrease the likelihood of bowel gas; however, the exam should still be attempted even if the patient has eaten. Although morbid obesity can make abdominal imaging difficult due to the depth of penetration necessary, it rarely precludes adequate IVC visualization. In surgical patients, open abdominal wounds can encroach on the areas of the abdomen typically used to place the ultrasound probe. These patients may require alternative probe placement and the assistance of the nursing staff to achieve a complete ultrasound exam.

PATIENT POSITIONING

The exam begins with the patient in a supine position and with the sonographer standing to the patient's right side. The height of the bed or stretcher should be adjusted so that the level of the patient's abdomen is slightly lower than the sonographer's waist. In this configuration, the sonographer can extend his or her scanning arm downward and ergonomically apply pressure to the patient's abdomen. The ability to easily and comfortably apply pressure with the probe often allows the sonographer to

TABLE	21-1
IVC Venous Tributaries	
Hepatic veins	
Renal veins	
Common iliac veins	
Right adrenal vein	
Right ovarian vein or testicular vein	
Inferior phrenic vein	
Four lumbar veins	
Medial sacral vein	

disperse bowel gas and obtain better images of deep abdominal structures. The amount of force exerted on the transducer must be regulated because excessive pressure will also compress the IVC, making it difficult to visualize.

SCANNING TECHNIQUE

Achieving adequate penetration usually requires a 1- to 4-MHz probe; however, a 5-MHz probe may be more appropriate for thin patients. A complete exam requires a longitudinal and transverse survey of the IVC from the diaphragm to the confluence of the common iliac veins. The exam begins with the probe perpendicular, at the midline of the body, and just distal to the xiphoid process of the sternum. Angling the transducer to the patient's left allows visualization of the proximal abdominal aorta posterior to the liver. After identifying this landmark, the transducer can be angled to the patient's right side to obtain a longitudinal image of the IVC posterior to the liver (Fig. 21-1). The hepatic veins, which are anterior tributaries of the proximal IVC, should be recognized and evaluated. The transducer can then be slowly moved inferiorly using a rock-and-slide motion. By slightly rocking to the right and then to the left, each side of the IVC is scanned while sliding the probe inferiorly.[5] Rotating the transducer may be required to keep the IVC in view. This technique uses the sagittal plane to obtain longitudinal images of the proximal, mid, and distal IVC to the common iliac vein confluence (usually at the level of the umbilicus).

To scan in the transverse plane, the transducer is returned to the anterior, subxiphoid location, and angled superiorly. Once the heart is visualized, the transducer should be slowly straightened to look for the IVC just to the right of the midline. In the transverse plane, the IVC will appear oval (Fig. 21-2). While keeping the IVC in view, the transducer is moved inferiorly with

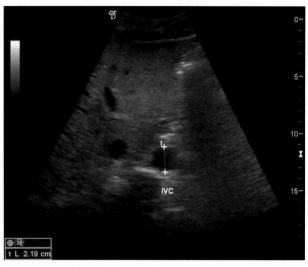

Figure 21-2 Grayscale image of a transverse view of the inferior vena cava (IVC) with a diameter measurement.

the rock-and-slide motion, as previously described. The renal veins, which are lateral tributaries of the IVC, should be noted and evaluated. The exam continues inferiorly through the level of the common iliac veins until they can no longer be visualized.

The coronal plane may offer better imaging of the distal IVC and the confluence of the common iliac veins. With the patient in the left lateral decubitus position, the probe is placed superior to the iliac crest in the mid-coronal plane. The inferior pole of the right kidney provides a landmark, and the IVC bifurcation is usually medial and inferior to it. Although scanning in the coronal plane is possible with the patient in supine position, the left lateral decubitus position offers an ergonomic advantage and may produce superior images in patients who have bowel gas that obscures an anterior acoustic window.

A portion of the common iliac veins will most likely be identified and evaluated during the IVC survey. For the rest of the iliac venous exam, the patient should be supine with the bed or stretcher in a reverse Trendelenburg position. The same 1- to 4-MHz probe can be used, or a 5-MHz probe may be more appropriate for thin patients. Starting at the groin, the common femoral vein can be followed proximally to identify and examine the distal external iliac vein. When the external iliac begins to dive deep into the pelvis, the exam continues using an anterolateral approach with the transducer placed lateral to the rectus muscle.[6] The external and common iliac veins are then followed proximally to their confluence. Imaging the entire iliac venous system can be challenging. The confluence of the external and common iliac veins often cannot be definitively identified, and the deep location of the iliac veins can compromise image quality.

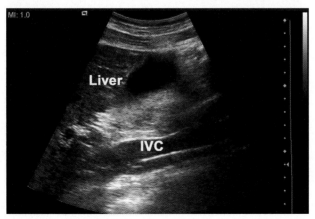

Figure 21-1 Grayscale image of a longitudinal view of the inferior vena cava (IVC).

TABLE 21-2		
Required Images for IVC and Iliac Veins		
Image Plane	Anatomic Level	Landmarks
Longitudinal	Proximal IVC	Diaphragm and hepatic vein(s)
	Middle IVC	Head of the pancreas
	Distal IVC	
	Common iliac vein confluence	Common iliac veins
	External iliac veins	
Transverse	Proximal IVC	Hepatic veins
	Middle IVC	Renal veins
	Distal IVC	
	Common iliac vein confluence	Common iliac veins
	External iliac veins	

The efficiency of the exam can be improved by minimizing the number of times the patient changes position. With the patient supine, the IVC survey to obtain longitudinal and transverse images should be performed, followed by the iliac vein evaluation. The patient can then be turned to the left lateral decubitus position for scanning in the coronal plane to obtain images of the distal IVC and the common iliac confluence. The required images for the IVC and iliac venous exam are listed in Table 21-2.

DIAGNOSIS

The normal IVC and iliac veins have echogenic, muscular walls. The lumen of these vessels should appear anechoic. With quiet respiration, the diameter of the IVC may appear to change with the phasic changes in abdominal pressure produced during respiration. The grayscale image can be evaluated for various pathology including thrombosis, intraluminal tumors, and extrinsic compressions.

THROMBOSIS

Thrombosis that results from propagation of a lower extremity venous thromboembolism represents the most common pathologic finding. Grayscale imaging may reveal a distended IVC or iliac vein with echogenic material within the lumen. A recently formed thrombus can be virtually anechoic and undetectable by grayscale imaging. This situation highlights the importance of a color flow and Doppler examination to evaluate IVC and iliac vein patency (Fig. 21-3). The echogenicity of a thrombus increases as it ages over the course of several days and weeks.

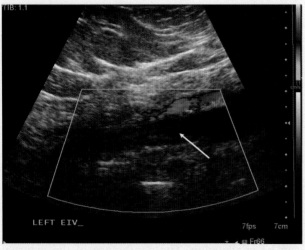

A

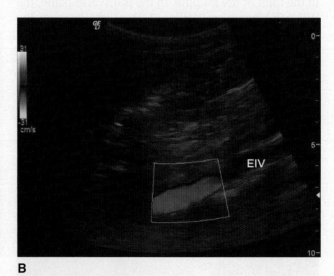

B

Figure 21-3 A: The external iliac vein (EIV) has a homogenous, hypoechoic appearance and no color flow is detected. These findings are consistent with acute deep venous thrombosis of the external iliac vein. **B:** A normal external iliac vein with an anechoic lumen on grayscale imaging and complete filling to the vessel walls on color flow imaging.

A thrombus that does not obstruct flow may only be detected by grayscale imaging demonstrating free floating echogenic material within the IVC or iliac vein lumen.

NEOPLASTIC OBSTRUCTION

Compared to thrombotic occlusion, neoplastic obstruction of the IVC and iliac veins is rare. Grayscale imaging reveals an intraluminal tumor or an extrinsic mass. Intraluminal tumors typically arise from hepatic or renal veins and may secondarily obstruct or thrombose the IVC.[7] Extrinsic tumors may completely or partially obstruct the IVC or iliac veins, resulting in dilated collateral veins and distention of the distal IVC and iliac veins. An intraluminal tumor is typically moderately echogenic and will demonstrate flow within the mass on color flow imaging. Small vessels can be seen within the tumor itself.

INFERIOR VENA CAVAL INTERRUPTION

Sonography of the IVC may demonstrate the presence of an IVC filter, a device used to protect patients from pulmonary emboli. IVC filters are typically placed just distal to the renal veins in order to trap lower extremity venous thromboemboli before they

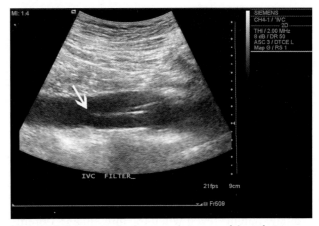

Figure 21-5 Longitudinal, grayscale image of the inferior vena cava with a filter in place. The *arrow* points to the superior tip of the filter.

can travel to the heart and lungs. Most IVC filters consist of thin metal struts joined at one end to form the shape of a cone (Fig. 21-4). In longitudinal views of the IVC, a filter's metal struts appear as echogenic lines that converge to a point near the level of the renal veins (Fig. 21-5). In transverse view, the filter appears as a central echogenic dot with lines radiating to the IVC wall. The patency of the IVC proximal and distal to the filter should be evaluated. Echogenic material within and around the filter represents a trapped thrombus and should be considered an abnormal finding.[8] Rarely, an IVC filter strut may perforate the IVC, causing a hematoma. In most cases, ultrasound can only visualize the hematoma, not the penetrating strut.[9] Computerized tomography (CT) scans usually prove to be more useful for diagnosing this condition.

COLOR AND POWER DOPPLER

Color Doppler provides a useful method for evaluating the patency of the IVC. Although a complete IVC survey requires imaging in the longitudinal and transverse planes, longitudinal images prove to be more informative in the assessment of color flow. Color flow may be difficult to demonstrate in the transverse plane because blood flow is perpendicular to the ultrasound beam. The entire IVC should be evaluated with color flow including the suprahepatic, intrahepatic, and infrahepatic IVC, as well as the IVC proximal and distal to an IVC filter, if present.

Color Doppler can also detect caval fistulas, which are abnormal connections between the IVC and surrounding vessels. Caval fistulas may occur spontaneously or they may be surgically created. Spontaneous aortocaval fistulas represent a rare complication of large abdominal aortic aneurysms. Color flow demonstrates visible tissue bruit and pulsatile flow in the IVC above

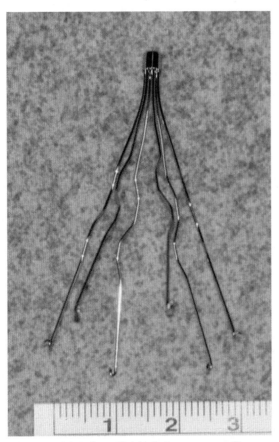

Figure 21-4 Greenfield inferior vena cava filter.

the fistula. Directly imaging the connection between the aorta and the IVC may be difficult. Surgically created portacaval fistulas usually involve a side-to-side connection between the portal vein and the IVC. The fistula creates a tissue bruit, and optimal visualization often requires using the liver as an acoustic window with the patient turned onto his or her left side.

The deep location and relatively low flow state of the IVC and iliac veins stress the limits of the color Doppler exam. Power Doppler offers a complementary assessment that can overcome these imaging challenges. Because power Doppler functions independent of the ultrasound angle of incidence, it can evaluate patency even when the only images obtainable are in the transverse plane. Power Doppler can also detect slow flow better than color Doppler. This increased sensitivity allows power Doppler to detect extremely low flow in the IVC or iliac veins, which could otherwise result in a false-positive diagnosis of venous thrombosis based on the color Doppler findings alone. The use of power Doppler to detect and define low flow conditions such as intrahepatic portacaval shunts has also been reported.[10]

SPECTRAL DOPPLER CHARACTERISTICS

Blood flows slowly through the IVC, and the caval waveform varies with respiration and the cardiac cycle. During quiet respiration, the diaphragm descends, creating positive pressure in the abdomen and negative pressure in the chest. Blood therefore flows from the abdomen to the chest during inspiration and the reverse occurs during expiration. Superimposed on this respiratory variation are the rapidly cycling pressure waves transmitted from the heart, specifically the right atrium (Fig. 21-6). The prominence of cardiac pulsatility in the IVC depends on the fluid status of the patient. Normally, the proximal IVC near the heart has a pulsatile waveform pattern, whereas flow in the

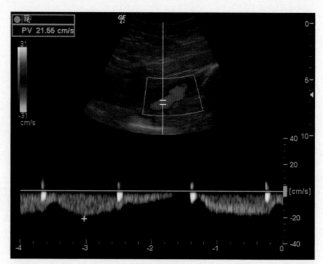

Figure 21-7 Color flow and spectral waveform analysis of the external iliac vein showing respiratory phasicity.

distal IVC and iliac veins remains phasic, resembling the pattern seen in lower extremity veins. Severe fluid overload may allow cardiac pulsations to be detected as far distally as the iliac veins. Partial obstruction of the IVC eliminates the normal respiratory and cardiac variation in the IVC and iliac veins. In this case, spectral analysis demonstrates continuous Doppler signals with a uniform flow velocity.

Spectral Doppler analysis plays an important role in detecting iliac vein thrombosis. Unlike lower extremity veins, the patency of iliac veins cannot be evaluated with compression maneuvers, and direct grayscale imaging may not be possible deep in the pelvis. In these circumstances, the diagnosis of an iliac vein thrombosis relies on indirect evidence from the spectral Doppler analysis (Fig. 21-7). Loss of respiratory phasicity and an inability to augment the signal with distal thigh compression indicate a proximal obstruction consistent with iliac veins thrombosis. These findings are usually absent in the setting of nonocclusive thrombosis, and ultrasound duplex cannot detect thrombosis of the internal iliac veins.

Iliac Vein Compression Syndrome

Iliac vein compression syndrome (IVCS) occurs when the left common iliac vein is compressed between the overlying right common iliac artery and the underlying vertebral body. Also known as May-Thurner syndrome, this condition most commonly presents as a left iliofemoral deep venous thrombosis; however, it may also cause chronic left lower extremity pain and edema secondary to venous insufficiency. Grayscale imaging can localize the point at which the right common iliac artery crosses the left common iliac vein. A Doppler examination can then determine if this crossing point causes significant compression. Monophasic

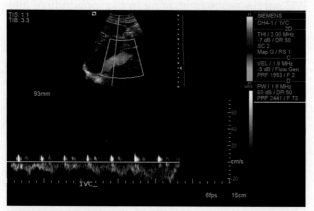

Figure 21-6 Color flow and spectral waveform analysis of the proximal inferior vena cava showing cardiac pulsatility superimposed on respiratory phasicity.

flow without respiratory variation distal to the compression and increased flow velocity at the point of compression are signs of a localized iliac vein stenosis consistent with IVCS.[11] Definitive imaging studies including venography with intraluminal pressures, intravascular ultrasonography, CT, or magnetic resonance imaging may be required to confirm the diagnosis. Pathology Box 21-1 lists the common pathology encountered during the ultrasound examination of the inferior vena cava and the iliac veins.

DUPLEX ULTRASOUND GUIDANCE FOR IVC FILTER PLACEMENT

The utility of duplex ultrasound has expanded beyond the diagnosis of a thrombus to now include guidance during IVC filter placement. Percutaneous IVC filter placement has traditionally been performed with contrast venography in an operating room or interventional radiology suite. Duplex ultrasound guidance can transform IVC filter placement into a bedside procedure that does not require exposure to radiation or intravenous contrast.[12]

PATIENT PREPARATION AND POSITIONING

Imaging the IVC for filter placement follows the same basic preparation and techniques outlined in the previous sections. The sonographer stands on the patient's right side, and the ultrasound machine is positioned on the same side toward the head of the bed so that it can be viewed by the sonographer and the physician performing the procedure. Ideally, the filter should be placed just distal to the level of the renal veins. In some patients, the right renal vein can be visualized during grayscale imaging of the IVC. However, in most cases, the right renal artery is easier to locate and provides a dependable and consistent marker for the level of the renal veins. With the IVC in a longitudinal projection, the right renal artery is easily identified in cross section as it passes posterior to the IVC (Fig. 21-8). Doppler interrogation can confirm the identity of the right renal artery by demonstrating the characteristic spectral waveform tracing of a renal artery.

SCANNING TECHNIQUE

While the physician gains percutaneous access to the right or left common femoral vein, the sonographer maintains a longitudinal image of IVC with the right renal artery in cross section. Maintaining this grayscale image allows real-time visualization of the wire and delivery sheath as the physician advances them into the IVC. The tip of the delivery catheter should then be identified and advanced with

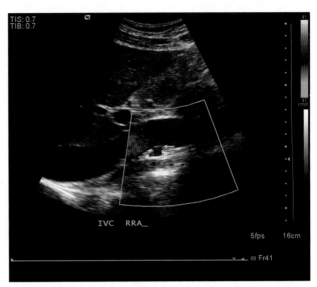

Figure 21-8 In a longitudinal view, the right renal artery *(arrow)* is identified posterior to the inferior vena cava *(IVC)*.

ultrasound guidance so that its tip is just below the level of the right renal artery. Flushing saline through the sheath can create echogenic turbulence at the sheath tip, which can often aid in its identification.

Once the sheath tip is in a satisfactory infrarenal location, the IVC filter is advanced through the sheath and into the IVC. Once the filter tip is at the level of the right renal artery, the physician deploys it under real-time sonographic visualization (Fig. 21-9). The grayscale image will show the filter quickly expanding and engaging the IVC sidewalls. A transverse image should then be obtained and recorded to confirm that the filter is completely expanded with its struts apposed to the sidewalls of the IVC.

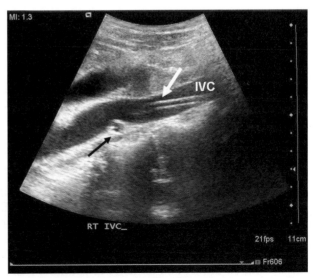

Figure 21-9 The tip of the filter delivery catheter *(white arrow)* is advanced in the inferior vena cava *(IVC)* to the level of the right renal artery *(black arrow)*.

PATHOLOGY BOX 21-1

Common Pathology of the Inferior Vena Cava and Iliac Veins

Condition	Sonographic Findings		
	Gray Scale	Color	Doppler
Thrombus (occlusive)	Distended vein with echogenic material within lumen	Absent flow	No signal
Thrombus (partially occlusive)	Echogenic material that appears partially free floating and partially attached to the vessel wall	Present or diminished	Continuous signal; loss of respiratory and cardiac variation
Neoplastic obstruction	Intraluminal tumor originating from renal or hepatic veins or extrinsic mass	Absent; collateral veins may be detected	No signal or continuous signal in partial obstruction; look for arterial flow with tumor
IVC filter with thrombus	Echogenic metal struts of filter; echogenic material within lumen	Absent	No signal or continuous signal with partial obstruction
Left-sided IVC	Paired IVC or IVC on left side only	Anomalous IVC drains into left renal vein or azygos vein	Normal
Absent intrahepatic IVC	Intrahepatic IVC not visualized	Hepatic veins drain directly into right atrium	Normal
Caval fistulas	Dilated vein	Tissue bruit	Pulsatile flow cephalad to fistula
Iliac vein compression syndrome (May-Thurner)	Left iliac vein compressed by right common iliac artery	Increased velocity and possible turbulent flow at compression point	Monophasic waveform distal to compression point

SUMMARY

Ultrasonography of the IVC and iliac veins offers several advantages over other imaging modalities. It is a noninvasive exam that does not require radiation exposure or contrast administration. As a diagnostic tool, ultrasonography provides an accurate anatomic and physiologic assessment of the IVC and iliac veins. Optimizing the sonographic exam requires adequate patient preparation and positioning, as well as knowledge of the pathophysiology of the IVC and iliac veins.

Critical Thinking Question

1. You receive a request for an ultrasound exam of the inferior vena cava and iliac veins in an obese patient who has at breakfast 2 hours ago. How should you proceed? What, if anything, can be done to optimize the quality of the exam?

2. During an ultrasound of the IVC, you note that the IVC appears distended; however, the lumen appears to be anechoic. You cannot detect a color

Doppler signal in the IVC, and the spectral Doppler signal in the common iliac veins is continuous without respiratory variation. What is the likely clinical scenario to explain these findings?

3. You are performing an ultrasound of the IVC on a patient who has had an IVC filter and now presents with bilateral lower extremity edema. You note that the echogenic struts of the filter extend to the vena caval wall. The filter appears to be located above the level of the renal veins, and there is echogenic material within and cephalad to the filter. Which of these findings are abnormal and why?

REFERENCES

1. Mintz GS, Kotler MN, Parry WR, et al. Real-time inferior vena caval ultrasonography: normal and abnormal findings and its use in assessing right-heart function. *Circulation.* 1981;64:1018–1025.
2. Skyes AM, McLoughlin RF, So CBB, et al. Sonographic assessment of infrarenal vena caval dimensions. *J Ultrasound Med.* 1995;14:665–668.
3. Allan PL. The aorta and inferior vena cava. In: Allan PL, Dubbins PA, Pozniak MA, et al., eds. *Clinical Doppler Ultrasound.* 2nd ed. Philadelphia, PA: Churchill Livingstone Elsevier; 2006:127–140.
4. Moore KL. *Clinically Oriented Anatomy.* 3rd ed. Baltimore, MD: Williams & Wilkins; 1992.
5. Tempkin BB. Inferior vena cava scanning protocol. In: Tempkin BB, ed. *Ultrasound Scanning Principles and Protocols.* 2nd ed. Philadelphia, PA: W.B. Saunders; 1999:41–52.
6. Zwiebel WJ. Extremity venous examination: technical considerations. In: Zwiebel WJ, ed. *Introduction to Vascular Ultrasonography.* 4th ed. Philadelphia, PA: W.B. Saunders; 2000:311–328.
7. Pussell SJ, Cosgrove DO. Ultrasound features of tumor thrombus in the IVC in retroperitoneal tumours. *Br J Radiol.* 1981;54:866–869.
8. Asward MA, Sandager GP, Pais SO, et al. Early duplex scan evaluation of four vena caval interruption devices. *J Vasc Surg.* 1996;24:809–818.
9. Mohan CR, Hoballah JJ, Sharp WJ, et al. Comparative efficacy and complications of vena caval filters. *J Vasc Surg.* 1995;21:235–246.
10. Oquz B, Akata D, Balkanci F, et al. Intrahepatic portosystemic venous shunt: diagnosis by colour/power Doppler imaging and three dimensional ultrasound. *Br J Radiol.* 2003;76:487–490.
11. Oguzkurt L, Ozkan U, Tercan F, et al. Ultrasonographic diagnosis of iliac vein compression (May-Thurner) syndrome. *Diag Interv Radiol.* 2007;13:152–155.
12. Connors MS, Becker S, Guzman RJ, et al. Duplex scan-directed placement of inferior vena cava filters: a five year institutional experience. *J Vasc Surg.* 2002;35:286–291.

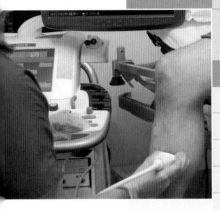

22 The Hepatoportal System

Wayne C. Leonhardt and Ann Marie Kupinski

OBJECTIVES

Identify normal hepatoportal anatomy

Describe normal hepatoportal Doppler waveforms

List the causes of portal hypertension

Describe portosystemic collateral pathways associated with portal hypertension

List sonographic findings associated with portal hypertension

KEY TERMS

hepatic artery | hepatic vein | hepatofugal | hepatopetal | portal hypertension | portal vein | TIPS

GLOSSARY

ascites an accumulation of fluid within the peritoneal cavity

Budd-Chiari syndrome hepatic vein thrombosis

hepatofugal away from the liver, usually referring to blood flow away from the liver

hepatopetal toward the liver, usually referring to the normal direction of portal vein flow

portal hypertension elevated pressure within the portal vein

TIPS transjugular intrahepatic portosystemic shunt

Duplex sonography is the most common imaging technique used to evaluate the portal and hepatic venous systems. This important noninvasive tool is paramount in determining the presence of flow, direction of flow, blood velocity, and in characterizing flow hemodynamics. A variety of vascular disorders alter blood flow into, within, and out of the liver. Duplex with color Doppler is particularly useful in the detection of an intraluminal thrombus, a hepatofugal flow, collateral circulation, an arterio-portal fistula, absent flow, and increased or decreased flow in both portal and hepatic venous systems. This chapter will review the sonographic duplex findings and the hemodynamics of the normal hepatoportal system as well as various pathological conditions.

ANATOMY

The liver receives a dual blood supply from the hepatic artery and portal vein. These two vessels constitute the hepatic inflow. The hepatic artery supplies approximately 30% of incoming blood. It carries oxygenated blood through branches in the portal triad and enters the sinusoids (capillaries) to reach the central veins

within the liver. The portal vein supplies the remaining 70% of hepatic blood flow.[1] It carries nutrient-rich blood from the gastrointestinal tract to the portal triad, where it enters the sinusoids to reach the central veins. Central veins are the actual beginnings of the hepatic venous system. They enter sublobular veins, which unite and converge to form three hepatic veins that drain into the inferior vena cava (IVC). The hepatic veins comprise the primary hepatic outflow vessels.

PORTAL VENOUS SYSTEM

Just slightly to the right of midline, the main portal vein (MPV) begins the junction of the splenic vein (SV) and superior mesenteric vein (SMV). The MPV courses cephalad approaching the porta hepatis and lies anterior to the IVC. The porta hepatis is the transverse fissure on the visceral surface of the liver between the caudate and quadrate lobes where the portal vein and hepatic artery enter the liver and the hepatic duct leaves the liver.[2] Figure 22-1 illustrates the normal portal venous anatomy and flow direction. Entering the portal hepatis, the MPV divides into a smaller, more anterior, and cranial left portal vein (LPV) and a larger, more posterior, and caudal right portal vein

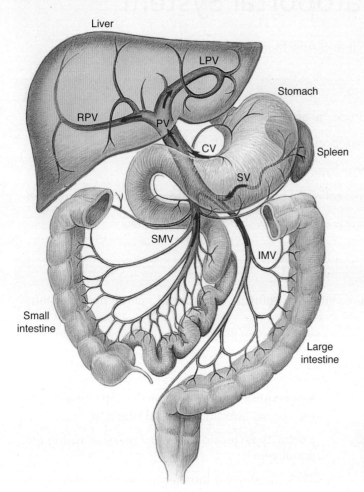

Figure 22-1 A diagram illustrating the normal portal vascular anatomy. The *red arrows* depict normal direction of blood flow. PV, portal vein; RPV, right portal vein; LPV, left portal vein; CV, coronary vein; IMV, inferior mesenteric vein; SMV, superior mesenteric vein; SV, splenic vein.

(RPV).[3] The portal veins then branch into medial and lateral divisions on the left, and anterior and posterior divisions on the right. Portal veins contain no valves and have bright echogenic walls due to thick collagenous tissue. They course within the liver segments (intrasegmental) and emanate from the porta hepatis.

HEPATIC VEINS

Hepatic veins are anatomically separate from the portal venous system. Unlike the portal veins, hepatic veins are thin-walled structures that run between the lobes of the liver (intersegmental) and increase in caliber as they approach the diaphragm. Three main hepatic veins (right, middle, and left) provide the primary outflow route of blood from the liver. They drain into the IVC close to the right atrium and contain no valves.[2] The right hepatic vein (RHV) is usually the largest. In 96% of individuals, the middle hepatic vein (MHV) and left hepatic vein (LHV) join to form a common trunk before entering the IVC. Accessory hepatic veins are common, but are seldom identified sonographically. Of note, the caudate lobe of the liver drains directly into the IVC with the caudate vein being the largest draining vein of this lobe.[4] This is important in the presence of venous outflow diseases, which will be discussed later in the chapter.

HEPATIC ARTERY

The hepatic artery branches off the celiac trunk to the right. At this level, the hepatic artery is known as the common hepatic artery. It continues over the anterior superior edge of the pancreas where it gives rise to the gastroduodenal artery. At this point, the common hepatic artery becomes the proper hepatic artery, terminating at the porta hepatis giving off right and left branches. In the majority of patients, the hepatic artery lies anteromedial to the portal vein. The hepatic artery branches accompany the portal veins.

SONOGRAPHIC EXAMINATION TECHNIQUES

There are various indications for hepatoportal duplex ultrasound. Table 22-1 lists several indications for hepatoportal scanning. Any of these conditions can alter the blood flow patterns within the inflow and outflow vessels in the liver.

TABLE 22-1
Indications for Hepatoportal Duplex Ultrasound
Liver cirrhosis both alcoholic and viral, hepatitis B and C
Portal hypertension, ascites of unknown etiology or esophageal varices
Thrombosis of the portal, splenic, and superior mesenteric veins
Budd-Chiari syndrome (hepatic vein thrombosis)
Preinterventional/postinterventional procedures and monitoring of portosystemic shunts
Abdominal trauma
Sudden onset of ascites, acute abdominal pain, elevated D-dimer
Patients with a history of abdominal malignancy

PATIENT PREPARATION

Patients should fast for 8 to 12 hours. Patients are instructed to abstain from smoking and chewing gum as these activities introduce air into the stomach.

PATIENT POSITIONING

The patient can be examined while supine as well as in the left posterior oblique (LPO), left lateral decubitus (LLD), and right posterior oblique positions. A combination of sagittal, transverse, and oblique scanning planes and various acoustic windows are necessary to assess the portal and hepatic vessels. Primary scanning planes include right coronal oblique, transverse epigastric, transverse right costal margin, left coronal oblique, and sagittal left lobe.

Right Coronal Oblique

The right coronal oblique scanning plane using an intercostal approach provides a window that provides excellent visualization of the porta hepatis. When patients present with large amounts of ascites and bowel gas, this increases abdominal girth, making it very difficult to image the liver and hepatoportal venous anatomy. The intercostal approach results in the following: Doppler angles varying from 0° to about 60°, decreases the anterior posterior distance, uses the liver as an acoustic window, and facilitates diagnostic imaging when patients are not compliant with holding their breath. To obtain this scanning plane, position the patient in the LPO or LLD positions. Place the transducer in the interspace parallel to the rib margins, aimed at the hepatic hilum.

Transverse Epigastric

With the patient supine or in the LPO position, place the transducer over the left lobe of the liver. Angle the transducer cephalad at the level of the diaphragm. This will provide visualization of the hepatic venous confluence. Next, angle the transducer caudad at the level of the left lobe of the liver. Here, the ascending branch of the left portal vein and accompanying hepatic artery are visualized. Finally, angle the transducer caudad to detect the splenic vein and portal confluence.

Right Transverse Costal Margin

Position the patient supine and, with the transducer in the transverse plane, place it over the right costal margin at the midclavicular line. The transducer is then angled superior to inferior until a transverse view of the porta hepatis is obtained. Here, the main portal and right anterior and posterior branches are seen together with accompanying hepatic artery.

Left Coronal Oblique

Place the patient in the right posterior oblique position with the transducer between the left lateral intercostal spaces. Aim the transducer toward the splenic hilum. This window can be used to image the splenic vein.

Sagittal Left Lobe

Position the patient supine and place the transducer in a longitudinal plane midline over the left lobe of the liver. This scanning approach demonstrates the left hepatic vein, ascending branch of the left portal vein, and accompanying artery. The left hepatic vein is seen in the long axis draining into the IVC.

SCANNING TECHNIQUE

The ultrasound examination begins with the patient in the supine position. As the examination progresses, multiple views and patient positions are used to obtain the various required images.

Very often, the ultrasound evaluation of the hepatoportal circulation also includes imaging of the liver itself and the surrounding area. The size, echogenicity, and surface contour of the liver are documented. The liver is examined for masses and cysts. The spleen is evaluated for splenomegaly. The abdomen is scanned to identify the presence of any ascites.

Grayscale and color images are obtained of the extrahepatic portal vein, intrahepatic portal veins, hepatic veins, and IVC. These images should

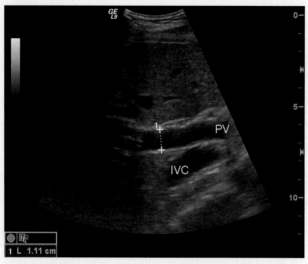

Figure 22-2 Portal vein diameter measured near where portal vein (PV) crosses the inferior vena cava (IVC).

include clear views of the adjacent liver parenchyma. The main portal vein diameter is measured during quiet respiration where this vessel crosses the IVC (Fig. 22-2).

Spectral Doppler waveforms and velocity measurements should be documented from the following:
- Main, right, and left portal vein
- Right, middle, and left hepatic veins
- Splenic vein
- Superior mesenteric vein
- IVC
- Hepatic artery proper (angle-corrected velocity)

TECHNICAL CONSIDERATIONS

When scanning the abdominal vasculature, imaging parameters such as depth, field of view, frame rate, and flow sensitivity are very important. Although imaging depths vary based on patient body habitus, transducer frequencies between 2 and 4 MHz may be required to penetrate depths of up to 20 cm. Higher transducer frequencies between 4 and 5 MHz are used in thin adults and children. Selection of the transducer should be made such that adequate depth penetration is achieved while selecting the highest transducer frequency because the higher frequencies provide better resolution. Most often, a 3-6 MHz pulsed Doppler is required for spectral analysis of abdominal vessels. Electronic phased sector transducers with 13- to 20-mm scan heads are more effective in obtaining acoustic windows using the intercostal approach. High-resolution convex (4-8 MHz) and linear (5-15 MHz) transducers are useful when imaging anterior abdominal wall varices and assessing the liver surface for nodularity.

PITFALLS

The ability to complete a hepatoportal examination depends, in part, on the experience of the technologist or sonographer as well as the patient. Major limitations affecting the success of the examination include patient obesity, diffuse liver disease, ascites, and bowel gas. Patients with severe abdominal pain, those unable to remain still, those unable to breathe quietly or vary their depth of respiration, and combative patients also present limitations to the examination.

DIAGNOSIS

There are multiple criteria to assess when evaluating the hepatoportal system. Major diagnostic characteristics are summarized as follows.

PORTAL VEIN

Portal veins have bright, echogenic borders due to collagenous tissue within the walls. Respiration and ingestion of food affect portal vein diameter and velocity flow. In normal patients, the portal vein diameter is ≤13 mm in quiet respiration and may increase to 16 mm with deep inspiration.[5] Portal vein diameter is increased in patients with portal hypertension, congestive heart failure, constrictive pericarditis, and portal vein thrombosis.

Portal venous flow is normally directed toward the liver with constant antegrade flow throughout the cardiac cycle. This is referred to as "hepatopetal" flow. Portal vein velocity does vary with cardiac activity and respiration. During inspiration, it decreases and increases during expiration. This is due to the diaphragm descending during inspiration, resulting in an increase in intra-abdominal pressure. This also impedes venous return to the right atrium, thus decreasing flow in the IVC and its tributaries, including the hepatic veins. Portal venous flow and velocity also decrease during exercise (related to the significant reduction in mesenteric arterial blood flow that occurs with exercise) and changes in posture (from supine to sitting or standing) attributed to venous pooling in the legs. It increases with expiration and ingestion of food, as a result of splanchnic vasodilatation and hyperemia. Postprandially, flow velocity increases 50% to 100%. Resting peak systolic velocities range from 10 to 30 cm/s. Mean flow velocity is approximately 15 to 18 cm/s. The Doppler spectral waveforms are monophasic and are slightly pulsatile or undulating (Fig. 22-3). Increased pulsatility has been described, particularly in thin patients. Principle determinants attributing to portal vein pulsatility may include

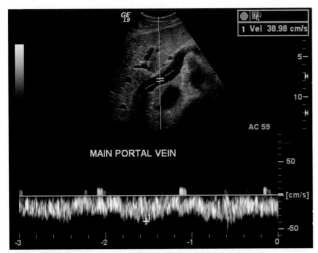

Figure 22-3 Normal portal vein Doppler waveforms with flow directed toward the liver.

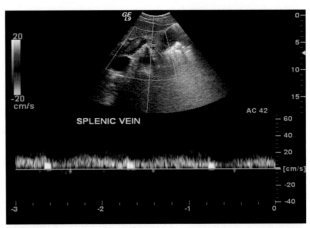

Figure 22-4 Normal splenic vein Doppler waveforms.

trans-sinusoidal transmission of atrial pulsations, the respiratory cycle, and the transmission of vena cava, hepatic arterial, or splanchnic pulsations.

SPLENIC VEIN

In normal patients, the diameter of the splenic vein (in the transverse view at the level of the superior mesenteric artery [SMA]) measures up to 10 mm (inner wall to inner wall) and increases by 20% to 100% from quiet respiration to deep inspiration. An increase in caliber of less than 20% indicates portal hypertension with 80% sensitivity and 100% specificity.[6]

Normal splenic vein flow direction is hepatopetal (toward the liver). As seen in the portal vein, respiration and cardiac activity can also affect splenic vein velocity. Flow velocity decreases during inspiration and increases during expiration. Peak systolic velocity in the splenic vein normally ranges from 9 to 30 cm/s. The mean velocity ranges from 5 to 12 cm/s. The Doppler spectral waveforms of the normal splenic vein display a monophasic waveform with slight pulsatility (Fig. 22-4).

SUPERIOR MESENTERIC VEIN

In normal patients, the diameter of the SMV can measure up to 10 mm at the trunk (inner wall to inner wall) and increases by 20% to 100% from quiet respiration to deep inspiration. As with the splenic vein, an increase in caliber of less than 20% indicates portal hypertension.[6]

Normal SMV flow is hepatopetal (toward the liver). Peak systolic velocity in the SMV normally ranges between 8 and 40 cm/s. The mean velocity range is 9 to 18 cm/s. Doppler spectral analysis of

the SMV shows a monophasic waveform with slight pulsatility (Fig. 22-5). Flow in the portal confluence is turbulent as the splenic vein joins the SMV to form the portal vein. Respiratory maneuvers and ingestion of food affect flow velocity. Flow velocity decreases during inspiration and increases with expiration, similar to that of the portal and splenic veins. Postprandially, SMV velocity increases 50% to 100%.

HEPATIC VEINS

The normal diameter of the RHV is less than 6 mm. The thin walls of the hepatic veins are less reflective as compared to the portal veins. In patients with congestive heart failure, the RHV diameter increases to a mean diameter of 9 mm or greater.[7]

The hepatic veins normally exhibit a pulsatile triphasic waveform with both antegrade and retrograde flow (Fig. 22-6). This waveform corresponds to cyclic pressure changes within the heart. The initial wave is termed the S wave and is directed toward the

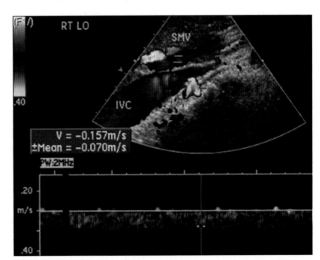

Figure 22-5 Normal superior mesenteric vein Doppler waveforms.

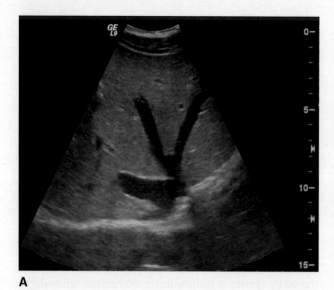

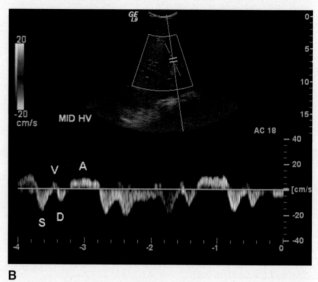

A

B

Figure 22-6 A: Normal B-mode appearance of the three hepatic veins. **B:** Normal hepatic vein Doppler waveforms with the initial S wave directed toward the heart, the V trough, the D wave again directed toward the heart, and the A wave directed toward the liver.

heart. It occurs during the filling of the right atrium in systole. The next component of the waveform is referred to as the V trough, which is due to the right atrium overfilling just before the opening of the tricuspid valve. The next waveform is again directed toward the heart and is called the D wave. This occurs with filling of the right atrium during diastole. The last feature of the waveform, the A wave, is flow toward the liver, which is produced by the contraction of the right atrium. The color flow imaging will display both red and blue filling, representing the multiphasic flow within the vessels. Hepatic vein PSV ranges between 22 and 39 cm/s. Normal respiratory variations can augment waveforms with inspiration, causing a slight decrease in the systolic wave and expiration increasing the systolic wave. The Valsalva maneuver diminishes waveform pulsatility.

HEPATIC ARTERY

The hepatic artery can be readily distinguished from the adjacent portal vein because the hepatic artery demonstrates a higher velocity and is smaller in diameter. Both the hepatic artery and portal vein exhibit flow in the same direction—hepatopetal. Doppler spectral waveforms exhibit a low-resistance flow pattern with antegrade flow throughout the cardiac cycle (Fig. 22-7). This is similar to the pattern observed within the internal carotid artery or renal arteries. Hepatic circulation differs from that of other arterial beds. When portal blood flow increases, hepatic arterial blood flow decreases, and vice versa. This phenomenon has been described as the "hepatic buffer response." Studies have shown an increase in the buffer index in normal patients

postprandially. With the ingestion of food, portal vein velocity increases and hepatic arterial diastolic flow diminishes, exhibiting increased pulsatility in healthy individuals with a normal liver. The peak systolic velocity in the hepatic artery ranges from 70 to 120 cm/s. The normal resistance index (RI) is between 0.50 and 0.70.[8]

INFERIOR VENA CAVA

Normal blood flow within the IVC is toward the right atrium. The Doppler waveform of the IVC near the heart is pulsatile and triphasic due to reflected right atrial pulsations (Fig. 22-8). The flow pattern becomes more phasic with respiration when sampling velocity flow in the lower abdomen. Peak systolic velocities range from 44 to 118 cm/s.

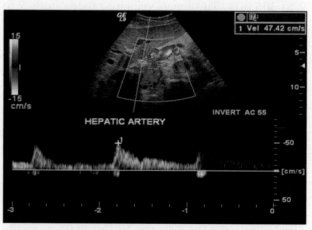

Figure 22-7 Normal hepatic artery Doppler waveforms illustrating a low-resistance pattern with forward flow throughout diastole.

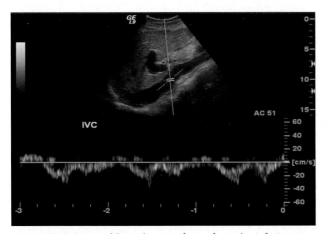

Figure 22-8 Normal Doppler waveforms from the inferior vena cava *(IVC)*. At this level, the flow within the IVC demonstrates slight pulsatility due to the proximity of the heart.

The size of the IVC varies markedly with respiration and the cardiac cycle. It ranges from 15 to 25 mm in diameter. Deep inspiration limits venous return to the chest, increasing the IVC diameter. Expiration improves venous return, decreasing its diameter. The Valsalva maneuver blocks venous return and flow is temporarily reversed in the IVC, causing it to dilate to its maximum diameter. When the IVC is obstructed, it tends to dilate below the level of obstruction. Respiratory changes are decreased or absent below the obstructed segment. The IVC diameter is also dependent on patient size, right atrial pressure, and fluid overload or heart failure.

DISORDERS

As with any organ system, there are a multitude of pathologic conditions that can occur. Diseases of the hepatoportal system often produce significant changes, which are evident on ultrasound examination. Some of the more commonly encountered disorders are described in the following sections.

PORTAL HYPERTENSION

Portal hypertension is defined as an abnormal increase in portal venous pressure as a result of obstruction of blood flow through the liver. In portal hypertension, hepatopetal flow is rerouted away from the liver through collateral channels to low-pressure systemic vessels. True portal pressure is defined as the portal pressure gradient, which is obtained by subtracting the pressure in the IVC (venous outflow) from the portal vein (venous inflow). Normal pressure is between 5 and 10 mm Hg. When the pressure gradient exceeds 15 mm Hg, the condition becomes clinically significant.[2] Life-threatening complications

of variceal hemorrhage associated with portal hypertension account for more than 15,000 hospital admissions per year in the United States.

Etiology

Portal hypertension results when venous blood flow is obstructed within the liver or in the extrahepatic hepatoportal venous system. The most common etiology for portal hypertension in North America is sinusoidal obstruction due to cirrhosis. Until recently, the most common cause of cirrhosis was alcohol abuse. Because of the rapid increase of hepatitis C virus infection, hepatitis C is now the leader (26%), with alcohol abuse falling second (21%).[9] Other causes include hepatitis B, primary biliary cirrhosis, autoimmune hepatitis, and hereditary hemochromatosis. Seventy-five percent of deaths attributable to alcoholism are caused by cirrhosis. In cirrhosis, most of the normal liver architecture is replaced by distorted vascular channels that provide increased resistance to portal venous blood flow and obstruction to hepatic venous outflow. The primary complication of portal hypertension is gastrointestinal bleeding from ruptured esophageal and gastric varices. Etiologies of hypertension are divided into three levels: prehepatic (inflow), intrahepatic (liver, sinusoids, and hepatocytes), and posthepatic (outflow). Disease processes associated with each level are listed in Table 22-2.

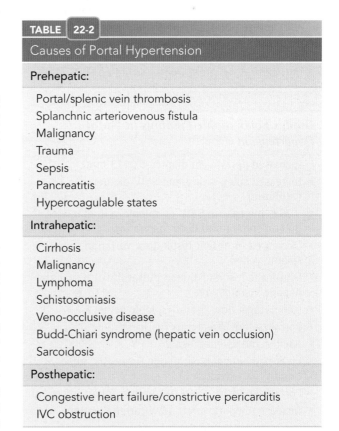

TABLE 22-2
Causes of Portal Hypertension
Prehepatic:
Portal/splenic vein thrombosis
Splanchnic arteriovenous fistula
Malignancy
Trauma
Sepsis
Pancreatitis
Hypercoagulable states
Intrahepatic:
Cirrhosis
Malignancy
Lymphoma
Schistosomiasis
Veno-occlusive disease
Budd-Chiari syndrome (hepatic vein occlusion)
Sarcoidosis
Posthepatic:
Congestive heart failure/constrictive pericarditis
IVC obstruction

Duplex Sonographic Findings in Portal Hypertension

Several sonographic findings are associated with portal hypertension. Pathology Box 22-1 lists the duplex sonographic findings.[10]

With the development of portal hypertension, the main portal vein initially increases due to increasing portal venous pressure (Fig. 22-9). In cases of severe portal hypertension, the diameter of the portal vein may decrease (decompression) due to portosystemic collaterals. An increased portal vein diameter >13 mm indicates portal hypertension with a high degree of specificity (100%) but with low sensitivity (40%).[11] Reversed or hepatofugal portal flow is generally associated with a significant reduction in the diameter of the portal vein because more blood is diverted to portosystemic collaterals. Hepatofugal flow in the MPV has been reported in the literature with an overall prevalence of 8.3% in patients.[6] Other studies have reported hepatofugal flow in the portal venous system (portal, splenic, and superior mesenteric veins) in 3% to 23% of patients with cirrhosis.[12] In some patients with cirrhosis, hepatofugal flow is identified in isolated intrahepatic portal vein branches only. Hepatofugal flow can change to hepatopetal flow after ingestion of a meal because of a postprandial increase in splanchnic venous flow. This phenomenon may be blunted in cirrhotic patients. Also, hepatofugal flow can revert to hepatopetal flow if the patient's condition improves after medication.

With severe portal hypertension, flow velocity within the portal vein generally decreases due to increased

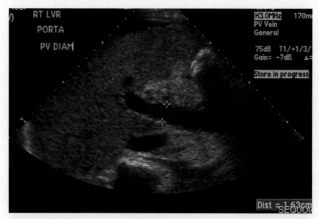

Figure 22-9 A portal vein with an increased diameter (1.63 cm) associated with portal hypertension.

resistance. Spectral Doppler demonstrates continuous (losing normal fluctuations), biphasic (to and fro in some patients), and eventually, reverse flow (hepatofugal) in patients with advanced disease (Fig. 22-10).

Although several studies advocate decreased portal vein flow as an indicator of portal hypertension, collateral pathways can augment portal vein hemodynamics. For example, a recanalized paraumbilical vein can increase portal vein velocity, whereas splenorenal collaterals can reduce and reverse flow.

An increased splenic vein diameter >10 mm with reduced flow or retrograde (hepatofugal) flow and no detectable thrombus is an indicator for portal hypertension. In this situation, the mesenteric venous blood is transported to the vena cava through

PATHOLOGY BOX 22-1

Duplex Sonographic Findings in Portal Hypertension

- Increased portal vein diameter (>13 mm)
- Increased splenic vein and SMV diameters (>10 mm)
- <20% increase in SMV or splenic vein diameter, quiet respiration to deep inspiration
- Decreased or absent respiratory variation (portal/splenic veins)
- Diminished, static, altered pulsatility of portal and hepatic venous flow
- Hepatofugal flow (portal/splenic veins)
- Portosystemic collaterals (varices)
- Ascites and splenomegaly
- Liver parenchymal pathology (cirrhosis, tumor, Budd-Chiari syndrome)
- Portal vein obstruction (thrombus, tumor invasion)
- Increased hepatic artery flow (arterialization)

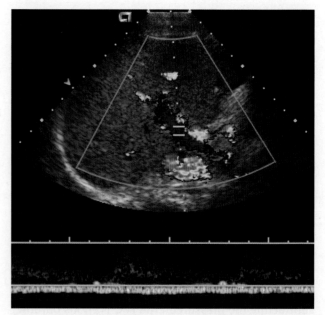

Figure 22-10 Abnormal hepatofugal Doppler waveforms from a portal vein in a patient with portal hypertension. The abnormal portal venous flow is displayed below the baseline and is color-coded in *blue* within the image. Normal antegrade hepatic artery flow is displayed above the baseline.

portosystemic collaterals. In the splenic hilum, dilated veins sometimes show anastomoses to veins of the stomach or esophagus.

Portosystemic Collateral Anatomy

Detection of portosystemic collateral veins (varices) is the most specific finding of portal hypertension. Varices are reported to occur in approximately 39% of patients with biopsy-proven cirrhosis and are more common in patients with advanced disease.[13] Color duplex sonography visualizes approximately 65% to 90% of collateral shunts.[14] Commonly seen collaterals include the paraumbilical vein, the coronary vein, the gastroesophageal veins, and the splenorenal vein (Fig. 22-11). The most common collateral shunt is the coronary-gastroesophageal route (80% to 90%); when dilated, these cause esophageal varices.[14] Pathology Box 22-2 describes various portosystemic collateral pathways.[2,10]

PATHOLOGY BOX 22-2
Portosystemic Collateral Pathways

Collateral	Features
Coronary vein (left gastric vein)	• Most often joins the portal system at the splenoportal confluence • With portal hypertension, diameter >7 mm • Can demonstrate hepatofugal flow, which often leads to esophageal varices
Gastroesophageal veins	• Located posterior to left lobe of liver • Can be large and tortuous
Recanalized paraumbilical vein	• Located in the fissure for the ligamentum teres • Diameter >3 mm is diagnostic for portal hypertension
Splenorenal	• Prominent varices at splenic hilum • Enlarged left renal vein
Gallbladder varices	• Portosystemic shunts between the cystic vein branch of the portal vein and either anterior abdominal wall veins or portal vein branches within the liver • Found in 30% of patients with portal hypertension • 3–8 mm in diameter • Tortuous vessels along gallbladder wall

Arterialization (Increased Hepatic Artery Flow)

When portal venous pressure increases, portal vein flow decreases and hepatic artery flow increases as a homeostatic mechanism to maintain hepatic perfusion. Enlargement, increased flow, and a tortuous "corkscrew" appearance are commonly seen in patients with cirrhosis, portal hypertension, portal vein thrombosis, and inflammation related to chronic active hepatitis. Color duplex imaging demonstrates an enlarged hepatic artery with high velocity turbulent flow (mixed color flow) referred to as "arterialization."

Arteriovenous Fistulae

Hepatic arterial–portal fistulae may cause life-threatening portal hypertension. Causes of arterial–portal fistulae include penetrating trauma, iatrogenic trauma secondary to liver biopsies, transhepatic cholangiography, and transhepatic catheterization of the bile ducts or portal veins. Profuse collateral flow typically accompanies severe portal hypertension in patients with hepatic artery to portal vein communications. With an arterial–portal fistula, the resulting pressure gradient causes blood to flow from the artery to the vein. Duplex sonography demonstrates arterialized hepatofugal flow in the portal vein. Large anechoic spaces are seen within the liver in the area of the communication. Color Doppler shows a turbulent high-velocity flow "color bruit" detected between the communication of the artery and the vein.

Another type of fistula can arise between the portal vein and a hepatic vein. The causes responsible for venovenous fistulae are trauma, surgery, organ punctures, perforated aneurysms, and idiopathic causes. The pressure gradients associated with venovenous fistulae cause blood to flow from the portal vein to the hepatic vein. In cases of hepatic vein to portal vein fistulae, the triphasic spectral pattern of the hepatic veins is reflected back to the portal system, producing increased pulsatility in the portal vein waveform.

Transjugular Intrahepatic Portosystemic Shunts

The treatment of portal hypertension involves techniques designed to decrease the pressure or decompress the portal venous system. In the past, surgical shunts were created that connected the portal vein to the IVC (portocaval shunt), the superior mesenteric vein to the IVC (mesocaval shunt), or the splenic vein to the left renal vein (splenorenal shunt). These all reduced flow into the liver and thus helped lessen the pressure in the portal venous system. Current therapy involves a percutaneously created shunt, which avoids

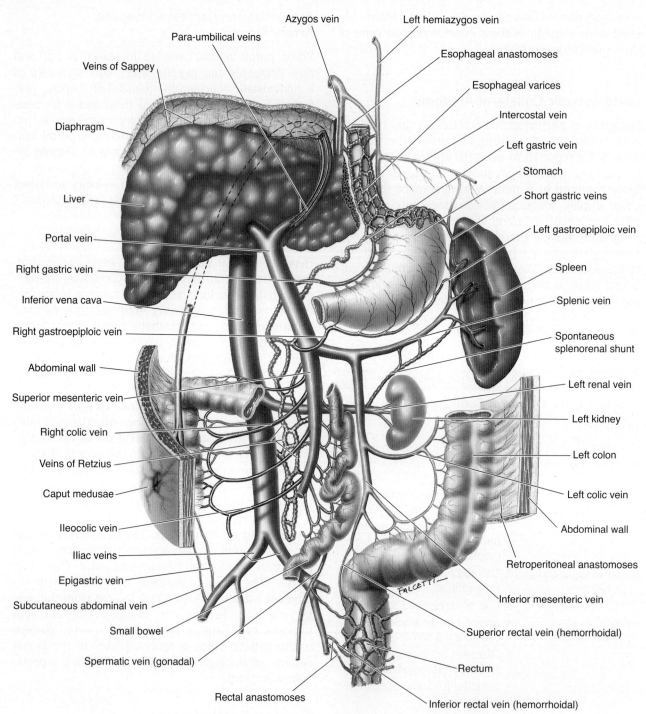

Figure 22-11 A diagram depicting the various portosystemic collaterals.

the risks of surgery and general anesthesia. The transjugular intrahepatic portosystemic (also known as portocaval) shunt or TIPS procedure has replaced the need for surgically created shunts in most patients.

Via jugular vein cannulation, a stent is deployed connecting one of the portal veins (often the right portal vein) with one of the hepatic veins (often the right hepatic vein). This has the effect of rerouting blood flow away from the liver, out through the stent, into the hepatic vein, and back to the heart. The stents employed had been bare metal stents but many are now created using partially covered stents.[15]

The ultrasound techniques employed to evaluate a patient with a TIPS are much the same as a conventional evaluation of the native portal system. These include the same transducers and scanning approaches, as well as the same patient preparation of having the patient fast prior to the ultrasound.

Velocities are recorded from the main portal vein, the portal vein end of the shunt, the mid shunt, the hepatic vein end of the shunt, and the IVC or outflow hepatic vein. The direction of flow should be noted within these vessels in addition to adjacent intrahepatic portal veins, the splenic vein, and the superior mesenteric vein. The presence of ascites or varices should be noted.

In a patient with a well-functioning TIPS, hepatofugal flow may be present within the intrahepatic portal veins beyond the site of the stent connection with the portal vein. Color flow imaging should reveal hepatopetal flow in the main portal vein with flow directed into the stent. The flow should continue in the direction of the hepatic vein and then out via the IVC. Color should be observed completely filling the stent (Fig. 22-12). If a covered stent is used, acoustic shadowing may be present in the immediate postprocedural period. This is a result of air being trapped within the layers of the material used to cover the stent. After a brief period of time (usually 2 to 3 days), the air dissipates and the stent will be able to be completely insonated.

The velocity findings vary between patients depending on several factors, including the severity of the portal hypertension, the diameter of the stent, pressure gradients of the system, and patient respiration. Normal velocities within the stent range from 90 to 190 cm/s.[16] A baseline study of each patient is important to gauge further follow-up examinations. Flow velocities will be high within the stent and should not vary significantly along the course of the stent (Fig. 22-13). Within the main portal vein and hepatic artery, flow velocities are increased. Portal vein velocities may increase to 37 to 47 cm/s, greater than the pre-TIPS velocities.[2] Hepatic artery peak systolic velocity may exceed 130 cm/s.[2] Splenic vein velocities are also observed to increase post-TIPS placement.

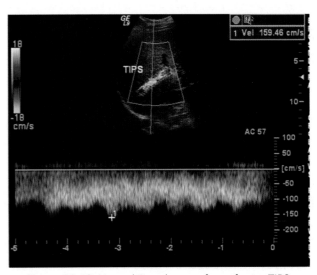

Figure 22-13 Normal Doppler waveforms from a TIPS.

Multiple duplex ultrasound changes have been associated with TIPS stenosis.[14] Pathology Box 22-3 lists criteria commonly employed in cases of suspected stenosis. Figure 22-14 illustrates a TIPS stenosis.

No single ultrasound criterion has yielded a strong predictive value or sensitivity in detecting stenosis. When multiple criteria are used, sensitivity in identifying TIPS stenosis improves.

TIPS occlusion should be suspected if echogenic material is observed within the stent and no flow is detected on spectral Doppler or color flow imaging techniques (Fig. 22-15). Care should be taken to optimize Doppler and color imaging techniques to avoid a false-positive finding of thrombosis. Multiple scanning planes should be used as well as appropriate

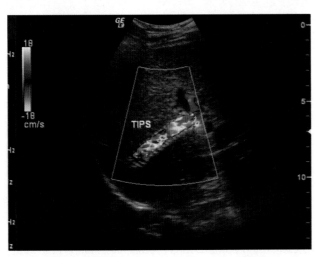

Figure 22-12 Color image of a normal TIPS.

PATHOLOGY BOX 22-3

Duplex Ultrasound Criteria for TIPS Stenosis

A change in the direction of flow within the main portal, right, or left portal veins as compared to baseline studies

Retrograde flow within the hepatic vein serving as the outflow for the shunt

A velocity of less than 50 cm/s within the stent

A velocity less than 30 cm/s within the main portal vein

A focal increase in stent velocity greater than 200 cm/s

An increase or decrease in velocity of greater than 50 cm/s within the same portion of the stent as compared to previous studies

A velocity gradient greater than 50 cm/s from one portion of the stent to another

Recurrent ascites, varices, or splenomegaly

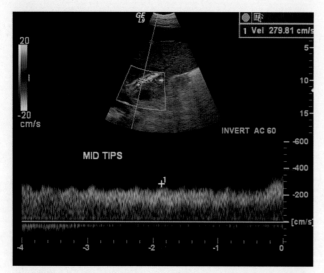

Figure 22-14 An image from a TIPS with a stenosis. Note the elevated velocity of 280 cm/s.

Doppler and color frequencies, color priority settings, and Doppler and color scale or pulse repetition frequencies.

PORTAL VENOUS THROMBOSIS

Thrombosis within the portal, splenic, and superior mesenteric veins can result from flow stasis secondary to cirrhosis and subsequent portal hypertension. As portal venous flow to the liver decreases, arterial flow increases. This is a homeostatic mechanism to maintain hepatic perfusion. Other etiologies of portal vein thrombosis (PVT) include inflammatory processes (such as pancreatitis, appendicitis, and diverticulitis), various hypercoagulable states (including protein C or S deficiencies, antithrombin deficiency, and polycythemia vera), surgical intervention, abdominal malignancy (hepatocellular or pancreatic carcinomas), sepsis, and trauma.[1] Patients with hepatocellular

carcinoma (HCC) are at greater risk of developing malignant thrombus (intravascular tumor) due to direct invasion of the portal vein. Pancreatitis and pancreatic carcinoma are frequent causes of thrombosis and tumor infiltration in the portal, splenic, and superior mesenteric veins. A sudden onset of ascites, acute abdominal pain, and elevated D-dimer in patients may indicate the presence of PVT.

Because the main portal vein is easily visualized in most patients, when a normal appearing portal vein is not readily seen, portal vein occlusion should be suspected. Diagnostic sonographic findings supporting the diagnosis of acute PVT are the absence of flow by spectral, color, or power Doppler accompanied by faintly echogenic material (a thrombus or tumor) within the portal vein lumen (Fig. 22-16). The portal vein diameter is larger than 15 mm in 38% of cases. Acute PVT may appear anechoic and go undetected when performing grayscale imaging. With complete obstruction of the portal vein, reverse flow in the splenic vein is often detected. A tumor in the portal vein may present identical to that of thrombosis. A tumor thrombus may be partial or complete and be mixed with a bland, avascular thrombus. Color Doppler imaging can aid in differentiating a thrombus from tumor infiltration by identifying small vascular channels that exhibit low-resistance pulsatile arterial signals within a soft-tissue mass in the portal veins.[17] Color Doppler imaging also helps to distinguish complete versus partial PVT.

A thrombosis of the SMV and splenic veins is more difficult to identify with duplex imaging than PVT. Sonographic duplex findings are the same in these veins as in the portal vein.

If PVT persists (up to 12 months) without substantial lysis, this leads to the development of periportal collateral veins known as "cavernous transformation."[2] With cavernous transformation,

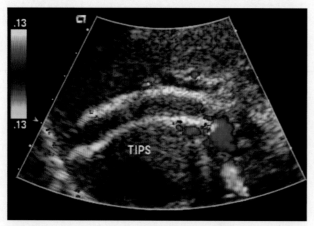

Figure 22-15 An occluded TIPS with no filling on color flow imaging and echogenic material within the shunt itself.

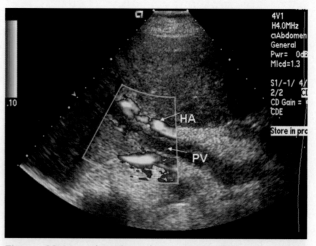

Figure 22-16 A thrombosed portal vein (PV) with no flow present using power Doppler techniques. Flow is seen in the adjacent hepatic artery (HA).

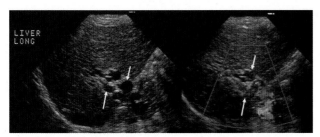

Figure 22-17 A thrombosed portal vein with cavernous transformation (*arrows* indicate the periportal collateral veins).

multiple serpiginous vessels are seen in and around the occluded portal vein. They can appear within 6 to 20 days after acute occlusion to reestablish portal flow. The thrombosed portal vein has a sponge-like mass appearance on grayscale, representing numerous venous recanalizing channels. Color duplex imaging demonstrates absent flow in the main portal vein and recanalizing hepatopetal portal venous flow (2 to 7 cm/s) within periportal collateral veins (Fig. 22-17). Because cavernous transformation results from long-standing portal vein occlusion, it is more likely to be caused by benign processes. The sonographic findings for PVT are listed in Pathology Box 22-4.

CONGESTIVE HEART FAILURE

Edema of the liver secondary to vascular congestion is a complication related to congestive heart failure. Impedance of flow into the right side of the heart

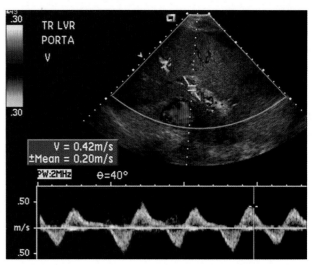

Figure 22-18 A portal vein image demonstrating markedly pulsatile flow from a patient with congestive heart failure.

due to cardiac or pulmonary disorders causes secondary dilatation and absence of vein wall motion with respiratory maneuvers both within the hepatoportal venous system and the IVC. Increased right heart pressure will impact the portal and hepatic waveforms. Portal vein flow becomes markedly pulsatile, corresponding to pressure transmitted from the right atrium (Fig. 22-18). Hepatic vein waveforms demonstrate a highly pulsatile inverted "**W**"-type pattern, showing flow reversal during systole secondary to tricuspid regurgitation. Two distinct findings that help differentiate between congestive heart failure and "true" portal hypertension are as follows: (1) In congestive heart failure, both portal and hepatic veins exhibit increased pulsatility, and (2) the IVC is dilated. Neither of these findings is indicative of portal hypertension related to liver disease.

BUDD-CHIARI SYNDROME

Obstruction of the hepatic venous outflow tract due to a thrombus and or a tumor with concomitant clinical features including right upper quadrant pain, jaundice, ascites, hepatomegaly, and liver function abnormalities suggesting hepatocellular dysfunctions are collectively known as Budd-Chiari syndrome.[1] There are many causes of Budd-Chiari syndrome, and these are related to the primary site of obstruction. Primary hepatic vein occlusion results from a thrombus or tumor infiltration. A thrombus can occur with cirrhosis, hypercoagulable disorders, the use of oral contraceptives, and abdominal trauma.[10] Tumor invasion is most often associated with hepatocellular carcinoma. IVC occlusion or stenosis cephalad to the hepatic veins can cause Budd-Chiari syndrome

PATHOLOGY BOX 22-4

Sonographic Characteristics of PVT

- Increased portal vein caliber (>15 mm) with intraluminal echoes (38%) of cases (acute)
- Massive portal vein caliber (>23 mm) with intraluminal echoes suggests tumor thrombus not specific
- Failure to visualize the portal vein (acute)
- Absent flow by color and power Doppler within a completely obstructed portal vein
- Hepatofugal pulsatile arterial waveform within a soft tissue mass in the main portal vein (tumor thrombus)
- Small vascular arterial channels within a soft tissue mass in the main portal vein (tumor thrombus)
- Increased hepatic arterial flow (arterialization)
- Small echogenic/fibrotic portal channels with intraluminal echoes (chronic)
- Cavernous transformation; periportal collaterals (chronic)
- Gallbladder varices

by creating hepatic vein congestion. Obstruction of the IVC may be caused by congenital stenosis or occlusion, thrombosis from hypercoagulable states, or tumor invasion.

Hepatic venous obstruction is often accompanied by stenosis or obstruction of the IVC. When the IVC is involved, lower extremity edema maybe present. With severe obstruction, collateral channels are formed as follows: portal vein collaterals via enlarged paraumbilical veins, reversed hepatic venous flow to systemic or capsular veins, and intrahepatic venous to hepatic venous collaterals. Flow in the portal vein maybe slow or reversed. The caudate lobe enlarges due to blood volume overload as the other lobes of the liver will try to drain out via the caudate veins, which empty directly into the IVC.[4] The sonographic findings of Budd-Chiari syndrome are listed in Pathology Box 22-5.

> **PATHOLOGY BOX 22-5**
>
> ### *Sonographic Findings in Budd-Chiari Syndrome*
>
> - Dilatation of the IVC with intraluminal echoes
> - Dilatation of the hepatic veins with intraluminal echoes
> - Stenosis or occlusion of the hepatic veins and IVC
> - Absence of hepatic vein and IVC flow
> - Continuous, turbulent, and reversed flow in the nonoccluded portions of hepatic veins and IVC
> - Enlarged caudate lobe (greater than 3.5 cm in anteroposterior diameter)
> - Enlarged caudate vein >3 mm in diameter
> - Slow or reversed flow in the portal vein
> - Ascites/hepatomegaly
> - Splenomegaly (25%)
> - Portosystemic collaterals

SUMMARY

Sonography provides important quantitative and qualitative information about the liver and hepatoportal venous dynamics. A thorough working knowledge of the anatomy, hemodynamics, instrumentation, and scanning windows, along with patience, are essential to best use this medical imaging tool. Furthermore, knowledge about abnormal vascular disorders and altered hemodynamics increases examination efficacy and sonographer knowledge, and contributes to quality patient care.

Critical Thinking Questions

1. A patient presents for an add-on portal system ultrasound examination. The patient has not fasted, is obese, and is known to have ascites. What scanning plane might you use to begin the scan and why?

2. Why is the breathing pattern of a patient important during a hepatoportal ultrasound examination?

3. You are asked to examine a patient who is 1-day postprocedure from a TIPS shunt being placed. You begin your ultrasound examination and observe a brightly reflective structure within the right lobe of the liver. However, a strong acoustic shadow is present. What is a likely explanation of this finding and what can be done?

REFERENCES

1. Leonhardt WC. Duplex sonography of the hepato-portal vascular system. *Vascular US Today.* 2005;10:129–180.
2. Wilson SR, Withers CE. The liver. In: Rumack CM, Wilson SR, Charboneau JW, et al., eds. *Diagnostic Ultrasound*. 4th ed. Philadelphia, PA: Elsevier Mosby Company; 2011:78–145.
3. Marks WM, Filly RA, Callen PW. Ultrasonic anatomy of the liver: a review with new applications. *J Clin Ultrasound.* 1979;7:137–146.
4. Bargallo X, Gilbert R, Nicolau C, et al. Sonography of the caudate vein: value in diagnosing Budd-Chiari Syndrome. *Am J Roentgenol.* 2003;181:1641–1645.

5. Weinreb J, Kumari S, Phillips G, et al. Portal vein measurements by real-time sonography. *Am J Roentgenol.* 1982;139:497–499.

6. Bolondi L, Galani S, Gebel M. Portohepatic vascular pathology and liver disease: diagnosis and monitoring. *Eur J Ultrasound.* 1998;7:S41–S52.

7. Henriksson L, Hedman A, Johansson R, et al. Ultrasound assessment of liver veins in congestive heart failure. *Acta Radiol.* 1982;23:361–363.

8. Al-Nakahabandi NA. The role of ultrasonography in portal hypertension. *Saudi J·Gastroentero.* 2006;12:111–117.

9. National Institute of Diabetes and Digestive and Kidney Diseases. *Cirrhosis of the Liver.* NIH Pub No 00-1134. Bethesda, MD: National Institutes of Health; 2000.

10. Zwiebel WJ. Vascular conditions. In: Ahuja AT ed. *Diagnostic Imaging: Ultrasound.* Philadelphia, PA: Elsevier Saunders; 2007:1–110.

11. Bolondi L, Gandolfi L, Arienti V, et al. Ultrasonography in the diagnosis of portal hypertension: diminished response of portal vessels to respiration. *Radiology.* 1982;142:167–172.

12. Wachsberg RH, Bahramipour P, Sofocleous CT, et al. Hepatofugal flow in the portal venous system: pathophysiology, imaging findings, and diagnostic pitfalls. *Radiographics.* 2002;22:123–140.

13. Andrew A. Portal hypertension: a review. *J Diag Med Sonog.* 2001;17:193–200.

14. Zwiebel WJ. Ultrasound assessment of the hepatic vasculature. In: Zwiebel WJ, Pellerito JS, eds. *Introduction to Vascular Ultrasonography.* 5th ed. Philadelphia, PA: Elsevier Saunders; 2005:585–609.

15. Vignali C, Bargellini I, Grosso M, et al. TIPS with expanded polytetrafluoroethylene-covered stent: result of an Italian multicenter study. *Am J Roentgenol.* 2005;185:472–480.

16. Kanterman RY, Darcy MD, Middleton WD, et al. Doppler sonography findings associated with transjugular intrahepatic portosystemic shunt malfunction. *Am J Roentgenol.* 1997;168:467–472.

17. Dodd GD, Memel DS, Baron RL, et al. Portal vein thrombosis in patients with cirrhosis: does sonographic detection of intrathrombus flow allow differentiation of benign and malignant thrombus? *Am J Roentgenol.* 1995;165:573–577.

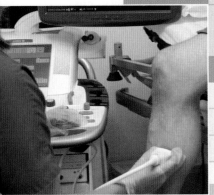

23 | Evaluation of Kidney and Liver Transplants

M. Robert De Jong, Leslie Millar Scoutt, and Monica Fuller

OBJECTIVES

Describe the types of transplant procedures and vascular anastomoses

Define the essential components of transplant ultrasound examinations

Define the vascular complications associated with transplants

KEY TERMS

arteriovenous fistula | liver transplant | pseudoaneurysm | rejection | renal transplant | vascular stenosis | vascular thrombosis

GLOSSARY

allograft any tissue transplanted from one human to another human

arteriovenous fistula a connection between an artery and a vein, usually posttraumatic in origin

immunosuppression drugs drugs used to inhibit the body's formation of antibodies to the allograft

orthotopic transplant a transplant that is placed in the same anatomic location as the native organ; a whole liver transplant is an orthotopic

transplant; renal transplants are not orthotopic in location

pseudoaneurysm develops secondary to a tear in the arterial wall, allowing extravasation of blood from the arterial lumen, which is contained by a compacted rim of surrounding soft tissue

transplant rejection the failure of a transplant occurring secondary to the formation of antidonor antibodies by the recipient; it can lead to loss of the transplant

Ultrasound evaluation of transplanted organs has become an established and important routine component of posttransplant patient follow-up. Modern advances in surgical techniques and in immunosuppression regimens have resulted in increased long-term survival of both allografts and transplant recipients. Renal and hepatic transplantation are the preferred treatment for patients with renal and hepatic failure, respectively. Pancreatic, small bowel, lung, and cardiac transplants are also increasingly performed. In most series, vascular complications are the second most common cause of graft loss, and ultrasound (US) is considered the initial screening modality of choice for the evaluation of a suspected vascular complication in a renal or hepatic transplant recipient. This chapter will review the ultrasound techniques and criteria for the US examination of kidney and liver transplants.

KIDNEY TRANSPLANTATION

The first successful kidney transplant was performed in 1954 at the Peter Bent Brigham Hospital in Boston, Massachusetts between identical twin brothers, which eliminated the potential for any adverse immune reaction.[1,2] However, kidney transplants continued to be very limited due to incompatibility issues until the early 1960s, when significant advances in tissue typing allowed for better matching of donor and recipients occurred. In addition, immunosuppression therapy was introduced in 1961, which dramatically improved graft survival, as these drugs helped the recipient accept the foreign tissue in the allograft. With immunosuppression therapy, transplantation of a cadaveric donor allograft became a realistic possibility and, in 1962, the first cadaveric kidney transplant was performed, again at the Peter Bent Brigham Hospital. In 1983, cyclosporine, a highly effective and relatively nontoxic immunosuppressant agent, was introduced and resulted in a significant improvement in patient outcomes by reducing the risk of rejection. Since then, continued evolution and refinement of immunosuppression protocols have even further decreased the rate of graft loss due to rejection in renal transplant recipients.

Currently, renal transplantation is considered the treatment of choice for the majority of patients with end-stage renal disease (ESRD), providing better quality of life and long-term survival when compared to either peritoneal dialysis or hemodialysis.[3-5] Common causes of ESRD include diabetes mellitus, autosomal dominant polycystic kidney disease, glomerulonephritis, hypertension, atherosclerosis, and systemic lupus erythematosus, with diabetes being the most common cause of kidney transplantation.

According to the Organ Procurement and Transplantation Network (OPTN) (http://optn.transplant.hrsa.gov), 16,829 kidney transplants (including both cadaveric and living-related donors) were performed in the United States in 2009. However, there were more than 86,000 people on the waiting list for a kidney transplant in 2010. In fact, it is estimated that a new name is added to the waiting list approximately every 13 seconds.[4] Thus, organ shortage is the major rate-limiting factor for patients awaiting renal transplantation. The current organ shortage has resulted in a loosening of the criteria for deceased donors (DDs), an increase in the use of living-related donors (LRDs), as well as other creative means of increasing organ availability.

There has been a steady increase in graft survival since the first kidney was transplanted in the 1950s due to significant advances in immunosuppression protocols, surgical techniques, and the improvement in rapid and efficient organ distribution of HLA-matched DD grafts by the United Network for Organ Sharing (UNOS). In 2010, the OPTN reported a 79.7% 5-year graft survival rate for living-related HLA-matched donors and a 66.5% 5-year graft survival rate for DD grafts.[4] Risk factors for graft loss include the number of HLA mismatches, the increased age of donors or recipients, African American race, cold ischemic time greater than 24 hours, and diabetic nephropathy as the cause of the recipient's renal failure.[6]

Once a person has received a transplant, they are closely monitored for any signs of graft failure or complication. Patients with graft failure most commonly present with anuria or a rising serum creatinine level. Pain, tenderness, fever, chills, or elevated white blood cell (WBC) count may also indicate graft dysfunction. However, these are all quite nonspecific signs and symptoms. Hence, imaging, particularly Doppler ultrasound, plays a vital role in the clinical assessment of graft dysfunction following renal transplantation by helping to differentiate anatomic and/or vascular problems that may require surgical intervention from functional abnormalities such as acute tubular necrosis (ATN), drug toxicity, and rejection, which are all treated medically.

THE OPERATION

In adults, renal transplants are most commonly placed extraperitoneally in the right iliac fossa. The right iliac fossa is preferred over the left simply because the sigmoid colon usually occupies more space than the right colon, thereby making the vascular anastomoses slightly technically more difficult on the left. In children, the transplanted kidney may be placed intraperitoneally. For DD transplants, the donor's main renal artery is harvested along with a surrounding cuff or patch of the aortic wall called the Carrel patch. This oval piece of the donor's aortic wall typically is anastomosed in an end-to-side fashion with the recipient external iliac artery (EIA) (Fig. 23-1). If the donor kidney has multiple renal arteries, either a larger Carrel patch surrounding the ostia of all the main renal arteries is harvested or multiple separate patches are obtained. Alternatively, the donor renal arteries may be grafted together in a "Y" graft with only a single anastomosis to the recipient EIA. For an LRD graft, the donor main renal artery is directly anastomosed either in an end-to-side fashion with the recipient EIA or end-to-end with the recipient internal iliac artery. Because the harvesting and use of a Carrel patch results in a larger anastomosis without direct suturing into the renal artery ostium, the incidence of renal artery stenosis is believed to be reduced in DD transplants in comparison to LRD renal transplants. The donor main

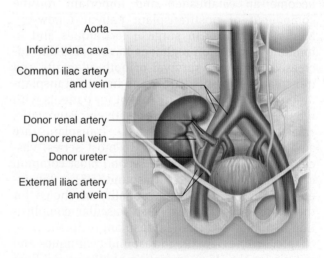

Figure 23-1 Diagram illustrating the most common surgical anatomy for renal transplantation.

renal vein is typically anastomosed to the recipient external iliac vein in an end-to-side approach. The ureteral anastomosis is most commonly made by creating an ureteroneocystostomy—implanting the donor ureter into the dome of the bladder above the native ureteral orifice (UVJ).

Rarely, two pediatric donor kidneys may be transplanted en bloc into an adult recipient. In such cases, the donor aorta with the main renal arteries attached is harvested along with the two kidneys, and a direct end-to-side anastomosis between the donor aorta and the recipient external artery is created. Similarly, the donor inferior vena cava (IVC) receiving both the right and left main renal veins is implanted end to side with the recipient iliac vein.

Although practice varies nationwide, placement of an external drain next to the kidney is believed to decrease the incidence of lymphoceles formation, a relatively common postsurgical complication that can cause graft dysfunction by compressing the renal parenchyma or vascular/ureteral anastomoses. Superinfection may also occur. Ureteral stents from the intrarenal collecting system into the bladder are commonly placed to reduce the likelihood of ureteral scarring or necrosis as well as extravasation of urine, which may lead to the development of urinomas. In most patients, the native kidneys are left in place.

SONOGRAPHIC EXAMINATION TECHNIQUES

PATIENT PREPARATION

Typically, no patient preparation is needed to evaluate a renal transplant. It may be helpful for the patient to have some urine in the bladder. It is important for the sonographer to review the surgical notes or speak to the surgeon before the initial or baseline ultrasound is obtained. The sonographer should know the following information at a minimum: location of the kidney, if a single kidney or two pediatric kidneys were placed, which native vessels were used to anastomose with the main renal artery and vein, any vascular anomalies such as duplicated vessels, and any additional information that may affect the ultrasound examination. The sonographer should also review any recent studies, especially if pathology was present as well as to review the vascular anatomy and anastomotic sites.

PATIENT POSITIONING

The patient is examined in the supine position. If bowel or gas is obscuring part of the kidney, the patient may be turned into an oblique or decubitus position to try to improve visualization of the kidney.

EQUIPMENT

A 3- to 5-MHz curved linear array transducer can be used. This will provide an aperture to allow for insonation of the entire kidney. The transducer can be gently rocked to push bowel gas out of the way to improve visualization of the kidney. Varying the imaging depth will be necessary due to the superficial placement of most transplanted kidneys. In thin patients, a higher transducer frequency or harmonic imaging may improve resolution.

SCANNING TECHNIQUE

Imaging protocols must be based on current accreditation guidelines and should be reviewed annually. These guidelines can be found at http://www.icavl. org, http://www.aium.org, and http://www.acr.org.

A baseline sonogram is usually obtained within 48 hours postoperatively. It is usually not necessary to evaluate the native kidneys, which are typically left in situ. The lie of the kidney will vary depending on the patient's anatomy. Usually, the kidney is superficial and runs with the axis of the incision site, with the hilum oriented inferiorly and posteriorly. The kidney will also be in a plane parallel to the skin surface, although sometimes the kidney will be tilted with either the upper or lower pole closer to the skin and the other pole deeper in the body. This gives the appearance of the kidney almost being in a plane perpendicular to the skin surface. The length and width of the kidney should be accurately measured (Figs. 23-2 and 23-3). Some protocols may require a volume

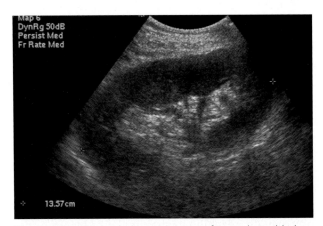

Figure 23-2 Grayscale long-axis view of transplanted kidney (calipers). The renal cortex is relatively hypoechoic, homogeneous, and symmetric in thickness. Mild dilatation of the intrarenal collecting system within the echogenic central renal sinus is a normal finding.

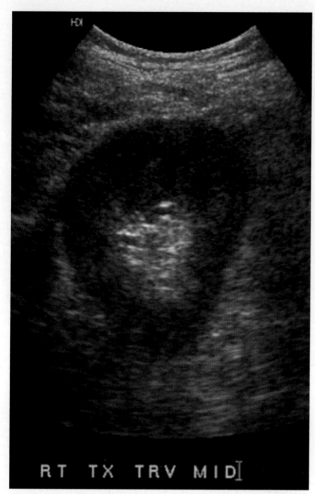

Figure 23-3 Grayscale transverse view of a transplanted kidney.

plane) are obtained. Many laboratories obtain transverse views superior to the kidney, through the upper pole, mid-pole with transverse and AP measurements, lower pole, and finally, inferior to the kidney. The superior and inferior transverse views are used to evaluate for any perinephric fluid collections. However, a general survey should also be performed to look for fluid collections. Multiple longitudinal and transverse images of the bladder, or the bladder area if the patient has a Foley catheter in place, should be obtained. An oblique view showing the lower pole of the kidney and the bladder in the same image can also be recorded. This is a helpful image to evaluate for the presence of a urinoma. Any fluid collection seen near the bladder will require further investigation either by having the patient void or by instilling appropriate fluid through the patient's catheter to distend the bladder.

Color and Spectral Doppler

After obtaining the requisite grayscale images, the sonographer should now perform the Doppler component of the examination. Color and spectral Doppler signals are obtained from the main renal artery, including angle-corrected peak systolic velocity measurements at the anastomosis, proximal, and distal (hilar) segments (Figs. 23-4 and 23-5). A color image and spectral Doppler signal is also obtained from the EIA superior to the anastomosis. A color Doppler image of the main renal artery is

measurement of the kidney, which would require measuring the kidney in all three planes: length, width, and anterioposterior (AP) dimensions. The transplanted kidney will look like a normal kidney in shape and echotexture. A comparison view with the liver or spleen cannot be obtained as the kidney is now located in the pelvis.

Grayscale

Grayscale imaging should be performed first. Documented images should include views of the long axis of the kidney in the mid-axis to measure the length of the kidney as well as longitudinal views of the lateral and medial aspects of the kidney. Renal length is variable but is often slightly larger than the native kidney as the kidney will hypertrophy, usually reaching its maximal size by 6 months postop. Increase or decrease in renal length from one exam to the next is a nonspecific indicator of graft dysfunction. Next, views that are 90° to the long axis of the kidney (i.e., in the transverse

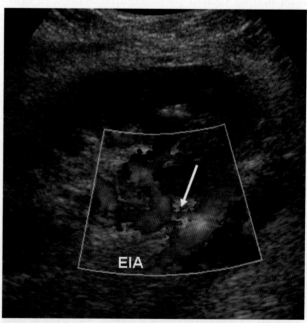

Figure 23-4 Color Doppler image of the main renal artery anastomosis (arrow).

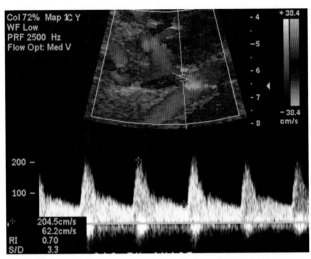

Figure 23-5 Normal spectral Doppler tracing from the origin of the main renal artery. Note the sharp systolic upstroke and continuous forward diastolic flow with an RI = 0.70. Mild elevation of the PSV in the main renal artery (204 cm/s) is common secondary to the acute angle of take off from the external iliac artery and increased blood flow through the single vessel.

essential to evaluate for kinking or torquing. Color and spectral Doppler signals are obtained from the main renal vein including the venous anastomosis with the external iliac vein (EIV) (Figs. 23-6 and 23-7). A color image and Doppler signal is also obtained from the EIV at the level of the anastomosis. Spectral tracings should be obtained from the intraparenchymal renal veins at the upper and lower poles. Note that the intraparenchymal renal veins will be found immediately adjacent to the intraparenchymal renal arteries. Color Doppler images demonstrating perfusion of the entire kidney should be obtained with power Doppler images as needed (Fig. 23-8). Perfusion of the renal cortex should be symmetric and homogenous throughout the transplant. Spectral Doppler signals from the segmental and interlobar arteries are obtained from the upper, mid, and lower poles, with angle-corrected peak systolic velocity measurements and calculation of the resistive index (RI). Some laboratories require sampling of the arcuate arteries as well. The normal arterial waveform has a low-resistance pattern characterized by continuous forward diastolic flow, an RI less than 0.7, and a sharp systolic upstroke with an acceleration time less than 70 to 80 ms (Fig. 23-9). The RI is a ratio that compares the amount of systolic and diastolic flow.

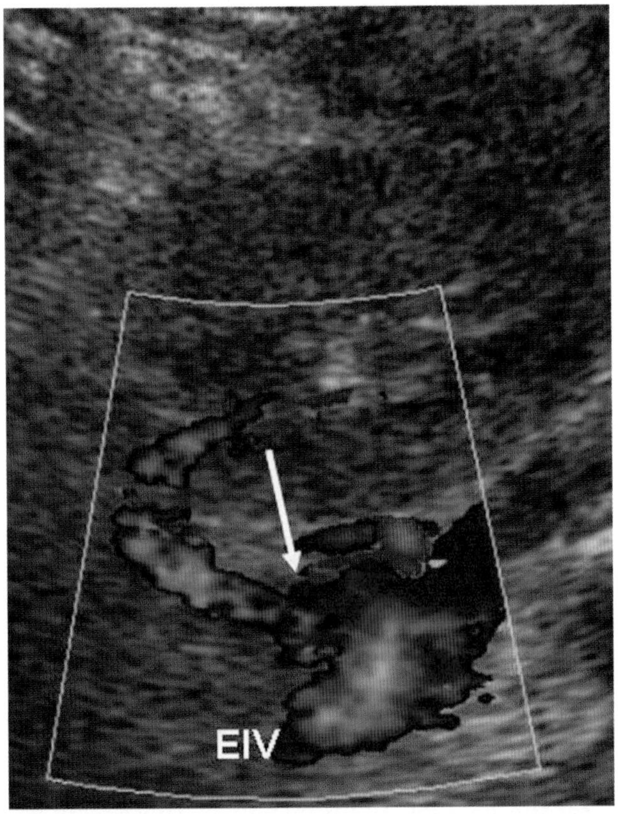

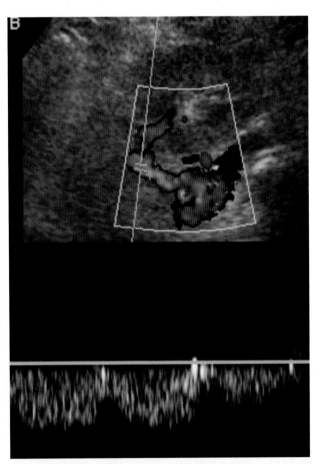

Figure 23-7 Normal spectral Doppler tracing from the origin of the main renal vein. Note the slight respiratory phasicity. Pulsatility of the venous tracing is due to close proximity to the main renal artery.

Figure 23-6 Color Doppler image of the renal vein anastomosis (arrow).

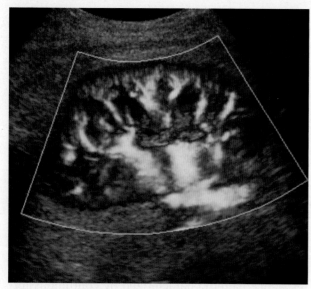

Figure 23-8 Power Doppler image demonstrating normal cortical perfusion of the kidney. Note the homogeneous perfusion of the renal cortex from the small interlobular arteries arising from the arcuate arteries, which course behind the renal pyramids parallel to the renal capsule.

The RI is angle independent, and angle correction is not needed. The formula is as follows:

$$\frac{(\text{Peak systolic velocity} - \text{end-diastolic velocity})}{\text{peak systolic velocity}}$$

In order to calculate the RI, it is critical to accurately measure end-diastolic velocity, which should be measured at the end of diastole right before the next systolic upstroke. It is important that the sonographer not mistake overlying venous flow, flow due to mirror artifact, or noise in the signal for true diastolic flow. By observing the amount of color in the interlobar arteries during diastole, the sonographer can subjectively estimate the RI. If the artery minimally diminishes, then there is good diastolic flow and the RI will be <0.7. However, if there is hardly any signal left by the end of diastole, then the RI will likely be >0.8. If the color is flashy and pulsatile and the artery completely disappears during end diastole, then there is no end-diastolic flow and the RI will be 1.0. A normal RI is between 0.6 and 0.8. In general, end-diastolic velocity should equal at least 25% of peak systolic velocity.

TECHNICAL CONSIDERATIONS

Typically, a curved linear array transducer is used with a frequency range of 3 to 5 MHz. If improvement in image quality is needed, harmonics and/or compound imaging may improve image quality and resolution as well as reduce artifacts. A proper color Doppler velocity scale should be chosen to allow for proper vessel fill-in. The scale may need to be adjusted as needed when changing from evaluating the arterial and venous signals. The color gain should be increased until color speckles appear in the background of the image and then reduced until the color speckles are erased. The color box should be kept to a size that allows a good frame rate.

The spectral Doppler baseline should be adjusted such that flow above as well as below the baseline can be assessed. Because the intraparenchymal renal arteries and veins are so small and close together, arterial and venous waveforms may both be displayed on the same image. The spectral Doppler scale should be adjusted such that the waveform fills the entire area available for the tracing. This will allow for better evaluation and measurement of the waveform. The Doppler spectral speed should be adjusted to allow visualization of three to five waveforms. The Doppler gain should be increased until noise or speckle artifacts appear in the background behind the Doppler waveform and then reduced until the speckles are gone.

PITFALLS

A variety of Doppler settings may be required to demonstrate the presence of vascular pathology. For example, due to the high velocity within an arteriovenous fistula (AVF) (see the following), the color velocity scale will need to be greatly increased to reduce color aliasing and blooming so that just the area of the AVF is seen. Before thrombosis of a vessel is diagnosed, Doppler settings should be maximized for the detection of low velocity blood flow.

DIAGNOSIS

After the baseline US examination, subsequent renal transplant duplex US examinations are ordered to evaluate potential causes of graft dysfunction.

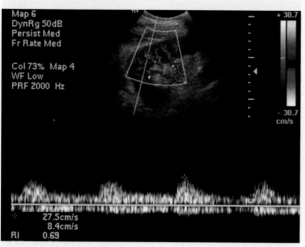

Figure 23-9 Normal spectral Doppler tracing from an interlobar renal artery. Note the sharp systolic upstroke and continuous forward diastolic flow. The amount of diastolic flow should equal approximately 25% of systolic flow with an RI <0.70.

Patients with graft dysfunction most commonly present with nonspecific signs and symptoms such as renal failure, pain, or evidence of infection. The goal of the US examination is to differentiate between causes of graft failure that are best managed medically, such as acute tubular necrosis, pyelonephritis, drug toxicity, or rejection, from etiologies that require intervention such as hydronephrosis, symptomatic fluid collections, and vascular thromboses or stenosis. Unfortunately, many of the US findings in such patients, such as increase in renal length, loss of or increase in corticomedullary differentiation, striation of the uroepithelium, and increased RI are also nonspecific findings of graft dysfunction and diagnosis may ultimately require US-guided renal biopsy. However, Doppler criteria are highly specific for most vascular complications following renal transplantation.

TRANSPLANT REJECTION

Rejection is one of the most common causes of graft loss and is the result of an attack by the immune system on the transplanted organ just as the immune system would combat any foreign object or virus. There are three types of renal transplant rejection: hyperacute, which occurs immediately postop due to the presence of preformed antibodies to the allograft; acute, which usually begins approximately 2 weeks posttransplantation, with most cases occurring in the first 3 months; and chronic. Fortunately, adjusting the immunosuppression protocol can effectively treat most episodes of rejection.

Rejection is suspected when one or more of the following clinical signs are detected: sudden cessation of urine output called anuria, decreased urine output called oliguria, increase serum creatinine, protein or lymphocytes in the urine, hypertension, or swelling or tenderness of the graft. One of the earliest signs of rejection is oliguria, with an associated rise in serum creatinine and blood urea nitrogen (BUN). Serum creatinine and BUN determine how well the kidney is functioning because these waste products are normally removed from the blood by the kidneys. However, a rise in creatinine is a nonspecific finding and may indicate a variety of underlying renal pathologies. A biopsy should be performed in patients with a high level of creatinine that persists or continues to increase.

ACUTE TUBULAR NECROSIS

Another common cause of graft dysfunction is ATN. ATN is caused by ischemia and is more common in DD transplants than in LRD. Risk factors for the development of ATN include prolonged ischemic time, hypotension or blood loss during surgery, prolonged ICU time or severe illness of the donor, and harvest from a non-heart–beating donor. ATN occurs in the early postoperative period usually beginning day 2 or 3 and may be a cause for delayed function of the renal transplant. The patient may require dialysis until the kidney starts to function properly.[7,8] Some investigators have used diminished diastolic flow in the segmental arteries as an indicator of ATN, whereas most use biopsy as the definitive diagnosis for ATN.[9,10]

FLUID COLLECTIONS

The most common perinephric fluid collections found in postrenal transplantation are hematomas, urinomas, and lymphoceles. The size and location of the collection should be documented on each ultrasound examination.

Hematomas are found immediately postoperatively or postbiopsy. Their size, echotexture, and location will vary. Postoperative hematomas may be located anywhere surrounding the transplant. Hematomas that develop postbiopsy are typically found near the biopsy site, usually at the lower pole. Acutely, hematomas will be echogenic, becoming more heterogeneous and complex with anechoic liquefied areas (Figs. 23-10, 23-11, and 23-12). These collections should be followed to ensure that they are decreasing in size.

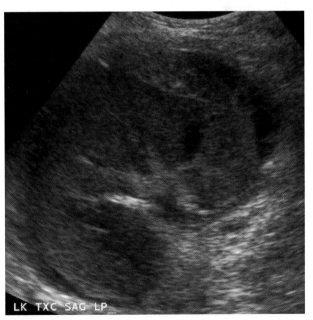

Figure 23-10 A postoperative perinephric hematoma. The grayscale sagittal image demonstrates a heterogeneous hypoechoic fluid collection surrounding the kidney. The cortex of the lower pole appears compressed by this collection. The echogenicity or perinephric hematomas are variable, depending on the time since the hemorrhage occurred.

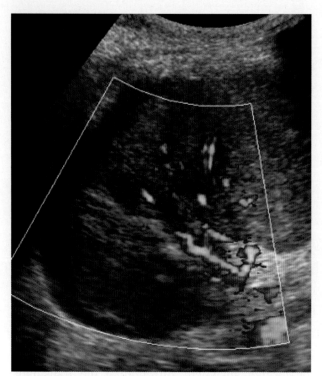

Figure 23-11 A postoperative perinephric hematoma (same patient as in Fig. 23-10). A color Doppler image demonstrates decreased cortical perfusion due to pressure from the surrounding fluid hematoma.

Urinomas form when urine leaks from either the ureteral anastomosis or a focal area of ureteral necrosis. These are usually discovered in the first few weeks posttransplant. Clinically, suspicion is raised when urine output decreases, especially in the absence of renal failure, or if there is leakage of urine from the surgical incision. Ultrasound will demonstrate a fluid collection, usually located between the kidney and the bladder. Urinomas are typically anechoic unless superinfection has occurred, but some may contain septations (Fig. 23-13).

Lymphoceles occur when there is surgical disruption of the lymphatic chain. These collections usually appear 4 to 8 weeks postoperatively. Typically, these collections are discovered incidentally. However, lymphoceles can compress the ureter causing obstruction of the collecting system or become superinfected, both of which require percutaneous drainage or surgical marsupialization. On US, lymphoceles are well-defined, anechoic fluid collections, which may demonstrate multiple thin septations (Fig. 23-14). It is important not to confuse a urinoma with a lymphocele. Remember that urinomas will occur within the first few weeks posttransplant, whereas lymphoceles will be seen in a later time frame, usually after the first month.

HYDRONEPHROSIS

Mild pelvicaliectasis (hydronephrosis) is a normal finding postrenal transplantation because the denervated kidney loses its autonomic tone, allowing the intrarenal collecting system to dilate. Patients are typically asymptomatic. However, true hydronephrosis may develop secondary to ureteral stricture from postsurgical scarring, ischemia, or rejection; a blood clot in the ureter; bladder distension; decreased ureteric tone or compression from surrounding lymphoceles or other fluid collections; and posttransplant lymphoproliferative disorder. The sonographer should attempt to discover the cause and the level of the obstruction.

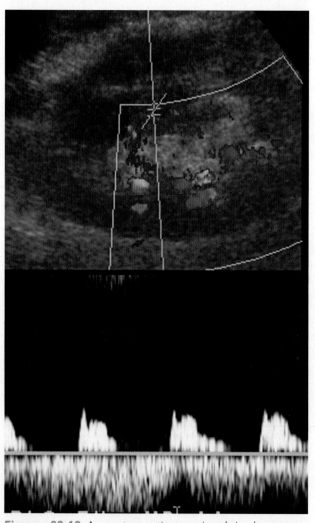

Figure 23-12 A postoperative perinephric hematoma (same patient as in Fig. 23-10). A duplex Doppler image with a waveform obtained from an interlobular artery demonstrates no diastolic flow (RI = 1.0) due to increased peripheral vascular resistance from compression of the renal cortex by the surrounding hematoma, the so-called page kidney physiology. Note the venous flow below the baseline.

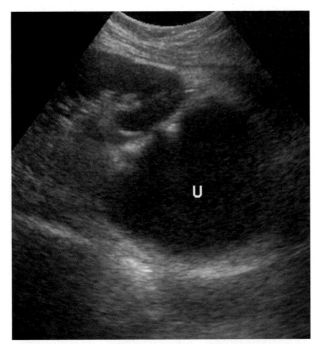

Figure 23-13 A urinoma. Grayscale images demonstrating an anechoic large fluid collection (U) at the lower pole of the kidney between the transplanted kidney and the bladder (not visualized on this image).

VASCULAR COMPLICATIONS

Vascular complications may occur immediately postoperatively or may have a delayed presentation. In the immediate postoperative period, venous or arterial thrombosis is suspected when there is sudden anuria or acute inset of pain in the region of the transplant. This is an emergent situation and the diagnosis must be made quickly to allow for the appropriate percutaneous or surgical intervention to salvage the kidney.

Arterial Thrombosis

Predisposing risk factors for renal artery thrombosis (RAT) include hypercoagulable states, hypotension, intraoperative trauma, mismatch of vessel size, and vascular kinking. Severe acute rejection and, rarely, emboli may result in occlusion or thrombosis of the intraparenchymal renal arteries. An intrarenal arterial thrombus may propagate to involve the main renal artery. RAT is estimated to occur in less than 1% of patients. Sonographic findings of RAT include intraluminal echoes and an absence of arterial and venous flow on color, power, or spectral Doppler interrogation of the intrarenal or main renal arteries and veins (Figs. 23-15 and 23-16). The sonographer should ensure that all color Doppler controls, such as color velocity scale, color gain, color wall filter, and output power, are optimized for the detection of slow flow before making the diagnosis of RAT.

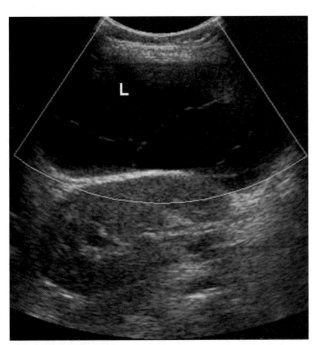

Figure 23-14 A lymphocele. A grayscale longitudinal image demonstrating an anechoic fluid collection (L) with several fine septations anterior to the kidney. Despite the large size of this collection, there is no mass effect on the kidney.

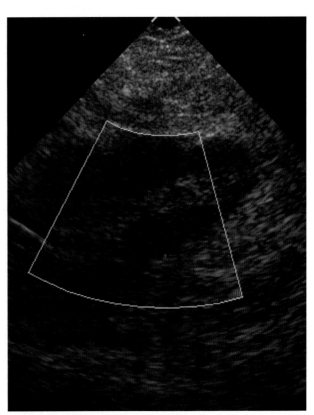

Figure 23-15 A renal artery thrombosis. A color Doppler image of a newly transplanted kidney demonstrating a complete absence of both venous and arterial flow in the kidney.

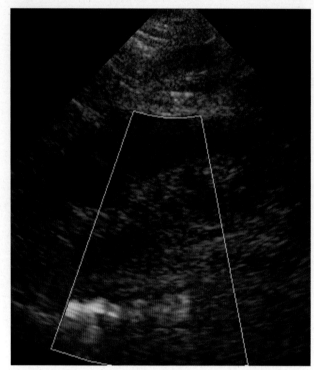

Figure 23-16 A renal artery thrombosis (same patient as in Fig. 23-15). A power Doppler image confirms the lack of flow. An arterial thrombosis from a hyperacute rejection was found in surgery.

Venous Thrombosis

Renal vein thrombosis (RVT) is also a rare event, occurring in less than 4% of renal transplants. RVT most commonly occurs within the first 24 to 48 hours postop. Patients with RVT may complain of pain or discomfort over the transplant due to the kidney swelling. Causes of RVT include surgical complications, compression by a lymphocele or other pelvic fluid collection, propagation of an iliac vein thrombus, hypotension, hypercoagulable states, or torquing of the vascular pedicle. Sonographic findings include enlargement of the kidney, decreased renal cortical echogenicity, an enlarged main renal vein that may or may not contain low-level echoes, and an absence of flow on color, power, or spectral Doppler interrogation of the main renal vein. A very helpful finding confirming this diagnosis is the presence of reversed flow in the renal arteries, resulting in a biphasic waveform (Fig. 23-17). However, reversed diastolic flow in the main renal artery is not a specific finding of RVT and may be seen in other clinical scenarios (see Table 23-1). However, in these other clinical situations, flow in the main renal vein will be observed.

Renal Artery Stenosis

Renal artery stenosis (RAS) is the most common vascular complication following renal transplantation, occurring in approximately 10% of patients. Patients

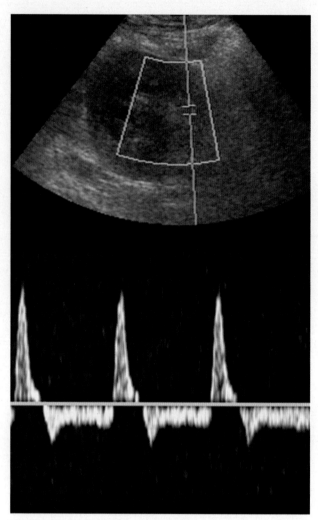

Figure 23-17 A renal vein thrombosis. A spectral Doppler waveform from a segmental renal artery in the renal sinus demonstrates reversed diastolic flow in this patient who presented with abrupt anuria 3 hours postsurgery. Thrombosis of the main renal vein was found at surgery.

will present with severe uncontrolled hypertension. Causes of RAS include postsurgical scarring or dissection, intimal hyperplasia, progressive atherosclerosis, or rejection. Vessel diameter mismatch or complex arterial reconstructions are predisposing risk factors. RAS occurs more commonly in LRD and pediatric renal

TABLE 23-1
Causes for Reversed Diastolic Arterial Flow in Renal Transplants
Renal vein thrombosis
Severe ATN
Hyperacute rejection
Page kidney (compression by surrounding fluid collection)

ATN, acute tubular necrosis.

transplantation than following DD renal transplantation. RAS may also occur secondary to twisting or kinking of the main renal artery. Excessive length of the renovascular pedicle predisposes a patient to vascular torsion.

To diagnose RAS on US examination, the entire length of the main renal artery and the anastomotic site must be carefully evaluated. Color Doppler should be optimized for assessing relatively high arterial velocities. The sonographer should use color Doppler to look for areas of aliasing with possible narrowing along the course of the main renal artery as well as for sharp bends or kinking of the artery. Any area of narrowing or aliasing should be sampled with spectral Doppler with an angle <60° and a sample volume just large enough to encompass the width of the renal artery. Doppler criteria for the diagnosis of RAS greater than 50% to 60% in a renal transplant include elevated peak systolic velocities greater than 200 to 250 cm/s, renal artery to external iliac artery ratio >2.0 to 3.0, plus poststenotic turbulence. In some patients, the distal arterial signal from the intraparenchymal renal arteries may have a tardus–parvus waveform pattern (Figs. 23-18 through 23-21).

Postbiopsy Vascular Complications

Patients who have had a renal biopsy may develop either an AVF or a pseudoaneurysm (PSA). An AVF is an abnormal connection between an artery and a vein.

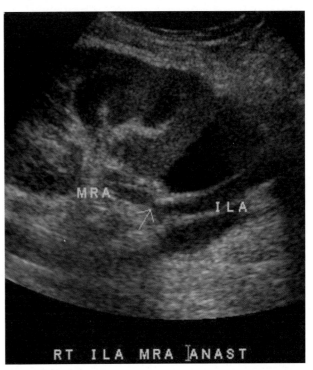

Figure 23-19 A renal artery stenosis (same patient as in Fig. 23-18). A grayscale image demonstrating narrowing (arrow) of the main renal artery (MRA) above the anastomosis, which was due to kinking of the vessel. Excessive length of the donor main renal artery predisposes to kinking of the vascular pedicle. ILA, external iliac artery.

This causes the arterial blood to empty directly into the vein, thus bypassing the capillary bed and creating a low-resistance gradient. Color Doppler will detect the presence of an AVF by demonstrating an area of color aliasing as well as a soft tissue color bruit (Fig. 23-22). A color bruit is caused by vibration of the surrounding soft tissue, which reflects back toward the transducer

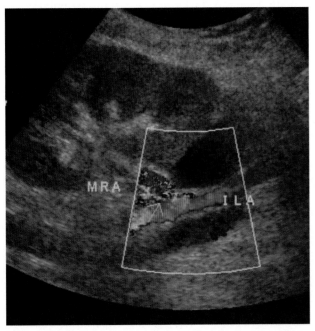

Figure 23-18 A renal artery stenosis. A color Doppler image of a renal artery anastomosis demonstrates focal color aliasing and a soft tissue color bruit (arrow). MRA, main renal artery; ILA, external iliac artery.

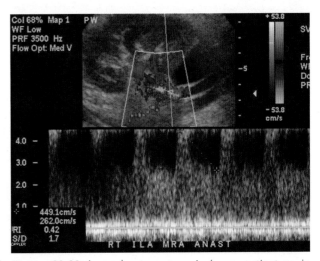

Figure 23-20 A renal artery stenosis (same patient as in Fig. 23-18). A pulsed Doppler tracing obtained at the area of narrowing demonstrating increased PSV >440 cm/s.

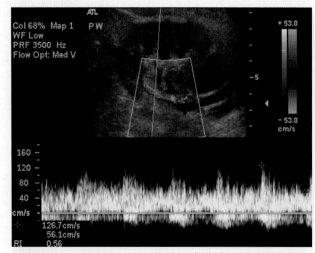

Figure 23-21 A renal artery stenosis (same patient as in Fig. 23-18). A pulsed Doppler tracing demonstrating distal poststenotic turbulence.

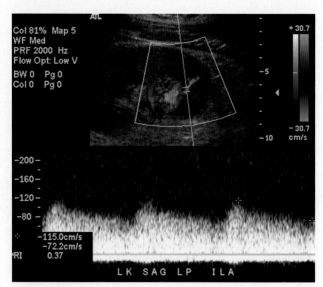

Figure 23-23 An arteriovenous fistula (AVF). A duplex Doppler image from another patient status postrenal biopsy demonstrating an enlarged feeding artery in the renal sinus, color aliasing in an interlobar artery at the lower pole, and increased systolic and diastolic flow, resulting in an abnormally low RI = 0.37.

a low velocity signal. The Doppler signal of the artery feeding the AVF will have high velocity in both systole and end diastole, whereas the draining vein will demonstrate a pulsatile, relatively high velocity waveform that may even resemble an arterial signal close to the AVF (Fig. 23-23).

A PSA will be visualized on grayscale imaging as an anechoic rounded area within the renal parenchyma, which will fill in with color in a swirling pattern (termed the "yin-yang" sign), which is flow heading toward the transducer as it enters the PSA in half the PSA and with reversed flow seen exiting the PSA in the other half (Figs. 23-24 through 23-26). A Doppler tracing obtained from the neck of the PSA where it joins the native artery will display a typical "to-and-fro" Doppler pattern with flow heading toward the PSA during systole and away from the PSA during diastole. If the neck is wide, more random, bizarre waveform patterns may be observed.

Most AVFs or PSAs are incidental benign findings and can be safely followed by sonography until they resolve. If they affect renal function, are larger than 2 cm, are expanding, or extrarenal in location, the patient is referred to interventional radiology to have the AVF or PSA treated with either embolization or stent exclusion.

Pathology Box 23-1 summarizes the vascular complications in renal transplant patients. The pathology along with the ultrasound appearance is described.

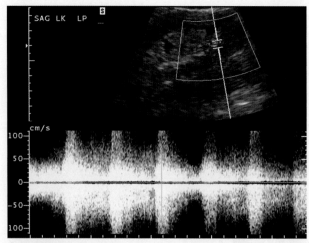

Figure 23-22 An arteriovenous fistula (AVF). A duplex Doppler image from a patient status postrenal biopsy demonstrating a soft tissue color bruit, increased systolic and diastolic flow, as well as turbulence from an AVF at the lower pole of the transplanted kidney.

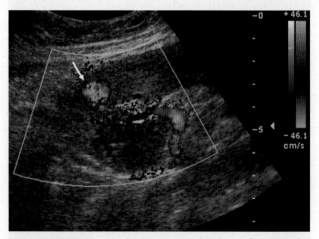

Figure 23-24 A pseudoaneurysm (PSA). A color Doppler image from a patient status postrenal biopsy demonstrating a soft tissue color bruit and large round area of color flow compatible with a PSA (arrow) in the cortex of the upper pole of the transplanted kidney. Note the significantly decreased flow in the surrounding renal cortex.

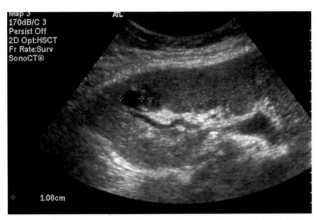

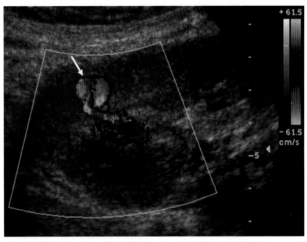

Figure 23-25 A pseudoaneurysm (PSA) (same patient as in Fig. 23-24). A grayscale image demonstrates an anechoic cystic area *(calipers)* in the upper pole cortex corresponding to the area that fills in with color in Figure 23-24, proving that this is a PSA and not a renal cyst.

Figure 23-26 A pseudoaneurysm (PSA) (same patient as in Fig. 23-24). A color Doppler image of the PSA *(arrow)* with the color velocity scale increased, demonstrating the "yin-yang" color flow pattern typical of a PSA. This patient was taken to interventional radiology to have the PSA coiled because it was shunting blood away from the rest of the kidney.

PATHOLOGY BOX 23-1

Vascular Complications in Renal Transplant Recipients

Pathology	Sonographic Appearance		
	B-Mode	**Color Doppler**	**Spectral Doppler**
Renal artery thrombosis (RAT)	Intraluminal echoes Hypoechoic, swollen kidney Loss of corticomedullary differentiation	Absence of color flow	Absence of spectral Doppler signal in main renal artery and vein as well as in the intraparenchymal renal arteries and veins
Renal artery stenosis (RAS)	Narrowing of vessel Poststenotic dilatation	Narrowing of vessel Focal color aliasing	↑ PSV >250 cm/s PSV ratio >2.0 to 3.0 Tardus–parvus waveform in intraparenchymal renal arteries AT >70–80 ms
Renal vein thrombosis (RVT)	Intraluminal echoes Hypoechoic, swollen kidney Loss of corticomedullary differentiation	Absence of color flow Color void if thrombus is nonocclusive	No spectral Doppler signal in main or intraparenchymal renal veins Reversed diastolic flow in renal arteries
Renal vein stenosis (RVS)	Focal narrowing Poststenotic dilatation	Narrowing Focal color aliasing	↑ velocity at site of stenosis Clinical significance likely if 3-4× increase in velocity in comparison to proximal renal vein or EIV
Pseudoaneurysm (PSA)	New anechoic round area in renal parenchyma Outpouching from main artery	"Yin-Yang" color pattern +/− intraluminal thrombus Color aliasing in neck	"To-and-fro" flow pattern in neck of PSA, if narrow A more disorganized flow pattern will be seen in wider necks
Arteriovenous fistula (AVF)	Tangle of tubular anechoic channels Draining vein may focally dilate and mimic PSA	Spectrum of findings from tangle of vessels to rounder area of color flow Focal color aliasing	↑ PSV and ↑ EDV in feeding artery Pulsatile, high-velocity flow in draining vein

LIVER TRANSPLANTATION

The first successful liver transplant was performed by Dr. Thomas Starzl in 1967. Since then, the liver has become the second most common organ to be transplanted after the kidney. It is estimated that about 6,000 liver transplants are performed every year in the United States, and that there are approximately 17,000 patients on the liver transplant waiting list. Approximately 104,000 liver transplants have been performed since 1988.[1]

For patients with either acute or chronic end-stage liver failure who are unresponsive to medical therapy, liver transplantation is the only available option. For such patients, organ availability is the rate-limiting factor. US is the initial imaging modality of choice for the evaluation of complictions following liver transplantation. US is portable, readily available, without risk or contraindications, and is a very sensitive test for the detection of vascular complications and postop fluid collections and biliary complications. However, US is also extremely user dependent and requires an in-depth knowledge of the principles of vascular technology, abdominal anatomy, and general liver transplant physiology. Liver transplant ultrasound is performed bedside in the immediate perioperative/postoperative phase for routine surveillance or when there are clinical indications of suspected graft failure or vascular complications.

There are several conditions that can lead to liver failure and, subsequently, liver transplantation. Table 23-2 lists the most common indications for liver transplantation.

Patients with life-threatening liver disease are only placed on the transplant waiting list if they meet the established Model for End-Stage Liver Disease (MELD) criteria or have a high Child-Pugh score. The Child-Pugh score is used routinely by gastroenterologists to assess liver disease. These criteria are used to rank patients on the waiting list for liver transplants based on the severity of illness and the eligibility of a patient. These criteria evaluate critical markers such as serum bilirubin, which indicates how well the liver excretes bile; international normalized ratio (INR) clotting time, which assesses adequacy of liver function; creatinine, which assesses kidney function; and mental function. There are a few pathologies for which the MELD criteria does not apply, such as hepatocellular carcinoma, hepatopulmonary syndrome, familial amyloidosis, and primary oxaluria. In the event that a patient's medical urgency does not fall under the MELD score, one can apply for a MELD exception.[1]

There are criteria used to exclude patients from liver transplantation. Table 23-3 lists several of the contraindications for liver transplantation.

TABLE 23-3
Contraindications or Exclusion Criteria for Liver Transplantation
Extrahepatic malignancy
Untreated infection
Anatomic abnormaltiy
Hepatocelluar carcinoma that has metastasized or is larger than 5 cm
Advanced cardiopulmonary disease
Active substance abuse
End-stage hepatitis B
Advanced age
Cholangiocarcinoma

TABLE 23-2
Most Common Indications for Liver Transplantation
Hepatitis C
Alcoholic liver disease
Cryptogenic cirrhosis
Primary biliary cirrhosis
Primary biliary sclerosing cholangitis
Budd-Chiari syndrome
Hemachromatosis
Wilson's disease
Autoimmune hepatitis
Acute or fulminant liver failure
Hepatocellular carcinoma (early stage)

THE OPERATION

Most commonly, the liver transplant recipient receives a whole liver from a DD. This is referred to as an orthotopic liver transplant (OLT), which means that an organ is transplanted into its normal anatomic position in the recipient. Due to organ shortage, partial liver transplants from an LRD are now increasingly performed. Usually, the right lobe is transplanted. Occasionally, a liver from a DD is divided between two recipients—one receiving the right lobe and the other the left lobe. Children, in particular, often undergo partial or split liver transplantation.

The precise vascular and biliary anastomoses created depend on the type of transplant as well as the donor and recipient anatomy (Fig. 23-27). Congenital anomalies of the hepatic vasculature and biliary tree are relatively common. Hence, there is wide variation in postsurgical anatomy. Most vessels

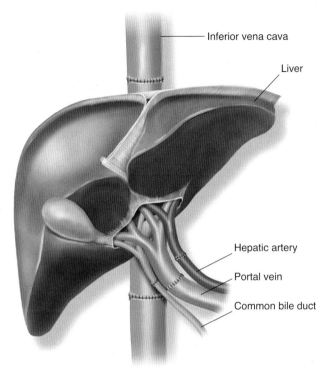

Figure 23-27 A diagram demonstrating the most common surgical anatomy following orthotopic liver transplantation with an interposition IVC graft.

and the common bile duct (CBD) in an OLT are anastomosed in an end-to-end fashion. During the OLT, once it is decided that the liver is suitable for donation, the organ procurement team will harvest the whole liver from a DD including the extrahepatic vessels and CBD. The liver is transported to the recipient on ice in a preservative solution. The implantation team then removes the recipient's native liver and gallbladder, called the anhepatic phase. The donor's CBD is preferentially anastomosed to the recipient's common hepatic duct in an end-to-end fashion. If the recipient's common hepatic duct is deformed or diseased, a choledochojejunostomy will be created, whereby the biliary system will drain directly into the jejunum. The choledochojejunostomy is usually made by the Roux-en-Y (i.e., end-to-side) surgical method. The biliary anastomosis is sometimes reinforced with a stent that can be seen sonographically as a linear echogenic structure in the vicinity of the proximal bile duct.

The arterial anastomosis is usually made between the donor's common hepatic artery or celiac artery and the recipient's common hepatic artery where it branches into the right and left hepatic artery or the common hepatic artery at the level of the gastroduodenal artery. The hepatic arterial anastomosis is created with a "fish mouth" technique, whereby the smaller vessel's walls are split and sewn over the larger, usually the donor, vessel. This technique

helps prevent the development of postsurgical stenosis at the hepatic artery anastomosis. If the donor or recipient vessels are diseased, the surgeon may use the donor's iliac vessels to patch or bypass part of a stenotic vessel. When evaluating the vessels, one should remember that there are several anatomic variations of the hepatic arterial system, and the course that the artery takes may not necessarily be the expected one. Complete evaluation of the hepatic artery may require a great deal of scanning and numerous acoustic windows.

The portal vein is typically anastomosed in an end-to-end fashion between the donor and the recipient main portal vein. If the donor's portal vein is scarred or thrombosed, a venous "jump" graft will have to be created to bypass the thrombus. The IVC may be "interposed" following resection of the donor IVC, requiring both a suprahepatic and infrahepatic end-to-end IVC anastomosis. However, in many centers, a "piggyback" technique is now preferred that leaves the recipient's IVC in place, attaching the suprahepatic donor IVC to the recipient's hepatic confluence (Figs. 23-28 and 23-29).

Single-lobe LRD transplants have become more common in recent years. The donor usually heals easily, as the liver is one of the few organs that can regenerate quickly. The adult donor provides the right portion of his or her liver to an adult recipient and the left portion to a child. The donated right liver will have a right hepatic vein, a right portal vein, a right hepatic artery, and the right hepatic bile duct.

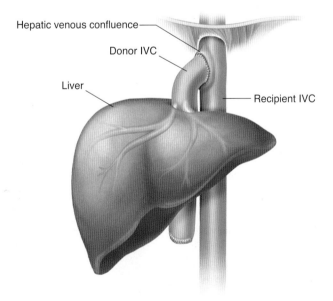

Figure 23-28 A diagram demonstrating the piggyback technique for performing an IVC anastomosis. (Reprinted with permission from Pellerito JS, Polak JF, ed. *Introduction to Vascular Ultrasonography*. 6th ed. Philadelphia, PA: Elsevier Saunders. In press.)

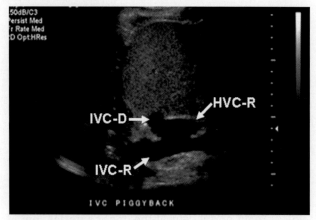

Figure 23-29 A grayscale ultrasound of a piggyback IVC anastomosis. IVC-R, recipient IVC; HVC-R, recipient hepatic vein confluence; IVC-D, donor IVC.

This is reversed if the left lobe is donated (Figs. 23-30 and 23-31). The middle hepatic vein may travel with the donated liver or remain with the donor depending on the surgical plane and whether the medial segment of the left lobe is also harvested. The pediatric patient will often have a choledochojejunostomy and no gallbladder.

Because patients undergoing liver transplantation are extremely ill and because the surgery is complicated, perioperative morbidity is relatively high. OPTN reports a 1-year graft survival rate of 82% for cadaveric liver transplants and 82.5% for living donor transplants. The 5-year graft survival rate is 65.1% and 66.1% for cadaveric and LRD transplants, respectively.[6]

SONOGRAPHIC EXAMINATION TECHNIQUES

Proper patient positioning and optimizing the controls are essential for the proper evaluation of a patient with a liver transplant. It is important for the sonographer to review operative notes so that he or she knows what type of transplant the patient received and can understand all the various anastomotic sites, as previously described. Any prior studies should also be reviewed.

PATIENT PREPARATION

An overnight fast may help minimize intestinal gas. A fasting state may also be needed to evaluate the size of the bile ducts.

PATIENT POSITIONING

The patient is usually positioned supine. The transplanted liver may also be examined in the left lateral decubitus position.

EQUIPMENT

A 3.5-MHz curved linear array transducer can be used to adequately insonate the transplanted liver. If intercostal scanning is needed, the sonographer may consider using a phased array transducer because this will allow better access between the ribs.

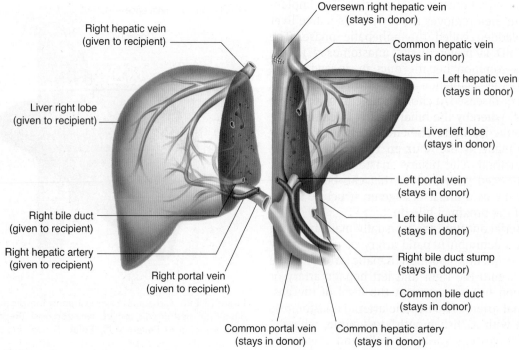

Figure 23-30 A diagram demonstrating the surgical technique for dividing a liver for a partial or split liver transplantation.

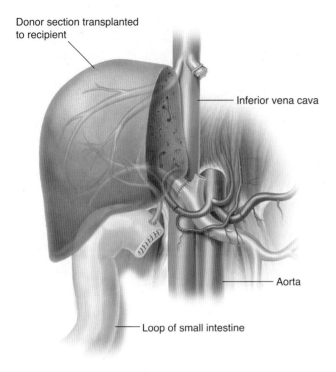

Donor section transplanted to recipient

Inferior vena cava

Aorta

Loop of small intestine

Figure 23-31 A diagram demonstrating the surgical placement of a partial liver transplant in the recipient.

Harmonic imaging may be used to help improve resolution and reduce artifacts. Varying imaging and Doppler frequencies can be helpful depending on the depth and position of the transplant's vessels.

SCANNING TECHNIQUE

Before performing the study, the sonographer must consult the surgeon or surgical report to determine if a full liver was transplanted or just a single lobe. Also, any vascular anomalies should be determined such as a piggyback IVC or an unusual anastomosis of the hepatic artery or portal vein. The most common cause of transplant loss is graft failure/rejection followed by biliary complications. Some complications are related to surgical technique or the amount of time the liver was handled before transplantation. Vascular causes are second only to rejection as a cause of transplant failure. After the initial postoperative baseline scan, physicians can use liver function tests to determine if there are any abnormalities or signs of failure. Serial US examinations may be performed to ensure that there are no early signs of failure that are being overlooked. There are some complications related to rejection that often may not surface for years. Patients may present with abnormal liver function tests (LFTs), ascites, pleural effusions, varices, sepsis, fever, biliary obstruction, leakage,

infection, or splenomegaly. Because symptoms are so varied and nonspecific, imaging plays a critical role in the evaluation of the symptomatic liver transplant patient, especially in the immediate postoperative period. Biliary tract pathology, however, is often associated with hepatic artery stenosis or occlusion because the hepatic artery is the sole supply of blood flow to the biliary tree in the transplanted liver.[11,12]

Grayscale

Standard scanning techniques are used to assess the transplanted liver. All portions of the transplant should be examined. The normal transplant is usually homogenous in appearance and appropriately sized depending on the type of transplant. There should be a normal appearing biliary tree that is free of dilatation, but the duct walls can appear thickened if biliary stents are in place. It is often possible to see surgical drains or stents that have been surgically placed to drain fluids from the cavities, and a small amount of perihepatic fluid is normal in the early postoperative period. This fluid should resolve within days or be drained (Fig. 23-32).

Color and Spectral Doppler

The Doppler examination of the transplant patient may be requested immediately postop depending on how challenging the surgery was. The basic liver transplant duplex consists of grayscale images

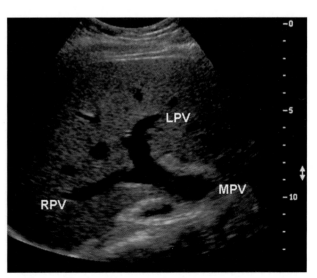

Figure 23-32 A grayscale image of a normal orthotopic (deceased donor, complete) liver transplant. MPV, main portal vein; RPV, right portal vein; LPV, left portal vein.

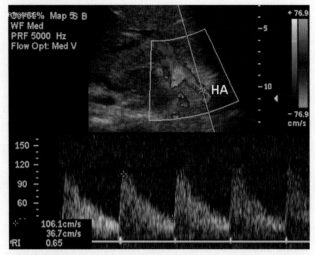

Figure 23-33 A duplex Doppler image of the normal main hepatic artery *(HA)*. Note sharp systolic upstroke and continuous forward diastolic flow with an RI = 0.65.

and angle-corrected velocity measurements of the intrahepatic main, right, and left hepatic arteries (Fig. 23-33). The main, right, and left portal vein with the anastomotic site are interrogated with color and spectral Doppler as well as waveforms of the IVC, and all three branches of the hepatic veins are recorded (Figs. 23-34 and 23-35). If vascular complications are detected intrahepatically, the recipient's native vessels may additionally be assessed with color and Doppler to determine the level of dysfunction. With the exception of the IVC and hepatic veins, all waveforms should also include an RI measurement.

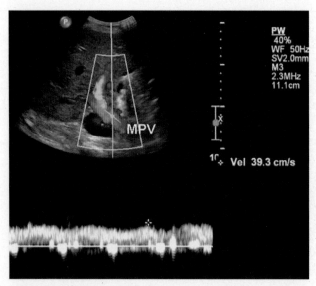

Figure 23-34 A duplex Doppler image of the normal main portal vein *(MPV)*. Note the hepatopetal flow with a slight respiratory variation.

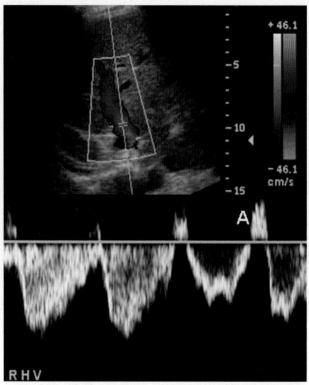

Figure 23-35 A duplex Doppler image of the normal right hepatic vein in a patient with a right lobe transplant. Flow is hepatofugal—heading away form the liver. The pulsatility of the waveform reflects right heart pressure. The transient reversal of flow, labeled the "A" wave, is produced by the contraction of the right atrium.

TECHNICAL CONSIDERATIONS

Due to the limitations described earlier, perhaps all of the Doppler measurements and images will have to be taken from the intercostal approach. This is actually an ideal method for evaluating the portal system, as the natural angle of the portal vein courses toward the transducer from this window, and will greatly enhance the Doppler shift and color fill-in.

PITFALLS

One pitfall is the presence of a high resistance signal immediately in the postoperative period. This is thought to be due to the liver being swollen, causing an increase in the intrahepatic pressure due to increased peripheral vascular resistance. In these patients, daily Doppler examinations of the hepatic artery with clinical correlation is essential to ensure that the RI improves daily as opposed to leading to an arterial thrombosis (Figs. 23-36 through 23-38).

The postoperative abdominal scan may be very challenging because it will likely be a portable exam,

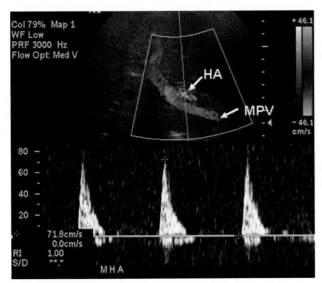

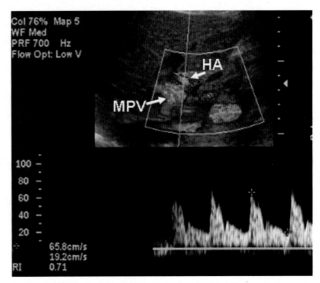

Figure 23-36 A duplex Doppler image of the main hepatic artery (HA) immediately posttransplantation demonstrates complete absence of diastolic flow and an RI = 1.0. This high resistance waveform pattern is likely secondary to increased peripheral vascular resistance, which is secondary to edema of the hepatic parenchyma. Within 48 hours posttransplantation, such a waveform pattern is not indicative of impending hepatic artery thrombosis. MPV, main portal vein.

Figure 23-38 A spectral Doppler tracing of the main hepatic artery (HA) from the same patient as in Figure 23-36 now 4 days postop, demonstrating a normal waveform pattern with normal diastolic flow. The RI is now 0.71. MPV, main portal vein.

and the scanning environment may be suboptimal. Also, the patient will likely be using an automated breathing apparatus, have multiple lines, and will likely have a completely bandaged abdomen. Often, vacuum-assisted closure devices with foam centers are used for very large body cavity openings. An intercostal scanning technique may be the only method for sonographically evaluating the

transplant. Occasionally, there will be residual air in the peritoneal cavity from the surgery, adding to the difficult nature of seeing the abdominal structures from a midline approach.

DIAGNOSIS

Vascular complications are easily detected by the presence, direction, and quantitative measurement of the blood flow to and from the allograft. Table 23-4 lists normal findings for a liver transplant. US examinations have an important role in evaluating the patient with suspected graft dysfunction. Although there is no role for US in the diagnosis of rejection following liver transplantation, US is the procedure of choice for the initial evaluation of potential fluid collections, abnormalities of the biliary tree, and vascular complications.

NONVASCULAR POSTOPERATIVE COMPLICATIONS

There are several nonvascular posttransplant complications that can occur. Table 23-5 lists several of such complications. There are several postoperative complications that are nonvascular in nature that must be documented. One type is a biloma, which is leakage of bile from the biliary anastomotic site (Fig. 23-39). The standard grayscale US evaluation includes sagittal and transverse images with appropriate measurements of the pancreas, right kidney, biliary tree, and liver parenchyma. Any pathologies,

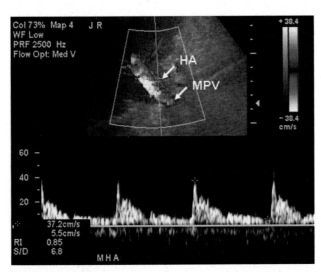

Figure 23-37 A spectral Doppler tracing of the main hepatic artery (HA) 2 days later from the same patient as in Figure 23-36, demonstrating an increase in the amount of diastolic flow. The RI has dropped to 0.85. MPV, main portal vein.

TABLE 23-4		
Normal Doppler Findings Post–Liver Transplantation[11,12]		
Vessel	**Direction/Color**	**Normal Doppler Values**
Main portal vein	Hepatopetal/above baseline/red	>125 cm/s = stenosis, respiratory variations
Right portal vein	Hepatofugal/below baseline/blue	Forward, continuous flow
Left portal vein	Hepatopetal/above baseline/red	Forward continuous flow
Main hepatic artery	Hepatopetal/above baseline/red	RI >0.50, AT <80 ms, velocity <200 cm/s
Right hepatic artery	Hepatofugal/below baseline/blue	Same
Left hepatic artery	Hepatopetal/above baseline/red	Same
IVC	Can be bidirectional/pulsatile hepatofugal/below baseline/blue (can also be slightly pulsatile due to proximity of heart)	Velocity not measured
Hepatic veins		Velocity not measured

such as free abdominal fluid, periadrenal collections, and hematomas, are also documented. Indirect sonographic signs of vascular complications may be seen in the liver parenchyma. These are frequently infarcts due to vascular insufficiency.

COMMON POSTOPERATIVE VASCULAR COMPLICATIONS

Table 23-6 lists the common vascular complications following liver transplantation. Using duplex techniques, one may see color filling defects when a thrombus is present, color aliasing and spectral broadening with stenosis, or a complete or partial absence of flow with thrombi. The presence of vascular findings on a US examination may precipitate further imaging studies such as angiography, computerized tomography, and subsequent interventional procedures. Hepatic artery complications are a cause for immediate surgical intervention because the hepatic artery is the sole blood supply to the bile ducts after transplantation and a lack of blood flow will lead to biliary necrosis and loss of the transplant.

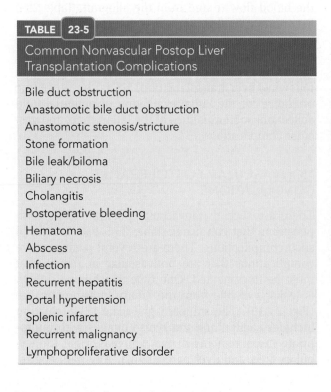

TABLE 23-5
Common Nonvascular Postop Liver Transplantation Complications
Bile duct obstruction
Anastomotic bile duct obstruction
Anastomotic stenosis/stricture
Stone formation
Bile leak/biloma
Biliary necrosis
Cholangitis
Postoperative bleeding
Hematoma
Abscess
Infection
Recurrent hepatitis
Portal hypertension
Splenic infarct
Recurrent malignancy
Lymphoproliferative disorder

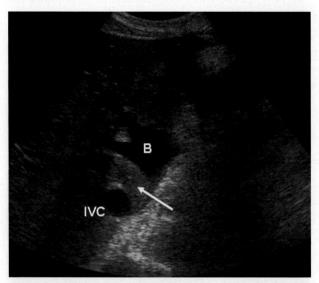

Figure 23-39 A biloma (*B*). Note the anechoic fluid collection anterior to the IVC and caudate lobe (*arrow*). Percutaneous aspiration proved this to be a biloma. This result should prompt immediate evaluation of the integrity of the biliary tree as well as evaluation of the hepatic artery to rule out thrombosis or stenosis.

TABLE	23-6
Common Vascular Postop Liver Transplantation Complications	

Hepatic artery thrombosis
Hepatic artery stenosis
Pseudoaneurysm
Portal vein thrombosis
Portal vein stenosis
IVC thrombosis
IVC stenosis
Hepatic vein thrombosis
Hepatic vein stenosis
Biliary ischemia due to hepatic artery stenosis

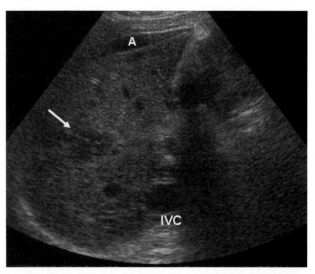

Figure 23-41 A hepatic artery thrombosis (same patient as in Fig. 23-40). A grayscale image of the liver demonstrating a peripheral wedge-shaped hypoechoic area *(arrow)* compatible with infarct due to hepatic artery thrombosis. Note the perihepatic ascites *(A)*. IVC, inferior vena cava.

Hepatic Artery Thrombosis

HAT is the most common vascular complication of the OLT. It occurs in 2% to 12% of liver transplants.[11] The risk factors of developing HAT are rejection, prolonged transport time of the organ, and use of an end-to-end surgical technique of the hepatic artery. Usually, the US examination will reveal absent or weak hepatic arterial flow. Postsurgically, a completely patent artery may be difficult to visualize due to vasospasm or parenchymal swelling (Figs. 23-40 and 23-41). Because of the impact on patient care, HAT usually requires imaging with other modalities.

Hepatic Artery Stenosis

HAS occurs in up to 11% of OLT patients.[12] The clinical symptoms are poor liver function tests or biliary ischemia. HAS is usually seen at the anastomotic site and is due to surgical technique, clamp injuries, perfusion catheter injuries to the intimal lining, and interruption of the vasa vasorum. Areas of narrowing will display higher velocities and a disturbed color flow. Lower RIs may be present, as well as tardus–parvus waveforms that would be reflected by a prolonged acceleration time. The intrahepatic waveforms can appear very similar to those of HAS. If an interparenchymal tardus–parvus waveform is seen, it is likely due to HAS versus HAT (Figs. 23-42 through 23-45).

Hepatic Artery Pseuodaneurysm

A PSA is an abnormal dilatation or ballooning of the hepatic artery that is either within the liver or is extrahepatic. Usually, extrahepatic PSAs are caused by disruption of the intimal lining of the artery, causing a dilation that can easily rupture. Intrahepatic PSAs are generally thought to be caused by core needle biopsy or infections that can damage the integrity of the vessel wall. Hepatic artery pseudoaneurysms are a rare finding but are more commonly seen at anastomotic sites. The patient usually presents with

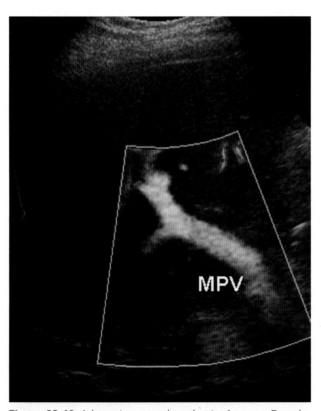

Figure 23-40 A hepatic artery thrombosis. A power Doppler image at the porta hepatis demonstrates normal flow in the main portal vein (MPV). However, the hepatic artery is not visualized. A power Doppler should always be used to show an absence of a vessel because it is more sensitive to slow flow than color Doppler and is not as angle dependent.

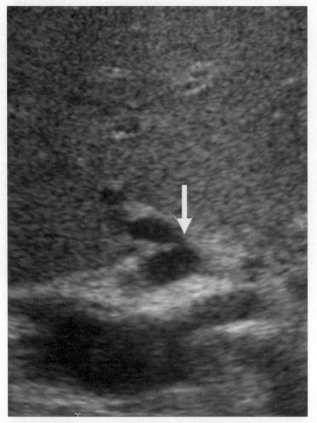

Figure 23-42 A hepatic artery stenosis. A grayscale image of the porta hepatis demonstrating narrowing of the hepatic artery (arrow). This was believed to be due to poor surgical technique.

fever, biliary colic, or signs of hemorrhage. The Doppler waveform is often disorganized, showing a typical mix of arterial and venous signal. There is a high risk of hemorrhage and resulting organ failure, so an interventional procedure must be performed to correct the PSA.

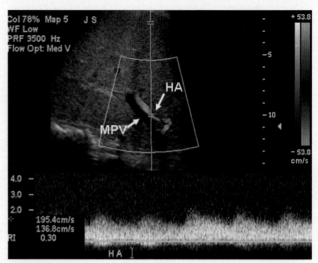

Figure 23-44 A hepatic artery stenosis (same patient as in Fig. 23-42). A spectral Doppler waveform from the distal main hepatic artery (HA) demonstrates poststenotic turbulence. Notice that there is no color fill in of the portal vein (MPV). However, the absence of flow in the portal vein is artifactual due to the high color velocity scale used to eliminate the color aliasing where velocity is increased at the site of the hepatic artery stenosis.

Portal Vein Thrombosis

PVT is also another relatively rare finding and usually involves the extrahepatic portion of the portal vein. Clinically, the patient may have early liver failure and signs of portal hypertension. The causes can be a surgical injury, vessel length, or hypercoagulable states. PVT will display complete or partial flow voids with color Doppler and an echogenic thrombus can be seen inside the lumen of the portal vein. A low-velocity scale setting must be used to ensure that failure to see color inside the portal vein is not due to technical issues. Power Doppler

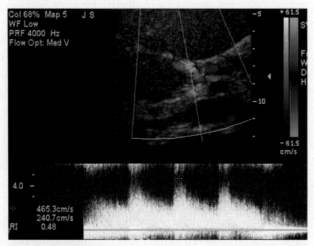

Figure 23-43 A hepatic artery stenosis (same patient as in Fig. 23-42). A spectral Doppler tracing demonstrates increased PSV = 465 cm/s and turbulent flow. Notice the use of the color aliasing to guide placement of the Doppler cursor.

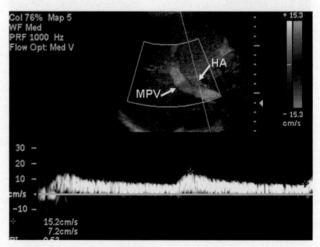

Figure 23-45 A hepatic artery stenosis. A spectral Doppler tracing demonstrates a tardus–parvus waveform pattern distal to the proximal hepatic artery (HA) stenosis in another patient. MPV, main portal vein.

should also be used to verify absence of flow. An intervention is required to save the transplant and the bowel.

Portal Vein Stenosis

PVS is likely seen at the anastomotic sites and is often related to surgical injury. The patient may present with signs of worsening hepatic function that correlates with the degree of stenosis. On color and Doppler, an area of narrowing is easily identified in this large vessel. Also, a peak velocity at the area of greatest stenosis will be >125 cm/s or will have an anastomotic-to-preanastomotic velocity ratio of 3:1. An angioplasty or stent placement will be required.

IVC Thrombosis/Stenosis

Although rare, thrombosis or stenosis of the IVC is also a finding that is particularly relevant to the surgical technique used to connect the recipient and donor IVCs. This finding is also associated with mechanical compression from fluid collections, hypercoagulability, vessel length, and retransplantation. The patient will often present with hepatic failure. It is helpful to know the technique used so that all portions of the IVC can be sampled. A thrombus can be seen inside the lumen, as well as visible signs of narrowing and velocity changes.

Pathology Box 23-2 summarizes the vascular complications in liver transplant patients. The pathology along with the ultrasound appearance are described (Pathology Box 23-2).

PATHOLOGY BOX 23-2

Vascular Pathology in Liver Transplant Recipients

Pathology	Sonographic Appearance		
	B-Mode	Color Doppler	Spectral Doppler
Hepatic artery thrombosis (HAT)	Intraluminal echoes	No flow in main or intraparenchymal hepatic arteries	No spectral Doppler signal in main or intraparenchymal hepatic arteries
Hepatic artery stenosis (HAS)	Narrowing of main HA May be obscured by overlying bowel gas	Focal narrowing and color aliasing at stenosis Poststenotic dilatation	PSV >200 cm/s at stenosis Tardus–parvus waveform in intraparenchymal HAs AT >80 ms RI <0.5–0.6
Portal vein thrombosis (PVT)	Intraluminal echoes Distension of PV	No color flow—if occlusive Focal color void with peripheral flow—if nonocclusive	Absence of Doppler signal— if occlusive ↑ velocity and tortuosity of main HA
Portal vein stenosis (PVS)	Narrowing of main PV Poststenotic dilatation	Narrowing of PV Focal color aliasing	↑ velocity at narrowed segment Velocity >125 cm/s May be clinically significant if velocity increases 3–4×
Inferior vena cava thrombosis	Intraluminal echoes May extend into HVs Distension of IVC	No color flow—if occlusive Focal color void—if nonocclusive May involve HVs	Absence of Doppler signal—if occlusive ↑ velocity if small residual lumen Flat waveforms in proximal HVs
Inferior vena cava stenosis	Narrowing of IVC	Narrowing of IVC Focal color aliasing	↑ velocity relative to proximal IVC May be clinically significant if velocity increases 3–4×
Pseudoaneurysm (PSA)	New anechoic round area in hepatic parenchyma Outpouching from main HA	"Yin-yang" color fill in +/− intraluminal thrombus Color aliasing in neck	"To-and-fro" flow in neck—if narrow A more disorganized flow pattern seen in wider necks
Arteriovenous fistula (AVF)	Tangle of tubular anechoic channels Focal dilatation of draining vein mimicking PSA	Spectrum of findings from tangle of vessels to rounder area of color fill in Focal color aliasing	↑ PSV and ↑ EDV in feeding artery Pulsatile, high velocity flow in draining vein

SUMMARY

Sonography plays an important part in evaluating both renal and liver transplants and is usually the initial imaging modality of choice for evaluating the transplant patient. It is important for the sonographer to review the operative notes or to talk to the surgeon so that the anatomy and anastomotic sites encountered during the examination are understood. The sonographer should adjust the various Doppler controls to optimize the detection of flow for each specific vessel, changing controls as needed according to the flow dynamics of the specific vessel being interrogated. Performing an adequate and thorough examination is vital for the care of these patients and has enormous impact in both graft and patient survival.

Critical Thinking Questions

1. The transplant surgeon calls down requesting a STAT ultrasound on his patient who now has decreased urinary output. Is this really an emergency? Why or why not?

2. A patient returns to ultrasound for a follow-up renal transplant sonogram. The patient informs you that he had a renal transplant biopsy 2 days ago. What should the sonographer be looking for as he or she obtains the images?

3. What is the significance of an elevated RI in a renal transplant?

4. Why is it important for the sonographer to review the operative notes before performing an examination of any transplanted organ?

5. Why is it normal to have an elevated RI in the hepatic artery in the immediate postop liver transplant patient?

6. What would be some unusual vascular findings of the portal vein in a patient with a liver transplant as opposed to a patient with a nontransplanted liver?

REFERENCES

1. Hricik D, ed. *Primer on Transplantation*. 3rd ed. Hoboken, NJ: Wiley-Blackwell; 2011
2. Kidney transplantation: past, present, and future. History. Stanford.edu Web site. http://www.stanford.edu/dept/HPS/transplant/html/history.html. Updated . Accessed June 11, 2011.
3. Vollmer WM, Wahl PW, Blagg CR. Survival with dialysis and transplantation in patients with end-stage renal disease. *N Engl J Med*. 1983;308:1553–1558.
4. Cecka JM. The OPTN/UNOS renal transplant registry. *Clin Transpl*. 2005:1–16.
5. Rao PS, Merion RM, Ashby VB, et al. Renal transplantation in elderly patients older than 70 years of age: results from the Scientific Registry of Transplant Recipients. *Transplantation*. 2007;83:1069–1074.
6. The Organ Procurement and Transplantation Network. U.S. Department of Health & Human Services Web site. http://optn.transplant.hrsa.gov/. Updated . Accessed June 11, 2011.
7. Irshad A, Ackerman SJ, Campbell AS, et al. An overview of renal transplantation: current practice and use of ultrasound. *Semin Ultrasound CT MR*. 2009;30:298–314.
8. Umphrey HR, Lockhart ME, Robbin ML. Transplant ultrasound of the kidney, liver and pancreas. *Ultrasound Clin*. 2008;3(1):49–65.
9. Cosgrove D, Chan K. Renal transplants: what ultrasound can and cannot do. *Ultrasound Q*. 2008;24:77–87.
10. Kolonko A, Chudek J, Wicek A. Prediction of the severity and outcome of acute tubular necrosis based on continuity of Doppler spectrum in the early period after kidney transplantation. *Nephrol Dial Transplant*. 2009;24:1631–1635.

11. Singh AK, Nachiappan AC, Verma HA, et al. Postoperative imaging in liver transplantation: what radiologists should know. *Radiographics.* 2010;30(2):339–351.
12. Crossin JD, Muradali D, Wilson SR. US of liver transplants: normal and abnormal. *Radiographics.* 2003;23:1093–1114

RECOMMENDED READING

Danovitch G. *Handbook of Kidney Transplantation.* Baltimore, MD: Lippincott Williams & Wilkins; 2009.
Hricik D, ed. *Primer on Transplantation.* 3rd ed. Hoboken, NJ: Wiley-Blackwell; 2011.
Rumack CM, Wilson SR, Charboneau J, et. al. *Diagnostic Ultrasound.* 4th ed. Philadelphia, PA: Elsevier Mosby; 2010.
Zwiebel WJ, Pellerito JS. *Introduction to Vascular Sonography.* 5th ed. Philadelphia, PA: Elsevier Saunders; 2005.

24 Intraoperative Duplex Sonography

Steven A. Leers

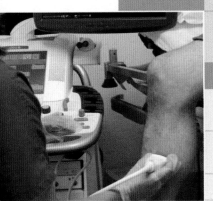

OBJECTIVES

List the types of vascular reconstructions where intraoperative ultrasound is helpful

Describe the setup and preparation of the ultrasound equipment and transducer for use during an operative procedure

Define the duplex ultrasound criteria applied to intraoperative data

KEY TERMS

endarterectomy | infrainguinal reconstruction | intraoperative | sterile technique

GLOSSARY

autologous/autogenous self-produced or from the same organism; in the case of a bypass, using the patient's own tissue (e.g., saphenous vein)

endarterectomy removal of plaque, intima, and part of the media of an artery to restore normal flow through the diseased segment

infrainguinal below the inguinal level; in the case of a bypass, procedures done from the groin down (outflow procedures)

prosthetic a device replacing an absent or damaged part; in the case of a bypass, a man-made

tube used for the bypass procedure; (e.g., Dacron and polytetrafluoroethylene [PTFE])

revascularization restoration of blood flow to an organ or area by way of bypass, endarterectomy, or angioplasty and stenting

sterile technique means by which a surgical field is isolated from nonsterile or contaminated materials

surveillance keeping a watch over; in the case of revascularizations, it suggests periodically monitoring patency and functioning by some means

visceral Pertaining to the viscera; in this case, the intestines or kidneys

Vascular surgery is unique in its requirement for intraoperative documentation of the technical success of revascularizations. In most surgical specialties, visual inspection and palpation are adequate to demonstrate this, but the meticulous nature of vascular surgery and the devastating result of technical errors demand more from the vascular surgeon. For decades, the necessity of documenting technical results has been acknowledged by vascular surgeons. Not only in lower extremity bypass but also in carotid

endarterectomy, this has led to the suggestion of routine angiography at the completion of the procedure, before closing the wound, and leaving the operating room. Color duplex scanning is the natural extension of this routine, avoiding contrast exposure and offering the advantage of anatomic and physiologic information not provided by angiography. This chapter will review current applications of duplex scanning in the operating room and the results of such an approach.

TABLE 24-1

Common Applications for Intraoperative Vascular Ultrasound

Surgical Procedure	Anatomy Examined	Potential Complications
Carotid endarterectomy	Common carotid artery Internal carotid artery External carotid artery	Intimal flap Residual plaque Platelet aggregate Suture line abnormalities Dissection
Infrainguinal revascularization	Inflow artery Outflow artery Anastomotic regions Entire conduit	Retained valves AV fistulae Platelet aggregate Anastomotic or suture line abnormalities
Renal and mesenteric artery bypass	Anastomotic regions Renal artery Celiac artery Mesenteric artery	Residual plaque Platelet aggregate Dissection Anastomotic or suture line abnormalities

SONOGRAPHIC EXAMINATION TECHNIQUES

Vascular reconstructions, which lend themselves to intraoperative application of duplex scanning, include carotid endarterectomy and infrainguinal and visceral bypass. Results of carotid endarterectomy are already consistently excellent, so improvements are likely to be in small increments. Lower extremity bypass results are plagued by problems related to the inflow, outflow, and conduit. Duplex bypass surveillance has been shown to enhance patency and limb salvage, and beginning the surveillance in the operating room is a natural extension of that policy. Renal and visceral bypass patency depends on technical excellence, which is easily assessed with duplex scanning. Table 24-1 summarizes the common vascular applications for intraoperative ultrasound and abnormalities that can be encountered.

SCANNING TECHNIQUE

Intraoperative ultrasound can be performed using a portable duplex ultrasound system with a transducer specifically designed for vascular applications such as a "hockey stick" type linear array transducer. This transducer has a small footprint to allow for easy access into the surgical areas. A sterile sheath with a latex tip is filled with sterile gel and used to isolate the transducer while being careful to remove any bubbles from the probe cover. The length of the probe cover allows a significant length of transducer and cord to be brought onto the sterile field. The wound is filled with saline, the overhead lights in the

operating room are extinguished to make viewing of the image easier, and the scan is begun (Figs. 24-1 through 24-4). The scanning protocol is simple, with the surgeon holding the transducer and the sonographer or vascular technologist optimizing the image and controlling the other components on the ultrasound console. In general, long axis imaging is used alone. Grayscale images are first obtained to best visualize small defects not well seen with color scanning. Color is added to facilitate placement of the pulsed spectral Doppler gate. Images and waveforms are stored in cine loops, as well as still images, to allow for careful interpretation. If an abnormality is identified that prompts revision, the scan process is repeated after revision. In infrainguinal

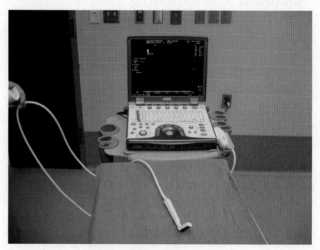

Figure 24-1 Portable color duplex scanner with "hockey stick" transducer.

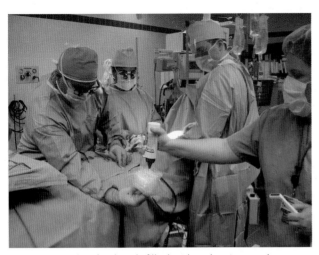

Figure 24-2 Sterile sheath filled with gel, prior to placement of the ultrasound transducer.

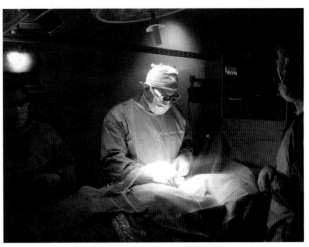

Figure 24-4. Scanning done with the operating room lights down.

revascularization, instillation of papaverine into the bypass is helpful to minimize the effects of vasospasm frequently seen in these procedures.

TECHNICAL CONSIDERATIONS

Intraoperative assessment during a vascular reconstruction requires a team that is comfortable with the techniques described as well as the equipment necessary for the procedure. Modern color duplex scanners are available in many shapes and forms, with many new and easily portable machines enclosed in a simple laptop computer configuration. As noted in the preceding section, specific ultrasound transducers for intraoperative use have been developed for vascular applications in multiple anatomic areas. Operating rooms with extensive experience with this technology frequently have dedicated ultrasound machines kept in the operating room at all times.

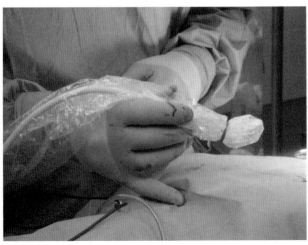

Figure 24-3 Ultrasound transducer brought onto the surgical field.

The vascular surgeon must be adept not only with the interpretation of vascular sonograms, but also with the application of the transducer to maximize image acquisition. In procedures where a prosthetic material is used, this can be challenging because many such materials absorb air in their interstices, which makes obtaining a meaningful image a challenge. In the case of prosthetic bypasses, this renders intraoperative scanning virtually impossible, but prosthetic patches on carotid endarterectomy usually allow adequate imaging by "working around" the patch. It is critical that the surgeon is directly involved in the scanning process along with the sonographer or vascular technologist to ensure accurate and dependable information. The sonographer or vascular technologist is key to a successful intraoperative sonography program. Familiarity with operating room sterile technique is critical to the safe application of duplex scanning, allowing the "nonsterile" sonographer to interact with the sterile team and field. Once the probe is sheathed and dispensed to the sterile field, the sonographer must work with the surgeon to maximize image acquisition as well as to coordinate pulse spectral analysis, color imaging, and grayscale imaging.

CAROTID ENDARTERECTOMY

Almost 60 years after its introduction, carotid endarterectomy remains one of the most frequent operations performed by vascular surgeons, and admirable stroke rates below 3% are expected. With such excellent results, one would expect that intraoperative assessment would not be particularly fruitful. On the contrary, early large reviews using a variety of techniques identified residual defects in between 5% and 43% of examined arteries. Although the majority of defects were found in the blindly endarterectomized external carotid artery, 6.5% of the collected cases had abnormalities in the internal carotid artery, usually at the distal end of the endarterectomy.[1]

Routine intraoperative angiography offers the advantage of visualizing the intracranial carotid artery, as well as the cervical area. Lesions proximal in the common carotid artery are usually not assessed, however, and no physiologic data is identified. In an early study using routine completion angiography, Donaldson et al. found 71 defects in a series of 410 carotid endarterectomies, warranting correction in 16% of cases. These corrections did not add to morbidity, as the stroke rate remained below 2%.[2] Zannetti et al. evaluated 1,305 carotid endarterectomies with completion angiography in 77% and identified 9% defects, 4% of which were revised. There was an increased stroke rate in this group despite revision. Nevertheless, the overall stroke rate was less than 1%; this raises questions regarding the advantage of routine imaging.[3] Westerband et al. reported a 19% incidence of defects requiring repair, with no postoperative occlusions in this group.[4]

CURRENT INTRAOPERATIVE EVALUATION

Currently, continuous wave Doppler interrogation alone is the most commonly used assessment during carotid endarterectomy. This method has been shown to be quite sensitive, but not specific, identifying abnormalities in 4.3% in early studies.[5] Although this modality is simple and fairly reliable in experienced hands, it usually requires a confirmatory study such as an angiography to justify re-exploration. B-mode ultrasound has also been used in completion studies to determine which findings signal the need for revision. Again, the incidence of complications is so low it is difficult to make recommendations based on these smaller studies.[6]

Bandyk et al. applied pulse Doppler spectral analysis to carotid endarterectomy sites and reported on 250 procedures using this technique.[7] In a follow-up study of 461 endarterectomies studied with duplex scanning, less than 6% required intraoperative revision, and the permanent stroke rate was 1.3%. Patients with normal scans had a lower incidence of late postoperative stroke.[8] The Mayo Clinic reported results in 87 patients using routine duplex scanning. In the study, 9% had significant findings requiring immediate revision. Stroke rates were 1.9% and were equal between normal and repaired groups. Two of three patients with significant common carotid lesions that were not addressed suffered strokes. These data suggest the safety and efficacy of routine duplex scanning.[9] Numerous other small studies have shown similar advantages of intraoperative duplex sonography.[10,11]

Although completion duplex sonography is intuitively beneficial, caution must be exercised in interpreting

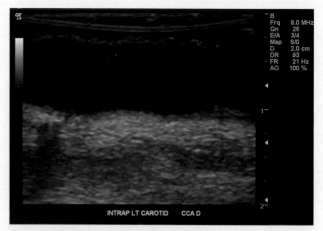

Figure 24-5 Normal grayscale image CCA.

the results of these studies. Excellent results with endarterectomy without any monitoring have been established, and the possibility that re-exploration carries risk to the patient is real. In fact, a review of a large database of New York State carotid endarterectomies demonstrated no difference in outcomes regardless of the type of intraoperative monitoring used.[12] The ease of application, the lack of risk, and the benefit of a normal intraoperative duplex study still argue for some application of this modality. How to interpret and react to abnormal studies remains controversial.

Intraoperative duplex scanning after carotid endarterectomy still remains routine for some, but not all, surgeons. Scanning protocols include the examination of the entire portion of the common, external, and internal carotid arteries that are accessible to the ultrasound transducer. Velocities are recorded from all the vessels, and the B-mode image is closely examined for any wall irregularities. Those surgeons using the technique are comfortable with the scanning process and are reassured by the findings of a normal intraoperative study (Figs. 24-5 through 24-8).

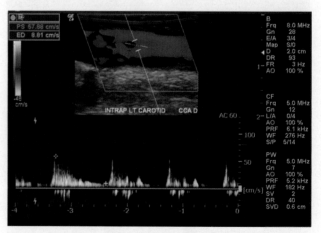

Figure 24-6 Normal CCA spectral analysis. Note the components of low-resistance ICA and high-resistance ECA in waveform.

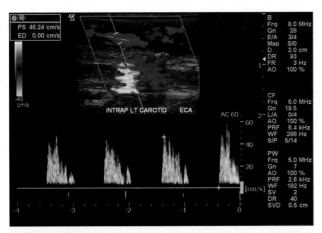

Figure 24-7 ECA spectral analysis. Normal velocity and high resistance waveform.

DIAGNOSIS

Diagnostic criteria used may vary between institutions and are often simplified versions of normally applied standards. In fact, many of the abnormalities noted are in the common or external carotid arteries where criteria are poorly established. Still, the abnormalities found in these vessels are usually so compelling that there is little disagreement about how to handle them. Abnormalities on the B-mode image can include residual plaque or a "shelf" lesion. Plaque remaining in the proximal common carotid artery or distal internal carotid artery, which appears as an abrupt edge or outcropping, is often referred to as a shelf lesion. If this residual plaque is greater than 2-mm thick, a revision may be performed. A piece of residual plaque can sometimes appear mobile and moves within the blood stream, thus necessitating a prompt revision. An intimal flap is another complication that may be apparent. If a flap is in excess of 2 mm, revision is usually performed. Less common is a dissection that occurs as a result of

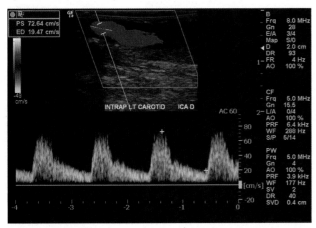

Figure 24-8 Normal ICA spectral analysis. Note the normal diastolic flow.

a vascular clamp injury, which may be present and would require attention.

A focal peak systolic velocity (PSV) increase in the internal carotid artery can identify a significant complication. Reexamination or revision of the surgical site is warranted if the PSV exceeds 180 cm/s or the internal carotid to common carotid PSV ratio is greater than 2.5. In some patients, this may be associated with a fresh platelet aggregate, which is often unable to be identified on the B-mode image due to its anechoic

PATHOLOGY BOX 24-1

Common Vascular Pathology Observed Intraoperatively

Pathology Observed	Ultrasound Characteristics
"Shelf" lesion/ residual lesion	• Hyperechoic plaque projecting into the vessel lumen • May display an abrupt edge
Intimal flap	• Small projection into the vessel lumen, usually a few millimeter in length • Disturbed flow or aliasing may be present
Dissection	• Linear object seen parallel to vessel walls • Turbulent or disturbed flow present
Platelet aggregate	• Hypoechoic or anechoic material adjacent to vessel wall • Focal elevation in PSV • Increased Vr
Stenosis: carotid or lower extremity bypass graft	• PSV >180 cm/s • Vr >2.5
Stenosis: renal or celiac artery	• PSV >200 cm/s
Stenosis: superior mesenteric artery	• PSV >275 cm/s
Arteriovenous fistula	• Patent branch may be seen arising from an in situ bypass • Turbulence and aliasing present in area of side branch • Elevated diastolic velocities in bypass graft proximal to side branch
Retained valve	• Hyperechoic structure protruding into lumen of vein bypass graft; may be associated with slight dilation of valve sinus • Turbulence or aliasing may be present

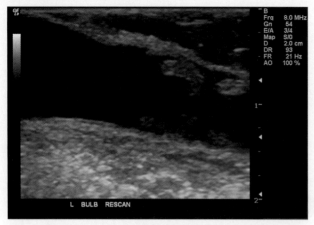

Figure 24-9 Grayscale image of residual plaque in proximal CCA.

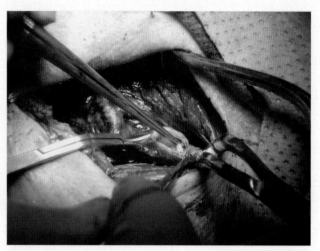

Figure 24-11 Dissected plaque being removed from CCA.

nature. Pathology Box 24-1 describes the ultrasound characteristics of common pathology observed during intraoperative ultrasound examinations.

Figures 24-9 through 24-13 demonstrate an abnormal finding in the common carotid artery, the intraoperative findings, and the repeat scan following revision. This is an excellent example of the benefit of direct clinical application of this policy.

INFRAINGUINAL REVASCULARIZATION

Infrainguinal revascularization can be performed for claudication or critical limb ischemia (CLI) and can be performed via percutaneous endovascular means or via open surgical bypass using either autogenous (vein) or prosthetic (Dacron or PTFE) material. Although carotid endarterectomy is a fairly standardized procedure, there are almost infinite variations in the performance of an infrainguinal reconstruction. Issues abound, such as assessing and obtaining adequate arterial inflow, choice of an appropriate conduit for bypass depending on the level of the bypass and available autogenous material, and the choice of adequacy of an outflow target. Any or all of these issues can result in success or failure of the procedure and the number of steps in these often tedious operations creates many opportunities for failure. Despite these significant obstacles to success, the results in terms of patency and limb salvage continue to be quite admirable.

Early in the experience with infrainguinal revascularization, the superiority of autologous material over prosthetic material in terms of bypass patency was demonstrated.[13] Adopting an all-autologous approach has introduced using arm veins, small saphenous veins, deep veins, and even radial arteries. These "alternative" veins are more prone to abnormalities that

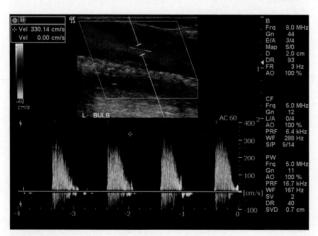

Figure 24-10 Elevated-velocity CCA consistent with severe stenosis.

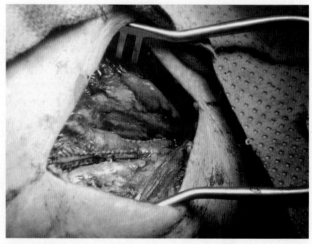

Figure 24-12 Carotid bifurcation after an endarterectomy and revision.

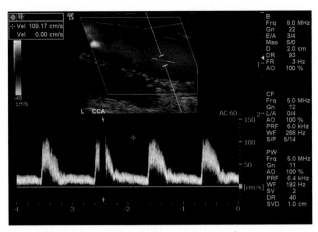

Figure 24-13 Normal spectral analysis CCA after revision.

can result in failure. Concomitantly, imaging advances and surgical techniques have allowed bypasses to very distal arteries. This combination has compounded the already significant obstacles to success in the surgical treatment of infrainguinal occlusive disease.

CURRENT INTRAOPERATIVE EVALUATION

Surveillance of infrainguinal bypass has been well-established as a means of enhancing autogenous bypass patency and resulting limb salvage.[14,15] Given the myriad of intraoperative issues previously described, it is intuitive that surveillance most appropriately should begin in the operating room. Methods of assessing bypasses in the operating room include palpation, continuous wave Doppler, angiography, angioscopy, and duplex ultrasound scanning. Although the "gold standard" has been arteriography, there are many drawbacks to the technique, such as an inability to assess inflow, difficulty in visualizing the entire length of the conduit, and the lack of physiologic information provided. Still, completion angiography has been liberally used, demonstrating between 6% and 12% of defects requiring immediate revision.[16]

Duplex scanning during lower extremity bypass offers unique advantages. The evaluation may begin with the imaging of the donor artery with pulsed spectral analysis, which allows for the characterization of adequate inflow. The entire length of the bypass conduit along with the anastomotic regions can be interrogated to identify retained valves, scarred areas, arteriovenous fistulae, or platelet aggregation. Technical adequacy of the often miniscule distal anastomosis can be ensured. Abnormally low graft velocities may identify problems with poor outflow vessels. Thus, the entire circuit from inflow artery, through the conduit and distally into the outflow vessel, should be examined. Repeated scanning after the repair of defects adds no risk.

DIAGNOSIS

Some institutions have championed the application of duplex scanning in the operating room at the time of bypass. Compared to carotid endarterectomy and renal bypass, infrainguinal bypass had the highest incidence (14%) of corrected defects identified by duplex scanning. Furthermore, a normal duplex scan was predictive of success and unrepaired defects were strong predictors of failure.[17,18] Findings that prompted revision included a PSV >180 cm/s and a velocity ratio (Vr) >2.5. In areas of elevated velocities, retained valves may sometimes be apparent on the ultrasound image. Occasionally, platelet aggregate may form at the site of vessel wall injury. This is usually anechoic in nature but will demonstrate an increased velocity shift. In a small conduit vein graft, a PSV of 150 to 200 cm/s may be recorded as result of hyperemic bypass flows rather than a focal stenosis. The Vr in these small caliber grafts will remain less than 2.0. Lastly, arteriovenous fistulae may be identified within in situ grafts. Turbulent flow will be present in the region of the fistula with elevated diastolic flow velocities proximal to the fistula.

It should be noted that the technique of scanning in these instances is more complex and requires more time than scans done during a carotid endarterectomy. Again, the interaction of the surgeon and sonographer or vascular technologist is of paramount importance in making such a system successful.

INTRA-ABDOMINAL REVASCULARIZATION

Aortoiliac reconstructions involve vessels much larger than carotid or lower extremity procedures; therefore, small technical defects that threaten graft patency are much less common. Assessment is usually by palpation or continuous wave Doppler. In the case of visceral (renal or mesenteric) revascularizations, however, minor technical defects can result in graft failure with catastrophic consequences. As a result, routine arteriography or duplex scan has been liberally applied. Here, duplex sonography has distinct advantages because these small anastomoses are deeply located and more easily accessible with small intraoperative probes. In addition, renal bypass is frequently performed for salvaging renal function, and contrast exposure is avoided if possible. Evaluation of the proximal anastomosis by angiography would require large volumes of contrast under high flow rates—another reason to adopt sonography.

Large studies have documented the feasibility and advantages of intraoperative visceral duplex scanning. Hansen and associates applied sonography to 800 renal bypasses, using a velocity of 200 cm/s as an indication to revise. Sensitivity was 86% and specificity was 100%.[19,20] Seventy-five percent of these reconstructions are performed in patients with some degree of renal insufficiency, underlining the advantages of avoiding contrast material. The consequences of failure in mesenteric revascularization are so catastrophic that intraoperative assessment is a natural adjunct to the procedure. In a study from the Mayo Clinic, 68 visceral reconstructions were monitored with intraoperative duplex scanning. A normal scan was predictive of long-term patency, and an abnormal study was associated with early reintervention, graft failure, and death.[21] Their normal criteria includes a PSV <200 cm/s for the celiac artery and a PSV <275 cm/s for the superior mesenteric artery, a Vr = 2.0, and no technical defects (such as vessel narrowing, a thrombus, a dissection, or an intimal flap).

PROCEDURES FOR VENOUS DISEASE

Although arterial reconstructions have received great attention with regard to operative monitoring with duplex sonography, venous interventions are done much more commonly, and duplex scanning is no less useful in this important area. Along with mapping varicose or incompetent veins, sonography is used for monitoring during endovenous laser therapy (EVLT). Sonographic localization for central venous catheterization has also become the standard of care. These applications of ultrasound with venous procedures are reviewed in other chapters within this text.

SUMMARY

Success in vascular reconstructions is dependent on excellent preoperative imaging, careful operative planning, technical perfection in the operating room, and careful surveillance and follow-up. Intraoperative duplex sonography offers a unique opportunity to maximize the technical outcomes of surgical revascularization. It requires a commitment to excellence and a team approach, which relies heavily on the interaction of the surgeon and the sonographer or vascular technologist. Applying these techniques will continue to improve the care of vascular patients.

Critical Thinking Questions

1. You are asked to bring equipment down to the operating room to assist with an intraoperative ultrasound on a patient undergoing a carotid endarterectomy. You have multiple ultrasound systems in your department. Which do you select and why?

2. In the operating room, the surgeon has the ultrasound transducer directly over the site of a completed carotid endarterectomy. In one area, there is a strong acoustic shadow and no image of the vessel. The surgeon moves the transducer slightly distally, and a normal carotid artery image is obtained. What is a likely explanation of this artifact?

REFERENCES

1. Barnes RW, Nix ML, Wingo JP, et al. Recurrent versus residual carotid stenosis. Incidence detected by Doppler ultrasound. *Ann Surg.* 1986;203:652–660.
2. Donaldson MC, Ivarsson BL, Mannick JA, et al. Impact of completion angiography on operative conduct and results of carotid endarterectomy. *Ann Surg.* 1993;217:682–687.
3. Zannetti S, Cao P, DeRango P, et al. Intraoperative assessment of technical perfection in carotid endarterectomy: a prospective analysis of 1305 completion procedures. *Eur J Vasc Endovasc Surg.* 1999;18:52–58.

4. Westerband A, Mill JL, Berman SS, et al. The influence of routine completion arteriography on outcome following carotid endarterectomy. *Ann Vasc Surg.* 1997;11:14–19.
5. Seifert KB, Blackshear WM Jr. Continuous-wave Doppler in the intraoperative assessment of carotid endarterectomy. *J Vasc Surg.* 1985;2:817–820.
6. Sawchuk AP, Flanigan DP, Machi J, et al. The fate of unrepaired minor technical defects detected by intraoperative ultrasonography during carotid endarterectomy. *J Vasc Surg.* 1989;9:671–676.
7. Bandyk DF, Kaebnick HW, Adams MB, et al. Turbulence occurring after carotid bifurcation endarterectomy: a harbinger of residual and recurrent carotid stenosis. *J Vasc Surg.* 1988;7:261–274.
8. Kinney EV, Seabrook GR, Kinney LY, et al. The importance of intraoperative detection of residual flow abnormalities after carotid artery endarterectomy. *J Vasc Surg.* 1993;17:912–923.
9. Panneton JM, Berger MW, Lewis BD, et al. Intraoperative duplex ultrasound during carotid endarterectomy. *Vasc Surg.* 2001;35:1–9.
10. Steinmetz OK, MacKenzie K, Nault P, et al. Intraoperative duplex scanning for carotid endarterectomy. *Eur J Vasc Endovasc Surg.* 1998;16:153–158.
11. Mullenix PS, Tollefson DF, Olsen SB, et al. Intraoperative duplex ultrasonography as an adjunct to technical excellence in 100 consecutive carotid endarterectomies. *Am J Surg.* 2003;185:445–449.
12. Rockman CB, Haim EA. Intraoperative imaging: does it really improve perioperative outcomes of carotid endarterectomy? *Semin Vasc Surg.* 2007;20:236–243.
13. Veith FJ, Gupta SK, Ascer E, et al. Six-year prospective randomized comparison of autologous saphenous vein and expanded polytetrafluoroethylene grafts in infrainguinal reconstructions. *J Vasc Surg.* 1986;3:104–114.
14. Mills JL Sr. Is duplex surveillance of value after leg vein bypass grafting? Principal results of the vein graft surveillance randomized trial. *Perspect Vasc Surg Endovasc Ther.* 2006;18:194–196.
15. Lundell A, Lingblad B, Bergqvist D, et al. Femoropopliteal-crural graft patency is improved by an intensive surveillance program: a prospective randomized study. *J Vasc Surg.* 1995;21:26–34.
16. Mills JL, Fujitani RM, Taylor SM. Contribution of routine intraoperative completion arteriography to early infrainguinal bypass patency. *Am J Surg.* 1992;164:506–511.
17. Bandyk DF, Mills JL, Gahtan V, et al. Intraoperative duplex scanning of arterial reconstructions: fate of repaired and unrepaired defects. *J Vasc Surg.* 1994;20:426–433.
18. Johnson BL, Bandyk DF, Back MR, et al. Intraoperative duplex monitoring of infrainguinal bypass procedures. *J Vasc Surg.* 2000;31:678–690.
19. Hansen KJ, Reavis SW, Dean RH. Duplex scanning in renovascular disease. *Geriatr Nephrol Urol.* 1996;6:89–97.
20. Hansen KJ, O'Neil EA, Reavis SW, et al. Intraoperative duplex sonography during renal artery reconstruction. *J Vasc Surg.* 1991;14:364–374.
21. Oderich GS, Panneton JM, Macedo TA, et al. Intraoperative duplex ultrasound of visceral revascularizations: optimizing technical success and outcome. *J Vasc Surg.* 2003;38:684–691.

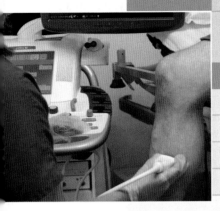

25 The Role of Ultrasound in Central Vascular Access Device Placement

Gail Egan Sansivero, Gary Siskin, and David Singh

OBJECTIVES

Describe the different types of vascular access device options

List the various veins that can be accessed for placement of a central line

Describe the ultrasound techniques used to obtain venous access

Define the potential complications of central venous access

KEY TERMS

basilic vein | jugular vein | peripherally inserted central catheter | superior vena cava | vascular access device

GLOSSARY

air embolism inadvertent release of air or gas into the venous system

collateral veins preexisting veins that enlarge to take flow from neighboring but occluded vessels

fistula an abnormal connection or passageway between two organs or vessels; may be created due to trauma, or intentionally for therapeutic purposes

gain the brightness of an ultrasound image, which can be manipulated on most devices

glidewire a hydrophilic guidewire

guidewire a Nitinol or stainless steel wire used to support sheath or catheter exchanges and to predict vessel patency; measured in diameter and length

infiltration leaking of IV fluid from a catheter into the tissue surrounding the vein

intima innermost layer of a vein or artery; composed of one layer of endothelial cells in contact with blood flow; also known as the tunica intima

microintroducer small needles and wires used to make the initial access into a target

peel away sheath a sheath that is perforated along the long axis, allowing the device to be split for removal from a catheter

PICC a peripherally inserted central catheter; a type of vascular access device that is typically inserted into a vein of the upper extremity and threaded to achieve a tip location in the distal third of the superior vena cava

pneumothorax a collection of air in the pleural space (between the lung and chest wall)

sheath a thin-walled, hollow plastic tube through which wires and catheters can be advanced; measured in French size according to the size of catheter it can accommodate (e.g., a 5-Fr sheath will allow a 5-Fr catheter to be passed through it)

stenosis narrowing of a vein or artery due to disease or trauma

Central venous access plays a vital role in the care of critically ill patients as well as in patients requiring intravenous antibiotic therapy, central venous pressure monitoring, and sampling, hemodialysis, chemotherapy, and total parenteral nutrition. Vascular access devices (VADs) are catheters that allow clinicians to infuse medications and blood components, obtain blood samples, and deliver other exchange therapies. Some patients may require only short-term access, whereas others are dependent on central vascular access for a lifetime. Central VADs are catheters placed so that the terminal tip of the catheter resides in a central vein, most often the superior vena cava. There are many different types of central VADs, each with varying characteristics. The goal for device selection is to match the right device to the right patient, with consideration given to therapy duration, number and type of infusions and patient lifestyle and activity issues. A thorough assessment prior to device placement is critical in selecting the right device and placing it in the right location for the right therapy.

Today, it is virtually the standard of care to use ultrasound guidance to assess potential target sites for VAD placement and to guide the initial venous puncture as the first step in device placement. The Agency for Healthcare Research and Quality has recommended the use of ultrasound as one of their 11 practices to improve patient care in their landmark 2001 publication, "Making Health Care Safer: A Critical Analysis of Patient Safety Practices."[1,2] This chapter will focus on the role ultrasound imaging plays in the placement of central vascular access devices.

ANATOMY

Central vascular access devices may be placed into a variety of target veins. These most commonly include peripheral; upper extremity veins, such as the basilic, brachial, and cephalic veins; and central veins, such as the subclavian and internal jugular veins. No matter where the initial puncture site is, the catheter typically passes through the brachiocephalic vein on its way to the superior vena cava (SVC) (Fig. 25-1). The catheter tip typically resides in the distal third of the SVC (Fig. 25-2). This is also known as the atriocaval junction. This is a desirable location for the tip of a VAD because a flow rate of 2,000 mL/min of venous blood flow is present here. From this location, blood flows directly into the right atrium, then to the right ventricle, and then into the pulmonary circulation. Given the high blood flow in this location, infusates are rapidly dispersed and diluted in this area of high flow. Aspiration for blood return, exchange transfusions, and dialysis or apheresis is also easily accomplished when the VAD tip is accurately located.

CENTRAL VASCULAR ACCESS DEVICE OPTIONS

There are a variety of vascular access devices available. Each of these devices has different characteristics, which confer different advantages and disadvantages. VADs may be divided into three categories: nontunneled devices, tunneled devices, and implanted ports.

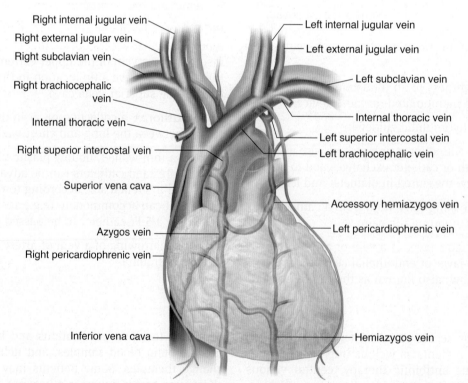

Figure 25-1 This anatomic drawing demonstrates the central veins, including the internal jugular and brachiocephalic veins in addition to the superior vena cava, all of which are important for placement of vascular access devices. (Image courtesy of Michael Ciarmiello, Albany, NY.)

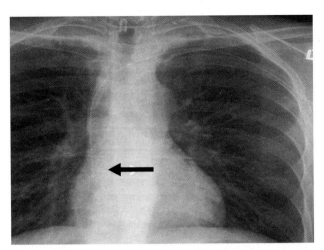

Figure 25-2 This single frontal x-ray of the chest demonstrates a left-sided peripherally inserted central catheter (PICC) placed under ultrasound guidance with the tip of the PICC at the RA-SVC junction *(arrow)*.

NONTUNNELED CENTRAL VASCULAR ACCESS DEVICES

Nontunneled central VADs are placed percutaneously into a central or peripheral vein, with the device's tip residing at the atriocaval junction or distal third of the SVC. These devices include critical care catheters, temporary dialysis and apheresis catheters, small-bore polyurethane catheters, and peripherally inserted central catheters (PICCs). They may have one to five lumens, depending on the patient's infusion needs. Nontunneled VADs are secured at the puncture site with sutures or adhesive securement devices. They are typically used for patients requiring access for days to weeks, although they may remain in place longer if needed.

TUNNELED CENTRAL VASCULAR ACCESS DEVICES

Tunneled VADs are placed via a central vein with their tip residing at the atriocaval junction or in the distal third of the SVC. These devices differ from the devices listed previously because they are tunneled under the skin to the puncture site. The point at which the catheter exits the skin from the tunnel is known as the exit site. The exit site is usually several centimeters from the puncture site, but the device cannot be seen because it is tunneled under the skin. The tunnel helps provide stability for the device and reduces the risk of device-related infection. These devices are often more comfortable for the patient, as the exit site is not in the neck or clavicle area, and may be hidden for cosmetic reasons. Tunneled VADs may be used for infusions and long-term dialysis or apheresis. They are available in one to three lumen configurations and may remain in place for years.

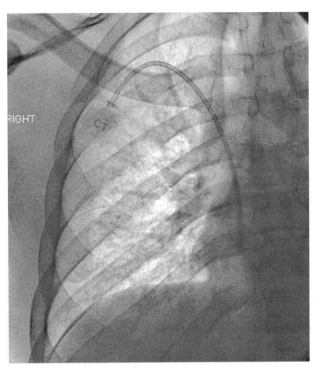

Figure 25-3 This single frontal image shows an implanted port that is compatible with a high-flow contrast injection. (The letters "CT" seen on the body of the port can confirm this.)

IMPLANTED PORTS

Implanted ports are VADs with a catheter segment attached to a plastic or titanium reservoir. The entire system is placed under the skin. The reservoir has a silicone septum, which is accessed with a noncoring needle when infusion or sampling is needed. Ports are most often used for patients who require intermittent therapy, such as weekly or monthly treatment. Because the device is under the skin, patients do not need to keep a dressing on the site or perform frequent maintenance when not in use. Newer ports are now available that are able to used for contrast injections during performance of computed tomography (CT) scans (Fig. 25-3).

PERIPHERAL VAD PLACEMENT

Venous access can be achieved by placing small caliber catheters (also known as peripheral cannulas) via the superficial veins of the upper and lower extremities. Use of the upper extremities is by far more common, with lower extremity access typically limited to use in infants and patients with few access site options. The basilic vein is the dominant superficial vein of the upper extremity and is located on the medial aspect. With a blood flow of approximately 80 mL/min, it is the vein of first choice for the placement of

PICCs. The basilic vein drains directly into the axillary vein, which becomes the subclavian vein as it enters the chest. The brachial veins are also located medially in the upper extremity and are paired veins in proximity to the brachial artery. Typically smaller than the basilic vein, they are a good choice for initial access as well. Their location adjacent to the brachial artery imparts a higher risk of inadvertent arterial puncture than other upper extremity veins. The cephalic vein is the smallest of the named upper extremity veins with a blood flow of approximately 30 mL/min and is thus the least preferred choice for VAD placement. It is positioned more laterally on the arm, making it easy to access. It joins the subclavian vein just past the shoulder.

Lower extremity veins, such as the saphenous vein or veins of the feet, may be used when there are no suitable upper extremity veins for access. This is more common in neonates and children. Although most peripheral veins are palpable and visible, ultrasound may be useful to place peripheral cannulas in challenging patients and in the brachial or saphenous veins. Use of peripheral cannulas should be limited to very short-term therapies (less than 1 week). Peripheral cannulas are changed every 72 hours if possible to reduce the risk of vein damage and infiltration of infusates. Only infusates that are nonirritating and lack vesicant properties should be administered via peripheral cannulas.

CENTRAL VAD PLACEMENT

The most common sites for central venous access are the internal jugular veins (IJVs) and the subclavian veins (SCVs). The IJVs are relatively superficial, facilitating assessment and cannulation. The right IJV approach is preferred over the left because it has a straighter course to the heart, making the procedure technically easier. In proximity to the internal jugular veins are the smaller external and anterior jugular veins, which drain blood from the face and neck. The external jugular veins are superficial and often tortuous. They join the IJV at the confluence of the subclavian and brachiocephalic veins. Because of their size, they are not preferred for central venous access and are more often used in the setting of IJV occlusion.

SONOGRAPHIC EXAMINATION TECHNIQUES

Ultrasound allows for the anatomical assessment of the IJV prior to the procedure, as well as dynamic guidance during vein puncture. The IJV can be cannulated blindly using an anatomical landmark approach, which was and still is a common method for performing this procedure. However, compared with the landmark method, real-time ultrasound guidance has been shown to be both a quicker and safer way to accomplish this goal. Two-dimensional ultrasound guidance can reduce the failure of catheter placement and complication rates related to insertion by 86% and 57%, respectively.[3] When using ultrasound, it is important to assess the depth of the vessel from the skin, the vessel patency, vessel diameter, variations in diameter with respiration, and the relationship of the vein to the common carotid artery (CCA). It is important to identify the CCA prior to attempted cannulation of the IJV. Typically, the IJV is located anterior and lateral to the CCA (Fig. 25-4). However, there are several variations of this relationship that can be encountered. In a prospective evaluation of 869 patients who had undergone real-time ultrasound-guided cannulation of the IJV, five anatomical arrangements of the IJV and CCA were found in 659 patients. In 328 cases (49.8%), the IJV was anterolateral to the CCA, whereas in an additional 146 cases (22.2%), it was lateral to the CCA. In 148 cases (22.5%), the vein lay directly anterior to the artery. In the remaining cases, the IJV was anteromedial to the CCA in 30 cases (4.5%) and directly medial to the artery in seven cases (1.0%).[4]

The subclavian veins are commonly used to attain central venous access. The SCVs are located in the chest, adjacent to the subclavian arteries. They usually lie directly under the clavicle. Because of this location, they are more difficult to visualize with ultrasound than other target veins. SCVs are typically large and thus suitable for cannulation with larger bore central VADs, such as dialysis and apheresis catheters. They terminate in the brachiocephalic veins, at the confluence with the internal jugular veins. Ultimately, the right and left brachiocephalic veins join to form the SVC. Neither the subclavian nor the upper extremity

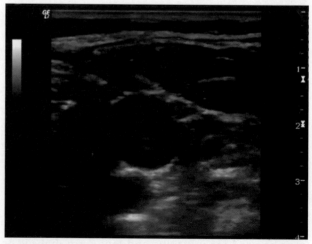

Figure 25-4 This transverse image of the left side of the neck shows both the larger internal jugular vein anterior and slightly lateral to the smaller common carotid artery.

veins should be used for cannulation in patients with chronic renal insufficiency or chronic kidney disease. Because use of these veins for VAD placement may be associated with thrombus and stenosis, avoidance of these veins preserves them for use as a permanent access for hemodialysis (arteriovenous fistula or graft formation) in the future.[5]

The common femoral veins (CFVs) are located in the groin, medial to the common femoral artery. The common femoral veins drain blood from the lower extremities into the external iliac veins. These ultimately become the common iliac veins, which join to form the inferior vena cava. The CFVs are most often used for central venous access in emergent situations and in patients in whom other potential access veins are occluded. VAD placement via the CFV is associated with a higher rate of mechanical and infectious complications, and therefore should be avoided unless necessary.

SCANNING TECHNIQUE

Ultrasound imaging is used to both assess potential access sites for VAD placement, as well as to guide the initial needle puncture into the access site. Initial assessment includes the evaluation of available patent vessels, their location in relation to other structures (e.g., arteries, other implanted devices), and the ability to access the target. The specific target vein is assessed for size and patency. A stenotic (or scarred) vein will appear smaller than expected. Patency is determined by a test of vessel compressibility, similar to that used in the assessment of a patient for deep venous thrombosis. Gentle pressure is applied on the skin overlying the vein using the transducer. A patent vein should compress easily under pressure and should re-expand once pressure is released. A thrombosed vein will not compress using this technique and, in addition, its lumen will appear more echogenic than that of a patent vein (Fig. 25-5). In comparison, compression of an artery will result in less reduction of vessel diameter, and pulsation will be visible. Clearly differentiating venous vessels from arterial vessels is a key factor in reducing the risk of inadvertent arterial puncture. Vessel caliber should also be assessed using ultrasound. The target vein must be of adequate diameter to accommodate the selected VAD, so that complete occlusion of the vein can be avoided.

Ultrasound guidance is used to guide the initial needle puncture into the target vessel. Once the patient is positioned, the skin is prepped with antiseptic solution, and sterile barrier drapes are applied. The skin is anesthetized with a local anesthetic. Additionally, systemic sedation or anesthesia may be used depending on the type of device placed and the patient's overall clinical condition. Sterile ultrasound gel is then applied to the skin overlying the target

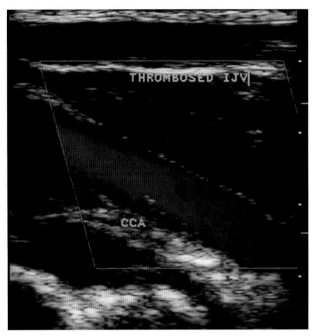

Figure 25-5 This longitudinal image of the neck shows a noncompressible internal jugular vein and its relationship to the common carotid artery.

vessel. A sterile sheath is used to cover the transducer. The ultrasound probe is positioned on the patient's skin in either a longitudinal or transverse position, depending on the preference of the clinician (Fig. 25-6). A needle guide may be attached to the probe depending on clinician preference as well. The depth of the probe is adjusted to accommodate for the size of the target vessel and its depth below the skin. Typically, a small (21 g) hyperechoic needle is used to attain access. The needle should be visualized once it enters the skin, as it approaches the

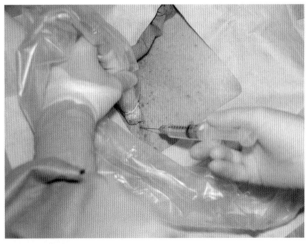

Figure 25-6 This single image during VAD placement shows the longitudinal approach to venous access.

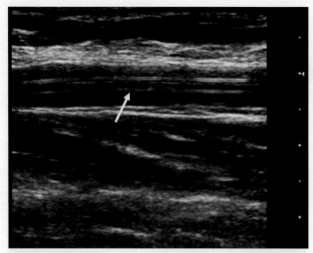

Figure 25-7 A sagittal image of a basilic vein with a PICC line in place *(arrow)*.

target vessel, and as a successful puncture has been attained. Confirmation of successful access is noted by flashback of blood in the needle hub or by aspiration for blood return with an attached syringe. Upon confirmation of accurate access, a small guidewire is advanced into the target vessel. A small skin incision is typically performed to allow the VAD to pass through the skin with minimal resistance. The needle is exchanged for a small venous sheath. Smaller VADs may be advanced into position directly through this sheath. Larger, guiding wires are often inserted for placement of larger VADs. Some VADs may be advanced directly over these wires, whereas others are advanced through a larger sheath following a series of exchange maneuvers. Once the VAD is in place, confirmation of an appropriate tip placement is made with fluoroscopy or chest x-ray. On ultrasound, the VAD is easily observed within the vein, producing a parallel hyperechoic linear structure (Fig. 25-7).

TECHNICAL CONSIDERATIONS

Complications associated with central venous access device placement include vein damage, nontarget puncture, bleeding, air embolism, and cardiac arrhythmias (Pathology Box 25-1). Each can be minimized with careful assessment of the target vein coupled with ultrasound guidance to attain access. Expert placement of VADs, along with minimizing additional venous interventions, serve to reduce and preserve access sites for future use. Consideration should be given to the assessment of a patient's access needs early in the patient's entry into the health care system. If the correct vascular access is placed in the right location early in the patient's therapy, other potential access sites are preserved. It should be noted that the presence of collateral veins does not constitute a neovascularization process. Rather, collateral veins are small veins that have enlarged to divert venous flow in the presence of a stenosis or thrombosis. Their presence on physical exam or ultrasound assessment should alert the clinician to potential difficulties in successfully placing a VAD.

Vein Damage

Vein damage occurs each time a vein is accessed, whether for sampling purposes or for placement of a vascular access device. Veins are composed of three layers: the intima, the media, and the adventitia. The innermost lining of the vein is the intima, composed of a single layer of endothelial cells. Each time a vein is accessed, this layer is disrupted. This disrupted surface allows platelets to adhere to its surface, thus beginning the clotting cascade. An arteriovenous fistula is another form of vein damage that can occur with device placement. This is most likely to occur when the initial needle is placed

---

PATHOLOGY BOX 25-1

Complications Associated with VAD Placement

Complication	Ultrasound Appearance
Vein damage	Irregular intimal surface
	Anechoic to hypoechoic area indicating extravascular accumulation of blood
	Arteriovenous fistula with flow evident between vein and companion artery on color or spectral Doppler
Nontarget puncture	Anechoic to hypoechoic area indicating extravascular accumulation of blood
	Expanding hematoma indicated by an enlarging extravascular mass
Bleeding	Anechoic to hypoechoic area indicating extravascular accumulation of blood; may be diffuse within tissue
Air embolism	Rounded hyperechoic structure in the blood stream producing an acoustic shadow
Cardiac arrhythmia	Uneven, irregularly spaced cardiac cycles displayed on arterial spectral analysis

through both walls of the vein into a neighboring artery. When recognized, the device should be removed and pressure applied to the site. An arteriovenous fistula may close on its own or may require intervention to close.

Nontarget Puncture

Nontarget puncture occurs when the access needle is directed to a neighboring structure such as an artery or lung. Careful identification and differentiation of arteries from veins prior to and during initial puncture will minimize the likelihood of inadvertent arterial puncture. Use of a small access needle will minimize the risk of bleeding should a nontarget puncture occur. In the event of arterial puncture, the needle should be immediately removed and gentle pressure should be applied to achieve hemostasis. A sterile occlusive dressing should be applied once hemostasis is achieved, and the patient's vital signs should be monitored. The site should be assessed frequently for an expanding hematoma, which could compromise venous blood flow or respiratory status, particularly with a carotid artery puncture. Inadvertent puncture of the lung may result in pneumothorax, or a collapsed lung. Pneumothorax is one of the most serious and potentially life-threatening complications of central venous catheterization. The complication rate varies from 0% to 6% but has been reported as high as 12.4% with inexperienced practitioners.[6] Pneumothorax accounts for 25% to 30% of all reported complications of central vein catheter insertion.[7,8] The internal jugular vein approach has been shown to have a lower risk of pneumothorax compared to subclavian vein cannulation.[9,10,11] The failure of the first attempt at catheter insertion is also associated with a significant increase in pneumothorax risk. A small pneumothorax can be treated conservatively with observation. If the patient is symptomatic, or the pneumothorax enlarges, placement of a pleural drainage catheter may be required.

Bleeding

Bleeding with or following VAD placement may occur because of traumatic or difficult VAD insertion, comorbid conditions such as a coagulopathy or other hematologic disorders, and concurrent treatment with certain medications. Medications that increase the likelihood of bleeding include clopidogrel, warfarin, aspirin and other nonsteroidal anti-inflammatory drugs, and heparin. When possible, these medications may be discontinued prior to device placement. If discontinuation is not clinically feasible, other measures can be taken to reduce the risk of bleeding. These include the use of hemostatic dressing materials, a change in VAD selection to a less invasive device, and administration of blood components or reversal agents.

Air Embolism

Air embolism during central VAD placement occurs when air enters the venous system via the needle, sheath, or device. Although unusual, it is a serious complication that can result in respiratory compromise and even death. The risk of air embolism can be minimized by using valved sheaths, performing exchange maneuvers efficiently, and ensuring that catheter lumens are flushed, secured, and locked. If the patient is symptomatic, the patient should be treated symptomatically with oxygen and supportive care. Air emboli are not often seen within the target vessel as these emboli move quickly within the blood stream.

Cardiac Arrhythmias

Cardiac arrhythmias during VAD placement typically occur when guidewires are advanced into the heart, triggering the heart's conduction system. This is often transient, and patients are often asymptomatic. In the absence of symptoms, arrhythmias are detected through use of intraprocedure cardiac monitoring.

SUMMARY

Ultrasound imaging has allowed clinicians to improve assessments and decision making prior to device placement by helping to identify target vessels and determining their suitability for use. Coupled with optimal device selection and the development of an infusion plan, ultrasound imaging is an integral component of access planning and placement. Real-time ultrasound imaging helps minimize placement complications by allowing the clinician to visualize venous access, avoid neighboring structures, and guide devices into position. Once thought to be a useful tool for access-limited or challenging patients, ultrasound imaging is now the standard of practice for central vascular access device placement.

Critical Thinking Question

1. While examining the subclavian vein of a patient with a peripherally inserted central vein access device, you notice the bright acoustic reflections of the catheter within the vein. A colleague who is observing the ultrasound asks if that is the catheter tip. What is your answer?

2. You are assisting during the placement of a central venous line via the internal jugular vein. Following the procedure, a hematoma is observed in the area of the puncture. Is this a normal occurrence and what could be done next?

REFERENCES

1. Rothschild JM. Ultrasound guidance of central vein catheterization. http://www.ahrq.gov/clinic/ptsafety/chap21.htm. Published 2001. Accessed June 4, 2007.
2. Markowitz JD, ed. Making health care safer: a critical analysis of patient safety practices. http://archive.ahrq.gov/clinic/ptsafety/. Published July 2001. Accessed June 4, 2007.
3. Lameris JS, Post PJ, Zonderland HM. Percutaneous placement of Hickman catheters: comparison of sonographically guided and blind techniques. *Am J Roentgenol.* 1990;155(5):1097–1099.
4. Gordon AC, Saliken JC, Johns D, et al. US-guided puncture of the internal jugular vein: complications and anatomic considerations. *J Vasc Interv Radiol.* 1998;9:333–338.
5. National Kidney Foundation Kidney Disease Outcomes Quality Initiative. Clinical practice guidelines and recommendations: vascular access. http://www.kidney.org/professionals/kdoqi/guideline_uphd_pd_va/index.htm. Published 2006. Accessed June 2011.
6. Seneff MG. Central venous catheters. In: Rippe JM, Irwin RS, Alpert JS, et al., eds. *Intensive Care Medicine.* 2nd ed. Boston, MA: Little Brown and Co.; 1991:17–37.
7. Sofocleous CT, Schur I, Cooper SG, et al. Sonographically guided placement of peripherally inserted central venous catheters: review of 355 procedures. *Am J Roentgenol.* 1998;170:1613–1616.
8. Funaki B. Central venous access: a primer for the diagnostic radiologist. *Am J Roentgenol.* 2002;179:309–318.
9. Lefrant JY, Muller L, De La Coussaye JE. Risk factors of failure and immediate complication of subclavian vein catheterization in critically ill patients. *Intensive Care Med.* 2002;28:1036–1041.
10. Chimochowski GE, Worley E, Rutherford WE, et al. Superiority of the internal jugular over the subclavian access for temporary dialysis. *Nephron.* 1990;54:154–161.
11. McGee DC, Gould MK. Preventing complications of central venous catheterization. *N Engl J Med.* 2003;348:1123–1133.

26 Hemodialysis Access Grafts and Fistulae

Michael J. Singh and Cheryl Sura

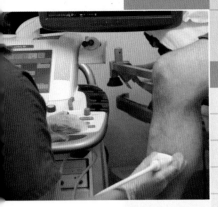

OBJECTIVES

Describe the difference between an arteriovenous fistula and graft

Identify the duplex findings of a normal arteriovenous fistula

Define normal venous and arterial anatomy in the upper extremity

Describe the venous Doppler findings in an occluded axillary vein

Demonstrate proper probe positioning for imaging a radiocephalic fistula

Differentiate a forearm graft from a brachiocephalic fistula

Quantify the degree of stenosis based on Doppler findings

KEY TERMS

arteriovenous fistula | arteriovenous graft | hemodialysis access

GLOSSARY

arteriovenous fistula an abnormal connection between an artery and vein; this may be congenital or acquired; one type of acquired arteriovenous fistula is surgically created to allow for hemodialysis

arteriovenous graft a type of hemodialysis access that uses a prosthetic conduit to connect an artery to a vein to allow for dialysis

hemodialysis access also known as vascular access; a surgically created connection between an artery and vein to allow for the removal of toxic products from the blood by dialysis

Due to various factors, the incidence of chronic kidney disease and end-stage renal disease are becoming more prevalent in the United States. In 2005, the Renal Data System determined that more than 106,000 patients began hemodialysis and the total number of people undergoing hemodialysis had reached 341,000. The National Kidney Foundation Kidney Disease Outcomes Quality Initiative was published in 1997 and recommended that 50% of future hemodialysis access be constructed with autogenous arteriovenous access. In 2005, the Centers for Medicare and Medicaid Services (CMS) promoted the Fistula First Breakthrough Initiative. The goal of this was to expand the creation of new autogenous access to 66% by 2009.[1]

The goal of arteriovenous (AV) access is to provide long-term hemodialysis access with a low frequency of reintervention and a low complication rate. The tenet for hemodialysis access is to create an autogenous fistula as far distally as possible in the nondominant arm. This technique preserves the proximal vessels for future access and allows the individual to carry out normal daily activities. Autogenous access has been the preferred first line of therapy because it has superior patency rates and lower complication rates compared to prosthetic grafts.[2] Upper extremity access is preferred; it maintains a lower infection rate and provides easier access for hemodialysis. A native AV fistula is a surgically created anastomosis between an artery and a vein. When fistula creation is not possible, a prosthetic graft is often used to connect the two vessels. These prosthetic grafts are made of polytetrafluoroethylene (PTFE) and tunneled in the subcutaneous tissue.

Failure of an AV fistula to mature and thrombose are frequent indications for reintervention.

393

AV fistulae have 2-year primary patency rates of 40% to 69%. In comparison, 2-year primary patency rates for prosthetic grafts range from 18% to 30%. Secondary patency rates for fistulae range from 62% to 75% at 2 years. For prosthetic grafts, secondary patency rates are 40% to 60% in the same time frame. The trade-off for higher long-term AV fistula patency rates is a lower maturation rate and higher early thrombosis rate. More often, maturation failure is due to the use of small or suboptimal veins.[2]

PREOPERATIVE EVALUATION

SONOGRAPHIC EXAMINATION TECHNIQUE

Given the importance of a proper conduit, preoperative evaluation of the arterial and venous systems is essential for the successful creation of long-term access and fistula maturation. Vascular Technology Professional Performance Guidelines have been established by the Society for Vascular Ultrasound.[3] Preoperative vein mapping is performed to determine suitability of the superficial veins of the upper extremity for placement of dialysis access (Fig. 26-1). This may be performed on patients who have yet to start hemodialysis or in those who have undergone previous access procedures and require a secondary intervention or access creation.

PATIENT PREPARATION

The technologist should introduce himself or herself and explain why the vein mapping is being performed. An explanation of the technique and duration of study is essential. Questions and concerns from the patient should be addressed before initiating the study. The room should be comfortably warm to avoid vasospasm.

PATIENT ASSESSMENT

The patient assessment must be complete prior to initiating the procedure. A comprehensive history should document the patient's ability to tolerate the imaging study and determine any contraindications to the procedure. Obtaining a current medical history is essential. This includes all previous access procedures, trauma history, medications, and arm dominance. Specifically inquire about any risk factors that may preclude fistula creation, such as the placement of central venous catheters, pacemakers, defibrillators, or prior mastectomy with lymph node dissection. The focused physical examination should include bilateral arm blood pressure measurements; a quantitative pulse exam of the brachial, radial, and ulnar arteries; an Allen test to demonstrate an intact

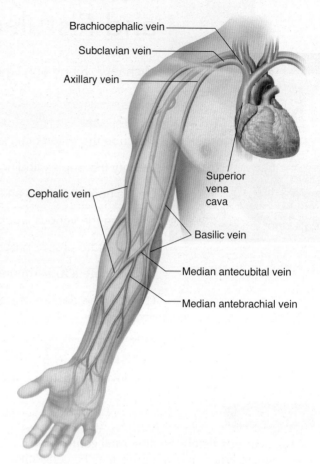

Figure 26-1 Diagram of normal venous anatomy of the upper extremity.

palmar arch; and an assessment of the superficial venous system using tourniquets (Fig. 26-2). Findings suggestive of a central venous stenosis or occlusion include arm edema, prominent chest wall veins, or arm collaterals. For those with any clinical abnormality, noninvasive imaging is necessary.

PATIENT POSITIONING

Optimal patient positioning may either be in the supine or sitting positions. The goal is to promote venodilation, and thus, positioning the arms in gravity dependent position is ideal.

SCANNING TECHNIQUES

During the procedure, sonographic characteristics of vessels, tissue, and blood flow must be observed and analyzed in order to ensure that the appropriate data are documented for the interpreting physician. The assessment of the upper extremity venous system includes direct imaging of the superficial and deep systems with appropriate instrumentation. Spectral analysis with or without color Doppler imaging

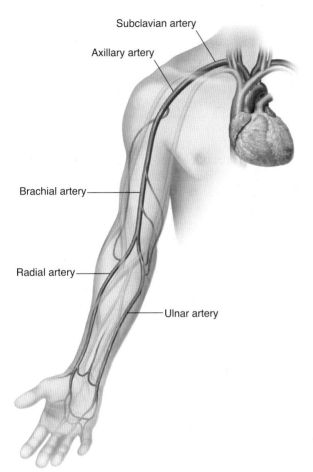

Figure 26-2 Diagram of normal arterial anatomy of the upper extremity.

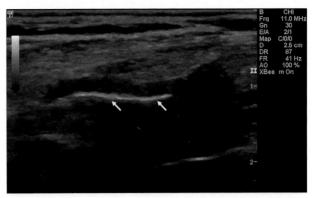

Figure 26-3 Ultrasound image of a calcified brachial artery. Note the bright white reflectors along the vessel wall.

should be performed using a high-resolution linear transducer of at least 5 to 10 MHz. These frequencies are ideal for imaging relatively superficial structures. Following a standard protocol, start with the arterial system in the nondominant arm. If the arteries have an acceptable size of >2 mm, proceed to imaging the venous system. If an abnormality is discovered or if the arteries or veins in the nondominant arm are suboptimal, move to the contralateral arm.

The preoperative assessment of the arterial system includes direct imaging with ultrasound and, in select situations, indirect evaluation with physiologic testing. (Chapter 8 discusses the indirect evaluation of the upper extremity arterial system.) Studies are routinely performed only in the nondominant arm unless otherwise indicated by the referring physician.

B-mode grayscale imaging is used to assess the diameters of the ulnar and radial arteries. Measurements can be obtained at several locations along both vessels but often, a proximal and distal diameter measurement is adequate. Many laboratories also include a diameter measurement of the brachial artery in the event a more proximal fistula placement is planned. Arteries should also be assessed for

calcification, intimal thickness, stenosis, and compliance (Fig. 26-3). Studies have shown that the quality of the arterial wall determines the capacity of the artery to dilate and accommodate the increased flow. In cases where an atherosclerotic vessel is present, the vessel is unable to compensate by dilating and thus increased flow is entirely dependent on the native arterial diameter. Generally, atherosclerosis in the upper extremities is most often observed in the subclavian and axillary vessels. However, in diabetic patients and patients with chronic renal disease, the brachial, radial, and ulnar arteries may present with atherosclerotic disease.

B-mode grayscale imaging is also used to assess the superficial arm veins and their spatial relationships. This begins in the transverse plane with an evaluation of the cephalic, basilic, and median cubital veins starting at the wrist and moving proximally (Fig. 26-4). B-mode imaging should confirm that the vein walls are compressible and free of thrombus, webbing, and calcium (Fig. 26-5). Transverse compression of the vein should be performed every 2 cm, and the diameter of the veins should be recorded along their entire length. Close attention should be paid to the antecubital fossa and areas of prior

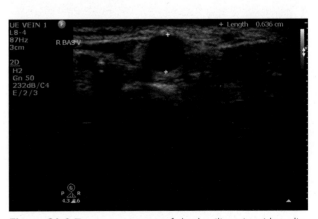

Figure 26-4 Transverse image of the basilic vein with a diameter measurement.

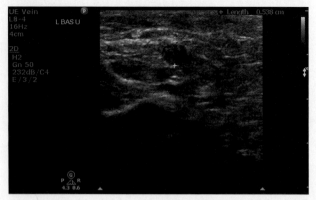

Figure 26-5 Increased intraluminal echoes consistent with occluding thrombosis in a basilic vein.

needle puncture. Documentation of vessel characteristics should include patency, depth, wall thickness, calcification, and location of a thrombus or fibrosis.

For maximal vein dilation, a double tourniquet technique can be used. One tourniquet should be placed on the forearm, which compresses the superficial vessels, and the other tourniquet should be placed in the axillary region to compress the deeper veins.

Spectral Doppler analysis is performed in a sagittal plane. All Doppler studies are performed at an angle of 60° or less with respect to the direction of flow. The actual venous velocity is not important; however, by using an angle of insonation of 60° or less, an adequate Doppler signal will be obtained. To complete the venous examination, spectral waveforms are performed while compressing the limb proximally or distally to demonstrate augmentation of venous flow. Patency of the proximal deep veins (brachial, axillary, and subclavian) should be confirmed. Doppler signals and spectral waveforms should be checked in the mid-subclavian vein and internal jugular vein (Fig. 26-6). Atypical

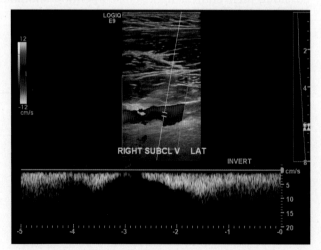

Figure 26-6 Doppler imaging of the mid-subclavian vein showing respiratory phasicity.

findings that may be life threatening (e.g., central vein thrombosis) should immediately be conveyed to a health care provider.

TECHNICAL CONSIDERATIONS

Upon completion of the examination, preliminary results should be recorded by the technologist. A technologist work sheet or summary will aid the interpreting physician while he or she reviews the diagnostic images. Proper documentation is essential and includes exam date, indications for the procedure, the technologist's name, the arm studied, and the patient's identification information. Any deviation from the protocol should be documented and explained on the work sheet.

The routine unilateral upper extremity vein mapping examination should take approximately 35 to 45 minutes. The goals are to provide an accurate high quality examination, thus appropriate time should be allowed for the completion of this examination.

PITFALLS

There are few contraindications to this ultrasound-guided assessment, and they include intravenous lines, dressings, open wounds, and limited patient positioning. Attempts should be made to use various approaches and scanning orientations to work around some of these obstacles.

DIAGNOSIS

For the assessment of the radial, ulnar, and brachial arteries, an arterial diameter greater than 2 mm is needed for fistula creation and maturation. Maturation is defined as a dilated, easily palpable, and usable fistula for hemodialysis at a flow rate of >350 mL/min.[4] Volume flow rates will be discussed later in this chapter. The grayscale image should demonstrate smooth walled vessels that are free of disease. Calcification will appear as bright white echoes along or within the vessel walls.

Venous criteria for acceptable conduit diameter varies between physicians. Although there is no consensus, a favorable vessel diameter for creation of AV access is greater than 2.5 mm. Using this diameter as a minimum, it has been shown that a 92% early maturation rate and an 83% 1-year patency rate can be obtained.[5] Vein walls should be completely compressible with light transducer pressure. A partially compressible or noncompressible vein suggests the presence of an occluding thrombus within the vein lumen, making it unusable as an autogenous conduit.

TABLE 26-1
Types of Autogenous Arteriovenous Access

Forearm:

Posterior radial artery to cephalic vein ("snuffbox" fistula)
Radial artery to cephalic vein (Brescia-Cimino fistula)
Radial artery to cephalic forearm vein transposition
Brachial artery to cephalic forearm vein looped transposition
Radial artery to basilic forearm vein transposition
Ulnar artery to basilic forearm vein transposition
Brachial artery to basilic forearm vein looped transposition

Upper arm:

Brachial artery to cephalic vein fistula
Brachial artery to basilic vein transposition
Brachial artery to brachial vein transposition

Venous Doppler signals from the central veins should display respiratory phasicity, cardiac pulsatility, and augmentation. These characteristics should be used to confirm patency of the central venous system.

HEMODIALYSIS ACCESS EVALUATION

The goal of hemodialysis access is to provide a durable site for cannulation, which is placed distally in the limb. This strategy allows for the option of creating a more proximal access should the distal AV fistula fail. There are numerous types of autogenous forearm AV access. Table 26-1 summarizes the various types of upper extremity AV access. A Brescia-Cimino fistula is most frequently performed and involves mobilizing the cephalic vein at the wrist and sewing it to the distal radial artery (Fig. 26-7). This type of fistula is ideal due to its distal location and the need for minimal dissection and vessel mobilization. On occasion, a "snuffbox" fistula may be created by connecting the posterior branch of the radial artery to the cephalic vein. In situations where the cephalic vein is unusable, the basilic vein is preferred. The medial location of the forearm basilic vein requires that it be transposed and juxtaposed to a distal artery (radial or ulnar) in order to create an AV fistula.

Upper arm autogenous AV access is necessary when more distal access options are unavailable or have failed. The most common upper arm access is a brachial artery to cephalic vein fistula, which is created in the antecubital fossa (Fig. 26-8). For

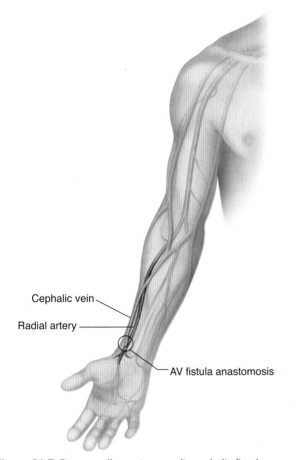

Figure 26-7 Diagram illustrating a radiocephalic fistula.

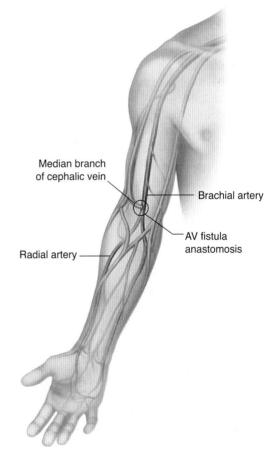

Figure 26-8 Diagram illustrating a brachiocephalic fistula.

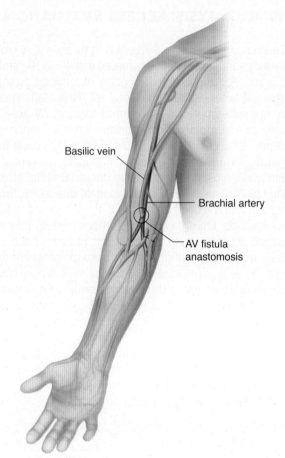

Basilic vein

Brachial artery

AV fistula anastomosis

Figure 26-9 Diagram illustrating a basilic transposition fistula.

those patients with suboptimal cephalic veins, the upper arm basilic vein can be used. Due to its deep location, transposition of this vessel is necessary. Possible sites for arterial inflow include the brachial, radial, and ulnar arteries (Fig. 26-9).

If the upper extremity vessels are unsuitable for the creation of a fistula, lower extremity vessels may be used. A hemodialysis access can be created using the common femoral or superficial femoral arteries along with the great saphenous or common femoral veins. These types of accesses are not very common.

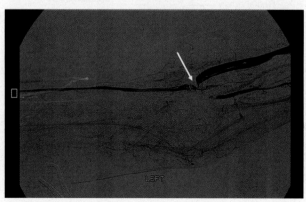

Figure 26-10 Venogram of an AV graft with a venous anastomotic stenosis indicated at the *white arrow*.

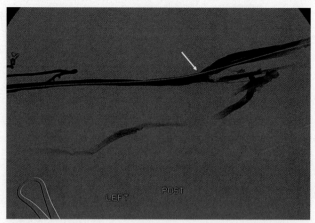

Figure 26-11 Venogram of the same AV graft in Figure 26-10 following endovascular venoplasty with resolution of anastomotic stenosis (*arrow*).

Approximately 8 to 12 weeks after the creation of an autogenous fistula, it should be mature and ready for needle cannulation. For those that fail to mature, they should be closely interrogated with ultrasound imaging. Low maturation rates correspond to the use of a small or suboptimal vein for fistula creation.[2] Berman and Gentile were able to demonstrate a 10% improvement in autogenous access use with close follow-up and early secondary interventions.[6] This includes open revision, branch ligation, endovascular intervention (Figs. 26-10 and 26-11), and vein superficialization.

The long-term follow-up of fistulae and grafts (Fig. 26-12) is essential for improved patency. Frequently, outflow vein segments, fistula anastomoses, and vein-to-graft anastomoses will develop a stenosis secondary to intimal hyperplasia. Other indications for close follow-up include pseudoaneurysm formation (Fig. 26-13), mid-graft stenosis, hematoma formation, and arterial stenosis. Vascular Technology Professional Performance Guidelines have been established by the Society for Vascular Ultrasound.[7] Indications for evaluation include pseudoaneurysm formation, peri-fistula mass, decreased thrill, pulsatile flow, difficult cannulation, elevated recirculation time (>12%), elevated venous pressure during dialysis (>200 mm Hg), low urea reduction rate (<60%), excessive bleeding following dialysis, arm edema, infection, and arterial steal symptoms. The same preoperative vein mapping contraindications are applied here.

SONOGRAPHIC EXAMINATION TECHNIQUE

PATIENT PREPARATION

As mentioned in the preceding section on preoperative scanning, the technologist should introduce himself or herself and explain why the dialysis access

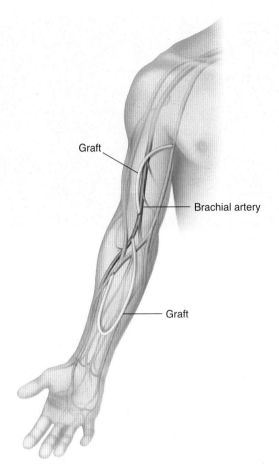

Figure 26-12 Diagram illustrating a forearm loop AV graft and an upper arm AV graft.

evaluation is being performed. An introduction and explanation of the technique, including the duration of study, is an essential component to all testing. During this time, any questions and concerns from the patient can be addressed. The room should be comfortably warm to avoid vasospasm.

PATIENT ASSESSMENT

The patient assessment is similar to that used for the preoperative testing and should be completed prior to initiating the procedure. A comprehensive medical and surgical history should be documented including the patient's ability to tolerate the imaging study. Any potential contraindications should be determined. The history should include all previous access procedures, trauma history, medications, and arm dominance. If available, reviewing access diagrams or operative notes will clarify the access type and location. Specifically, inquire about any risk factors that may preclude fistula maturation or use, such as central venous thrombosis or placement of central venous catheters, pacemakers, or defibrillators. The focused physical examination should include a quantitative exam of the fistula or graft. Assessment for the presence of a thrill, and the quality of the thrill throughout the entire access is important. Visual inspection of the arm and access site is necessary to assess for edema, redness, presence of collateral veins, rotation of access sites, and focal dilations.

PATIENT POSITIONING

Optimal patient positioning should be supine, with the arm extended and relaxed. Depending on the exact placement of the dialysis access site, the arm position may need to be adjusted during the course of the examination.

SCANNING TECHNIQUES

The patient and arm are placed in a comfortable position. Use minimal pressure and abundant ultrasound gel to optimize imaging. Characteristics of vessels, tissue, and blood flow must be observed and analyzed in order to ensure that appropriate data is documented

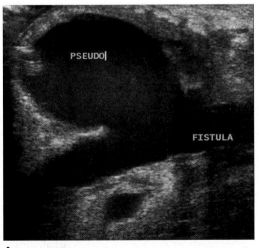

A

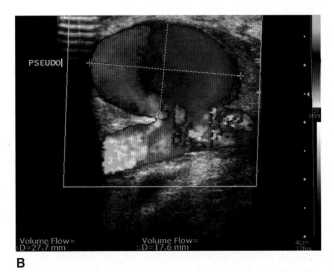

B

Figure 26-13 A: A grayscale image of a pseudoaneurysm. **B:** The same pseudoaneurysm with color flow imaging demonstrating the "yin-yang" appearance in the color pattern.

for the interpreting physician. Spectral analysis with or without color Doppler imaging should be performed using a carrier frequency of at least 7 to 12 MHz. System presets should be adjusted to the high flow settings, and decreasing color gain will minimize tissue bruit. Use B-mode to assess for various abnormalities such as perigraft masses, pseudoaneurysms, stenotic valves, and intimal flaps. Perigraft fluid collections and pseudoaneurysms can be differentiated using B-mode, color flow imaging, and Doppler imaging. The fistula diameter should be measured along its length. Scanning the fistula in a transverse view will locate side branches that can limit fistula maturation. Measure the branch vessel diameter and document the location.

Doppler evaluation is used to document patency of the fistula as well as to identify areas of stenosis. Doppler spectral analysis is performed in the sagittal plane. All Doppler samples must be performed at an angle of 60° or less with respect to the direction of flow. Doppler cursor alignment should be parallel to the vessel wall. When a stenosis is found, velocities should be measured proximal, distal, and within the area of interest. Arterial inflow is first assessed with duplex imaging. Peak systolic velocities (PSVs) should be recorded in the native artery proximal to the anastomosis, at the anastomosis, throughout the body of the fistula, and along the venous outflow. Scanning throughout the entire fistula or graft, obtaining spectral signals, and paying close attention to the needle puncture sites is essential. The examination must include the venous outflow and, in some cases, may extend into the chest for assessing the central veins. Color imaging is helpful in this location.

Volume flow measurements are useful when evaluating access function and are best accomplished with a wide-open sample gate. Volume flow calculations should be made in the mid-graft or fistula at a site of normal flow. The volumetric flow (millimeters per minute) is calculated as follows:

Flow = Time Average Velocity × Area × 60.
The area is calculated based on:
$(1/2 \text{ diameter})^2\pi$.

Most modern ultrasound systems are capable of measuring this automatically. The technologist manually measures the diameter, which the ultrasound system then uses to calculate the area. A Doppler spectrum is recorded from which the system calculates the time average velocity. The time average velocity should be measured over three to four cardiac cycles to obtain an accurate calculation (Fig. 26-14). Some laboratories choose to obtain triplicate measurements of volume flow and then average these three values to improve accuracy.

In select situations, the presenting symptoms may suggest an arterial steal syndrome. In these cases, it is imperative to know the orientation of the sound beam and the expected flow direction. Using color

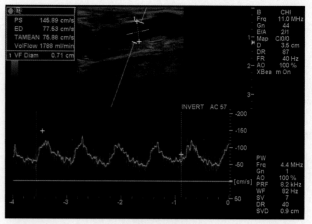

Figure 26-14 A duplex ultrasound of a fistula with volume flow calculated.

flow, check for retrograde flow in the distal native artery, compress the graft, and then reassess flow direction in the native artery. Measuring distal arterial velocity or flow with and without fistula compression is helpful. Absolute forearm pressures should also be obtained with and without compression. In situations when this is not possible, pulse volume recordings of the digits are an acceptable option.

TECHNICAL CONSIDERATIONS

Documentation should include the examination date, indications for the procedure, the technologist's name, the arm studied, and the patient's identification information. Vessel characteristics, including patency, wall thickness, calcification, and thrombus content, should be recorded. Documenting native vessel or fistula stenosis or thrombosis, anastomotic lesions, PSVs, and poststenotic turbulence is necessary. Any deviation from the protocol must be documented and explained. Similar to preoperative vein mapping for dialysis access, thorough surveillance imaging with direct and indirect components of these examinations will routinely require 35 to 45 minutes for a unilateral limb.

Pitfalls

The examination of a fistula or graft presents a few unique challenges. It is a very superficial structure and, as such, it is possible to inadvertently partially compress it if too much transducer pressure is applied by the technologist or sonographer. This transducer pressure can result in elevated velocities recorded during the examination. Care needs to be taken to avoid excess transducer pressure. Another factor related to the position of the fistula or graft involves scanning mature access sites. As both fistulae and grafts age, they dilate, can become aneurysmal, can develop pseudoaneurysms, and can become tortuous. All of these conditions make for an irregular scanning surface on the arm. The surface

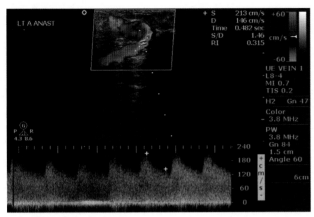

Figure 26-15 Color flow imaging and spectral Doppler of a normally functioning fistula.

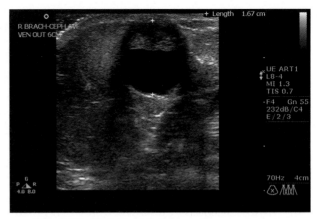

Figure 26-17 A B-mode image of venous stenosis.

irregularities require regular, large amounts of gel to maintain proper skin contact. Larger pseudoaneurysms may require scanning from various approaches to fully document all the findings. Occasionally, patients present with contraindications to scanning including dressings or open wounds or possibly decreased mobility leading to poor patient positioning.

DIAGNOSIS

The grayscale image should reveal an access free of a thrombus or calcifications. A thrombus may appear hypoechoic or anechoic depending on its age. Calcifications will appear as bright white reflectors with the vessel walls. In a fistula, the valves within the vein should not be evident and should appear to be adhered to the vessel wall. Any valve projecting into the lumen should be noted, as it can be a source for stenosis development.

A well-functioning fistula will have a PSV between 150 and 300 cm/s and end-diastolic velocities (EDVs) of 60 to 200 cm/s (Fig. 26-15).[8] High-grade stenoses are present with focal velocity elevations of 100%, thus producing a velocity ratio (Vr) >2 as compared to the adjacent segment.[9] A stenosis is also likely to be present within the fistula or the inflow/outflow vessels if the PSV of a fistula is <50 cm/s.[9] Marked spectral broadening, continuous forward diastolic flow, and a high velocity are expected to be seen throughout the fistula (Fig. 26-16). The inflow artery will have a low resistance flow, and increased PSV (30 to 100 cm/s) with pulsatility will be noted in the outflow vein.

DISORDERS

Anastomotic and vein stenoses account for the majority (80%) of access complications. Multiple stenoses are more commonly found in AV grafts. Venous stenosis is represented by a sonolucent intraluminal lesion, which has a luminal flow reduction on B-mode imaging (Fig. 26-17). A fistula or graft occlusion is represented by a high resistance signal, absent flow lumen, and an intraluminal echogenic thrombus (Fig. 26-18). Pathology Box 26-1 summarizes ultrasound findings within normal and abnormal AV fistulae.

A normal flow volume is >800 mL/min. A mild-to-moderate stenosis will decrease the volume of flow to 500 to 800 mL/min. A severe stenosis is represented by a volume of flow <500 mL/min.[9]

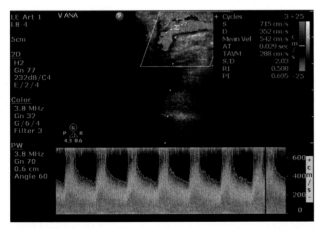

Figure 26-16 Image of an anastomotic stenosis with elevated velocities.

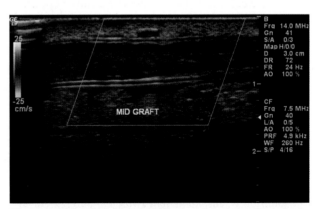

Figure 26-18 An occluded AV graft with no color filling and a thrombus present within the graft.

PATHOLOGY BOX 26-1

AV Fistula Ultrasound Findings

	B-mode	Color Flow	Doppler
Normal AV fistula	Compressible vessel	Phasic or nonphasic color flow pattern	Turbulent flow pattern with unelevated velocities PSV 150–300 cm/s EDV 60–200 cm/s
Stenotic AV fistula	Intraluminal echoes, thickened walls	Reduced flow lumen, disturbed color flow patterns	Elevated velocities in region of stenosis Vr >2
Occluded AV fistula	Intraluminal echogenicity, loss of flow lumen	No flow	Absent Doppler signal

AV, arteriovenous; PSV, peak systolic velocity; EDV, end-diastolic velocity; Vr, velocity ratio.

SUMMARY

Ultrasound imaging when used in conjunction with clinical examination has proven to be an extremely powerful tool in the evaluation and management of hemodialysis access. It is a highly sensitive and noninvasive technique that complements the physical examination. Preoperative imaging of both the arterial and venous systems should be performed to allow the surgeon to select the optimal hemodialysis access option. This technique has been shown to improve fistula maturation and has become the standard of care for preoperative vessel assessment. Ultrasonography has been shown to be extremely useful in access surveillance. Initial baseline examinations provide reference for follow-up studies. It has successfully been used to predict the maturation of fistulae. Criteria have been established to define threatened fistulae and grafts.

Critical Thinking Questions

1. B-mode imaging reveals a small (1.75 mm) calcified radial artery. What is the next step in the evaluation of this patient?

2. Dilated chest wall veins are seen during the examination of a patient with arm edema and a nonmaturing AV fistula. What noninvasive imaging study is recommended?

3. One week after the creation of a radiocephalic fistula, a patient presents with a cool, painful hand. What is the expected direction of flow in the distal native radial artery?

4. To assess fistula function, volumetric flow calculations are best measured in what part of the AV fistula?

REFERENCES

1. Sidawy AN. Arteriovenous hemodialysis access: the Society for Vascular Surgery practice guidelines. *J Vasc Surg.* 2008;48:1S–80S.
2. Macsata RA, Sidawy AN. Hemodialysis access: general considerations. In: Cronenwett JL, Johnston W, eds. *Rutherford's Vascular Surgery.* 7th ed. Philadelphia, PA: Saunders Elsevier; 2010:1104–1114.

3. The Society for Vascular Ultrasound. Upper extremity vein mapping for placement of a dialysis access. Vascular Technology Professional Performance Guidelines. http://www.svunet.org/files/positions/0809-upper-extrem-vein-map.pdf. Published August 10, 2009. Accessed June 2011.
4. Miller PE, Tolwani A, Luscy CP, et al. Predictors of adequacy of arteriovenous fistulas in hemodialysis patients. *Kidney Int.* 1999;56(1):275–288.
5. The Society for Vascular Ultrasound. Upper extremity arterial segmental physiologic evaluation. Vascular Technology Professional Performance Guidelines. http://www.svunet.org/files/positions/UpperExtremityArterialSegmentalPhysiologic%20Evaluation.pdf. Published October 10, 2010. Accessed June 2011.
6. Berman SS, Gentile AT. Impact of secondary procedures in autogenous arteriovenous fistula maturation and maintenance. *J Vasc Surg.* 2001;34:866–871.
7. The Society for Vascular Ultrasound. Evaluation of dialysis access. Vascular Technology Professional Performance Guidelines. http://www.svunet.org/files/positions/0409-Evaluation-of-Dialysis-Access.pdf. Published April 6, 2009. Accessed June 2011.
8. Robbin ML, Lockhart ME. Ultrasound evaluation before and after hemodialysis access. In: Zweibel W, Pellerito J, eds. *Introduction to Vascular Ultrasonography.* 5th ed. Philadelphia, PA: Elsevier Saunders; 2005:325–340.
9. Wellen J, Shenoy S. Ultrasound in vascular access. In: Wilson SE, ed. *Vascular Access Principles and Practice.* 1st ed. Philadelphia, PA: Lippincott Williams & Wilkins; 2010:232–240.

27 Vascular Applications of Ultrasound Contrast Agents

Daniel A. Merton

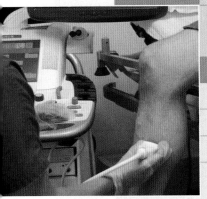

OBJECTIVES

Describe the basic characteristics of ultrasound contrast agents

Describe how ultrasound contrast agents enhance ultrasound images

List the most important characteristics of ultrasound contrast agents

Describe the basic concepts of contrast-specific ultrasound imaging technology

List the most common vascular applications of contrast-enhanced sonography

KEY TERMS

contrast-enhanced sonography | microbubbles | ultrasound contrast agent

GLOSSARY

contrast-enhanced sonography the use of medical ultrasound imaging after administration of an ultrasound contrast agent

microbubbles encapsulated gas-containing structures that are typically smaller than 8 μm in size

ultrasound contrast agent compositions that, after administration, alter the acoustic properties of body tissues (including blood), typically resulting in higher ultrasound signal reflectivity; also known as ultrasound contrast medium

The use of ultrasound (US) contrast agents in the United States is currently limited to echocardiographic applications. However, in other parts of the world, the use of contrast-enhanced sonography (CES) has been established as a valuable imaging procedure for many applications. The use of ultrasound contrast agents (UCAs) that are administered intravenously has been shown to improve the evaluation of blood flow through both large and small vessels as well as through cardiac chambers. CES has been shown to reduce or eliminate some of the current limitations of US imaging. These limitations include contrast resolution on grayscale (B-mode) US, as well as the detection of slow blood flow and flow in very small vessels using color flow imaging (CFI) or pulsed Doppler with spectral analysis. Advances in US equipment technology have resulted in contrast-specific imaging modes that, when combined with UCAs, markedly improve the capabilities of diagnostic sonography and expand its already impressive range of clinical applications.

TYPES OF ULTRASOUND CONTRAST AGENTS

The concept of using contrast agents to enhance the diagnostic potential of US dates back to 1968 when Gramiak and Shah injected agitated saline directly into the ascending aorta and cardiac chambers during echocardiographic examinations.[1] These and subsequent investigations revealed that microbubbles formed by agitation of saline resulted in strong reflections of the ultrasound beam arising from within the normally echo-free lumen of the aorta and chambers of the heart. Currently, intravenously administered agitated saline is used for the so-called bubble study echocardiography examinations, including the assessment of patients with suspected pulmonary hypertension or intracardiac shunts (Fig. 27-1).[2,3] However, microbubbles produced by simple agitation of saline are nonuniform in size, relatively large, and unstable. After peripheral venous

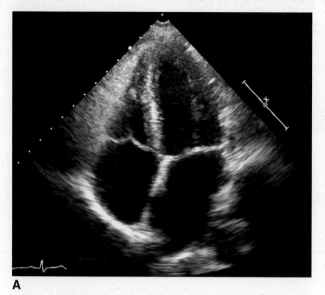

A

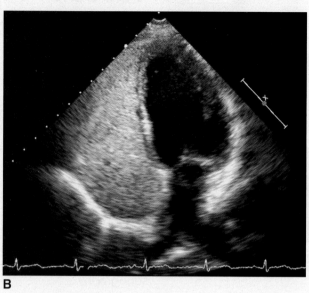

B

Figure 27-1 Use of agitated saline as an ultrasound contrast agent. This patient previously had a stoke and an echocardiogram and was ordered to rule out a patent foramen ovale (PFO). On the grayscale examination, **(A)** no obvious PFO was visualized. After intravenous injection of 10 mL of agitated sterile saline **(B)**, bubbles can be seen filling in the right heart but no bubbles were visualized on the left side of the heart. No PFO was identified. (Image courtesy of Kara Lopresti, RDCS, Thomas Jefferson University Hospital, Philadelphia, PA.)

administration, microbubbles within agitated saline do not persist through passage of the pulmonary and cardiac circulations, which makes this technique unsuitable for sonographic evaluations of the left heart and systemic circulation.

Numerous attempts have been made to encapsulate gas in order to make a more suitable microbubble-based UCA that can be administered intravenously for CES examinations. For a UCA to be clinically useful, it should be nontoxic; have microbubbles or microparticles that are small enough to traverse the pulmonary capillary beds (i.e., less than 8 μm in size) but large enough to reflect US signals; and be stable enough to provide multiple recirculations. A number of agents posses these desirable traits and are commercially available worldwide. Table 27-1 summarizes some of the current clinically available UCAs.

ULTRASOUND CONTRAST AGENT ADMINISTRATION

Typically, contrast is administered in small (<3mL) intravenous (IV) bolus injections via an upper extremity vein which, depending on the agent administered and the patient's characteristics, typically provide several minutes of enhancement. When necessary, a second administration of contrast can be performed. US contrast media can also be administered via slow IV infusion to provide prolonged enhancement. Albrecht and colleagues found that the infusion of contrast-provided enhancement lasting as much as 12 minutes or more compared to just over 2 minutes with a bolus injection.[4] The additional enhancement time provided by the infusion of contrast is useful for difficult and time-consuming evaluations of vessels, such as the renal arteries.

TABLE 27-1			
Ultrasound Contrast Agents			
Contrast Agent	**Manufacturer**	**Microbubble Shell**	**Microbubble Gas**
Optison	GE Healthcare, Princeton, NJ	Human serum albumin	Octafluoropropane (C_3F_8)
Definity	Lantheus Medical Imaging, N. Billerica, MA	Lipid	Octafluoropropane (C_3F_8)
SonoVue	Bracco Imaging SpA, Milan, Italy	Phospholipid	Sulfur hexafluoride (SF_6)

TISSUE-SPECIFIC AND TARGETED AGENTS

The kinetics of UCA microbubbles following an IV injection is complex, and each agent has its own unique characteristics.[5] In general, after an IV administration, blood pool UCAs are contained exclusively in the body's vascular spaces. When a vascular agent's microbubbles are ruptured or otherwise destroyed, the microbubble shell products are metabolized or eliminated by the body, and the gas is exhaled.

Tissue-specific UCAs differ from vascular agents in that the microbubbles of these agents are removed from the blood pool and are taken up by or have an affinity toward specific tissues; for example, a thrombus or the reticuloendothelial system (RES) in the liver and spleen. Thus, to be clinically effective, tissue-specific agents must possess two unique characteristics: an affinity for the targeted tissue and the ability to alter that tissue's sonographic appearance. By changing the signal impedance (or other acoustic characteristics) of normal and abnormal tissues, these agents improve the detection of abnormalities and can permit more specific sonographic diagnoses. Like blood-pool agents, tissue-specific UCAs are typically administered by an IV injection. Some tissue-specific UCAs also enhance the sonographic detection of blood flow so they can be used to improve the detection of flow as well as enhance targeted tissue. Because tissue-specific UCAs target specific types of tissues and their behavior is predictable, they are considered molecular imaging agents.[6]

One type of tissue-specific UCA that is of particular interest for vascular applications is a thrombus-specific agent.[7] Although the administration of a blood-pool UCA can be used to better delineate the functional lumen of both arteries as well as veins, blood-pool agents do not directly enhance the sonographic appearance of thrombi. However, research is ongoing to develop UCAs that attach to fibrin, platelets, or other components of blood clots to enhance their sonographic detection.[8]

THERAPEUTIC AGENTS

Investigations are also ongoing in the development of UCAs that can be used for a variety of therapeutic applications. Typically, therapeutic UCAs have a specific ligand or other binding moiety attached to their shell that has an affinity for a particular receptor (i.e., the target). Researchers have investigated the ability to enhance thrombolysis using acoustic energy with and without nontargeted UCA microbubbles. A significant amount of additional research has been performed using thrombus-targeting UCAs that, when insonated, enhance thrombolysis (referred to as sonothrombolysis).[9,10] This concept, if applied to the intracranial vessels, potentially offers a noninvasive therapy for patients who suffer from embolic stoke.

CONTRAST-SPECIFIC EQUIPMENT MODIFICATIONS

Although microbubble-based UCAs can be used with conventional grayscale US and spectral Doppler to enhance the detection of blood flow, the clinical utility of UCAs is vastly improved by the use of so-called contrast-specific US software. Numerous investigations have been performed to better understand the complex interactions between acoustic energy (i.e., the US beam) and UCA microbubbles, which have, in turn, resulted in modifications to US instrumentation that is specifically designed to exploit these interactions.

HARMONIC IMAGING

Harmonic imaging (HI) can be performed with the same transducers used for conventional US. In HI mode, the US system is configured to receive only echoes at the second harmonic frequency, which is twice the transmit frequency (e.g., 6 MHz for a 3-MHz transducer).[11,12] When subjected to the acoustic energy present in the US field, UCA microbubbles oscillate in size (i.e., they get larger and smaller). The reflected echoes from the oscillating microbubbles contain energy components at the fundamental frequency, as well as at higher and lower harmonics.[13] In HI mode, the echoes from the oscillating microbubbles have a higher signal-to-noise ratio than would be provided by using conventional US so that regions with microbubbles are more easily appreciated visually. Thus, contrast-specific HI provides a means to visualize contrast-enhanced blood flow and contrast-containing tissue using B-mode imaging. These modes obviate the need to use Doppler (which is susceptible to artifacts and other limitations) for the detection of blood flow. Most US equipment manufacturers now have available on their scanners some form of contrast-specific imaging modes, including simultaneous dual displays of the contrast-enhanced image and the conventional US image in real time (Fig. 27-2).

LOW MECHANICAL INDEX IMAGING AND INTERMITTENT IMAGING

During CES examinations, the energy present within the ultrasound beam can have a detrimental effect on contrast microbubbles.[14] Contrast-specific imaging modes are designed to use low acoustic output power (as defined by the mechanical index [MI]) to avoid or minimize microbubble destruction.

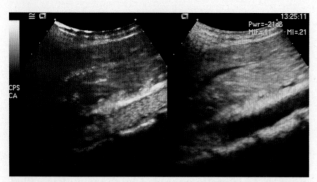

Figure 27-2 Combined conventional and contrast-specific imaging display. This dual image display of a normal aorta demonstrates the conventional grayscale ultrasound image on the *right* and the low-MI contrast-specific (pulse-inversion) mode on the *left*. The combination of contrast with contrast-specific imaging provides the ability to visualize blood flow within the aorta with a higher frame rate and better spatial resolution than is provided by contrast-enhanced color Doppler imaging.

Equipment manufacturers have incorporated intermittent imaging capabilities on their systems to provide an additional option to the user seeking to reduce microbubble destruction during CES examinations. Intermittent imaging reduces the exposure of contrast microbubbles to the acoustic energy and allows additional microbubbles to enter the field between pulses. The additional microbubbles then contribute to an even greater increase in reflectivity of the contrast-containing vessel or tissue than is possible by continuous real-time imaging.

In some situations, it is desirable to rapidly destroy contrast microbubbles in an organ and observe the reperfusion of contrast-containing blood flow into the tissue. Manufacturers have addressed this need by providing "flash echo" modes that, when activated, briefly increase the transmitted acoustic power. After the contrast microbubbles are destroyed, a low-MI imaging mode is used to observe reperfusion of the tissue over time.

CLINICAL APPLICATIONS

The use of CES has been investigated for virtually all clinical applications of sonography.[15-21] Contrast-enhanced sonography has been found to be beneficial for such diverse applications as transcranial Doppler (TCD) evaluations, enhanced assessment of abdominal trauma, and improved detection of vesicoureteral reflux in children.[22-24] Contrast agents have proven particularly valuable for echocardiographic examinations and are routinely used as a rescue tool to salvage otherwise nondiagnostic examinations. Thus, echocardiography remains the most common application of UCAs, and their use for evaluation of

the heart is considered indispensable as a means to improve the delineation of endocardial borders, assess regional wall motion, and detect intracavitary thrombi.[25,26]

The second-most common application of UCAs (after echocardiography) is for the evaluation of liver lesion detection and characterization.[27-31] The sensitivity of CES for the detection and characterization of focal liver lesions has been reported to be comparable to that of more expensive modalities, including contrast-enhanced computed tomography or magnetic resonance imaging.[32]

CES offers several benefits over many other imaging modalities; it does not require the use of ionizing radiation. UCAs have a good safety profile and CES has been found to be cost-effective. These traits are becoming more important in today's health care environment and will likely contribute to continued advances in the use of UCAs for screening, diagnosis, and therapy of a wide range of abnormalities.

Vascular applications of CES include the evaluation of peripheral vessels, the cerebrovascular system, as well as the abdominal and retroperitoneal vasculature.[33-35] Qualitative assessments (i.e., detecting blood flow or areas that lack blood flow) can be performed using conventional color flow imaging modes or, more commonly, contrast-specific imaging modes. When necessary, a characterization of blood flow can be accomplished using spectral Doppler analysis.

PERIPHERAL APPLICATIONS

Limitations to sonographic assessments of peripheral arteries and veins include poor visualization of deeply located and/or small vessels and low velocity or low volume blood flow (Fig. 27-3). The use of CES has been found to facilitate and improve assessments of the peripheral vasculature, including evaluations of patients before and after bypass surgery and increasing the diagnostic confidence level of examination interpretations.

Peripheral Arterial Applications

Signal attenuation resulting from atherosclerotic plaque, which in severe situations causes acoustic shadowing, can limit the visualization of arterial walls as well as blood flow detection and characterization. The addition of UCAs has been found to overcome some of these limitations. Even in cases where the vessel lumen is obscured by shadowing, CES has been found to be helpful in detecting flow in a vessel segment distal to the shadowed area so that a tight stenosis can be differentiated from a complete occlusion.

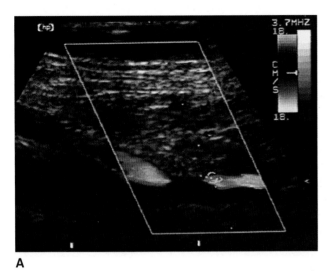
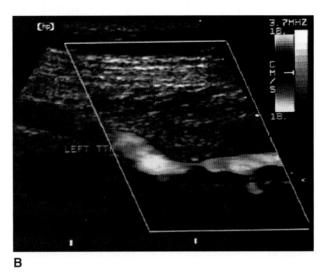

A **B**

Figure 27-3 Contrast-enhanced color Doppler imaging of calf vessel flow. The baseline image **(A)** demonstrates a vessel segment that does not contain detectable blood flow. In postcontrast injection **(B)**, there is continuity of flow through the vessel and a stenosis is seen. (Adapted with permission from Goldberg BB, Raichlen JS, Forsberg F, eds. *Ultrasound Contrast Agents.* 2nd ed. London, England: Informa Healthcare; 2001.)

The ability of UCAs to function as a rescue tool for nondiagnostic conventional Doppler evaluations was confirmed in a study by Langholtz et al.[36] These investigators studied 33 patients with iliac or lower extremity arterial disease. All of the CES examinations were considered adequate in answering the diagnostic question for the patients studied. The group particularly remarked on the improvement of flow visualizations in the iliac artery, which could be seen after contrast despite the presence of overlying bowel gas.

Several recent reports have described the use of CES for assessing patients with peripheral artery disease (PAD).[37,38] A report by Duerschmied et al. described the use of CES to evaluate calf muscle perfusion and vascular collateralization in patients with PAD. The authors concluded that CES could be used to detect perfusion deficits as well as the degree of arterial collateralization in symptomatic PAD patients.

Peripheral Venous Applications

The use of conventional compression sonography has been proven effective for evaluating patients with suspected venous thromboses. Thus, UCAs have not been widely used for peripheral venous applications.

In 1999, Puls et al. described their results using Levovist (administered via an upper extremity IV access site) in 31 patients who had suspected DVT and at least one vein segment that was inadequately imaged with color Doppler imaging.[39] All patients had a venogram for comparison. Baseline CDI was inadequate in 43 of 279 vessel segments and contrast-enhancement was seen in 40 of these 43 segments. Of the 27 vein segments that were confirmed to have

DVT, 18 were detected on baseline imaging, whereas CES identified 25. Five of the seven additional DVTs detected with CES were below the knee. Three iliac vein thromboses were identified with CES, but only one was detected at baseline. The overall diagnostic accuracy increased from 60% (26 of 43 vein segments) at baseline to 86% (37 of 43 vein segments) postcontrast administration.

CEREBROVASCULAR APPLICATIONS

The use of CES for evaluating the cerebrovascular system includes assessments of both the intracranial and extracranial vasculature. Color flow–guided duplex Doppler sonography has become a mainstay for the evaluation of the carotid and vertebral arteries and, in some cases, it is the only imaging examination performed before an endarterectomy. The use of CES for carotid and other relatively large vessel evaluations has the potential to permit direct assessments of the functional lumen and plaque morphology in a similar manner as other imaging modalities (Fig. 27-4). If CES were to be used routinely, it has the potential to reduce the need for additional, more expensive diagnostic imaging studies.

Extracranial Applications

The use of UCAs for evaluating the carotid arteries has been found to enhance Doppler signals and improve visualization of blood flow using contrast-specific imaging modes, resulting in improved delineation of the residual lumen. CES can also be used to differentiate tight stenoses from carotid artery occlusion (Fig. 27-5).

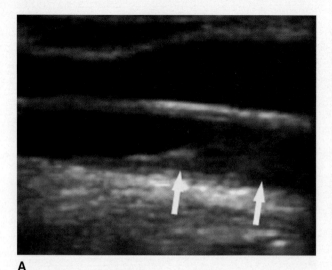

A

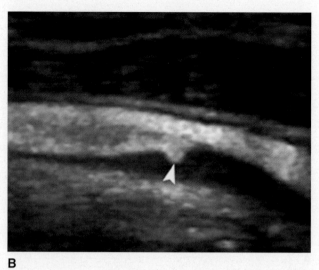

B

Figure 27-4 Improved delineation of plaque ulceration. The baseline scan **(A)** demonstrates an area of plaque along the deep wall of the common carotid artery *(arrows)*. After injection of contrast **(B)**, the functional lumen fills with contrast-containing blood, and an area of ulceration *(arrowhead)* in the plaque is identified. Unlike Doppler sonography, CES provides the ability to directly assess the functional lumen and plaque morphology in a manner similar to conventional angiography and CT angiography. (Image courtesy of Steven Feinstein, MD, Rush University Medical Center, Chicago, IL.)

A published study by Pfister et al. described the use of conventional Doppler US, three-dimensional (3D) US (with and without an UCA), and contrast-enhanced B-flow imaging (GE Healthcare, Waukesha, WI) for presurgical evaluations of the extent of internal carotid artery (ICA) stenosis in 25 patients.[40] The authors found that contrast-enhanced 3D B-flow had the highest correlation (93%) with surgical findings. They also reported that the use of 3D CES was particularly valuable in cases of circular calcifications with severe stenoses and that CES facilitated the assessment of the morphology of ICA plaque.

The use of CES to differentiate ICA stenoses from occlusions was the focus of a report by Hammond et al.[41] They compared the diagnostic accuracy of CES, time-of-flight magnetic resonance angiography (MRA), and contrast-enhanced MRA (CE-MRA) using digital subtraction angiography (DSA) as a reference standard in 31 patients with suspected carotid occlusion on conventional US. The authors concluded that in cases where occlusion is confirmed by either CES or CE-MRA, no additional imaging is required.

Intracranial Applications

Sonographic assessments of the intracranial vasculature is often limited by insufficient acoustic windows, low velocity flow, and signal attenuation through the calvarium. The use of CES for evaluating the intracranial circulation can overcome many problems related to vessel visualization and can expand the clinical utility of transcranial US examinations. The addition of UCAs has been found to improve the ability to evaluate intracranial blood flow, leading to fewer nondiagnostic studies and higher diagnostic confidence levels (Fig. 27-6).

Droste et al. used color flow imaging and pulsed Doppler with spectral analysis to evaluate 47 patients with insufficient acoustic windows before and after administration of SonoVue.[42] A total of 67 temporal windows provided insufficient acoustic access (both temporal windows in 20 patients and 27 unilateral studies). Contrast-enhanced TCD significantly improved the number of intracranial vessel segments that could be evaluated by pulsed Doppler and allowed color flow detection of flow in longer vessel segments. Only 26 middle cerebral arteries could be evaluated using noncontrast TCD compared to 65 with CES.

Specific indications for transcranial CES include assessing patients with arterial occlusions and stenoses, venous thrombosis, and detecting blood flow in solid brain tumors.[43-45] CES has also been used intraoperatively to improve the localization of the feeding arteries and draining veins of arteriovenous malformations.[46]

Evaluation of Carotid Artery Vasa Vasorum and Plaque Neovascularity

The use of CES to evaluate blood flow in the vasa vasorum and carotid artery plaque neovascularization is a new and intriguing area of investigation.[47-50] Some investigators have equated atherosclerotic plaque with a tumor because, like tumors, plaque requires a nutrient-rich blood supply in order to

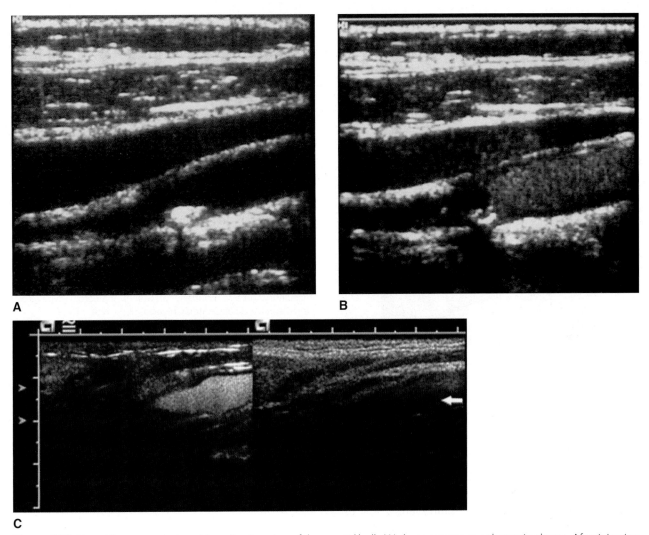

Figure 27-5 Carotid artery occlusion. A baseline imaging of the carotid bulb **(A)** demonstrates an echogenic plaque. After injection of contrast **(B)**, contrast-enhancement of flow is identified in the functional lumen of the common carotid artery, but no enhanced flow is seen distal to the plaque. A carotid occlusion was confirmed with digital subtraction angiography. In a different patient **(C)**, CES using a dual-display with low-MI contrast-specific imaging on the *left* and conventional US on the *right* demonstrates blood flow up to the location of an occlusion. Note that the presence of contrast causes acoustic shadowing on the conventional image *(arrow)*. (**A** and **B** Adapted with permission from Goldberg BB, Raichlen JS, Forsberg F, eds. *Ultrasound Contrast Agents.* 2nd ed. London, England: Informa Healthcare; 2001. **C** Courtesy of David Cosgrove, FRCR, Hammersmith Hospital, London, UK.)

grow. Studies have shown that plaque neovascularization is predominantly derived from the arterial wall vasa vasorum with changes to the vascular morphology preceding the development of obvious plaque and luminal narrowing. These early vascular changes can be identified using CES (Fig. 27-7).

In the future, the use of CES for evaluating the carotid artery vasa vasorum and plaque neovascularization may prove to be a valuable, noninvasive method to identify patients who have vulnerable plaques and to better determine a patient's risk of cardiovascular events. The use of CES for this application could also complement sonographic measurements of the intima-media thickness as a

means to monitor the response to antiatherosclerotic therapies.

ABDOMINAL AND RETROPERITONEAL APPLICATIONS

Abdominal vascular applications of sonography include the evaluation of the aorta and its branches, veins of the systemic as well as portal venous system, and blood flow in abdominal organs. The use of CES has been investigated for all of these applications and has been found to be highly beneficial in many. The use of CES has also improved the use of sonography for evaluating organ perfusion and tumor characterizations.

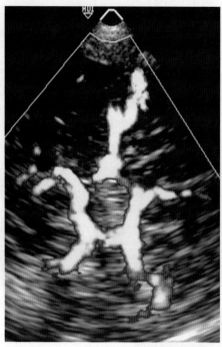

Figure 27-6 Contrast-enhanced color Doppler imaging of intracranial vessels. (Image courtesy of Jeff Powers, PhD, Philips Ultrasound, bothell, WA)

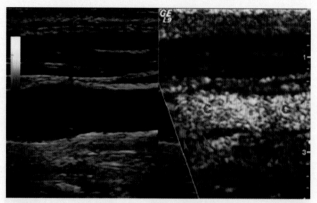

Figure 27-7 Neovascularization of the carotid artery vasa vasorum. This dual image display shows the conventional US image on the *left* and the low-MI contrast-specific image on the *right*. Contrast-enhanced blood flow is seen within the functional lumen of the carotid artery *(C)* and tiny vessels within the adventitial vasa vasorum *(arrowheads)* consistent with neovascularity. (Image courtesy of Steven Feinstein, MD, Rush University Medical Center, Chicago, IL.)

Hepatic Applications

Ultrasound contrast agents have shown the potential to improve the accuracy of hepatic sonography, including enhanced detection and characterization of hepatic masses and improved detection of intrahepatic and extrahepatic blood flow. Contrast-enhanced sonography has been shown to improve the detection of hepatic blood flow in normal subjects as well as in patients with liver disease and portal hypertension (PHT).[51–53] Contrast-enhanced sonography has also been used effectively for assessing flow through transjugular intrahepatic portosystemic shunt (TIPS) (Fig. 27-8).[54,55]

Renal Artery Stenosis

The sonographic evaluation of the main renal arteries and intrarenal vessels in patients with suspected renal artery stenosis (RAS) is limited by factors including the deep location of the vessels, the overlying bowel, and patient obesity. Furthermore, there may be limited sonographic windows to view the renal arteries, and these windows may not be in optimal locations from which to obtain adequate Doppler angles. A significant number of patients have anatomical variations of the renal vasculature, including duplicate or accessory renal arteries, and these variations can be very difficult to identify with conventional US. Thus, sonographic examinations for RAS are extremely operator dependent and are often time consuming.

By improving the signal intensity of Doppler flow signals and increasing the likelihood of obtaining adequate Doppler flow information, UCAs have been found to be helpful during examinations of patients with suspected RAS (Fig. 27-9).[56,57] Thus, in cases where the renal arteries are not well visualized or the spectral waveforms are of poor quality, administrating a UCA can potentially reduce the number of technically inadequate or otherwise nondiagnostic examinations, as well as reduce examination time.

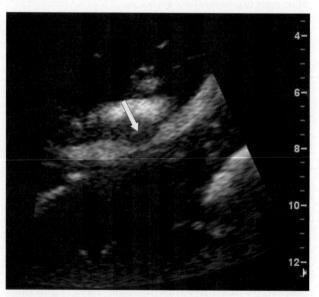

Figure 27-8 CES of a transjugular intrahepatic portosystemic shunt (TIPS). A stenosis *(arrow)* is identified in this TIPS using a contrast-specific grayscale CES. (Image courtesy of Antonio Sergio Marcelino, MD, Sirio-Libanes Hospital and Cancer Institute of University of Sao Paulo, Sao Paulo, Brazil.)

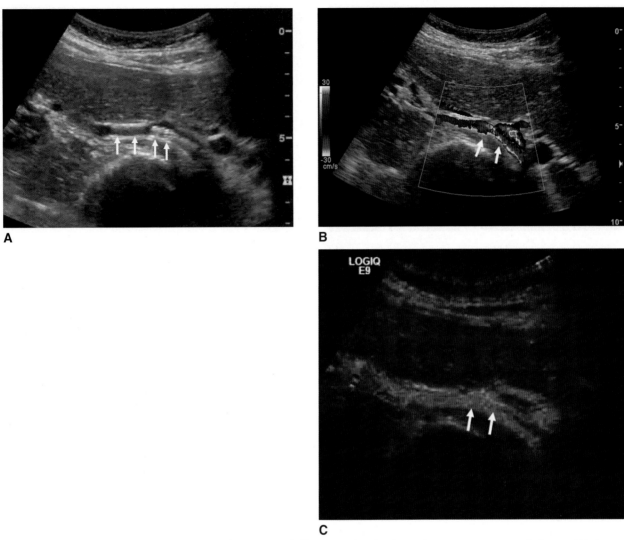

Figure 27-9 Renal artery stent evaluation in a patient with fibromuscular dysplasia. A precontrast grayscale image **(A)** demonstrates two echogenic stents *(arrows)* within this patient's right renal artery. Evaluation of blood flow through the stented vessel segment using color Doppler imaging **(B)** suggested the presence of disturbed flow; however, the CES evaluation **(C)** indicated no flow abnormality. (Images courtesy of Hans-Peter Weskott, MD, Klinikum Region Hanover, Hanover, Germany.)

Organ Transplants

Sonography is routinely used to evaluate renal, hepatic, and pancreatic transplants. The modality is often employed as a first-line examination in the immediate postsurgical period as well as for serial studies to assess organ viability. After organ transplantation, sonography is used to detect postsurgical fluid collections, to identify urinary or bile obstructions, and to assess blood flow to and from the transplanted organ. Conventional sonography is also useful in evaluating blood flow within the organ, but it does not have an adequate level of sensitivity to detect flow at the microvascular level (i.e., tissue perfusion). When a vascular abnormality is suspected, angiography or contrast-enhanced CT may be necessary to obtain a definitive diagnosis.[58] However, angiography is invasive, CT requires ionizing radiation, and the administration of contrast media required for these exams may be contraindicated in renal-compromised patients.

The enhanced detection of blood flow provided by CES improves the assessment of blood flow in the arteries and veins that supply the transplant, the host vessels to which these vessels are anastomosed, as well as the parenchyma of transplanted organs (Fig. 27-10). CES has also been found to improve the ability to detect ischemic regions within native and transplanted organs.[59-61]

Several published reports have described the use of CES for the evaluation of liver transplant recipients.[62,63] Sindhu et al. reported on the use of CES to examine 31 liver transplant patients with suspected hepatic artery thrombosis and compared the results to arteriography or follow-up US. They reported that

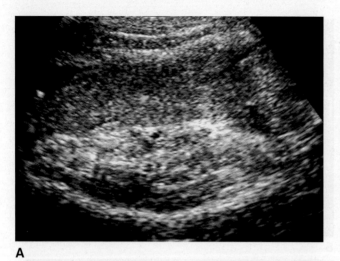
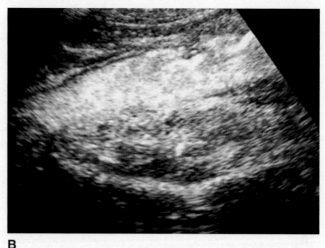

A   **B**

Figure 27-10 Pancreatic transplant evaluation. Baseline **(A)** and postcontrast **(B)** images of a transplanted pancreas. The homogeneous enhancement seen with the addition of contrast confirms normal vascularity in the gland. (Image courtesy of Antonio Sergio Marcelino, MD, Sirio-Libanes Hospital and Cancer Institute of University of Sao Paulo, Sao Paulo, Brazil.)

in approximately 63% of studies, CES could have obviated the need for arteriography.

Aortic Graft and Stent Surveillance

The use of CES is gaining attention as a viable alternative to other diagnostic imaging examinations used to evaluate patients after endovascular aneurysm repair (EVAR) of abdominal aortic aneurysms.[35,64-65] Endoleaks with persistent perigraft flow within the aneurysm sac are common complications of EVAR procedures. Thus, strict postprocedure surveillance of these patients is required to enable the early detection of endoleaks. Although CT angiography is

commonly used as a surveillance method, the use of CT contrast is contraindicated in some patients (e.g., those with chronic renal insufficiency), and repeated computed tomographic angiography (CTA) examinations cause high levels of radiation exposure. Because of the safety of UCAs and the lack of potentially harmful ionizing radiation, CES offers a viable alternative to conventional angiography and CTA, particularly when CTA is contraindicated and serial studies are required. Furthermore, the ability to assess blood flow in real time using CES has been found to improve the characterization of endoleaks (Fig. 27-11).

In one published study, CES was used for the surveillance of aortic stent grafts. Thirty patients were serially

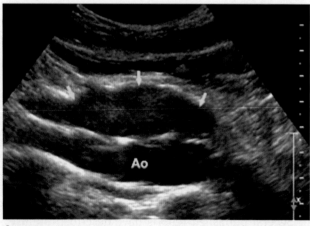
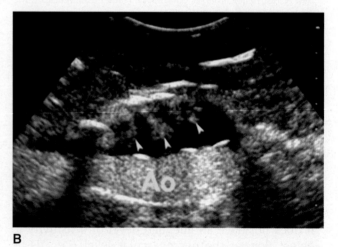

A   **B**

Figure 27-11 Aortic endograft evaluation. Using conventional grayscale US **(A)**, a fluid-filled region *(arrows)* anterior to the aorta (Ao) was identified, but it was difficult to determine the nature of this fluid. A CES study **(B)** demonstrated flow within the functional lumen and small amounts of contrast-containing blood *(arrowheads)* within the fluid pocket consistent with a small leak of the graft. (Image courtesy of Carlos Ventura, MD, Ultrasound Division, Albert Einstein Hospital and Radiology Institute of University of Sao Paulo, Sao Paulo Brazil.)

evaluated with CES, and the results were compared to either CTA or magnetic resonance angiography (MRA) as the gold standard. All CTA/MRA-detected endoleaks were detected by CES, yielding a 100% sensitivity.

Other Abdominal Applications

Other common abdominal/retroperitoneal applications of US include assessing flow in the mesenteric arteries for mesenteric ischemia; the aorta and iliac arteries to evaluate suspected aneurysms, stenoses, or dissections; and the inferior vena cava to evaluate filters or thromboses (Fig. 27-12). Often, these examinations are limited by the presence of overlying bowel and bowel gas, or the affects of signal attenuation due to the deep location of the vessels. Vascular UCAs have been used with success to improve assessments of the abdominal vasculature and blood flow.[66]

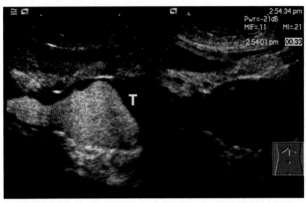

Figure 27-12 CES of an abdominal aortic aneurysm (AAA). The image on the *left*, obtained using low-MI contrast-specific imaging, demonstrates an area within the AAA that does not contain flow (T) consistent with intraluminal thrombus. The thrombus is not seen well on the conventional US image (*right*). (Image courtesy of David Cosgrove, FRCR, Hammersmith Hospital, London, UK.)

SUMMARY

Two UCAs are currently being marketed in the United States: Optison and Definity. However, as of this writing, they are approved by the Food and Drug Administration only for echocardiographic applications. In the future, additional agents and/or clinical applications of existing agents are likely to become available. US contrast agents have been shown to improve the detection of blood flow in large and small vessels throughout the body as well as to improve sonographic detection and characterization of tumors, inflammation, and other abnormalities in many anatomical areas.

The enhancement capabilities of UCAs have been shown to have the ability to salvage nondiagnostic US examinations and render them diagnostic. The use of UCAs has also resulted in new applications of the modality that were not possible without them. Improvements in US technology that exploit the acoustic behavior of contrast microbubbles are further improving the clinical capabilities of contrast-enhanced sonography. The use of CES is expected to increase as sonography becomes more omnipresent throughout medical disciplines.

Critical Thinking Questions

1. A hypertensive patient is referred to the noninvasive vascular laboratory to rule out renal artery stenosis. During the examination, the main renal arteries are not well visualized using color Doppler imaging, and the sonographer is having difficulty obtaining adequate spectral Doppler waveforms. How could the administration of an ultrasound contrast agent help in this examination?

2. A patient who received an aortic endograft presents to the emergency department 3-weeks postsurgery with a sudden onset of abdominal pain and an abdominal bruit. The emergency medicine physician is concerned that the patient's symptoms may be related to a complication from the recent aortic repair. A sonogram performed in the emergency department demonstrates a fluid collection with what appears to be color flow signals immediately adjacent to the aorta. However, the sonographer is having difficulty determining if the color signals are the result of flash artifacts from the pulsatile aorta or the result of true flow in the collection. How could the administration of an ultrasound contrast agent help in this important differentiation?

REFERENCES

1. Gramiak R, Shah PM. Echocardiography of the aortic root. *Invest Radiol.* 1968;3:356–366.
2. Lopes LR, Loureiro MJ, Miranda R, et al. The usefulness of contrast during exercise echocardiography for the assessment of systolic pulmonary pressure. *Cardiovasc Ultrasound.* 2008;6:51.
3. Harrah JD, O'Boyle PS, Piantadosi CA. Underutilization of echocardiography for patent foramen ovale in divers with serious decompression sickness. *Undersea Hyperb Med.* 2008;35(3):207–211.
4. Albrecht T, Urbank A, Mahler M, et al. Prolongation and optimization of Doppler enhancement with a microbubble US contrast agent by using continuous infusion: preliminary experience. *Radiology.* 1998;207:339–347.
5. Blomley MJK, Harvey CJ, Eckersley RJ, et al. Contrast kinetics and Doppler intensitometry. In: Goldberg BB, Raichlen JS, Forsberg F, eds. *Ultrasound Contrast Agents: Basic Principles and Clinical Applications.* 2nd ed. London, England: Martin Dunitz Ltd.; 2001;81–89.
6. Miller JC, Thrall JH. Clinical molecular imaging. *J Am Coll Radiol.* 2004;1(1 suppl):4–23.
7. Unger EC, Wu Q, McCreery T, et al. Thrombus-specific contrast agents for imaging and thrombolysis. In: Goldberg BB, Raichlen JS, Forsberg F, eds. *Ultrasound Contrast Agents: Basic Principles and Clinical Applications.* 2nd ed. London, England: Martin Dunitz Ltd.; 2001;337–345.
8. Takeuchi M, Ogunyankin K, Pandian NG, et al. Enhanced visualization of intravascular and left atrial appendage thrombus with the use of a thrombus-targeting ultrasonographic contrast agent (MRX-408A1): in vivo experimental echocardiographic studies. *J Am Soc Echocardiogr.* 1999;12:1015–1021.
9. Laing ST, McPherson DD. Cardiovascular therapeutic uses of targeted ultrasound contrast agents. *Cardiovasc Res.* 2009;83(4):626–635.
10. Molina CA, Barreto AD, Tsivgoulis G, et al. Transcranial ultrasound in clinical sonothrombolysis (TUCSON) trial. *Ann Neurol.* 2009;66(1):28–38.
11. Forsberg F, Liu JB, Rawool NM, et al. Gray-scale and color Doppler flow harmonic imaging with proteinaceous microspheres. *Radiology.* 1995;197(P):403.
12. Kono Y, Mattrey RT. Harmonic imaging with contrast microbubbles. In: Goldberg BB, Raichlen JS, Forsberg F, eds. *Ultrasound Contrast Agents: Basic Principles and Clinical Applications.* 2nd ed. London, England: Martin Dunitz Ltd.; 2001;37–46.
13. Forsberg F, Picolli CW, Merton DA, et al. Breast lesions: imaging with contrast-enhanced sub-harmonic US: initial experiences. *Radiology.* 2007;244(3):718–726.
14. Harvey CJ, Blomley MJK, Cosgrove DO. Acoustic emission imaging. In: Goldberg BB, Raichlen JS, Forsberg F, ed. *Ultrasound Contrast Agents: Basic Principles and Clinical Applications.* 2nd ed. London, England: Martin Dunitz Ltd.; 2001;71–80.
15. Lencioni R, ed. *Enhancing the Role of Ultrasound with Contrast Agents.* Milan, Italy: Springer-Verlag; 2006.
16. Quaia E, ed. *Contrast Media in Ultrasonography: Basic Principles and Clinical Applications.* Berlin, Germany: Springer-Verlag; 2005.
17. Zamorano JL, Fernandez MA. *Contrast Echocardiography in Clinical Practice.* Milan, Italy: Springer-Verlag; 2004.
18. Albrecht T, Thorelius L, Solbiati L, et al. *Contrast-Enhanced Ultrasound in Clinical Practice: Liver, Prostate, Pancreas, Kidney and Lymph Nodes.* Milan, Italy: Springer-Verlag; 2005.
19. Liu JB, Merton DA, Goldberg BB. Ultrasound contrast agents. In: McGahan JP, Forsberg F, Goldberg BB, ed. *Diagnostic Ultrasound: A Logical Approach.* 2nd ed. New York, NY: Informa Healthcare; 2008.
20. Merton DA. Abdominal Applications of Ultrasound Contrast Agents. In: Ansert SL, ed. *Textbook of Diagnostic Ultrasonography.* 6th ed. Philadelphia, PA: Mosby Elsevier Inc.; 2006.
21. Abramowicz JS. Ultrasound contrast media: has the time come in obstetrics and gynecology? *J Ultrasound Med.* 2005;24:517–531.
22. Llompart-Pou JA, Abadal JM, Velasco J, et al. Contrast-enhanced transcranial color sonography in the diagnosis of cerebral circulatory arrest. *Transplant Proc.* 2009;41:1466–1468.
23. Valentino M, Serra C, Zironi G, et al. Blunt abdominal trauma: emergency contrast-enhanced sonography for detection of solid organ injuries. *Am J Radiol.* 2006;186:1361–1367.
24. Papadopoulou F, Anthopoulou A, Siomou E, et al. Harmonic voiding urosonography with a second-generation contrast agent for the diagnosis of vesicoureteral reflux. *Pediatr Radiolol.* 2009;39:239–244.

25. Grayburn PA, Raichlen JS. Evaluation of the heart at rest. In: Goldberg BB, Raichlen JS, Forsberg F, ed. *Ultrasound Contrast Agents: Basic Principles and Clinical Applications*. 2nd ed. London, England: Martin Dunitz Ltd.; 2001:143–154.

26. Nathan S, Feinstein SB. Evaluation of the heart during exercise and pharmacologic stress. In: Goldberg BB, Raichlen JS, Forsberg F, ed. *Ultrasound Contrast Agents: Basic Principles and Clinical Applications*. 2nd ed. London, England: Martin Dunitz Ltd.; 2001:155–164.

27. Luo W, Numata K, Morimoto M, et al. Role of Sonazoid-enhanced three-dimensional ultrasonography in the evaluation of percutaneous radiofrequency ablation of hepatocellular carcinoma. *Eur J Radiol.* 2010;75:91–97.

28. Claudon M, Cosgrove D, Albrecht T, et al. Guidelines and good clinical practice recommendations for contrast enhanced ultrasound (CE-US)—update 2008. *Ultraschall Med.* 2008;29(1):28–44.

29. Burns P, Wilson S. Focal liver masses: enhancement patterns on contrast-enhanced images —concordance of US scans with CT scans and MR images. *Radiology.* 2007;242:162–174.

30. Strobel D, Raeker S, Martus P, et al. Phase inversion harmonic imaging versus contrast-enhanced power Doppler ultrasound for the characterization of focal liver lesions. *Int J Colorectal Dis.* 2003;18(1):63–72.

31. Catala V, Nicolau C, Vilana R, et al. Characterization of focal liver lesions: comparative study of contrast-enhanced ultrasound versus spiral computed tomography. *Eur Radiol.* 2007;17(4):1066–1073.

32. Trillaud H, Bruel JM, Valette PJ, et al. Characterization of focal liver lesions with SonoVue® enhanced sonography: international multicenter-study in comparison to CT and MRI. *World J Gastroenterol.* 2009;15(30):3748–3756.

33. Needleman L, Merton DA. *Vascular Applications of US Contrast Vascular applications of US contrast is the title of the chapter within this book.* In: Goldberg BB, Raichlen JS, Forsberg F, eds. *Ultrasound Contrast Agents: Basic Principles and Clinical Applications. 2nd ed.* London, England: Martin Dunitz Publishing; 2001.

34. Robbin ML. The utility of contrast in the extra-cranial carotid ultrasound examination. In: Goldberg BB, Raichlen JS, Forsberg F, ed. *Ultrasound Contrast Agents: Basic Principles and Clinical Applications.* 2nd ed. London, England: Martin Dunitz Ltd.; 2001:239–252.

35. Pfister K, Rennert J, Uller W, et al. Contrast harmonic imaging ultrasound and perfusion imaging for surveillance after endovascular abdominal aneurysm repair regarding detection and characterization of suspected endoleaks. *Clin Hemorheol Microcirc.* 2009;43:119–128.

36. Langholtz J, Schiel R, Schurman R, et al. Contrast enhancement in leg vessels. *Clin Radiol.* 1996;51:31–34.

37. Lindner JR, Womack L, Barrett EJ, et al. Limb stress-rest perfusion imaging with contrast ultrasound for the assessment of peripheral arterial disease severity. *JACC Cardiovasc Imag.* 2008;1(3):343–350.

38. Duerschmied D, Zhou Q, Rink E, et al. Simplified contrast ultrasound accurately reveals muscle perfusion deficits and reflects collateralization in PAD. *Atherosclerosis.* 2009;202(2): 505–512.

39. Puls R, Hosten N, Bock JS, et al. Signal-enhanced color Doppler sonography of deep venous thrombosis in the lower limbs and pelvis. *J Ultrasound Med.* 1999;18:185–190.

40. Pfister K, Rennert J, Greiner B, et al. Pre-surgical evaluation of ICA-stenosis using 3D power Doppler, 3D color coded Doppler sonography, 3D B-flow and contrast enhanced B-flow in correlation to CTA/MRA: first clinical results. *Clin Hemorheol Microcirc.* 2009;41(2):103–116.

41. Hammond CJ, McPherson SJ, Patel JV, et al. Assessment of apparent internal carotid occlusion on ultrasound: prospective comparison of contrast-enhanced ultrasound, magnetic resonance angiography and digital subtraction angiography. *Eur J Vasc Endovasc Surg.* 2008;35(4):405–412.

42. Droste DW, Boehm T, Ritter MA, et al. Benefit of echocontrast-enhanced transcranial arterial color-coded duplex ultrasound. *Cerebrovasc Dis.* 2005;20(5):332–336.

43. Kunz A, Hahn G, Mucha D, et al. Echo-enhanced transcranial color-coded duplex sonography in the diagnosis of cerebrovascular events: a validation study. *AJNR Am J Neuroradiol.* 2006;27:2122–2127.

44. Bogdahn U, Holscher T, Schlachetzki F. Transcranial color-coded duplex sonography (TCCS). In: Goldberg BB, Raichlen JS, Forsberg F, ed. *Ultrasound Contrast Agents: Basic Principles and Clinical Application.* 2nd ed. London, England: Martin Dunitz Ltd.; 2001:253–265.

45. Droste DW. Clinical utility of contrast-enhanced ultrasound in neurosonology. *Eur Neur.* 2008;59(S1):2–8.

46. Wang Y, Wang Y, Wang Y, et al. Intraoperative real-time contrast-enhanced ultrasound angiography: a new adjunct in the surgical treatment of arteriovenous malformations. *Neurosurg.* 2007;107:959–964.

47. Shah F, Balan P, Weinberg M, et al. Contrast-enhanced ultrasound imaging of atherosclerotic carotid plaque neovascularization: a new surrogate marker of atherosclerosis? *Vasc Med.* 2007;12(4):291–297.

48. Magnoni M, Coli S, Marrocco-Trischitta MM, et al. Contrast-enhanced ultrasound imaging of periadventitial vasa vasorum in human carotid arteries. *Eur J Echocardiogr.* 2009;10: 260–264.

49. Coli S, Magnoni M, Sangiorgi G, et al. Contrast-enhanced ultrasound imaging of intraplaque neovascularization in carotid arteries: correlation with histology and plaque echogenicity. *J Am Coll Cardiol.* 2008;52(3):223–230.

50. Staub D, Patel MB, Tibrewala A, et al. Vasa vasorum and plaque neovascularization on contrast-enhanced carotid ultrasound imaging correlates with cardiovascular disease and past cardiovascular events. *Stroke.* 2010;4(1):41–47.

51. Albrecht T, Blomley MJ, Cosgrove DO, et al. Non-invasive diagnosis of hepatic cirrhosis by transit-time analysis of an ultrasound contrast agent. *Lancet.* 1999;353:1579–1583.

52. Lee KH, Choi BI, Kim KW, et al. Contrast-enhanced dynamic ultrasonography of the liver: optimization of hepatic arterial phase in normal volunteers. *Abdom Imaging.* 2003;28(5): 652–656.

53. Sellars ME, Sidhu PS, Heneghan M, et al. Infusions of microbubbles are more cost-effective than bolus injections in Doppler studies of the portal vein: a quantitative comparison of normal volunteers and patients with cirrhosis. *Radiology.* 2000;217(P):396.

54. Skjoldbye B, Weislander S, Struckmann J, et al. Doppler ultrasound assessment of TIPS patency and function- the need for echo enhancers. *Acta Radiol.* 1998;39:675–679.

55. Uggowitzer MM, Hausegger KA, Machan L. Echo-enhanced Doppler sonography in the evaluation of transjugular intrahepatic portosystemic shunts: clinical applications of a new transpulmonary US contrast agent. *Radiology.* 1996;201(P):266.

56. Missouris CG, Allen CM, Balen FG, et al. Non-invasive screening for renal artery stenosis with ultrasound contrast enhancement. *J Hypertens.* 1996;14(4):519–524.

57. Needleman L. Review of a new ultrasound contrast agent: EchoGen emulsion. *Appl Rad.* 1997;26(S):8–12.

58. Karamehic J, Scoutt LM, Tabakovic M, et al. Ultrasonography in organs transplantation. *Med Arh.* 2004;58(1 suppl 2):107–108.

59. Benozzi L, Cappelli G, Granito M, et al. Contrast-enhanced sonography in early kidney graft dysfunction. *Transplant Proc.* 2009;41(4):1214–1215.

60. Boggi U, Morelli L, Amorese G, et al. Contribution of contrast-enhanced ultrasonography to nonoperative management of segmental ischemia of the head of a pancreas graft. *Am J Transplant.* 2009;9(2):413–418.

61. Faccioli N, Crippa S, Bassi C, et al. Contrast-enhanced ultrasonography of the pancreas. *Pancreatology.* 2009;9(5):560–566.

62. Leutoff UC, Scharf J, Richter GM, et al. Use of ultrasound contrast medium Levovist in aftercare of liver transplant patients: improved vascular imaging in color Doppler ultrasound. *Radiology.* 1998;38:399–404.

63. Sidhu PS, Shaw AS, Ellis SM, et al. Microbubble ultrasound contrast in the assessment of hepatic artery patency following liver transplantation: role in reducing frequency of hepatic artery arteriography. *Eur Radiol.* 2004;14(1):21–30.

64. Giannoni MF, Palombo G, Sbarigia E, et al. Contrast-enhanced ultrasound for aortic stent-graft surveillance. *J Endovasc Ther.* 2003;10(2):208–217.

65. Iezzi R, Cotroneo AR, Basilico R, et al. Endoleaks after endovascular repair of abdominal aortic aneurysm: value of CEUS. *Abdom Imaging.* 2010;35(1):106–114.

66. Oka MA, Rubens DJ, Strang JG. Ultrasound contrast agent in evaluation of abdominal vessels. *J Ultrasound Med.* 2001;20:S84.

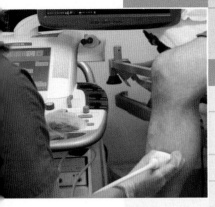

28 | Quality Assurance Statistics

Terrence D. Case

OBJECTIVES

Define the term "gold standard"

Describe the common statistical terms including sensitivity, specificity, and accuracy

Define other commonly used statistical parameters

Calculate basic statistical values using a chi-square test

KEY TERMS

accuracy | gold standard | negative predictive value | positive predictive value | sensitivity | specificity

GLOSSARY

accuracy the overall percentage of correct results

gold standard a well-established and reliable testing parameter, which for vascular disease, is often angiography

sensitivity the ability of a test to detect disease

specificity the ability of a test to correctly identify a normal result

---

Ultrasound is technology that is safe and reliable when used by well-trained sonographers in a department that is focused on quality assurance (QA). QA refers to a program for the systematic monitoring and evaluation of the various aspects of vascular testing to ensure that standards of quality are being met. However, it has taken years of research and development to convince physicians and other health care providers that ultrasound technology alone is accurate in the assessment of vascular disease. To achieve that confidence, the ultrasound profession relied on statistics to demonstrate the effectiveness of sonography and Doppler in the assessment of vascular disease.

STATISTICS

Statistics is the science of making effective use of numerical data relating to groups of individuals or experiments. It deals with all aspects of the collection, analysis, and interpretation of such data. In addition, statistics is used in the planning of the collection of data in terms of the design of surveys and experiments. This chapter will briefly review some of the common terminology and systems used to determine the accuracy of vascular ultrasound reports or studies.

COMPARING DIAGNOSTIC TESTS

The "Gold Standard"

Medical science has borrowed the term "gold standard" to compare one form of a newer diagnostic test with another that is well-established and reliable. The "gold standard" in vascular imaging typically refers to the angiogram (or in some cases, a venogram). The angiogram has a long history of accuracy and, therefore, all newer types of vascular imaging must be compared to it to determine the presence or absence of disease and the extent to which it presents. However, there are some risks with angiography, which may be as minimal as a hematoma at the insertion site to allergic reaction to the dye, which could end with either a stroke or even death. In medicine, the benefits must always outweigh the risks, and although ultrasound is considered safe and accurate now, it had to be first compared with the gold standard in order to establish accuracy. Ideally, a vascular ultrasound would match the gold standard 100% of the time, but this is often not the case. There are various common measurements employed to compare testing results to a gold standard.

True Positives

True positives (TPs) are the number of studies performed by ultrasound, which state that disease is present, and the gold standard agrees with the ultrasound findings. For example, an ultrasound shows a dilated noncompressible femoral vein with no flow. The venogram demonstrates an occluded femoral vein, and the physician's diagnosis is a deep venous thrombosis (DVT). All are in agreement that disease is present; therefore, a true positive.

True Negatives

True negatives (TNs) are the number of negative findings reported by ultrasound that were also reported negative by the gold standard. For example, the ultrasound indicates no evidence of echogenic plaque and normal flow velocities in the proximal internal carotid artery. An arteriogram does not identify any disease, and the physician's interpretation is no internal carotid artery disease. Thus, all are in agreement that no disease is present; therefore, a true negative.

False Positives

Unfortunately, there are some cases where the ultrasound and gold standard do not agree. When using arteriography as the gold standard, in almost every case, those findings represent the correct findings. There may be a situation where the duplex ultrasound demonstrates velocity elevations consistent with a stenosis, but the arteriogram finds no disease. Another example may be a case where the sonographer fails to properly compress a vein, which is then interpreted as an occluded vein. Subsequent venography demonstrates a patent, thrombus-free vessel. Fortunately, disagreements are relatively rare but statistics is necessary to help identify these inaccuracies. When these mismatches occur, studies can be carefully reviewed to determine the specific source of the error.

The examples in the preceding paragraph are false positive (FP) results. False positives are studies that are reported positive but found to be negative by the gold standard. Another variation of the FP result could occur when a carotid ultrasound study met the criteria for a 50% to 79% stenosis, but the arteriogram only detected a 40% stenosis. This is a false positive; however, it is important here for both radiology and ultrasound to be clear about what an FP constitutes. A difference of 5% error in velocity measurement could put the findings in one category or another. Although the categories are significantly different and could affect medical management, the actual difference is relatively small.

False Negatives

False negatives (FNs) state that a study was normal when the gold standard identifies disease. An example of a false negative would be if a normal aortic diameter is reported by ultrasound, but the arteriogram shows a tortuous aorta with a 3.0 cm abdominal aortic aneurysm (AAA). Some might argue that this may be a relatively minor error and would have little clinical significance. But a report stating "No DVT in femoral vein" that turns out to be a false negative may be life threatening. Clearly, the sonographer wants to have a high degree of true positives and true negatives, with no or very few false negatives and false positives.

ACCURACY

QA statistics use the calculations of TN, TP, FN, and FP in order to determine other indicators that describe the results of a test. Accuracy is one such indicator. Accuracy can be thought of as the degree of "closeness" of something to its actual value. For example, in the vascular laboratory, we gather imaging and Doppler data to identify carotid artery disease into a category such as 50% to 79%, or 80% to 99% stenosis. We typically then compare our results (duplex findings) with the gold standard (arteriogram results) to see how "close" the ultrasound findings are to the actual value (degree stenosis). Accuracy is the percentage of correct results. Not only is it important to be accurate in identifying disease when it is present, but also to identify normal vessels when disease is absent. Accuracy is calculated as the total number of correct tests divided by the total number of all tests.

SENSITIVITY

Sensitivity measures the proportion of actual positives studies, which are correctly identified. It is the ability to identify disease when disease is present. When positive ultrasound studies correlate closely with positive arteriogram findings, the test is said to have good sensitivity. Ultrasound is very good at determining if DVT is present in the lower extremities but is of no use in detecting pneumonia in the lungs. Here, one might say that ultrasound is very sensitive for DVT, but has no sensitivity for detecting pneumonia.

Sensitivity is calculated by taking the true positives results and dividing these by the all-positive results as determined by the gold standard.

SPECIFICITY

As sonographers, we know it is not only important to identify disease when it is present but also to be certain that when we fail to find disease, no disease truly exists. Physicians rely heavily on the ultrasound reports and, more often than not, manage the patient based on the sonographer's findings alone. However, in the early 1980s when duplex ultrasound was first used to assess the presence or absence of DVT, ultrasound studies were in almost every case followed up by a venogram. After time, the consistency of accuracy and reliability of duplex ultrasound to identify or rule out DVT eventually led to the virtual end of venograms. Using duplex ultrasound to rule out DVT is said to have good specificity. Specificity is the ability of a test to identify something as normal. It is calculated by dividing the number of true negative results by all the negative results as identified by the gold standard.

RELIABILITY

Reliability is the consistency of obtaining similar results under similar circumstances. In a sense, it is accuracy over a period of time. A laboratory or ultrasound department is reliable when the results of the tests produced are consistently accurate. Once the medical community determines that a department produces reliable results on a consistent basis, confidence in the department is ensured.

POSITIVE PREDICTIVE VALUE

The positive predictive value (PPV) is the proportion of patients with positive test results that are correctly identified. It is an important measure of a diagnostic method, such as ultrasound, that provides the probability that a positive test reflects the underlying disease for which the test is being conducted. In other words, of all the positive venous studies in a department, the PPV is the percentage that correctly predicted a DVT based on the gold standard. This is calculated as the number of true positive studies divided by all the positive studies (true positives plus false positives).

NEGATIVE PREDICTIVE VALUE

The negative predictive value (NPV) is the proportion of negative test results when there is no underlying disease present. It is an important measure of a diagnostic method, such as ultrasound, that provides the probability that a negative test reflects the absence of disease. If this test states that there is no arterial obstruction of the arteries in the lower extremity, one can be confident that there is no disease present if the negative predictive value is high.[1]

THE CHI-SQUARE TEST

The chi-square (pronounced "kye" as in sky) is a statistical test that, in sum, compares the difference between what you "expect" and what you actually "observe."[2] If velocities meet a criteria of 50% to 79%, that is what you would expect to see on the

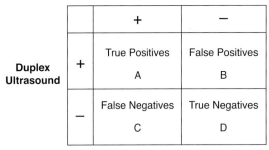

Figure 28-1 Basic design of a chi-square table comparing observed results (angiography) with expected results (duplex ultrasound). The cells of the chi-square are identified, indicating the appropriate placement of true positive, false positive, true negative, and false negative data.

arteriogram. What is observed is the arteriogram that either confirms or disproves your expectations.

The more tests that are performed that agree with the gold standard or the narrower the difference between what is expected and what is observed, the greater the accuracy of the studies. On the other hand, the more disagreements identified or the wider the difference between what is expected and observed, the lesser the accuracy of the studies.

The simplified chi-square is a table containing four letters (A through D). Each letter represents the results of what was expected and what was observed. We typically define the duplex ultrasound results as what is expected. The angiogram represents the gold standard or what was observed.

THE CHI-SQUARE EXERCISE

Before attempting to calculate some data using the chi-square, try this simple exercise. With a blank sheet of paper, draw a blank chi-square (a box containing four equal squares). Write in the correct identifiers for the vertical axis: Duplex Ultrasound, and for the horizontal axis: Angiogram (Fig. 28-1). Next, identify and write in A (True Positives), B (False Positives), C (False Negatives), and D (True Negatives) in the appropriate boxes. Now, take your finger and sweep it across boxes A and B (Fig. 28-2).

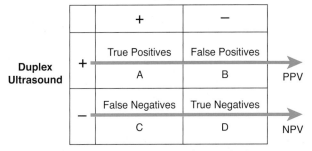

Figure 28-2 Using the chi-square table to calculate positive predictive value (PPV) and negative predictive value (NPV).

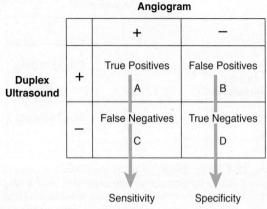

Figure 28-3 Using the chi-square table to calculate sensitivity and specificity.

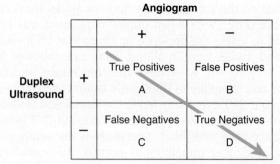

Figure 28-4 Using the chi-square table to calculate the overall accuracy.

These boxes represent all the studies (both duplex ultrasound and angiogram) that were reported as positive. Here we want many true positives and as few false positives as possible. These numbers will be used to calculate the PPV. Next, sweep your finger across boxes C and D. The sum of these two boxes represents all the studies that were reported as negative. Here we want to have as many true negatives and as few false negatives as possible. These numbers will be used to determine the NPV.

Now, sweep your finger down boxes A and C (Fig. 28-3). The numbers in these two boxes will be used to calculate the sensitivity of the study. Again, the fewer false negatives, the better the sensitivity. Then draw your finger down boxes B and D. These numbers are used to calculate the specificity of the test. As with the previous calculations, specificity is improved by a large

number of true negatives and a low number of false positives.

Finally, sweep your finger diagonally down the chi-square from right to left (Fig. 28-4). Here you will intersect the box containing the true positives (A) and the true negatives (D), the total of which will be divided by the sum of all four squares (A + B + C + D). This is the calculation of overall accuracy.[3,4]

Table 28-1 provides a summary of the statistical parameters of sensitivity, specificity, PPV, NPV, and accuracy. All of these parameters can be calculated from the chi-square.

By examining these calculations, it can be seen that the accuracy is both related to the ability to correctly find disease as well as to correctly identify the absence of disease.[5] Thus, the absolute value for accuracy must be between the values of sensitivity and specificity. The accuracy must also be between the negative and positive predictive values.

TABLE 28-1

Statistical Parameters Calculated Using a Chi-Square Table

Statistical Parameter	Chi-Square Table Variable	Actual Measurement
Sensitivity	$\dfrac{A}{A + C}$	$\dfrac{TP}{TP + FN}$
Specificity	$\dfrac{D}{D + B}$	$\dfrac{TN}{TN + FP}$
Positive predictive value (PPV)	$\dfrac{A}{A + B}$	$\dfrac{TP}{TP + FP}$
Negative predictive value (NPV)	$\dfrac{D}{C + D}$	$\dfrac{TN}{FN + TN}$
Accuracy	$\dfrac{A + D}{A + B + C + D}$	$\dfrac{TP + TN}{TP + FP + FN + TN}$

Labels A, B, C, and D refer to cell values of the chi-square table. Refer to Figure 28-1 TP, true positives; TN, true negatives; FP, false positives; FN, false negatives.

STATISTICS QUIZ

Applying the formulas already provided to the data presented in Figure 28-5, solve for the following questions.

1. What is the sensitivity of this study?
   A. 95%   B. 90%
   C. 60%   D. 85%
2. What is the specificity of this study?
   A. 92%   B. 96%
   C. 60%   D. 85%
3. What is the positive predictive value?
   A. 93%   B. 96%
   C. 60%   D. 85%
4. What is the negative predictive value?
   A. 33%   B. 96%
   C. 60%   D. 89%
5. What is the accuracy?
   A. 76%   B. 96%
   C. 91%   D. 85%

	Angiogram +	Angiogram −
Duplex Ultrasound +	88	7
Duplex Ultrasound −	10	84

Figure 28-5 A chi-square table with sample data filled in, comparing results of duplex ultrasound to angiography.

SUMMARY

Statistical values are an integral part of a QA program. A periodic review of ultrasound data and comparisons to gold standards will enable a vascular laboratory or ultrasound department to ensure reliable data. It is important for the vascular technologist or sonographer to understand the calculation and meaning of common statistical parameters. These statistics will serve to identify discrepancies, which in turn, can be used to adjust everyday work practices, thus maximizing the accuracy of duplex ultrasound testing results.

REFERENCES

1. Case T. *Primer of Non-invasive Vascular Technology*. 1st ed. Boston, MA: Little Brown; 1996.
2. Matthews DE, Farewell VT. *Using and Understanding Medical Statistics*. 2nd ed. Basel, Switzerland: Karger; 1988.
3. Rumwell C, McPharlin M. *Vascular Technology*. Pasadena, CA: Davies Publishing, 2009; 349-355.
4. Chi-Square Test. Independent Research Project, Penn State Web site. www2.lv.psu.edu/jxm57/irp/chisquar.html. Accessed June 11, 2011.
5. Ridgeway DP, Bean BS, Owen CA, et al. *Vascular Technology Review*. 1st ed. Pasadena, CA: Davies Review and Publishing Aids; 2001.

Index

Page numbers followed by *f*, *t*, and *b* indicate figures, tables, and boxes, respectively.

A

AAA. *See* abdominal aortic aneurysm
abdomen, vessels, major, 10–13, 10–13*f*
abdominal, retroperitoneal applications, ultrasound contrast agents (UCAs), 417–421
abdominal aorta, common iliac arteries, diagnosis, 319–320
abdominal aortic aneurysm (AAA) protocol, 282–283, 282*f*, 283*f*
abnormal color, spectral Doppler, lower extremity venous system, 227, 228*f*
ACA. *See* anterior cerebral artery
accessory renal arteries, identification, 318, 318*f*
accuracy, 427
    quality assurance (QA) statistics, 428
acute mesenteric ischemia, 307–308
acute stroke, transcranial Doppler (TCD), 119
acute thrombus, 211, 233
    determining presence, 223–224, 223*f*, 224*f*
acute tubular necrosis (ATN), kidney transplantation, 361
agent types, ultrasound contrast agents (UCAs), 411–412, 412*f*, 412*t*
   administration, 412
   therapeutic, 413
   tissue-specific, targeted, 413
air embolism, 391, 396–397
air plethysmography (APG), 275–276
aliasing, turbulence, flow direction, color feature use, mesenteric artery scanning, 302, 302*f*
Allen test, 123
allograft, 355
anastomosis, 169
anatomical approaches, intracranial cerebro- vascular examination, 97–98, 97*f*
anatomical variants
   inferior vena cava (IVC), iliac veins, 330
   mesenteric arteries, 299, 299*t*
anatomy
   hepatoportal system, 339
     artery, veins, 340
     portal venous system, 339–340, 340*f*
   inferior vena cava (IVC), iliac veins, 330, 330*t*
   intracranial cerebrovascular examination, 94, 94*f*
   lower extremity venous system, 212
   mesenteric arteries, 298–299, 298*f*
   renal vasculature, 312–314, 312*f*, 313*f*, 314*f*
   superficial venous system, 262–263, 262*f*, 263*f*, 264*f*
    cephalic, basilic veins, 250, 250*f*
    great saphenous vein (GSV), 246–249, 246–249*f*, 246*t*, 248*t*

small saphenous vein (SSV), 249–250, 250*f*
   upper extremity arterial duplex scanning, 157–159, 158*f*
aneurysm, 67, 143, 195, 281
   carotid, 74
   mesenteric arteries, 306–307, 307*f*, 307*t*
   upper extremity arterial duplex scanning, 163–164
angioplasty, 185
angle determination, scanning, mesenteric arteries, 301–302, 301*f*
ankle–brachial index, 123
   systolic pressures, 127, 127*t*, 128*f*
anterior accessory saphenous vein, 261
anterior cerebral artery (ACA), Doppler duplex imaging, 110, 110*f*
anterior tibial vein (ATV), scanning technique, 217–218
aorta, iliac arteries, 281–282
   diagnosis, 285–287, 285*f*, 286*f*, 287*f*
   sonographic examination techniques, 282
    equipment, 282
    patient preparation, positioning, 282
    pitfalls, 284
    scanning, 282–284
    technical considerations, 284
aorta, mesenteric, renal arteries, interrogation, 312*f*, 316–318, 317*f*, 318*f*
aortic arch, upper extremity arteries and, 3*f*, 6–7, 8*f*, 9*f*
aortic graft, stent surveillance, ultrasound contrast agents (UCAs), 420–421, 420*f*
aortoiliac duplex ultrasound following endovascular aortic stent graft repair (EVAR), 287–288
   diagnosis, 289–290, 290*f*, 291*f*, 292*b*
   EVAR devices, 288
   scanning technique, 288–289, 288*f*, 289*f*
aortoiliac protocol
   postintervention, 284, 284*f*
   preintervention, 282*f*, 283–284, 283*f*
APG. *See* air plethysmography
arterial aneurysms, evaluation, 206–207
arterial bypass grafts
   diagnosis, 175
    color flow imaging, 178, 179*f*
    grayscale findings, 175–178, 176–179*f*
    spectral analysis, 178–180, 179*f*, 180*f*, 181*f*, 182*b*
   failure mechanisms, 171
   sonographic examination techniques, 171
    equipment, documentation, 172
    patient preparation, position, 172
    pitfalls, 175
    scanning, 172–175, 172–175*f*